Reconstructive and Reproductive Surgery in Gynecology

This collective work reflects the current state of the art
in reconstructive and reproductive surgery in gynecology.
It is dedicated to those who will continue to advance
this exciting field.

Victor Gomel

With ineffable gratitude for my life partner and beloved wife,
Marla Joy

Andrew I. Brill

Reconstructive and Reproductive Surgery in Gynecology

Edited by

Victor Gomel, MD

Professor
Department of Obstetrics and Gynecology
Faculty of Medicine
University of British Columbia
and
BC Women's Hospital & Health Center
Vancouver, British Columbia
Canada

Andrew I. Brill, MD

Director of Minimally Invasive Gynecology and Reparative Surgery
Department of Obstetrics and Gynecology
California Pacific Medical Center
San Francisco, California
U.S.A.

informa
healthcare

New York London

First published in 2010 by Informa Healthcare, Telephone House, 69-77 Paul Street, London EC2A 4LQ, UK.

Simultaneously published in the USA by Informa Healthcare, 52 Vanderbilt Avenue, 7th Floor, New York, NY 10017, USA.

Informa Healthcare is a trading division of Informa UK Ltd. Registered Office: 37–41 Mortimer Street, London W1T 3JH, UK. Registered in England and Wales number 1072954.

A CIP record for this book is available from the British Library.

Library of Congress Cataloging-in-Publication Data available on application

ISBN-13: 9780415419550

Orders may be sent to: Informa Healthcare, Sheepen Place, Colchester, Essex CO3 3LP, UK
Telephone: +44 (0)20 7017 5540
Email: CSDhealthcarebooks@informa.com
Website: http://informahealthcarebooks.com/

For corporate sales please contact: CorporateBooksIHC@informa.com
For foreign rights please contact: RightsIHC@informa.com
For reprint permissions please contact: PermissionsIHC@informa.com

Typeset by Aptara, Delhi, India
Printed and bound in the United Kingdom

Preface

In the last three decades, the field of gynecology has undergone significant developments, resulting largely from scientific discoveries, technical innovations, and clinical research and applications. New treatment options have evolved to replace more radical measures. Pertinent information, increasingly and readily available through the Internet and other sources, has permitted our patients to become more knowledgeable and active participants in their health care decision making. Use of endoscopic access to perform gynecologic surgical procedures has reached maturity and has gained wide acceptance, replacing more invasive approaches.

These developments occurred while the world was experiencing dramatic demographic changes. Despite the ongoing rapid increase in world population, the industrialized countries have and continue to experience a significant decline in their birth rate. Coupled with the continuing rise of life expectancy, the proportion of elderly persons in our societies is expanding greatly. Women outlive men by 5 to 6 years and will require medical care during an increasingly longer postmenopausal lifespan. With improved well-being they will remain active, at work and at play, and require gynecologic care including reconstructive procedures. Another important demographic trend is the increasing delay in childbearing by a greater percentage of women, which will augment the demand for services of assisted reproduction and new techniques of fertility preservation.

Taking into account the great progress made in gynecologic surgery coupled with the demographic and social changes cited above, this textbook was thematically conceived to provide conservative surgical solutions for conditions commonly encountered in reproductive and postmenopausal aged women by the gynecologic surgeon; hence its title *Reconstructive and Reproductive Surgery in Gynecology*.

Authored by a group of international authorities, all widely recognized for their knowledge and surgical expertise, each chapter critically answers the practicing gynecologic surgeon's prerequisite for sound rationale and contemporary surgical techniques to treat women with benign and malignant pelvic conditions, and those who desire to enhance and/or preserve fertility.

Contents

Contributors

Annalisa Abbiati Department of Obstetrics and Gynecology, Istituto "Luigi Mangiagalli," University of Milan and Center for Research in Obstetrics and Gynecology, Milan, Italy

Mauricio S. Abrão Department of Obstetrics and Gynecology, Faculty of Medicine, São Paulo University, and SBE—the Brazilian Endometriosis and Minimally Invasive Society, São Paulo, Brazil

Leila V. Adamyan Scientific Center for Obstetrics, Gynecology and Perinatology, Moscow, Russia

Giorgio Aimi Department of Obstetrics and Gynecology, Istituto "Luigi Mangiagalli," University of Milan, Milan, Italy

Saad A. K. Amer Department of Obstetrics and Gynecology, Nottingham University Medical School, Nottingham, U.K.

Fabio Amicarelli Department of Obstetrics and Gynecology, Istituto "Luigi Mangiagalli," University of Milan, Milan, Italy

Giussy Barbara Department of Obstetrics and Gynecology, Istituto "Luigi Mangiagalli," University of Milan, Milan, Italy

Maria Mercedes Binda Department of Obstetrics and Gynaecology, KULeuven, Leuven, Belgium

Revaz Botchorishvili Departments of Obstetrics and Gynecology and Reproductive Medicine, CHU Estaing, Clermont Ferrand, France

Andrew I. Brill Department of Obstetrics and Gynecology, California Pacific Medical Center, San Francisco, California, U.S.A.

Mauro Busacca Department of Obstetrics and Gynecology, University of Milan, Milan, Italy

Michael Canis Departments of Obstetrics and Gynecology and Reproductive Medicine, CHU Estaing, Clermont Ferrand, France

Roberta Corona Departments of Obstetrics and Gynaecology, KULeuven, Leuven, Belgium

Benjamin Cotte Departments of Obstetrics and Gynecology and Reproductive Medicine, CHU Estaing, Clermont Ferrand, France

Geoffrey W. Cundiff Department of Obstetrics and Gynecology, Faculty of Medicine, University of British Columbia, Vancouver, British Columbia, Canada

Raffaella Daguati Department of Obstetrics and Gynecology, Istituto "Luigi Mangiagalli," University of Milan, Milan, Italy

Xavier Deffieux Université Paris-Sud and AP-HP, Service de Gynécologie-Obstétrique et Médecine de la Reproduction, Hôpital Antoine Béclère, Clamart, France

Jacques Donnez Department of Gynecology, Université Catholique de Louvain, Cliniques Universitaires Saint-Luc, Brussels, Belgium

Marie-Madeleine Dolmans Department of Gynecology, Université Catholique de Louvain, Cliniques Universitaires Saint-Luc, Brussels, Belgium

Jean-Bernard Dubuisson Department of Gynaecology and Obstetrics, University Hospitals of Geneva, Geneva, Switzerland

Hervé Fernandez Université Paris-Sud and Service de Gynécologie-Obstétrique et Médecine de la Reproduction, Hôpital Bicêtre, Le Kremlin Bicêtre, France

Gwenael Ferron Institut Claudius Regaud, Toulouse, France

Victor Gomel Department of Obstetrics and Gynecology, Faculty of Medicine, University of British Columbia, Vancouver, British Columbia, Canada

Celine Houlle Departments of Obstetrics and Gynecology and Reproductive Medicine, CHU Estaing, Clermont Ferrand, France

Fred M. Howard Division of Gynecologic Specialties, Obstetrics & Gynecology, University of Rochester Medical Center, Rochester, New York, U.S.A.

Pascale Jadoul Department of Gynecology, Université Catholique de Louvain, Cliniques Universitaires Saint-Luc, Brussels, Belgium

Grace Janik Reproductive Specialty Center, Milwaukee, Wisconsin, U.S.A.

Kris Jardon Departments of Obstetrics and Gynecology and Reproductive Medicine, CHU Estaing, Clermont Ferrand, France

Eva Jouve Institut Claudius Regaud, Toulouse, France

Philippe Robert Koninckx Department of Obstetrics and Gynaecology, KULeuven, Leuven, Belgium

Tin Chiu Li Department of Reproductive Medicine and Surgery, Sheffield Teaching Hospitals, Sheffield, U.K.

Gérard Mage Departments of Obstetrics and Gynecology and Reproductive Medicine, CHU Estaing, Clermont Ferrand, France

Peter F. McComb Department of Obstetrics and Gynecology, Faculty of Medicine, University of British Columbia, Vancouver, British Columbia, Canada

Carlos Roger Molinas Centre for Gynaecological Endoscopy (Cendogyn), Centro Médico La Costa, Asunción, Paraguay

David L. Olive Department of Obstetrics and Gynecology, University of Wisconsin, Madison, Wisconsin, U.S.A.

Recai Pabuccu Centrum Clinic and Department of Obstetrics and Gynecology, Ufuk University School of Medicine, Ankara, Turkey

William H. Parker Obstetrics and Gynecology, UCLA School of Medicine, Santa Monica, California, U.S.A.

Marc Possover Surgical Gynecology and Neuropelveology, Hirslanden Clinic, Zurich, Switzerland

Jean Luc Pouly Departments of Obstetrics and Gynecology and Reproductive Medicine, CHU Estaing, Clermont Ferrand, France

Elizabeth A. Pritts Department of Obstetrics and Gynecology, Faculty of Medicine, University of British Columbia, Vancouver, British Columbia, Canada

Denis Querleu Division of Gynecologic Oncology, Claudius Regaud Cancer Center, Toulouse, France and Division of Gynecologic Oncology, McGill University, Royal Victoria Hospital, Montreal, Quebec, Canada

Benoit Rabischong Departments of Obstetrics and Gynecology and Reproductive Medicine, CHU Estaing, Clermont Ferrand, France

Arash Rafii Institut Claudius Regaud, Toulouse, France

Cécile Rivoire Obstetrics and Gynecology and Reproductive Medicine, CHU Estaing, Clermont Ferrand, France

Robert M. Rogers, Jr. Kalispell Regional Medical Center, Northwest Women's Health Care, Kalispell, Montana, U.S.A.

Barry Sanders Department of Obstetrics and Gynecology, Faculty of Medicine, University of British Columbia, Vancouver, British Columbia, Canada

Jean Squifflet Department of Gynecology, Université Catholique de Louvain, Cliniques Universitaires Saint-Luc, Brussels, Belgium

Dingeman J. Swank Department of Surgery, Groene Hart Hospital, Gouda, The Netherlands

Elizabeth L. Taylor Department of Obstetrics and Gynecology, Faculty of Medicine, University of British Columbia, Vancouver, British Columbia, Canada

Richard H. Taylor Kalispell Regional Medical Center, Northwest Women's Health Care, Kalispell, Montana, U.S.A.

Anne-Sophie Van Eyck Department of Gynecology, Université Catholique de Louvain, Cliniques Universitaires Saint-Luc, Brussels, Belgium

Anne Van Langendonckt Department of Gynecology, Université Catholique de Louvain, Cliniques Universitaires Saint-Luc, Brussels, Belgium

Paolo Vercellini Department of Obstetrics and Gynecology, Istituto "Luigi Mangiagalli," University of Milan and Center for Research in Obstetrics and Gynecology, Milan, Italy

1

Reconstructive and reproductive surgery: an introduction

Victor Gomel

The last three decades have witnessed rapid and significant strides in various scientific and technological fields that have affected the current practice of medicine. In addition, there have been important demographic and social changes; these together with the continuing important scientific and technical discoveries will continue to significantly change the practice of our specialty. These changes will be influenced partly by forces internal to our discipline and partly by those external to our discipline (1).

Internally, there will always be the innovator who "pushes the envelope" with innovations, new approaches and techniques. It will continue to be imperative for those who practice the discipline to critically appraise the outcomes of new techniques and approaches. The external forces are far more important and include the effect of the dramatic demographic changes the world is experiencing, the influence of industry in our practices; the very significant progress in various scientific fields that will affect our own; and last but not the least the influence of the regulatory agencies and costs associated with medical care (1).

One of the major future changes may well be the separation of obstetrics and gynecology. This change will be triggered by many factors, one of which is the inability to train residents in both disciplines adequately. The training period for specialization has been significantly shortened—not in terms of years but in terms of working hours of the residents—because of markedly reduced weekly working hours and frequency of nights and weekends on call. The increasing trend of subspecialization augments the number of learners competing for the limited hospital and patient resources. In addition, there has been a dramatic change in the gender of applicants to obstetrics and gynecology—most applicants now are women. Once they go into practice, they tend to be much more rational in their working habits and work less hours per week than do their male counterparts. This will require the training of greater number of doctors to meet the demand. The increasing number of litigations and the very large awards decided by the courts for complicated obstetrical outcomes cause many of our specialist colleagues and those in general practice to abandon obstetrical practice, which decreases further the number of professionals in obstetrical practice. Separation of obstetrics and gynecology is in effect already occurring because of subspecialization; indeed, colleagues who have specialized in maternal fetal medicine rarely, if ever, practice gynecology.

We are witnessing very important demographic changes. The world population has increased 34%, from 5 billion to 6.7 billion, in the short span of 20 years, from 1987 to 2007, despite a significant decline in the birth rate in the industrialized countries. This rate of population growth has a significant impact on the environment, because each individual adds to the carbon print, an important current concern.

A fertility rate (number of children born per women in her childbearing years) of 2.1% is required to maintain a steady population in a given society. Yet this rate in the European Union has fallen to 1.5%. It is interesting to note that the European countries that had the highest fertility rates are those that currently have the lowest, 1.3% for Spain, Italy, Portugal, and Poland. Russia and Japan have similarly low fertility rates. China, in need to decrease population growth, introduced the policy of one child per couple: this resulted in the reduction of fertility rate to 1.7%. India continues to have a high fertility rate of 2.7%. But owing to the preference of male offspring in both these countries, and the practice of feticide of the females, tens of million young men in both these countries will not be able to find wives: a problem that has already become evident. The population explosion is occurring in the developing countries.

The number of children younger than 5 years has greatly declined in Europe, from 57 million in 1960 to 35 million in 2007. In Italy, there were 4.5 million children younger than 5 years in 1965—this number declined gradually to 4.3 million in 1975, 3.5 million in 1985, and 2.3 millions in 2007. In terms of percentage of total population, this represents a drop from 9% in 1965 to 4.3% in 2007. The life expectancy has reached 81 years for women and 75 to 76 years for men in the industrialized world; these are higher in Japan and much lower in Russia. The life expectancy will continue to increase: a woman who was 50 years of age in 2002 is expected to live, on the average, an additional 35 years. These are dramatic changes with important social, economic, and political consequences that will certainly trigger the intervention of national governments and even governments of national unions, such as the European Union.

Women will live increasingly longer, continue to stay in the work force longer, and likely continue to delay childbearing. These in themselves have important repercussions for medical practice in general and our specialty in particular: indeed, trends that are already becoming evident. Women will require medical care during a much longer postmenopausal lifespan; they will increasingly seek antiaging treatment and cosmetic surgery. There are already many gynecologists doing cosmetic surgery as part of their practice. There is an increasing use of cosmeceuticals (cosmetics that contain a pharmaceutical compound); this represented a business of $6.5 billion in the United States in 2004, an increase of 25% in the four years since 2000. Women leading a longer healthy and active life after menopause will require reconstructive surgery for various conditions such as stress incontinence and genital prolapse as well as for cosmetic reasons.

The demographic changes discussed above will require more women to join the work force, which may delay childbearing further and for a greater percentage of women. These trends are already clearly evident today: the proportion of U.S. women who had their first child over 30 years of age increased from 5% in 1975 to 22% in 1995, the number of women having their first child at age 35 and older increased by 50% between 1981 and 1999, and those having their first child between 40 and 45 years of age increased by 75%. Delay in childbearing will increase demand for services of assisted reproduction (ART; assisted reproductive technology). Already, 60% of those using ART are 35 years of age and older (2). ART services have become an industry and the number of clinics and cycles performed will continue to increase; this is already an annual business worth about $1.5 billion in the United States and more than €3 billion in the European Union. There will be an increasing demand for techniques to preserve fertility—embryo, oocyte, ovarian tissue, and stem cell banking are already in use. These techniques, and others, will undoubtedly be improved and expanded to respond to the significant increase in need.

Gynecologic practice, like medicine as a whole, will continue to change as a result of progress in other scientific fields: physics, mechanics, electronics, computer technology, robotics, cell and molecular biology, immunology, biochemistry, and DNA technology.

Technical innovations had a very important role in each of the steps of the development of endoscopy, in the initiation and acceptance of operative endoscopy, and in making possible for more complex procedures to be performed by this form of minimal access with greater efficiency and safety. Laparoscopy, as a diagnostic tool, gained universal acceptance only when it became possible to illuminate with a light source placed external to the peritoneal cavity. This technical advance was made possible by the invention of transmitting an intense light by means of a quartz rod, by Fourestier, Gladu, and Vulmière, and the application of fiberoptics to endoscopy by Hopkins and Kapany in the early 1950s. Gynecologists, in the 1960s, started to use the endoscope for surgical access to do simple procedures, such as tubal sterilization, with monocular vision, with an eye placed directly on the optic. Pioneers, in the early 1970s, demonstrated the value and safety of this approach in other procedures, such as excision of ectopic pregnancy, salpingectomy, oophorectomy, salpingo-ovariolysis, and salpingostomy (3).

The use of endoscopic access for increasingly more complex procedures became possible after many important technical developments that included the introduction of more sophisticated insufflators, endoscopes with improved optics, better and specialized instruments, etc. More important were the development of increasingly smaller, lighter, and more powerful television cameras and high-definition TV monitors (3). These miniaturized high-definition cameras become an integral part of the optic system. Their development was the result of the invention of an imaging semiconductor circuit (the CCD sensor), for which their innovators W.S. Boyle and G.E. Smith were the recipients of the 2009 Nobel Prize in physics. The ability to operate by viewing the operative field on TV monitors enabled the surgeon, surgical assistant, and operating room personnel to work as an efficient team. These innovations, introduced in the early 1980s, permitted the great evolution in minimal access surgery.

Indeed, many complex gynecological procedures are now being routinely and successfully performed by laparoscopy. The most telling of these developments has been the use of laparoscopic access for pelvic and para-aortic lymphadenectomy and radical hysterectomy for gynecologic malignancy (4,5).

In the 1970s, hysteroscopy was described as "a technique looking for an indication." The application of the technique, which at the time was purely diagnostic, remained limited. This was largely due to significant improvements in noninvasive imaging techniques, especially ultrasonography, and the use of a vaginal transducer for the assessment of the pelvic organs. Yet the impact of hysteroscopy in our specialty has been radical. This came about with the use of hysteroscopy as a means of surgical access into the uterus. It greatly simplified many procedures that previously required a laparotomy and a hysterotomy to access the uterine cavity: lysis of severe uterine synechiae, metroplasty for septate uterus, and excision of symptomatic intrauterine fibroids. These, after all, are common conditions; hysteroscopy has radically simplified these procedures and reduced their morbidity. It has also permitted the introduction of simple techniques of permanent tubal sterilization (6).

The industry also had a significant influence in the acceptance of endoscopic surgery, through the development and marketing of new equipment and instruments, the sponsoring of workshops, etc. The influence of industry in the acceptance of endoscopic surgery will continue to prevail in our medical and surgical practices, usually for the good. We now have greatly improved optics, even with smaller caliber endoscopes, more precise and specialized instruments for various procedures, high-definition mini cameras and television monitors, better insufflators for both laparoscopy and hysteroscopy, equipment and instruments that permit to secure hemostasis more effectively and safely, powerful morcellators that enable rapid removal of excised tissues (Fig. 1), etc. Production of small caliber, high-definition hysteroscopes has permitted hysteroscopy to be performed without anesthesia; this eventually led to the introduction of the so-called office hysteroscopy (Fig. 2). Improved optics, together with better equipment and instruments, allow hysteroscopic intrauterine procedures to be performed more easily and quickly and with greater safety. We can even have an integrated high-definition operative theater for endoscopic surgery, such as the OR1 developed by Storz (Fig. 3). While such impressive developments facilitate the work, improving safety and efficiency, they do have a cost factor that is frequently beyond many jurisdictions.

Marketing practices may also have negative outcomes, especially in increasing costs. For example, the use of disposable instruments may be helpful, even necessary, in certain circumstances; however, their routine use increases the cost

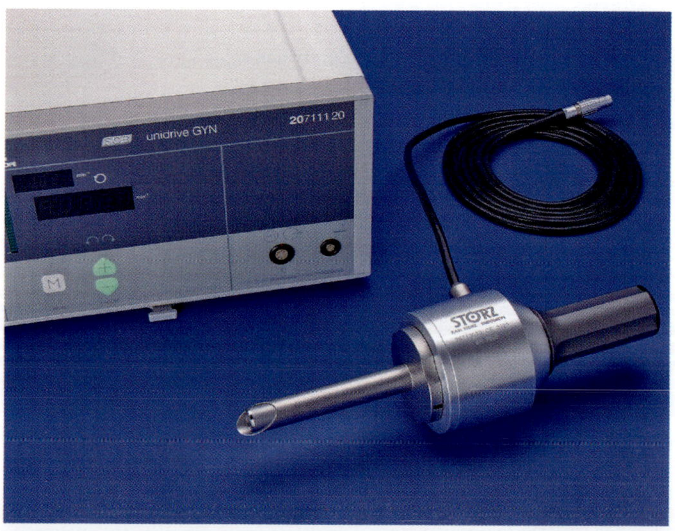

Figure 1 Rotocut G1 Morcellator: ergonomic and powerful morcellator for fast removal of myomas or uteri, after myoma enucleation or hysterectomy.

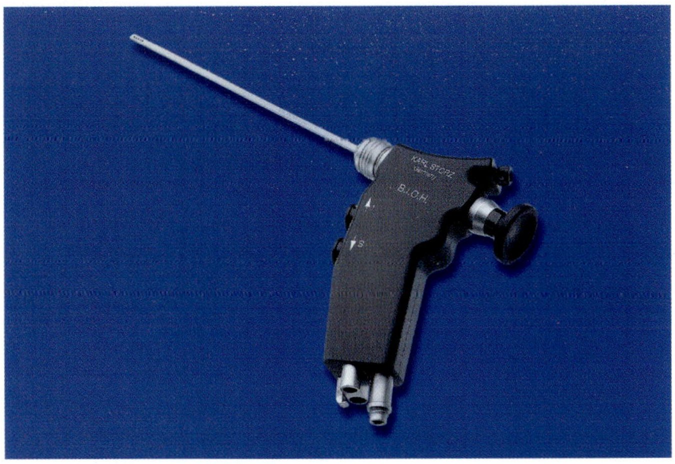

Figure 2 BIOH: integrated office hysteroscope, based on a 2.0-mm rod lense telescope with inflow/outflow and light cable connections from below.

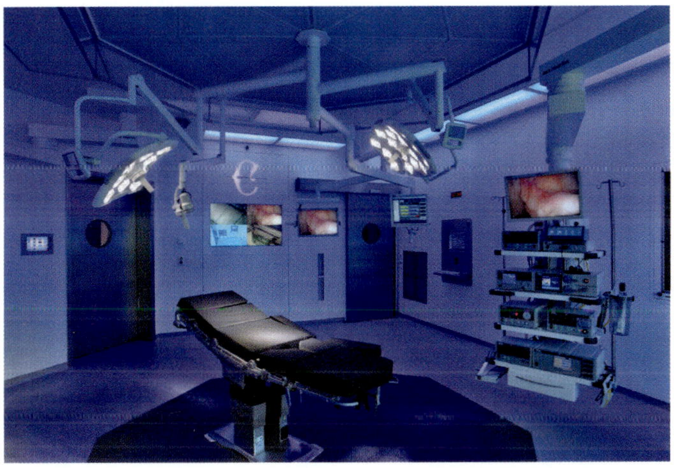

Figure 3 OR1: integrated operating theater with high-definition technology.

associated with each procedure. The same applies to major equipment. The development of a complex surgical robot such as the da Vinci® robot represents a major accomplishment (Fig. 4). Its effective use has a lengthy learning curve (7), but it facilitates performance of complex procedures, increasing the precision of the successive steps of the surgeon. Furthermore, it permits the surgeon to carry out the procedure by telesurgery, without even scrubbing, which is quite an accomplishment. However, the use of such equipment for routine surgical procedures has only a marketing value, as it increases the time frame in the operating room with the preparation and placement of the equipment and certainly increases costs. How many jurisdictions are able to afford the purchase of such expensive equipment for use in routine surgery? I wonder how the skills of the surgeon would be affected, over time, by the routine use of the robot for ordinary cases. Will his/her ability to operate on the patient directly, without the intermediary of the robot, diminish? What would happen when the robot is not available or in need of repairs?

There are simpler and much less expensive robots that hold the laparoscope and/or retracting instruments; some operate on command. They replace an assistant and are very useful for routine procedures. But they do not have the same marketing sex appeal! One of these is the "Lapman®," a dynamic laparoscope holder guided by a joystick clipped onto the laparoscopic instruments under the index finger of the operator (Figs. 5 and 6). It confers optimal control of the visual field, while operating, by smooth displacement of the laparoscope. The price of this simple robot is around €34,000; the remote control device that clips onto the instrument is disposable and costs around €50.

Another innovation that greatly facilitates intraperitoneal surgery is the LaparoTenser®. This is a new, subcutaneous abdominal lifting device that can be sterilized and is used to perform isobaric (gasless) laparoscopy (8). Isobaric laparoscopy was introduced to avoid the risks arising from blind introduction of the insufflating needle into the peritoneal cavity and from the effects of pneumoperitoneum on cardiac and respiratory function (9), as well as to enable the use of conventional surgical instruments along with laparoscopic instruments (8). Earlier equipment were cumbersome and required the placement of three blades into the peritoneal cavity. These blades were joined at the site of introduction into the peritoneal cavity: the distal extremities separated to form a triangle and, in this particular configuration, they were used to elevate the abdominal wall. But the system did not provide adequate exposure. With the LaparoTenser, two curved, multiplan, solid large-gauge needles with blunt tips are inserted subcutaneously through 2 mm skin incisions, one in each lower quadrant of the abdomen, and are passed superiorly in the subcutaneous tissue (Fig. 7A). The base of each needle is then attached to the lifting device that elevates the needles and the abdominal wall (Fig. 7B). Once the abdomen is

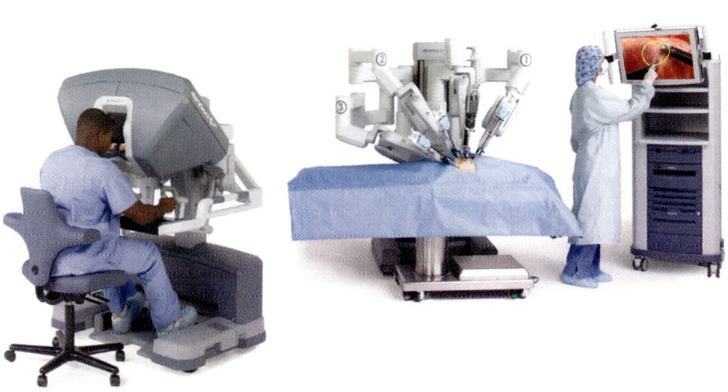

Figure 4 The da Vinci robot Si system: surgeon using console with nurse at vision cart. © 2010 Intuitive Surgical, Inc.

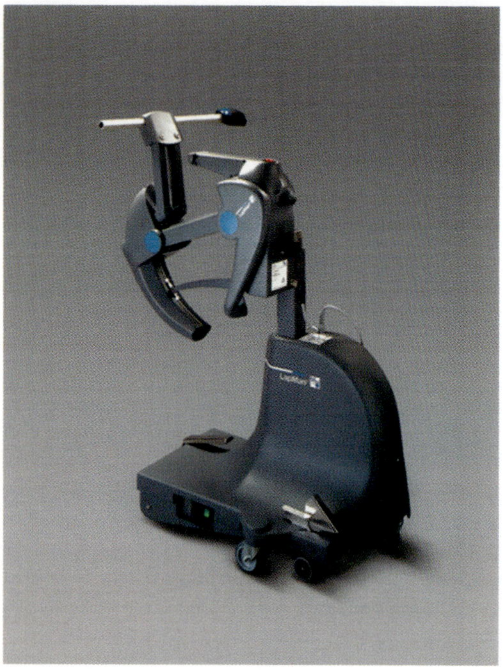

Figure 5 The Lapman: A dynamic laparoscope holder.

elevated, the primary trocar is inserted intraumbilically (or elsewhere, depending on the procedure), either through an open or an optical approach (Fig. 8A). The intraperitoneal laparoscopic view obtained is comparable to that obtained with pneumoperitoneum (Fig. 8B). Isobaric laparoscopy permits the use of conventional surgical instruments through a small incision, along with laparoscopic instruments through appropriate trocars (Fig. 9). The LaparoTenser has been used successfully to perform various gynecological, surgical, and oncologic procedures (10–13) (Fig. 10).

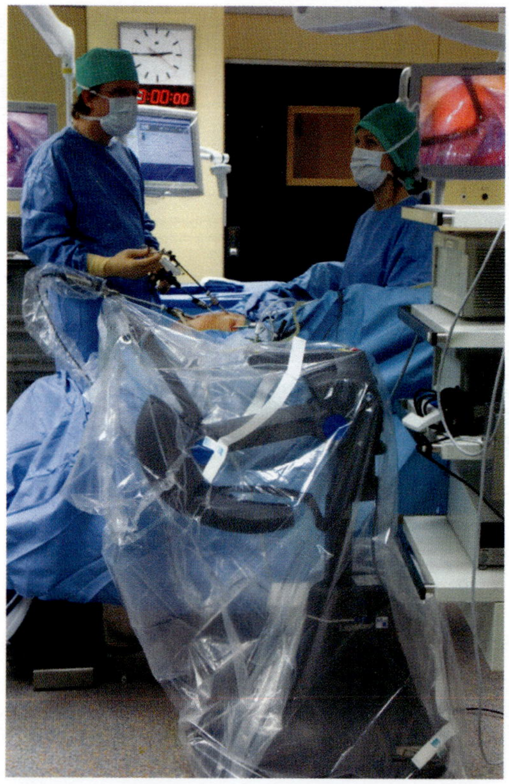

Figure 6 The Lapman in use.

Progress in imaging and interventional imaging, robotics, cell and molecular biology, immunology, biochemistry, and DNA technology will continue to influence and benefit our field of practice, as it did in the past. We can take tubal pregnancy as an example to illustrate this. Not too long ago, tubal pregnancy was a difficult diagnosis; it became simplified with the introduction of diagnostic laparoscopy, which

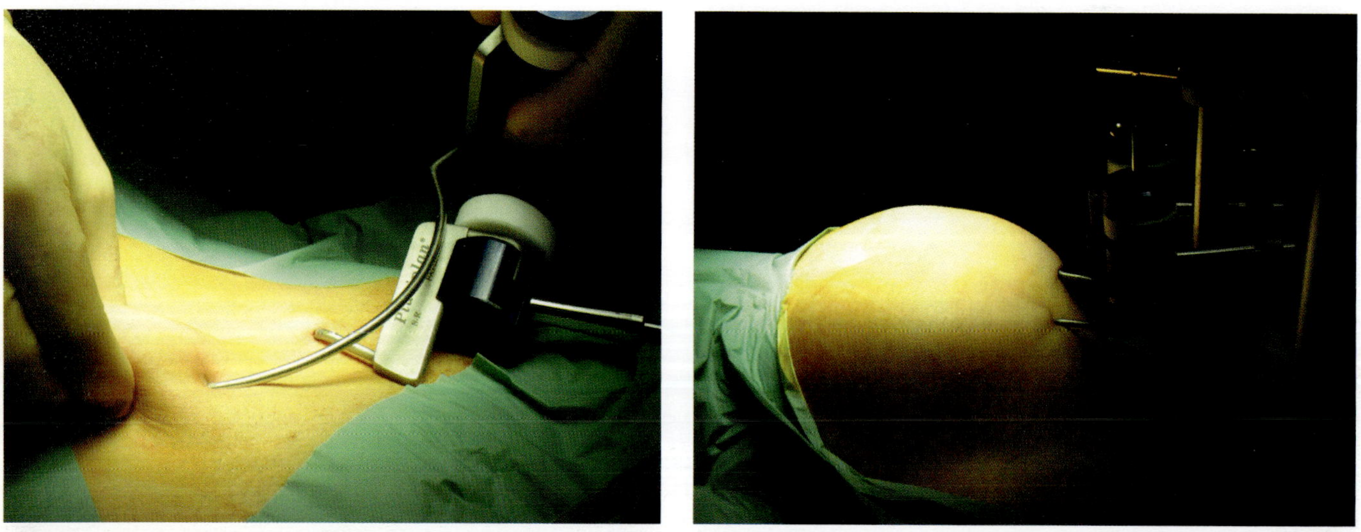

(A) (B)

Figure 7 LaparoTenser: **(A)** subcutaneous insertion of curved, multiplan needles; **(B)** the needles are each attached to the respective part of the lifter, and the abdominal wall is lifted.

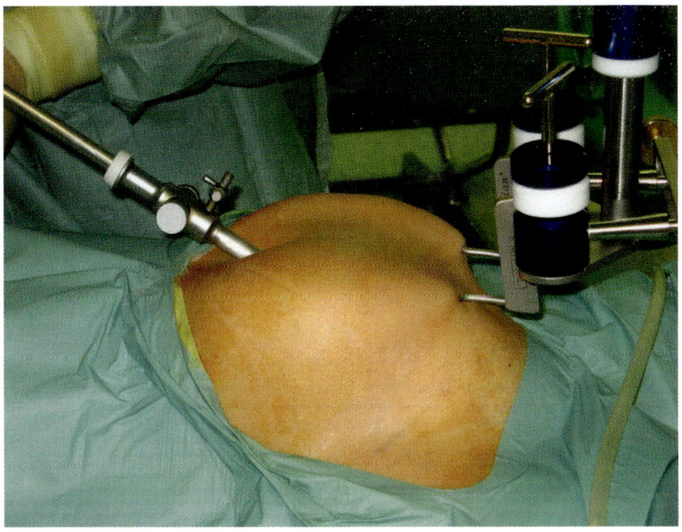

(A)

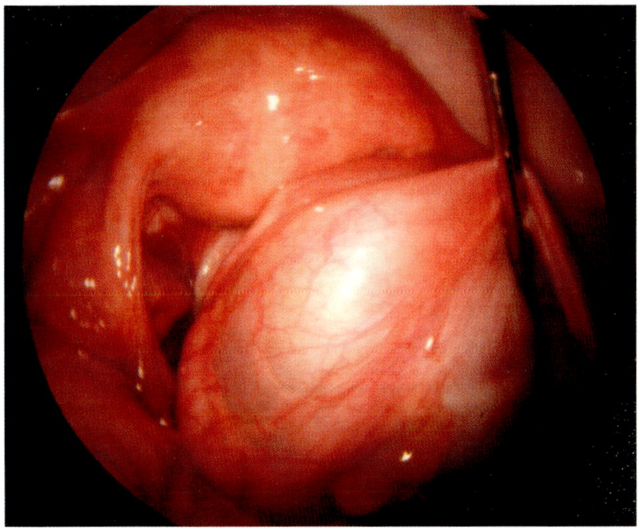

(B)

Figure 8 LaparoTenser: (**A**) the laparoscope is inserted through an appropriate cannula; (**B**) pelvic view (large, right tubo-ovarian cystic tumor).

permitted early diagnosis, provided, of course, the condition was suspected. In the early 1970s, pioneers in laparoscopy started to exploit the potential of surgical access into the peritoneal cavity that this instrument provided; they started to perform various procedures including excision of tubal pregnancy (3). The advantages of this approach as opposed to conventional laparotomy soon became clearly evident. These include shortened postoperative hospital stay and recovery period; reduced postoperative discomfort, which results in less analgesia requirements; frequently lesser costs; and the cosmetic gain associated with the avoidance of a laparotomy scar. But acceptance of this approach, and its use for more complex procedures, had to await another major technical development, the production of light-weight, mini video cameras and high-resolution television monitors, as discussed above. Continuing our example, the subsequent introduction of a sensitive and rapid βhCG assay, and the endovaginal ultrasound probe, together with improvements in ultrasound imaging made early diagnosis of tubal pregnancy possible in most cases, without recourse to laparoscopy. Laparoscopy became largely used to confirm and treat the ectopic pregnancy. The demonstration that early tubal pregnancies can be successfully treated medically, with single or more doses of methotrexate, was another important step of this evolution. Many such cases are now treated medically, in turn significantly reducing the number of surgical interventions for this condition.

Evolution and change will continue. Many of the conditions that are currently treated by surgery will be prevented or managed by medical or other less or noninvasive means. Hysterectomy is the most commonly performed major gynecological procedure (14), as evident from Table 1. The two major indications, which together account for nearly 80% of

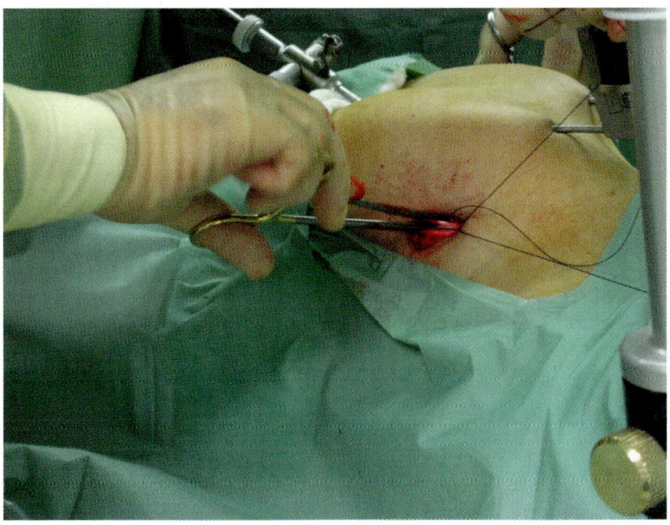

Figure 9 LaparoTenser: permits use of conventional surgical instruments through a small incision.

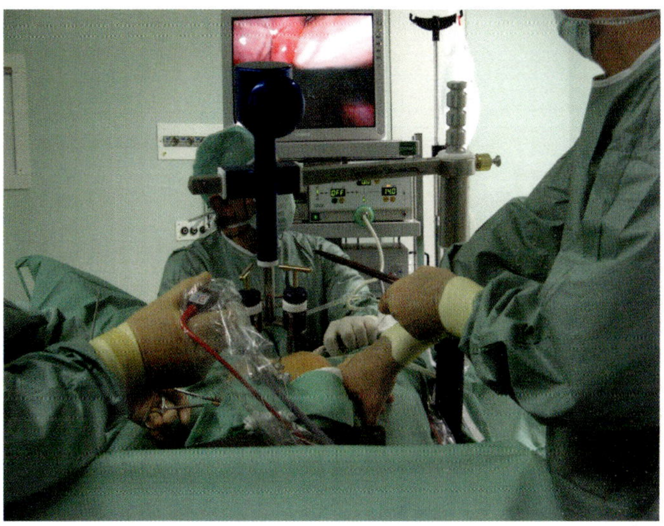

Figure 10 The LaparoTenser in use.

Table 1 Number of Hysterectomies Performed, in the Major Countries of the World, in 2003[a]

USA	636,973
France	131,067
Germany	178,788
Italy	125,933
Spain	87,373
Sweden	19,942
South Africa	96,413
Australia	43,193
Brazil	399,336
India	2,310,263
China	2,817,353
Total	6,846,184

[a]Data from "US Census Bureau, International Database, 2004."

the hysterectomies, are uterine bleeding and uterine fibroids (15). Increasingly, more effective medical and less-invasive surgical treatments are becoming available for both of these conditions. For dysfunctional uterine bleeding, endometrial excision was introduced first, followed by endometrial ablation, which simplified the technique. These did not attain general acceptance because of the level of skill required and the associated complication rate, including severe ones. Subsequent introduction of nonhysteroscopic, so-called Global, ablation devices greatly simplified the procedure, providing similar outcomes as hysteroscopic ablation. The Mirena® levonorgestrel-releasing intrauterine system, which proved to be an effective medical treatment, was added to the local surgical measures to treat dysfunctional uterine bleeding. The use of these measures decreased the use of hysterectomy significantly, by two-thirds, in the United Kingdom (16) (Fig. 11).

Another vivid example is cervical cancer. Radical hysterectomy was introduced by Wertheim who published results on 500 cases in 1907 (17). Radiotherapy became another treatment modality in the early 1960s. The demonstration of the effectiveness of the cervical smear (Papanicolaou test, also known as Pap smear) in the diagnosis of malignant and precancerous lesions offered the opportunity of mass screening of women. Mass screening was introduced in the Canadian province of British Columbia, through the Cancer

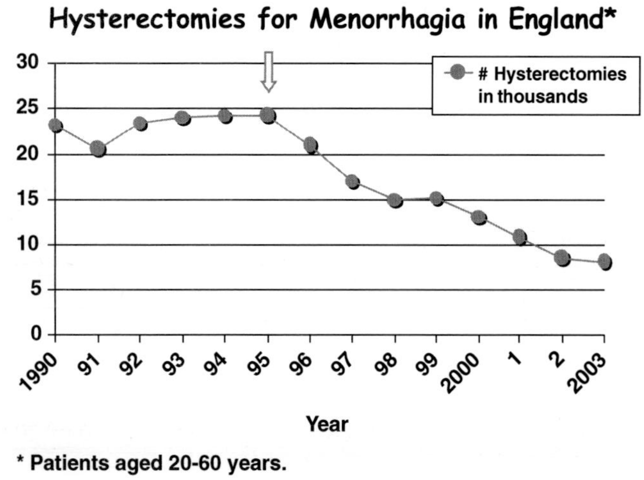

Figure 11 Hysterectomies for menorrhagia in the United Kingdom.

Control agency, by Boyes and Fidler (18). More than 500,000 cervical smears are being examined each year in the central laboratory. Through such screening in the province, between 1955 and 1985, 26,000 cases of carcinoma in situ of the cervix were detected and treated. Furthermore, the incidence of clinically invasive carcinoma of the cervix in the province decreased by 78% and the mortality from the same condition by 72%, as a result of treatment of precancerous lesions, diagnosed through the screening (19). The role of the human papilloma virus in the genesis of this condition has since been elucidated and a vaccine has been developed against it. Because of the cost associated with screening and treatment of precancerous lesions, both regional and national authorities will urge the use of this vaccine (20). Appropriate use of this vaccine will undoubtedly largely prevent development of this malignancy in the future (21).

Significant progress in imaging such as ultrasonography; computed tomography, helical or spiral CT; positive electron tomography; and magnetic resonance imaging have already reduced the need for more invasive methods to gain a diagnosis; they are permitting targeted biopsy of the lesions for diagnosis and treatment of many, by vascular embolization, ablation by cryotherapy, trackless ablation by various forms of energy such as focused ultrasound. Uterine artery embolization, in appropriate cases, has proven to be a good alternative for the treatment of symptomatic uterine fibroids (22). Focused ultrasound has been successfully used in several preliminary studies to ablate symptomatic uterine fibroids (23) and adenomyosis (24). Medical treatment of uterine fibroids, with mifepristone, has proven successful in reducing the size of the tumors and the various associated symptoms including the amount of bleeding, generally improving the patient's quality of life (25,26).

Increasing advances in robotics will result in increased use of robots in the community, as well as in health care: in surgery, anesthesia, and hospital services including pharmacy and distribution of medications to patients, etc.

Medical practice will continue to change and improve as a result of progress in modern biology, with cloning of pure antibodies; polymerase chain reaction, differential hybridization, and multiparameter flow cytometry; and the capability to clone and engineer genes. We have learned of the presence of cancer stem cells; they represent a minority of the cells within the tumor. Their biological properties are often very different from those of the major tumor cell population that responds to chemotherapy by virtue of its rapid division. Any treatment that does not eradicate these stem cells is bound to fail, because the malignancy is very likely to reoccur. Development of "biomarkers" is helping to identify these cells. This will eventually lead to the production of new and more effective therapies specifically targeted to cancer stem cells. Progress in prevention and specific chemotherapy for malignancies will reduce the role of surgery, as was the case, for example, for choriocarcinoma (27). *Performed for other than trauma, congenital defects, and cosmetics, surgery represents the failure of medicine, failure of having discovered the etiology of the disease, and consecutively developed specific and effective preventive and therapeutic measures.*

Many of the required surgical procedures will be performed without incisions (trackless surgery) using alternative forms of energy. Increased knowledge about stem cells and their use, application of proteomics, and the use of specific nanomolecules will change our current treatments for many conditions. As a result of the preceding evidence, the nature of our practice of gynecology, and the way we practice it, will dramatically change.

Stem cells, as we learn more, will increasingly be used in medical treatment (28). A recent study reported on 23 insulin-dependent diabetics who had transplantation of their own bone marrow stem cells. Subsequently, they did not require insulin administration from 14 to 52 months. It is not known, as yet, which of the bone marrow stem cells (HSC or MAPC) produce pancreatic β cells (29).

Another interesting and promising field is proteomics. This is a new "cutting-edge" field that looks at the proteins created by genes. Mass spectrometry maps a thousand or more protein peaks, in a pattern shared by patients with a particular disease. High-powered computing technology analyzes and compares the data with a control group, resulting in an algorithm that can predict disease. This technology is permitting development of new screening test to detect malignancies, even before occurrence of symptoms. During the next decades, it will likely be possible to identify and subclassify diseases and provide new screening tests and new markers for outcomes. A series of blood tests will provide a patient a profile of his/her disease risks. Use of specific nanomolecules will block specific pathways that control growth in tumor cells. A nanomolecule for endometrial cancer is currently being tested.

We can expect a dramatic progress in the way to prevent, diagnose, and treat diseases. These will result in significant changes in medical structures and ways of practice. Schopenhauer said it so well: "change alone is eternal, perpetual, immortal."

Technological and scientific advances are costly: Will we be able to afford it? What will be the influence of regional and central governing bodies on the practice of medicine? Will all of the technological and scientific advances be universally available and affordable? These questions will be answered in the future.

This book, all of the chapters of which have been authored by recognized authorities in their field, presents the current state of the art in both reconstructive and reproductive surgery in gynecology.

REFERENCES

1. Gomel V, Taylor PJ. Future directions. In: Gomel V, Taylor PJ, eds. Diagnostic and Operative Gynecologic Laparoscopy. Mosby: St. Louis, 1995:309–312
2. Centers for Disease Control and Prevention. CDC STD Surveillance Data, 2006. www.cdc.gov/std/stats/.
3. Gomel V, Taylor PJ. Introduction. In: Gomel V, Taylor PJ, eds. Diagnostic and Operative Gynecologic Laparoscopy. Mosby: St. Louis, 1995:1–4
4. Querleu D, Leblanc E, Castelain B. Laparoscopic pelvic lymphadenectomy in the staging of early carcinoma of the cervix. Am J Obstet Gynecol 1991; 164:579–581.
5. Querleu D, Leblanc E, Cartron G, et al. Audit of preoperative and early complications of laparoscopic lymph node dissection in 1000 gynecologic cancer patients. Am J Obstet Gynecol 2006; 195:1287–1292.
6. Gomel V. Foreword. In: Donnez J, ed. Operative Laparoscopy and Hysteroscopy. London, U.K.: Informa Healthcare, 2007.
7. Lenihan JP Jr, Kovanda C, Seshadri-Kreaden U. What is the learning curve for robotic assisted gynecologic surgery? J Minim Invasive Gynecol 2008; 15:589–594.
8. Gomel V. Isobaric laparoscopy. J Obstet Gynaecol Can 2007; 29:493.
9. Alijani A, Hanna GB, Cuschieri A. Abdominal wall lift versus positive-pressure capnoperitoneum for laparoscopic cholecystectomy: Randomized controlled trial. Ann Surg 2004; 239:388–394.
10. Damiani A, Melgrati L, Marziali M, et al. Laparoscopic myomectomy for very large myomas using an isobaric (gasless) technique. JSLS 2005; 9:434–438.
11. Sesti F, Capobianco F, Capozzolo T, et al. Isobaric gasless laparoscopy versus minilaparotomy in uterine myomectomy: A randomized trial [published online ahead of print August 20, 2008]. Surg Endosc 2008; 22(4):917–923.
12. Bossotti M, Bona A, Borroni R, et al. Gasless laparoscopic-assisted ileostomy or colostomy closure using an abdominal wall lifting device. Surg Endosc 2001; 15:597–599.
13. Ammori1 BJ, Davides D, Vezakis A, et al. Day-case laparoscopic cholecystectomy: A prospective evaluation of a 6-year experience. J Hepatobiliary Pancreat Surg 2003; 10:303–308.
14. Keshavarz H, Hillis SD, Kieke BA, et al. Hysterectomy surveillance—United States, 1994–1999. MMWR 2002; 51(SS05): 1–8.
15. Vessey MP, Villard-Mackintosh L, McPherson K, et al. The epidemiology of hysterectomy: Findings in a large cohort study. Br J Obstet Gynaecol 1992; 99:402–407.
16. Reid PC, Mukri F. Trends in number of hysterectomies performed in England for menorrhagia: Examination of health episode statistics, 1989 to 2002–3. BMJ 2005; 330:938–939.
17. Wertheim E. Die erweiterte abdominale Operation bei Carcinoma colli Uteri (auf Grund von 500 Fällen). Urban und Schwarzenberg: Berlin-Vienna, 1911.
18. Boyes DA, Fidler HK. Cervical cancer control program in British Columbia. Am J Obstet Gynecol 1963; 85:328–331.
19. Anderson GH, Boyes DA, Benedet JL, et al. Organisation and results of the cervical cytology screening programme in British Columbia, 1955–85. Br Med J Clin Res Ed 1988; 296:975–978.
20. Bergeron C, Breugelmans JG, Bouee S, et al. Cervical cancer screening and associated treatment costs in France. Gynecol Obstet Fertil 2006; 34:1036–1042.
21. Villa LL, Costa RL, Petta CA, et al. High sustained efficacy of a prophylactic quadrivalent human papillomavirus types 6/11/16/18 L1 virus-like particle vaccine through 5 years of follow-up. Br J Cancer 2006; 95:1459–1466.
22. Goodwin SC, Bradley LD, Lipman JC, et al. UAE Versus Myomectomy Study Group. Uterine artery embolization versus myomectomy: A multicenter comparative study. Fertil Steril 2006; 85: 14–21.
23. Stewart EA, Rabinovici J, Tempany CM, et al. Clinical outcomes of focused ultrasound surgery for the treatment of uterine fibroids. Fertil Steril 2006; 85:22–29.
24. Rabinovici J, Stewart EA. New interventional techniques for adenomyosis. Best Pract Res Clin Obstet Gynaecol 2006; 20:617–636.
25. Steinauer J, Pritts EA, Jackson R, et al. Systematic review of mifepristone for the treatment of uterine leiomyomata. Obstet Gynecol 2004; 103:1331–1336.
26. Fiscella K, Eisinger SH, Meldrum S, et al. Effect of mifepristone for symptomatic leiomyomata on quality of life and uterine size—A randomized controlled trial. Obstet Gynecol 2006; 108:1381–1387.
27. Hiramatsu Y, Masuyama H, Ishida M, et al. Term delivery choriocarcinoma patient with brain and lung metastases successfully treated by etoposide, methotrexate, actomycin D, cyclophosphamide and vincristine (EMA-CO) chemotherapy. Acta Med Okayama 2005; 59:235–238.
28. Gargett CE. Stem cells in gynaecology. Aust NZ J Obstet Gynaecol 2004; 44:380–386.
29. Couri CE, Oliveira MC, Stracieri AB, et al. C-peptide levels and insulin independence following autologous nonmyeloablative hematopoietic stem cell transplantation in newly diagnosed type 1 diabetes mellitus. JAMA 2009; 301:1573–1579.

2

Postoperative adhesions and their prevention

Philippe Robert Koninckx, Maria Mercedes Binda, Roberta Corona, and Carlos Roger Molinas

INTRODUCTION

The fact that adhesions can form following abdominal surgery has been known since the beginning of surgery. Yet during the early years of surgery, adhesion formation received little attention, the focus being on infection and survival. In the seventies clinical endocrinology developed explosively, driven by the introduction of oral contraceptives and by the introduction of radioimmunoassays—a technique that permitted for the first time the assay of reproductive hormones—and reproductive medicine and infertility became a subspecialty. Simultaneously, reproductive surgery developed and the prevention of postoperative adhesion formation became important. Microsurgery was introduced (1) first as a magnification tool permitting tubal reanastomosis and developing subsequently as a principle of surgery emphasizing the prevention of desiccation and gentle tissue handling (Fig. 1). Prevention of adhesion formation was mainly based upon careful observational medicine and common sense, and most of the principles became only much later experimentally confirmed. Some mistakes, however, were also introduced such as the free peritoneal graft to cover denuded peritoneal areas, a technique shown later to be strongly adhesiogenic (2).

The history of surgery and adhesion prevention cannot be viewed separately from the development of endometriosis and endometriosis surgery because cystic ovarian endometriosis is strongly associated with adhesion formation and also because endometriosis surgery is the most frequently performed fertility surgery. Diagnosis of infertility and of endometriosis and their treatment has driven the development of diagnostic laparoscopy complemented with minor laparoscopic surgical interventions and by microsurgery.

When lightweight endoscopic cameras were introduced in the mid-eighties, endoscopic surgery developed explosively replacing microsurgery and also laparotomy not only in gynecology but also in abdominal surgery and urology. This had important consequences for fertility and endometriosis surgery and for our awareness of adhesion formation. Until the early nineties, fertility surgery with prevention of adhesion formation had remained centralized in highly specialized fertility centers (3,4). We then witnessed in parallel the increasing use and success of IVF and the development of more advanced endoscopic surgery such as deep endometriosis and bowel, pelvic floor, and oncologic surgeries. With laparoscopic reproductive surgery becoming mainstream surgery, the microsurgical focus on the prevention of adhesion formation got lost. Indeed outside reproductive surgery, adhesion formation was widely considered as an unavoidable by-product of surgery, which could largely be prevented by good quality surgery. In retrospect, it is astonishing how fast the principles of microsurgery became by and large forgotten, with the overall belief that laparoscopic surgery was "minimal invasive" surgery and thus even better than microsurgery and that adhesion formation would rapidly become a minor problem (5,6).

With the realization that laparoscopic surgery was not the solution to prevent adhesion formation (7,8), laboratory research on and clinical interest in adhesion formation revived and new products were developed. Only in the last decade, we have become aware of the clinical importance of adhesion formation, mainly though the SCAR studies (9–11). These studies clearly demonstrated that the incidences of bowel obstruction and of reoperation due to postoperative adhesions keep increasing linearly for at least 10 years and are much higher than anticipated. In addition, the awareness of postoperative adhesions as a cause of infertility and pain grew. With the awareness of the clinical importance, we realized the associated costs, the market potential, and the necessity of randomized clinical trials for new products. "Quality of surgery" obviously being a key element in these trials, we realized that quality control of the individual surgical procedure was close to non-existent (12), and video registration was introduced as a monitoring aid for these trials. And simultaneously also came the awareness that quality of surgery might be variable—that good quality surgery cannot be considered as universal with obvious consequences for the interpretation of adhesion formation statistics.

In conclusion, postoperative adhesion formation has never received the attention it deserves as evidenced by the absence of adequate keywords to search the literature. Only very recently the clinical importance has been acknowledged (13–17), stimulating research and the foundation of a dedicated society, the PAX society, today called the Peritoneum and Surgery Society (P&S), spanning gynecology and surgery.

PATHOPHYSIOLOGY OF ADHESION FORMATION

The Mesothelial Cell and the Peritoneal Cavity

Mesothelial cells form a monolayer resting on a basal membrane and an underlying connective tissue lining the organs and the wall of the abdominal cavity, the pleura, and the pericardium. Mesothelial cells have been considered to be of mesothelial origin, but recent evidence has shown that both mesothelial cells and endothelial and hematopoietic cells are derived from a common progenitor cell originating embryologically in the splanchnic mesothelium (18). More recently mesothelial stem cells, which are able to differentiate to mesothelial cells, endothelial cells, smooth muscle cells, myofibroblasts, neuronal cells, adipocytes, chondrocytes, and osteoblasts, have been described. In culture these mesothelial cells behave as epithelial cells, expressing mainly cytokeratin, but under the influence of TGF-β, HGF, or EGF, they transform into spindle-shaped mesenchymal cells expressing mainly vimentin. The relationship between mesothelial stem cells and peritoneal repair following injury remains unclear:

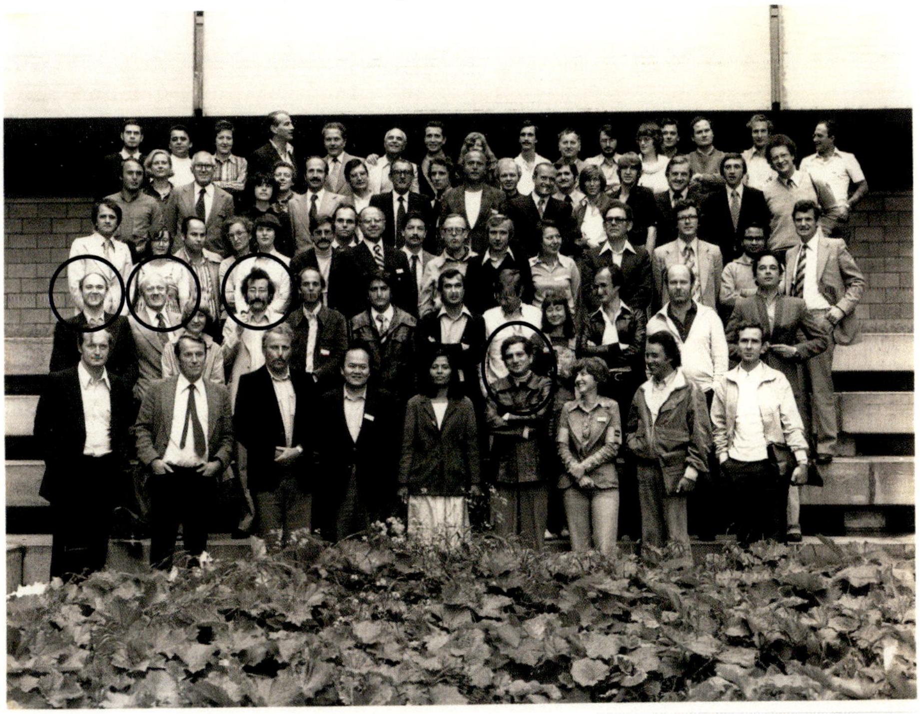

Figure 1 The pioneers of microsurgery at a workshop on microsurgery held in Leuven, Belgium, in 1978. (*From left to right*) Willy Boeckx, Ivo Brosens, Robert Winston, and Victor Gomel. Courtesy of I. Brosens.

Indeed it remains debated whether these cells derive from the peritoneal fluid, from the mesothelium, from the submesothelial connective tissue, from the vascular endothelium, or from blood cells. In any case, the concept of mesothelial stem cells is bound to be important for our understanding of peritoneal repair and of adhesion formation (19–21).

The roles of mesothelial cells in maintaining normal serosal membrane integrity and function is still only partially understood. They secrete glycosaminoglycans and surfactant to allow the parietal and visceral serosa to slide over each other. They actively transport fluids, cells, and particulates across the serosal membrane. They actively modulate gas resorption as CO_2 from the pneumoperitoneum (22,23). They synthesize and secrete mediators, which play important roles in regulating inflammatory, immune, and tissue repair responses, but we do not understand yet how these mesothelial cells communicate with each other and with surrounding cells as well as what the role of progenitor cells is (24).

In the absence of ovarian activity, peritoneal fluid is scanty. During the menstrual cycle, peritoneal fluid is mainly formed as an ovarian transudate arising mainly from the developing follicle or corpus luteum. Hence peritoneal fluid contains concentrations in steroid hormones that are much higher than in plasma. Mesothelial cells are highly specialized cells regulating the transport of fluid and proteins, especially those larger than 20 kDa, between the peritoneal cavity and the blood stream. For small molecules exchange is rapid by simple diffusion, but for larger molecules transfer is much slower. Thus concentrations of blood proteins such as albumin, LH, and FSH are more than 40% lower than in plasma, whereas locally secreted macromolecules as CA125 and glycodelins accumulate in peritoneal fluid with concentrations that are much higher than in plasma (25–31). Peritoneal fluid contains high amounts of macrophages, which secrete, especially when activated, such as in endometriosis, a large variety of cytokines and growth factors. Peritoneal fluid thus is a specific microenvironment with protein and hormone concentrations that are much different from plasma (32,33).

When the mesothelial cell becomes traumatized (Fig. 3), as demonstrated for hypoxia during CO_2 pneumoperitoneum, the large flat mesothelial cell retracts, known as "bulging of cells," and the highly specialized layer of contiguous peritoneal cells is transformed into a layer of individual cells and between these cells large areas of basal membrane is directly exposed (34–39). Similar effects are believed to occur in response to all types of trauma such as desiccation, mechanical, or chemical trauma. The repair of this mesothelial cell trauma is rapid, and the peritoneal lining becomes normal again within two to three days. The consequence of this effect is largely unknown. Disruption of this highly specialized membrane is bound to affect all those substances transport of which is actively regulated by the mesothelium layer. The resorption of CO_2 from a pneumoperitoneum increases (22,23), whereas diffusion of larger molecules probably is greatly enhanced. It remains unclear to what extend this is associated with an inflammatory reaction and what the role is of attraction and activation of macrophages and their secretion products as cytokines and growth factors.

The Classic Model of Adhesion Formation: A Local Phenomenon

A trauma of the peritoneum, involving besides the mesothelial cells also the basal membrane and the subendothelial connective tissue, is followed by a local inflammatory reaction, exudation, and fibrin deposition (Fig. 2). This fibrin is normally

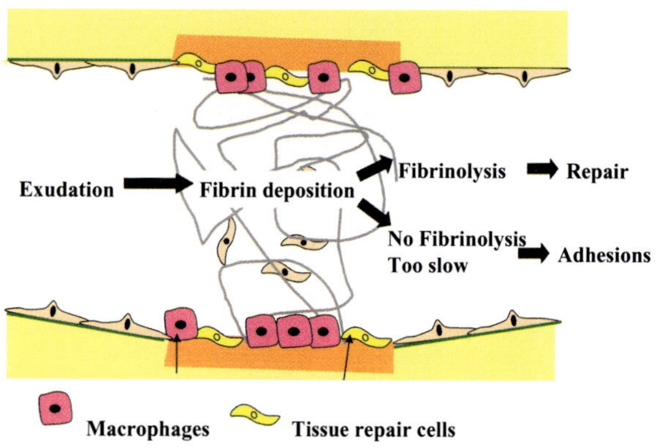

Figure 2 The classic model of adhesion formation as a local process with trauma, exudation and fibrin deposition, fibrinolysis, and rapid repair involving macrophages and tissue repair cells.

rapidly removed by fibrinolysis (40) while simultaneously the peritoneal repair process is started (41). Within hours of injury, the injured area is covered by what is believed macrophages and "tissue repair cells," which within three to four days differentiate into mesenchymal cells. Repair starts specifically from numerous small islands, and the repair of small and large areas therefore is similar. Given the concept of mesenchymal stem cells, the discussion about the exact nature of macrophages and tissue repair cells has acquired a new dimension, whereas the specific mechanism of repair starting from numerous small islands is easily understood (42). If the normal rapid repair of peritoneal lesions fails or when repair is delayed, other processes that were activated become dominant. Within four to six days, fibroblast proliferation invading the fibrin scaffold and angiogenesis starts, leading invariably to adhesion formation. The importance of the fibrin scaffold between two injured surfaces was elegantly demonstrated since separating these areas by Silastic membranes for up to 30 hours abolished adhesion formation (41). This type of experiments reinforced the belief that adhesion formation is a local process and that prevention should aim at separating the surfaces for at least two days. In addition, medical treatment given intravenously or intraperitoneally has been considered less important because this type of treatment would have difficulties reaching the injured zone because of local ischemia and it being shielded by the fibrin plug. The pathophysiology of this local process has been considered an inflammatory reaction, with players and mechanisms as fibrinolysis, plasmin activation, and PAIs, local macrophages and their secretion products and the overall oxygenation of the area or the absence thereof driving angiogenesis, fibroblast proliferation, and mesothelial repair. The focus on macrophages and tissue repair cells is changing rapidly given the actual concept to consider these stem cells.

Other arguments in favor of viewing adhesion formation as a local process are derived from the observations that some organs are more adhesiogenic than others and that this may be related to their fibrinolytic activity. A local process shielded from the rest of the peritoneal cavity seems also supported by the observation that normally peritoneal infection is kept localized by fibrin and adhesions. If not, a generalized peritonitis can become life-threatening.

Little is known about the mechanisms that determine whether adhesions will be velamentous, thick, and or vascularized and what factors determine innervations (43–45). Also adhesion remodeling is something that is poorly understood.

The Updated Model: The Peritoneal Cavity as a Cofactor

Studies published since mid-nineties have shown that the entire peritoneal cavity can be a cofactor in adhesion formation (7,8,22,23,46–60). Identified so far in laparoscopic rabbit and mouse models for adhesion formation are desiccation, hypoxia, reactive oxygen species (ROS), and manipulation (60), which increase adhesion formation at an injured area. Since CO_2 pneumoperitoneum–induced mesothelial hypoxia results in the entire exposed peritoneal area in retraction of mesothelial cells exposing directly the extracellular matrix (34–39), it is postulated that this results in the attraction into peritoneal fluid of substances of cellular elements and thus enhances adhesion formation and/or decrease repair, without causing adhesion formation outside the injured area. For hypoxia by CO_2 pneumoperitoneum, or for desiccation, one might argue that they also affect the injured site. The observation, however, of a similar dose-dependent effect following manipulation of the omentum and organs outside the injured area supports the concept that the entire peritoneal cavity can be a cofactor in adhesion formation (Fig. 3).

It seems logical to postulate that any trauma to the large and flat mesothelial cells will induce them to retract as a defense mechanism and that this effect is more pronounced when trauma is more severe. However, we do not know what the exact mechanisms are through which adhesion formation is further modulated. We only can speculate that macrophages and their secretion products, blood constituents, or other inflammatory products affect directly the repair process or the differentiation of stem cells at the injured area. Any postulated mechanism should explain that desiccation enhances

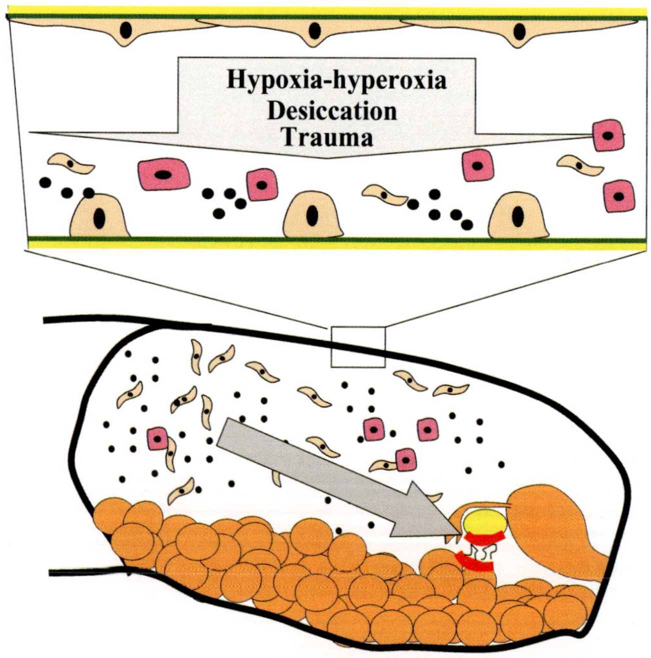

Figure 3 The updated model of adhesion formation. Flat mesothelial cells respond to trauma by retraction and bulging, exposing directly the extracellular matrix. The peritoneal fluid subsequently increases adhesion formation at the trauma site.

adhesion formation and that the effect is dose dependent. CO_2 pneumoperitoneum also enhances adhesion formation and the effect is pressure and duration dependent. The effect upon adhesions seems mediated through mesothelial hypoxia since the mesothelial layer stains hypoxic and since the increase in adhesions is prevented by the addition of 3% to 4% of oxygen (restoring the physiologic intraperitoneal partial oxygen pressure of 30–40 mm Hg) and is absent in mice partially deficient for hypoxia-inducible factor-1α and 2α (HIF1α and HIF2α) being the first to be activated by hypoxia. Similar effects are observed when partial oxygen pressures exceed 80 mm Hg, thus increasing ROS, and this effect can be prevented by ROS scavengers.

Pathophysiology of Adhesion Formation: Conclusions

The classic model, which views adhesion formation as a local phenomenon (Fig. 2), and the effect of the entire peritoneal cavity (Fig. 3) and its constituents should be considered as complementary. The importance of each effect might vary with the localization and the type of injury. Following severe traumas, large areas, e.g., the pelvic cavity, can become completely occluded by fibrinous adhesions and these areas probably escape from the influence of peritoneal fluid. In these circumstances, adhesion formation may follow mainly the classic model. For minor lesions, especially nonapposed lesions, such as those frequently occurring during fertility surgery, the effect of the peritoneal cavity probably is dominant.

Both models are also important for our understanding of adhesions prevention agents. A flotation agent will also dilute peritoneal fluid and any factor secreted locally by the denuded areas as well as will hamper the access of macrophages, which cannot swim. Barriers on the other hand might, in addition to keeping tissues separated, shield the injured area from the peritoneal fluid and its constituents, something that might be beneficial or detrimental according to circumstances.

To understand the role of the mesothelial cells in peritoneal repair, both models have to be considered simultaneously. Obviously, peritoneal repair and adhesion formation between injured areas is a local process. The repair cells, however, are at least partially derived from incorporation of free-floating mesothelial cells in the peritoneal fluid, which today could be considered partially differentiated stem or progenitor cells. Since repair can be accelerated and adhesion formation decreased, by intraperitoneal injection and transplantation of autologous mesothelial cells, any deleterious effect to the peritoneal cavity is bound to affect these free-floating cells. Today we can only speculate about endocrine or other factors affecting the function of these cells and even about the sheer number of cells available for repair. It is unclear whether, as a response to trauma of the peritoneal cavity by hypoxia or desiccation, the number of free-floating mesothelial cells/stem cells are expected to be increased by attraction or to be decreased because free-floating cells could attach to cover the denuded areas in between retracted mesothelial cells. The importance of mesothelial cell and their differentiation is also highlighted by the observation that the fibroblast cultured from adhesions are permanently differentiated from other mesothelial fibroblasts (61–63) and by the observation that recurrence rates after adhesiolysis are much higher than expected.

Clinically, some individuals form adhesions more easily after surgery than others—an observation supported by the fact that some mice strains form much more adhesions than others—while variability of adhesion formation is much lower in inbred strains (53). We also do not know why some adhesions are filmy and thin while other adhesions are dense; why some adhesions are vascular or avascular, or innervated or not.

PREVALENCE AND CLINICAL CONSEQUENCES OF POSTOPERATIVE ADHESION FORMATION

Following abdominal surgery, adhesions are formed in over 70% of women, and they have been considered as a cause of infertility, pain, and bowel obstructions (Fig. 4). The clinical importance of adhesion formation has been emphasized by the SCAR study (9–11) demonstrating in a 10-year follow-up of abdominal surgery in Scotland that the incidence of reoperation and of bowel obstruction kept rising almost linearly for a period of at least 10 years. Moreover, reinterventions occurred in some 30%, in many persons more than once, and at least 6% could be linked directly to adhesion formation. Repeat surgery was more difficult, more tedious, and associated with more complications because of adhesions. From these findings, models have been constructed, calculating cost of adhesions formation for society, and conversely the savings that could be realized by adhesion prevention assuming that reduction in adhesion formation could linearly be extrapolated to a reduction in pain, in infertility, and in repeat surgery or bowel obstructions.

The real clinical picture, however, is not so clear. The first confounding factor is quality of surgery, which is variable. Duration of surgery and complication rates decrease by training as demonstrated in a series of learning curves in both humans and animal models. Both the duration of endoscopic surgery and the extent of manipulation have been demonstrated to directly affect adhesion formation. It must be recognized that in contrast with medical therapy for which quality control is strictly organized, there is no quality control for surgery (12). Further, there are no data available permitting to judge the importance of adhesion formation for fertility, not even after fertility-promoting surgery. The results reported rather reflect centers of excellence and it is hard to judge whether differences in results are the consequence of techniques, indications, or surgeons. Finally, the introduction of laparoscopic surgery has probably decreased the overall quality of fertility surgery. Indeed, during the eighties fertility surgery was performed in specialized centers by surgeons highly trained in microsurgery, who had an important clinical interest in adhesion prevention and who had developed the concepts of gentle tissue handling and moistening. The introduction of endoscopic surgery, a surgical access route used by most general gynecologists, had as a consequence that generalists started performing fertility surgery, irrespective of training. That quality went down is difficult to prove given the absence of quality control in surgery, but the exponential rise in IVF cycles over the world might be due to some extent to the decrease in the training and hence to the use and to the quality of this type of surgery. If this is true, adhesion formation is a key factor.

That adhesions cause pain is widely believed based upon the observations that adhesions can be innervated (43,45) and that under local anesthesia, palpation of adhesions can cause pain (64,65). However, at present, we clearly cannot predict which adhesions cause pain or whether adhesiolysis would be beneficial. Given this variability in the relationship between pain and adhesions, and given the variable rate of adhesion reformation, it is not surprising that the results of adhesiolysis are still debated. Individual studies have reported pain reduction, but this could be due to placebo effect after surgery,

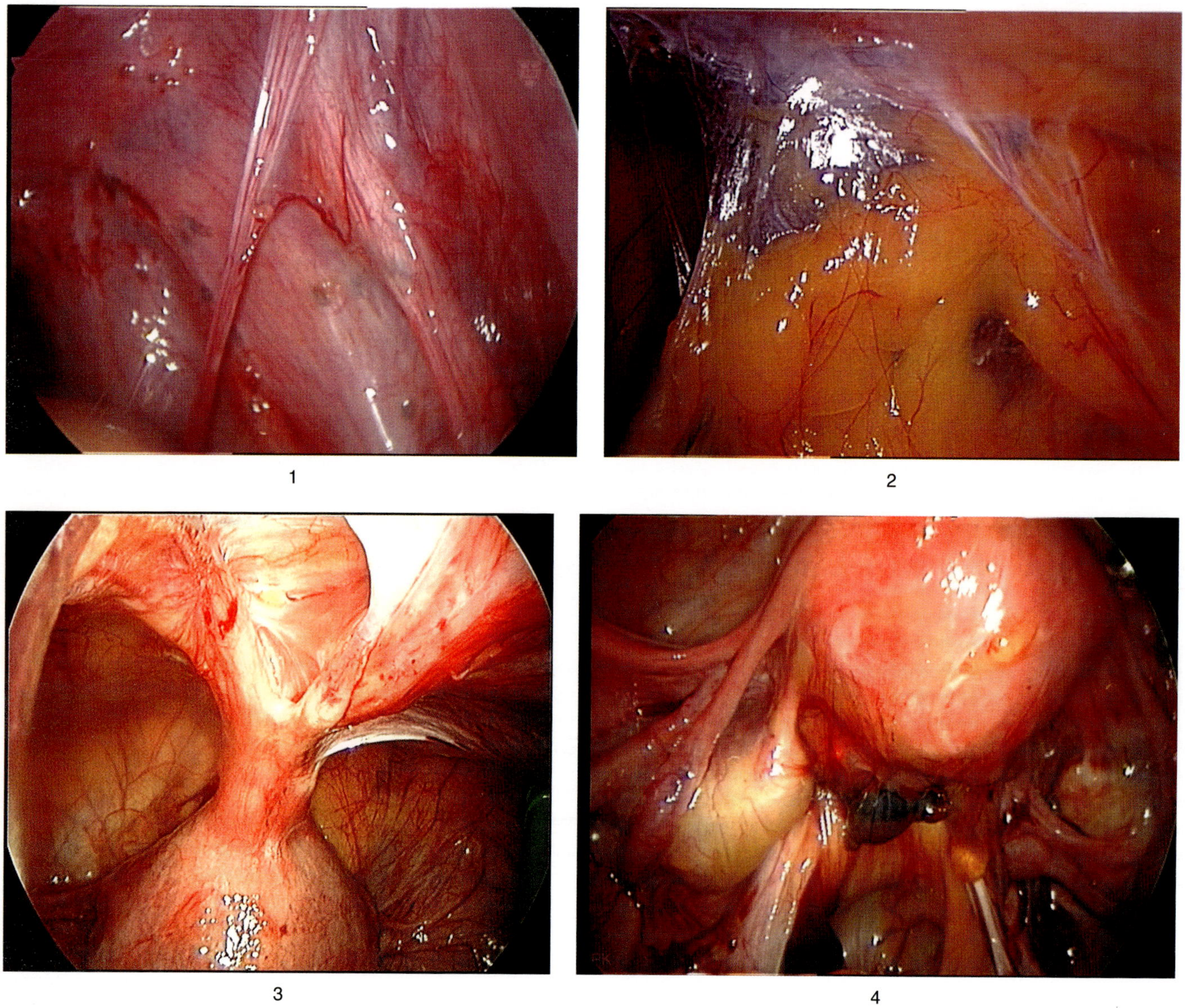

Figure 4 Adhesions vary from short but strong bands (**1**), causing eventually bowel obstruction, to filmy adhesions between omentum and the appendectomy scar (**2**) to dense vascularised adhesions between uterus and abdominal wall (**3**) to dense adhesions as seen in endometriosis (**4**).

whereas the only randomized control trials did not demonstrate a clear effect upon pain (66).

PREVENTION OF POSTOPERATIVE ADHESION FORMATION

Adhesion formation between opposing injured peritoneal surfaces are acknowledged to be different from adhesion reformation following lysis of adhesions and from *de novo* adhesion formation outside the areas of surgery. Since adhesion prevention has been investigated adequately only for the former, the following paragraphs will not discuss *de novo* adhesions and adhesion reformation.

Good Surgical Practice and Conditioning of the Peritoneal Cavity

Good surgical practice and gentle tissue handling have been introduced as an important tenet by the pioneers of microsurgery. This includes moistening of tissues by continuous irrigation, moistening of abdominal packs, glass or plastic rods for mobilization of tissues, and precise microinstruments. Reduction in adhesion formation was anticipated. However, it is only recently that the importance of prevention of desiccation and of gentle tissue handling have been proven, emphasizing how important and accurate clinical observation can be.

Key to good surgical practice today is whether the animal data can be extrapolated to humans. These data probably can be extrapolated because the effect of CO_2 pneumoperitoneum, the duration-dependent increased CO_2 resorption, observed in mice and in rabbits also occurs in women. Taking into account the findings in animal models, good surgical practice today should include the following. First, the insufflation gas should be conditioned in order to minimize hypoxia and desiccation; this requires humidification of the gas and the addition of 3% to 4% of oxygen to the CO_2. Moreover, cooling of the peritoneal cavity is important since it decreases both the effects of hypoxia and of desiccation, cells being more resistant to

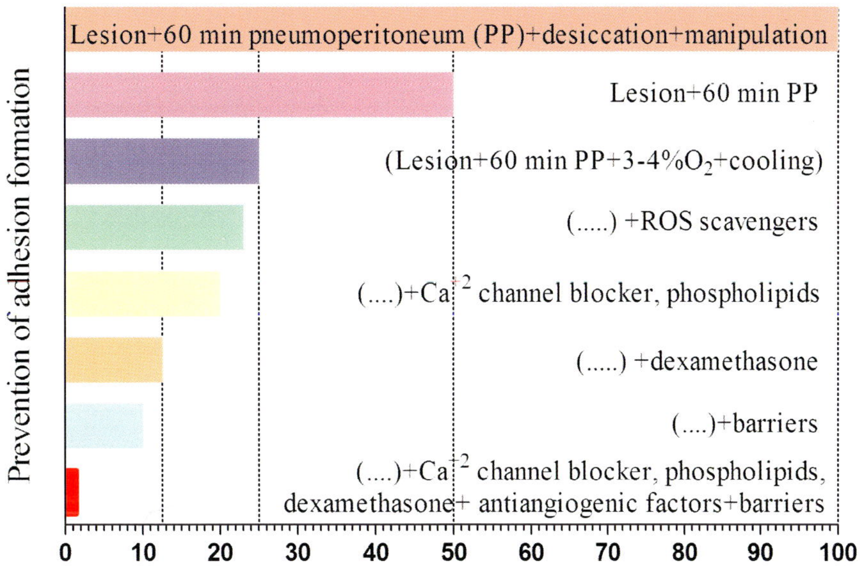

Figure 5 Prevention of adhesion formation in a laparoscopic mouse model. Minimizing mesothelial damage by preventing desiccation, gentle tissue handling, adding oxygen, and cooling decrease adhesion formation to some 25%. Adhesions decrease further by adding ROS scavengers, calcium channel blockers, phospholipids, or dexamethasone. In addition barrier gels can be used for over 90% reduction in adhesion formation. If in this model, calcium channel blockers, phospholipids, antiangiogenic monoclonal antibodies, and fibroblast manipulation would have additional effect, close to 100% adhesion reduction might be achieved.

metabolic damage at lower temperatures. Cooling of the peritoneal cavity makes it possible for the humidified and saturated insufflation gas to condense upon entrance to the pelvic cavity, thus preventing desiccation. Secondly, the duration of surgery should be kept to a minimum as well as the amount of bleeding and the extent of tissue manipulation. In summary, the surgeon should be experienced and well trained.

Observation of strict sterility remains mandatory to prevent any kind of infection. This simple statement should be balanced against the observation that it is difficult to completely disinfect the umbilicus and that each time the vagina is opened, at least some risk of infection occurs. This is even more likely with entry into the bowel. Good surgical practice therefore should begin by observing strict sterile conditions. This might sound obvious but it is not so evident, since in endoscopic surgery many surgeons no longer wear masks (endoscopic surgery being considered a semisterile intervention). Looking carefully at endoscopic interventions many minor mistakes are noticed if judged by the standards of open surgery. Whether extensive lavage following surgery might reduce adhesion formation or the risk of some minor infection is unknown. Following deep endometriosis surgery with full thickness resection and a bowel suture, extensive lavage with 8 L clearly decreased the postoperative inflammation as judged by CRP concentrations while preventing late bowel perforations (De Cicco C, unpublished observations). This has stimulated us to extend the use of extensive lavage to all surgical interventions with an increased risk of infection such as following hysterectomy or salpingostomy for hydrosalpinx. Interestingly, microsurgery also emphasized lavage for removing clots, foreign substances, and fibrin.

Taken together these measures of good surgical practice along with conditioning of the pneumoperitoneum, cooling and prevention of inflammation, should reduce adhesion formation by more than 60%.

Adhesion Prevention in Animal Models

A wide range of products have been shown to be effective in animal models. Efficacy of all products described so far has been extensively investigated in our laparoscopic mouse model. It should be realized that in this model all criteria of good surgical practice as described are fulfilled, with standardized lesions, controlled duration of surgery, strict control of temperature, and absence of desiccation (Fig. 5). It should also be realized that the laparoscopic mouse model is a model for three distinct pneumoperitoneum conditions: normoxia, hypoxia, and hyperoxia. The first model intends to minimize any peritoneal damage except for the lesions inflicted to induce adhesions. Thus, adhesions will form according to the classic model, with little or no effect of the peritoneal cavity. In this model, 4% of oxygen was added to the CO_2 pneumoperitoneum to prevent mesothelial hypoxia. The second model is the "hypoxia model" since adhesions are enhanced by CO_2 pneumoperitoneum–induced mesothelial hypoxia. In this model, pure CO_2 was used. In the third model, called hyperoxia model, 12% of oxygen was added to the CO_2 pneumoperitoneum, a concentration known to enhance adhesions probably by cell damage by ROS.

Dexamethasone decrease adhesions by some 30% in the hypoxia model (47), by 60% in the hyperoxia model (67), and, especially, by some 76% in the normoxia model when it is combined with low temperature (68). ROS scavengers decrease adhesions by 10% to 15% in both the hypoxia and hyperoxia models, an effect too small to be demonstrated in the normoxia model, with much less adhesions to start with. Calcium channel blockers decrease adhesion formation by some 35% of inhibition in both hypoxia (47) and hyperoxia models, and around 58% in the normoxia model when is combined with low temperature; recombinant plasminogen activator (rPA) decrease adhesion formation by 40% in the hypoxia (69) and normoxia models, whereas less inhibition, around 17%, was observed in the hyperoxia model. Ringers lactate as a flotation agent is marginally but significantly effective (51). The effects of other flotation agents such as carboxymethylcellulose (CMC) and Hyskon are marginal (46) and surfactants such as phospholipids give some 35% of inhibition in the hypoxia and hyperoxia models and 58% in the normoxia model when it is combined with low temperature. Icodextrin (Adept, 4% α (1-4) glucose polymer) unfortunately could not be evaluated since it is degraded enzymatically in mice. Barriers such as Hyalobarrier gel, Spraygel, and Intercoat are highly effective in all models with a reduction of 58% to 90% in adhesion formation.

Prevention of angiogenesis also reduces adhesion formation, as demonstrated in PlGF knockout mice and by the administration of anti-VEGF and anti-PlGF monoclonal antibodies (55,56,61–63,70,71).

The transplantation of cultured mesothelial cells into the peritoneal cavity also is effective in decreasing adhesion formation (72,73) and in remodeling the area of mesothelial denudation. More recently, mesothelial cells were used as transplantable tissue-engineered artificial peritoneum and research is focusing on the use of mesothelial progenitor cells (74).

Adhesion Prevention in Humans

Adhesion prevention in humans has been limited to barriers and flotation agents with a reduction of adhesion formation that ranges, for all products, between 40% and 50%. Most important is that for none of these products efficacy has been proven for endpoints that really matter, i.e., pain, infertility, bowel obstruction, or reoperation rate. We should also realize that large randomized controlled trials were needed because of the high intraindividual variability and that in these trials the surgical interventions were limited to rather simple and straightforward interventions as cystectomy and myomectomy. In addition, these trials have been performed during interventions performed by laparotomy or by laparoscopy under conditions of CO_2 pneumoperitoneum–enhanced adhesion formation and slight desiccation. It, therefore, is still unclear to what extend the available results of efficacy can be extrapolated to more severe or other types of surgery, and whether in the human the effect will be additive to good surgical practice and conditioning of the peritoneal cavity (46).

Sheet barriers such as Seprafilm (hyaluronic acid–carboxymethylcellulose) (75–77), Interceed (oxidized regenerated cellulose), (78,79) and Gore-Tex (expanded polytetrafluoroethylene) (80) are proven effective but did not become very popular for various reasons. Seprafilm is difficult to use during laparoscopy, Interceed requires the removal of any remaining bleeding to be efficacious, whereas Gore-Tex, being nondegradable, must be removed from the applied site during a second surgery.

Since Intergel (0.5% ferric hyaluronate gel) has been withdrawn from the market, only Hyalobarrier gel [auto-cross-linked hyaluronic acid gel (81)], Spraygel (polyethylenglycol), and Intercoat/Oxiplex (82,83) remain available for clinical use. Overall efficacy appears to be similar for all three products. A comparison between these three gels can unfortunately not be made since comparative trials do not exist. Also the strength of the available evidence varies and a Cochrane review of hyaluronic acid and Spraygel concluded that only for hyaluronic acid the evidence was solid (84).

While in humans the efficacy of Ringers lactate as a flotation agent has not been proven, Adept (Icodextrin) (85–87), a macromolecular sugar with a higher retention time in the peritoneal cavity, was expected and shown to be efficacious in adhesion reduction. A major advantage is the safety and absence of side effects, which were well established since this has been extensively used for peritoneal dialysis. The strength of the available evidence demonstrating efficacy was in a Cochrane review not considered very solid (84).

Strong arguments can be found in the literature to use LHRH agonist prior to surgery as adhesion prevention (88), but specific clinical trials are lacking.

DISCUSSION AND A LOOK INTO THE FUTURE

The concept of mesothelial cells as stem cells, which can be transplanted to peritoneal trauma areas to modulate repair and decrease adhesion formation in animal models, is actually stimulating research aimed at collecting large amounts of autologous mesothelial stem cells and at manipulating them in culture prior to transplantation. Simultaneously, the addition to the peritoneal fluid of factors known to stimulate resident mesothelial proliferation or mobilization or differentiation are investigated in order to decrease adhesion formation (89). Both the activation and multiplication of mesothelial cells is expected to be developed into new strategies to reduce postoperative adhesion formation (24,90,91). Also, the potential of using mesothelial stem cells derived from muscle is actively been investigated (92).

Immense progress has been made over the last 15 years in our understanding of the pathophysiology of adhesion formation and the mechanisms involved. Besides the traditional concept viewing adhesion formation as a local inflammation with fibrin deposition and removal, the peritoneal cavity has been demonstrated to have an important role. Hence good surgical practice, gentle tissue handling, prevention of desiccation, hypoxia and ROS production, and conditioning of the peritoneal cavity by cooling have become the first key aspects in prevention of adhesion formation. Since the mechanisms by which the peritoneal cavity influences adhesion formation remains unexplored we may reasonably expect that in the near future we will be able to decrease adhesion formation even further.

Inhibition of fibroblast proliferation obviously is an objective in adhesion prevention. The use of dexamethasone to reduce adhesion formation has been around since a long time but the efficacy has been debated and questioned. In our laparoscopic mouse model especially under conditions of minimal trauma to the peritoneal cavity the effectiveness was very pronounced. This was surprising, since other anti-inflammatory agents such as COX1 and COX2 inhibitors were not effective. Therefore, dexamethasone is suggested to be effective, and that not because it is an anti-inflammatory agent but because it inhibits mesothelial proliferation. This is also consistent with the observations that dexamethasone reduces cell proliferation, collagen deposition, and lung fibrosis (93). The hormonal factors modulating fibroblast proliferation are being extensively investigated and hepatocyte-derived growth factor (HGF) has been demonstrated to prevent peritoneal fibrosis. (94,95). That HGF is also effective in reducing adhesion formation was demonstrated by "painting" with adenovirus containing the HGF gene directly onto surface of the injured area (96).

Since we understand that during adhesion formation different mechanisms are sequentially involved, adhesion prevention strategies should aim no longer at only one mechanism but consider sequentially all different mechanisms. By doing so, we can decrease adhesion formation by more than 90% in animal models. Prevention of adhesions will start with good surgical practice, conditioning of the peritoneal cavity through cooling, and prevention of desiccation and of hypoxia by adding 3% to 4% of oxygen. This will reduce adhesion formation by over 50%. If all the last strategies are associated with products as ROS scavengers and dexamethasone, adhesion formation in mice drops by an additional 30% this means to an 80% to 85% of total adhesion reduction. If at the end of surgery, barriers are added, which by themselves are more than 50% effective, the cumulative adhesion formation reduction has been proven today to be more than 90%. Since the mechanisms through which the following products decrease adhesion formation are different from those listed before, we may expect that the effects will be additive. Indeed, effectivity between 30% and 40% was demonstrated for phospholipids and calcium channel blockers, whereas drugs preventing angiogenesis, by blocking PlGF of VEGF, are even more effective. This has not been demonstrated yet since in models in which adhesion formation is already reduced by more than 90%, it becomes statistically difficult to prove additional effects. In conclusion, it seems reasonable to expect virtually adhesion-free surgery in not too distant future.

SUMMARY

We have been aware for a long time that adhesions occur almost systematically in at least over 80% of women undergoing abdominal surgery. The widely held belief has been that adhesion formation increases with the severity of surgery and with infection but that this could largely be prevented by good quality surgery. Thus, postoperative adhesion formation has for many years been emotionally ignored by the "good surgeons." Only in the last decade, we have become aware of the clinical importance of adhesion formation, mainly though the SCAR studies, which have clearly demonstrated that the incidences of bowel obstruction and of reoperation due to postoperative adhesions keep increasing linearly for at least 10 years and are much higher than anticipated. That postoperative adhesions can cause infertility and pain is well known, although quantitative data are missing.

Adhesions formation between traumatized areas has traditionally been considered as a local process, i.e., an inflammatory reaction, exudation, and fibrin deposition followed by fibrinolysis and mesothelial repair. If the repair process is slowed down by infection, or very severe surgical trauma, locally insufficient blood supply, or foreign bodies such as sutures, a process of fibroblast proliferation together with angiogenesis starts and adhesions are formed. Key in this concept is that the fibrin is used as a scaffold for this process and that without prior fibrinous attachment between surfaces, adhesions do not occur. Over the last decade, awareness has grown that secretions and/or cells from the entire peritoneal cavity strongly influence this local phenomenon. The factors identified so far are desiccation, mesothelial hypoxia as it occurs during CO_2 pneumoperitoneum, ROS, which occurs during open surgery, and mesothelial trauma as a result of grasping and manipulation of intraperitoneal organs. If judged from animal models, this peritoneal effect is quantitatively much more important than the local phenomenon.

Prevention of adhesion formation therefore traditionally has focused upon good surgical practices and upon barriers or flotation agents or barriers preventing fibrinous attachments between injured surfaces. Flotation agents as Ringers lactate are marginally effective, whereas Adept has claimed 40% to 50% effectiveness explained by an increased retention time. Mechanical barriers produced as sheets (Seprafilm, Interceed, or Gore-Tex) and gels (Spraygel, Hyalobarrier gel, Intercoat) have also shown some 40% to 50% effectiveness albeit for specific interventions performed by recognized good surgeons only. Most importantly this is a highly variable efficacy and it remains unknown whether this variability in adhesions and in prevention is patient or intervention or surgeon dependent. In any case, for none of these products efficacy has been demonstrated for the clinically important endpoints such as pain, infertility, or reoperation rate.

The concept emphasizing the importance of the peritoneal cavity has opened new approaches to prevention. Gentle tissue handling is getting a new dimension: during surgery the peritoneal cavity should be conditioned by preventing hypoxia (adding 3% to 4% of oxygen to the pneumoperitoneum), by preventing desiccation (using humidified gas), and by cooling, when using laparoscopy as surgical access. In animal models these factors in combination are effective in reducing adhesions way over 80%. If used together with products such as dexamethasone and barriers, an overall efficacy over 95% maybe obtained.

We are at the beginning of understanding the mechanisms by which the peritoneal cavity affects adhesion formation. Although today the focus is on prevention of deleterious factors, we must also focus on increasing favorable factors and recognize the importance of peritoneal stem cells in the repair process.

ACKNOWLEDGMENTS

PRK wishes to thank his current collaborators, Jasper Verguts, Carlo De Cicco, Ron Schonman, Roberta Corona, and Adriana Bastidas, and his past collaborators, Jose Ordonez, Narter Yesidaglar, Osama Elkelani, Ospan Mynbaev, and Karina Mailova, for contributing actively to the concepts described. The authors also thank Marleen Craessaerts and Diane Wolput for their help.

REFERENCES

1. Gomel V. The impact of microsurgery in gynecology. Clin Obstet Gynecol 1980; 23:1301–1310.
2. Buckman RF Jr, Buckman PD, Hufnagel HV, et al. A physiologic basis for the adhesion-free healing of deperitonealized surfaces. J Surg Res 1976; 21:67–76.
3. Gomel V. Operative laparoscopy: Time for acceptance. Fertil Steril 1989; 52:1–11.
4. Gomel V, Yarali H. Infertility surgery: Microsurgery. Curr Opin Obstet Gynecol 1992; 4:390–399.
5. Gomel V. From microsurgery to laparoscopic surgery: A progress. Fertil Steril 1995; 63:464–468.
6. Gomel V, Urman B, Gurgan T. Pathophysiology of adhesion formation and strategies for prevention. J Reprod Med 1996; 41:35–41.
7. Molinas CR, Mynbaev O, Pauwels A, et al. Peritoneal mesothelial hypoxia during pneumoperitoneum is a cofactor in adhesion formation in a laparoscopic mouse model. Fertil Steril 2001; 76:560–567.
8. Molinas CR, Koninckx PR. Hypoxaemia induced by CO(2) or helium pneumoperitoneum is a co-factor in adhesion formation in rabbits. Hum Reprod 2000; 15:1758–1763.

9. Parker MC, Ellis H, Moran BJ, et al. Postoperative adhesions: Ten-year follow-up of 12,584 patients undergoing lower abdominal surgery. Dis Colon Rectum 2001; 44:822–829.
10. Lower AM, Hawthorn RJ, Ellis H, et al. The impact of adhesions on hospital readmissions over ten years after 8849 open gynaecological operations: An assessment from the Surgical and Clinical Adhesions Research Study. BJOG 2000; 107:855–862.
11. Ellis H, Moran BJ, Thompson JN, et al. Adhesion-related hospital readmissions after abdominal and pelvic surgery: A retrospective cohort study. Lancet 1999; 353:1476–1480.
12. Koninckx PR. Videoregistration of surgery should be used as a quality control. J Minim Invasive Gynecol 2008; 15:248–253.
13. Practice Committee of the American Society for Reproductive Medicine; Society of Reproductive Surgeons. Pathogenesis, consequences, and control of peritoneal adhesions in gynecologic surgery. Fertil Steril 2007; 88:21–26.
14. Parker MC, Wilson MS, van Goor H, et al. Adhesions and colorectal surgery – call for action. Colorectal Dis 2007; 9(suppl 2):66–72.
15. Moran BJ. Adhesion-related small bowel obstruction. Colorectal Dis 2007; 9(suppl 2):39–44.
16. van Goor H. Consequences and complications of peritoneal adhesions. Colorectal Dis 2007; 9(suppl 2):25–34.
17. Nappi C, Di Spiezio SA, Greco E, et al. Prevention of adhesions in gynaecological endoscopy. Hum Reprod Update 2007; 13:379–394.
18. Munoz-Chapuli R, Perez-Pomares JM, Macias D, et al. Differentiation of hemangioblasts from embryonic mesothelial cells? A model on the origin of the vertebrate cardiovascular system. Differentiation 1999; 64:133–141.
19. Herrick SE, Mutsaers SE. The potential of mesothelial cells in tissue engineering and regenerative medicine applications. Int J Artif Organs 2007; 30:527–540.
20. Lucas PA. Stem cells for mesothelial repair: An understudied modality. Int J Artif Organs 2007; 30:550–556.
21. Mutsaers SE, Prele CM, Lansley SM, et al. The origin of regenerating mesothelium: A historical perspective. Int J Artif Organs 2007; 30:484–494.
22. Mynbaev OA, Molinas CR, Adamyan LV, et al. Pathogenesis of CO(2) pneumoperitoneum-induced metabolic hypoxemia in a rabbit model. J Am Assoc Gynecol Laparosc 2002; 9:306–314.
23. Mynbaev OA, Molinas CR, Adamyan LV, et al. Reduction of CO(2)-pneumoperitoneum-induced metabolic hypoxaemia by the addition of small amounts of O(2) to the CO(2) in a rabbit ventilated model. A preliminary study. Hum Reprod 2002; 17:1623–1629.
24. Mutsaers SE, Wilkosz S. Structure and function of mesothelial cells. Cancer Treat Res 2007; 134:1–19.
25. Koninckx PR, Heyns W, Verhoeven G, et al. Biochemical characterization of peritoneal fluid in women during the menstrual cycle. J Clin Endocrinol Metab 1980; 51:1239–1244.
26. Koninckx PR, De Moor P, Brosens IA. Diagnosis of the luteinized unruptured follicle syndrome by steroid hormone assays on peritoneal fluid. Br J Obstet Gynaecol 1980; 87:929–934.
27. Koninckx PR, Renaer M, Brosens IA. Origin of peritoneal fluid in women: An ovarian exudation product. Br J Obstet Gynaecol 1980; 87:177–183.
28. Pattinson HA, Koninckx PR, Brosens IA, et al. Clotting and fibrinolytic activities in peritoneal fluid. Br J Obstet Gynaecol 1981; 88:160–166.
29. Cornillie FJ, Lauweryns JM, Seppala M, et al. Expression of endometrial protein PP14 in pelvic and ovarian endometriotic implants. Hum Reprod 1991; 6:1411–1415.
30. Koninckx PR. CA 125 in the management of endometriosis. Eur J Obstet Gynecol Reprod Biol 1993; 49:109–113.
31. Koninckx PR, Riittinen L, Seppala M, et al. CA-125 and placental protein 14 concentrations in plasma and peritoneal fluid of women with deeply infiltrating pelvic endometriosis. Fertil Steril 1992; 57:523–530.
32. Koninckx PR, Kennedy SH, Barlow DH. Endometriotic disease: The role of peritoneal fluid. Hum Reprod Update 1998; 4:741–751.
33. Koninckx PR, Kennedy SH, Barlow DH. Pathogenesis of endometriosis: The role of peritoneal fluid. Gynecol Obstet Invest 1999; 47(suppl 1):23–33.
34. Volz J, Koster S, Spacek Z, et al. Characteristic alterations of the peritoneum after carbon dioxide pneumoperitoneum. Surg Endosc 1999; 13:611–614.
35. Volz J, Koster S. Laparoscopy. To inflate or lift? Cancer 1999; 86:749–750.
36. Volz J, Koster S, Spacek Z, et al. The influence of pneumoperitoneum used in laparoscopic surgery on an intraabdominal tumor growth. Cancer 1999; 86:770–774.
37. Ordemann J, Jakob J, Braumann C, et al. Morphology of the rat peritoneum after carbon dioxide and helium pneumoperitoneum: A scanning electron microscopic study. Surg Endosc 2004; 18:1389–1393.
38. Suematsu T, Hirabayashi Y, Shiraishi N, et al. Morphology of the murine peritoneum after pneumoperitoneum vs laparotomy. Surg Endosc 2001; 15:954–958.
39. Obradovic MM, Stojimirovic BB, Trpinac DP, et al. Ultrastructural changes of peritoneal lining cells in uremia. Adv Perit Dial 2000; 16:26–30.
40. Holmdahl L. The role of fibrinolysis in adhesion formation. Eur J Surg Suppl 1997; 577:24–31.
41. DiZerega GS, Campeau JD. Peritoneal repair and post-surgical adhesion formation. Hum Reprod Update 2001; 7:547–555.
42. Mutsaers SE. Mesothelial cells: Their structure, function and role in serosal repair. Respirology 2002; 7:171–191.
43. Herrick SE, Mutsaers SE, Ozua P, et al. Human peritoneal adhesions are highly cellular, innervated, and vascularized. J Pathol 2000; 192:67–72.
44. Sulaiman H, Gabella G, Davis C, et al. Growth of nerve fibres into murine peritoneal adhesions. J Pathol 2000; 192:396–403.
45. Sulaiman H, Gabella G, Davis MC, et al. Presence and distribution of sensory nerve fibers in human peritoneal adhesions. Ann Surg 2001; 234:256–261.
46. Binda MM, Molinas CR, Bastidas A, et al. Efficacy of barriers and hypoxia-inducible factor inhibitors to prevent CO(2) pneumoperitoneum-enhanced adhesions in a laparoscopic mouse model. J Minim Invasive Gynecol 2007; 14:591–599.
47. Binda MM, Molinas CR, Bastidas A, et al. Effect of reactive oxygen species scavengers, antiinflammatory drugs, and calcium-channel blockers on carbon dioxide pneumoperitoneum-enhanced adhesions in a laparoscopic mouse model. Surg Endosc 2007; 21:1826–1834.
48. Binda MM, Molinas CR, Hansen P, et al. Effect of desiccation and temperature during laparoscopy on adhesion formation in mice. Fertil Steril 2006; 86:166–175.
49. Binda MM, Molinas CR, Mailova K, et al. Effect of temperature upon adhesion formation in a laparoscopic mouse model. Hum Reprod 2004; 19:2626–2632.
50. Mynbaev OA, Koninckx PR, Bracke M. A possible mechanism of peritoneal pH changes during carbon dioxide pneumoperitoneum. Surg Endosc 2007; 21:489–491.
51. Elkelani OA, Molinas CR, Mynbaev O, et al. Prevention of adhesions with crystalloids during laparoscopic surgery in mice. J Am Assoc Gynecol Laparosc 2002; 9:447–452.
52. Elkelani OA, Binda MM, Molinas CR, et al. Effect of adding more than 3% oxygen to carbon dioxide pneumoperitoneum on adhesion formation in a laparoscopic mouse model. Fertil Steril 2004; 82:1616–1622.
53. Molinas CR, Binda MM, Campo R, et al. Adhesion formation and interanimal variability in a laparoscopic mouse model varies with strains. Fertil Steril 2005; 83:1871–1874.
54. Molinas CR, Tjwa M, Vanacker B, et al. Role of CO(2) pneumoperitoneum-induced acidosis in CO(2) pneumoperitoneum-enhanced adhesion formation in mice. Fertil Steril 2004; 81:708–711.
55. Molinas CR, Binda MM, Carmeliet P, et al. Role of vascular endothelial growth factor receptor 1 in basal adhesion formation and in carbon dioxide pneumoperitoneum-enhanced adhesion

formation after laparoscopic surgery in mice. Fertil Steril 2004; 82(suppl 3):1149–1153.
56. Molinas CR, Campo R, Dewerchin M, et al. Role of vascular endothelial growth factor and placental growth factor in basal adhesion formation and in carbon dioxide pneumoperitoneum-enhanced adhesion formation after laparoscopic surgery in transgenic mice. Fertil Steril 2003; 80(suppl 2):803–811.
57. Molinas CR, Campo R, Elkelani OA, et al. Role of hypoxia inducible factors 1alpha and 2alpha in basal adhesion formation and in carbon dioxide pneumoperitoneum-enhanced adhesion formation after laparoscopic surgery in transgenic mice. Fertil Steril 2003; 80(suppl 2):795–802.
58. Molinas CR, Elkelani O, Campo R, et al. Role of the plasminogen system in basal adhesion formation and carbon dioxide pneumoperitoneum-enhanced adhesion formation after laparoscopic surgery in transgenic mice. Fertil Steril 2003; 80:184–192.
59. Molinas CR, Koninckx PR. CO_2 and helium pneumoperitoneum and the related anoxemia as a cofactor in adhesion formation. A prospective randomized trial in a rabbit model. In: Combined Meeting of the International Congress on Peritoneal Repair and Adhesions (PAX, Fifth Meeting) and International Mesothelioma Interest Group (IMIG, Fifth Meeting). October 5–8, 1999; Stoke Rochford, Grantham, Lincolnshire, UK.
60. Schonman R, Corona R, Bastidas A, et al. Effect of upper abdomen tissue manipulation on adhesion formation between injured areas in a laparoscopic mouse model. J Minim Invasive Gynecol 2009; 16(3):307–312.
61. Saed GM, Jiang Z, Fletcher NM, et al. Modulation of the BCL-2/BAX ratio by interferon-gamma and hypoxia in human peritoneal and adhesion fibroblasts. Fertil Steril 2008; 90(5):1925–1930.
62. Alpay Z, Ozgonenel MS, Savasan S, et al. Possible role of natural immune response against altered fibroblasts in the development of post-operative adhesions. Am J Reprod Immunol 2006; 55:420–427.
63. Saed GM, Zhao M, Diamond MP, et al. Regulation of inducible nitric oxide synthase in post-operative adhesions. Hum Reprod 2006; 21:1605–1611.
64. Demco L. Mapping the source and character of pain due to endometriosis by patient-assisted laparoscopy. J Am Assoc Gynecol Laparosc 1998; 5:241–245.
65. Demco L. Review of pain associated with minimal endometriosis. JSLS 2000; 4:5–9.
66. Swank DJ, Jeekel H. Laparoscopic adhesiolysis in patients with chronic abdominal pain. Curr Opin Obstet Gynecol 2004; 16:313–318.
67. Binda MM, Koninckx PR. Hyperoxia and prevention of adhesion formation: A laparoscopic mouse model for open surgery. BJOG 2010; 117(3):331–339.
68. Binda MM, Koninckx PR. Prevention of adhesion formation in a laparoscopic mouse model should combine local treatment with peritoneal cavity conditioning. Hum Reprod 2009; 24(6):1473–1479.
69. Binda MM. Pathophysiology and Prevention of Adhesion Formation in a Laparoscopic Mouse Model. Leuven, Belgium: Leuven University Press, 2008. http://hdl.handle.net/1979/1728.
70. Saltzman AK, Olson TA, Mohanraj D, et al. Prevention of postoperative adhesions by an antibody to vascular permeability factor/vascular endothelial growth factor in a murine model. Am J Obstet Gynecol 1996; 174:1502–1506.
71. Chiang SC, Cheng CH, Moulton KS, et al. TNP-470 inhibits intraabdominal adhesion formation. J Pediatr Surg 2000; 35:189–196.
72. Di Paolo N, Sacchi G, Vanni L, et al. Autologous peritoneal mesothelial cell implant in rabbits and peritoneal dialysis patients. Nephron 1991; 57:323–331.
73. Di Paolo N, Vanni L, Sacchi G. Autologous implant of peritoneal mesothelium in rabbits and man. Clin Nephrol 1990; 34:179–184.
74. Di Paolo N, Sacchi G, Del Vecchio MT, et al. State of the art on autologous mesothelial transplant in animals and humans. Int J Artif Organs 2007; 30:456–476.
75. Zeng Q, Yu Z, You J, et al. Efficacy and safety of Seprafilm for preventing postoperative abdominal adhesion: Systematic review and meta-analysis. World J Surg 2007; 31:2125–2131.
76. Beck DE. Seprafilm review and meta-analysis. World J Surg 2008; 32(8):1883–1884.
77. Mohri Y, Kusunoki M. Efficacy and safety of seprafilm: Systematic review and meta-analysis. World J Surg 2008; 32(8):1886–1887.
78. DiZerega GS. Use of adhesion prevention barriers in ovarian surgery, tubalplasty, ectopic pregnancy, endometriosis, adhesiolysis, and myomectomy. Curr Opin Obstet Gynecol 1996; 8:230–237.
79. Larsson B. Efficacy of Interceed in adhesion prevention in gynecologic surgery: A review of 13 clinical studies. J Reprod Med 1996; 41:27–34.
80. Baakdah H, Tulandi T. Adhesion in gynecology complication, cost, and prevention: A review. Surg Technol Int 2005; 14:185–190.
81. Carta G, Cerrone L, Iovenitti P. Postoperative adhesion prevention in gynecologic surgery with hyaluronic acid. Clin Exp Obstet Gynecol 2004; 31:39–41.
82. DiZerega GS, Coad J, Donnez J. Clinical evaluation of endometriosis and differential response to surgical therapy with and without application of Oxiplex/AP* adhesion barrier gel. Fertil Steril 2007; 87:485–489.
83. Lundorff P, Donnez J, Korell M, et al. Clinical evaluation of a viscoelastic gel for reduction of adhesions following gynaecological surgery by laparoscopy in Europe. Hum Reprod 2005; 20:514–520.
84. Metwally M, Watson A, Lilford R, et al. Fluid and pharmacological agents for adhesion prevention after gynaecological surgery. Cochrane Database Syst Rev 2006; CD001298.
85. Brown CB, Luciano AA, Martin D, et al. Adept (icodextrin 4% solution) reduces adhesions after laparoscopic surgery for adhesiolysis: A double-blind, randomized, controlled study. Fertil Steril 2007; 88:1413–1426.
86. Menzies D, Pascual MH, Walz MK, et al. Use of icodextrin 4% solution in the prevention of adhesion formation following general surgery: From the multicentre ARIEL Registry. Ann R Coll Surg Engl 2006; 88:375–382.
87. DiZerega GS, Verco SJ, Young P, et al. A randomized, controlled pilot study of the safety and efficacy of 4% icodextrin solution in the reduction of adhesions following laparoscopic gynaecological surgery. Hum Reprod 2002; 17:1031–1038.
88. Schindler AE. Gonadotropin-releasing hormone agonists for prevention of postoperative adhesions: An overview. Gynecol Endocrinol 2004; 19:51–55.
89. Mutsaers SE, Whitaker D, Papadimitriou JM. Stimulation of mesothelial cell proliferation by exudate macrophages enhances serosal wound healing in a murine model. Am J Pathol 2002; 160:681–692.
90. Mutsaers SE, Di Paolo N. Future directions in mesothelial transplantation research. Int J Artif Organs 2007; 30:557–561.
91. Herrick SE, Mutsaers SE. Mesothelial progenitor cells and their potential in tissue engineering. Int J Biochem Cell Biol 2004; 36:621–642.
92. Schultz SS, Abraham S, Lucas PA. Stem cells isolated from adult rat muscle differentiate across all three dermal lineages. Wound Repair Regen 2006; 14:224–231.
93. Dik WA, McAnulty RJ, Versnel MA, et al. Short course dexamethasone treatment following injury inhibits bleomycin induced fibrosis in rats. Thorax 2003; 58:765–771.
94. Warn R, Harvey P, Warn A, et al. HGF/SF induces mesothelial cell migration and proliferation by autocrine and paracrine pathways. Exp Cell Res 2001; 267:258–266.
95. Matsuoka T, Maeda Y, Matsuo K, et al. Hepatocyte growth factor prevents peritoneal fibrosis in an animal model of encapsulating peritoneal sclerosis. J Nephrol 2008; 21:64–73.
96. Liu HJ, Wu CT, Duan HF, et al. Adenoviral-mediated gene expression of hepatocyte growth factor prevents postoperative peritoneal adhesion in a rat model. Surgery 2006; 140:441–447.

3

Principles and practice of electrosurgery

Andrew I. Brill

The need to achieve hemostasis in surgery has been a concern of physicians from at least the days of ancient Egypt (1). Since that time various forms of cautery—to destroy tissue by burning or searing it—have long been used. The earliest known use of cautery described how the physician Imhotep treated medical cases in about 3000 B.C. Dr. William Gilbert, often referred to as the Father of Electrotherapy, began exploring the static electricity properties of amber in the late sixteenth century. The first to use the term "electricity," his studies laid the groundwork for the development of electrosurgical generators (2).

The first clinical use of electrosurgery was by French surgeon Joseph A. Riviere, who in the late 1800s used an electrical spark to treat an ulcer on a musician's hand (2). The potential for therapeutic uses of electricity increased significantly when William J. Morton later showed that current at a very high frequency does not produce pain and shock in tissues; neuromuscular stimulation by depolarization—known as the Faradic effect—ceases above a certain level (3). By the early 1900s, researchers were using electrical current in various forms to produce a number of different tissue effects, coining new terms such as "fulguration," "coagulation," and "desiccation" that are still in use today. In 1907, a patent was filed for the first electrosurgical generator unit (ESU) (4).

In the 1910s and 1920s, it was the work of William T. Bovie and Harvey Cushing that resulted in the worldwide acceptance and use of electrosurgery (5). Bovie, a biophysical engineer who worked with the Harvard Cancer Commission, believed that high-frequency current could heat tissue just as well as the radium that was then being used for cancer patients. The innovation and research that yielded this pioneering work is the foundation for today's electrosurgery, which is among the most widely used surgical technologies. Electrosurgery is now a universally accepted method of dissecting tissue and achieving hemostasis. In fact, it is estimated that electrosurgery is used in approximately 85% of all surgical procedures performed (6).

Appreciating the multiplicity of variables that can be proactively manipulated with electrosurgery will increase surgeon facility and serve to reduce excess thermal damage and risks inherent to electrosurgery. Moreover, a keen understanding of the biophysical principles that regulate electrosurgery will empower physicians' applications of electrosurgical techniques.

FUNDAMENTALS AND BIOPHYSICS OF ELECTRICITY

Two types of electrical current exist: direct current (DC) and alternating current (AC). With DC, the electrons flow in only one direction. With AC, the electrons constantly change direction, moving between positive and negative poles, as the current flows along a circuit (Fig. 1). The frequency at which AC

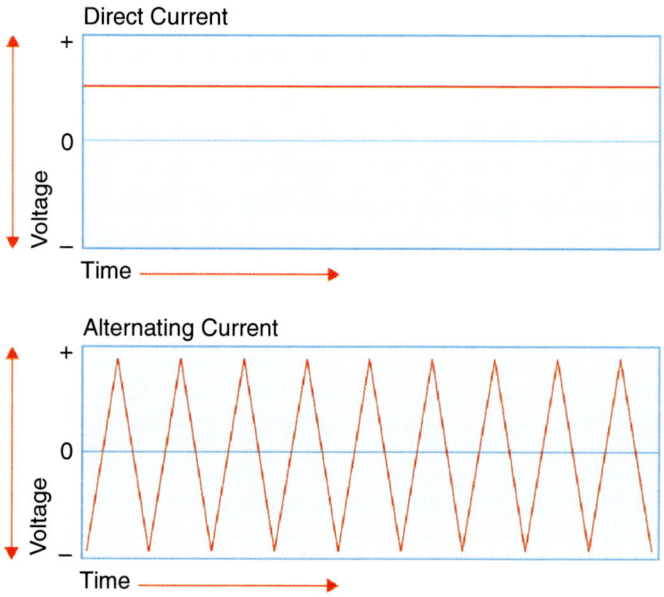

Figure 1 In direct current (*top*), electrons flow in only one direction. In alternating current (*bottom*), they move between positive and negative poles.

oscillates between the positive and negative poles is measured in Hertz (Hz), or cycles per second (1 Hz equals one cycle per second).

Accidental contact with household outlet current, which oscillates at 60 cycles per second (60 Hz), can cause tetanic skeletal muscle contraction due to depolarization of the neuromuscular junction (Faradic effect), burns, or electrocution. As Morton showed, however, depolarization of the neuromuscular junction by electricity can be prevented by using AC at a frequency significantly higher than household current (3). Contact with current above 100,000 cycles per second or 100 kilohertz (kHz) does not cause tetanic muscle contraction or pose any risk for electrocution, as the kinetic energy is simply dissipated in tissues as heat (7). The traditional electrosurgical generator (ESU) converts low-frequency AC from a standard electrical outlet (60 Hz) to very high-frequency AC (300–600 kHz range). Since the frequency used for electrosurgery includes that of both radio and television signal transmission (550–880 kHz), electrosurgery current is also referred to as radiofrequency (RF) current (Fig. 2).

Simply defined, electrosurgery is accomplished by the generation and delivery of a high-frequency AC between an active electrode, through living tissue, and to a dispersive (return) electrode. All electrosurgical tissue effects result from the conduction of electrons with sufficient concentration to create variable rates of tissue heating. Moving nearly at the speed

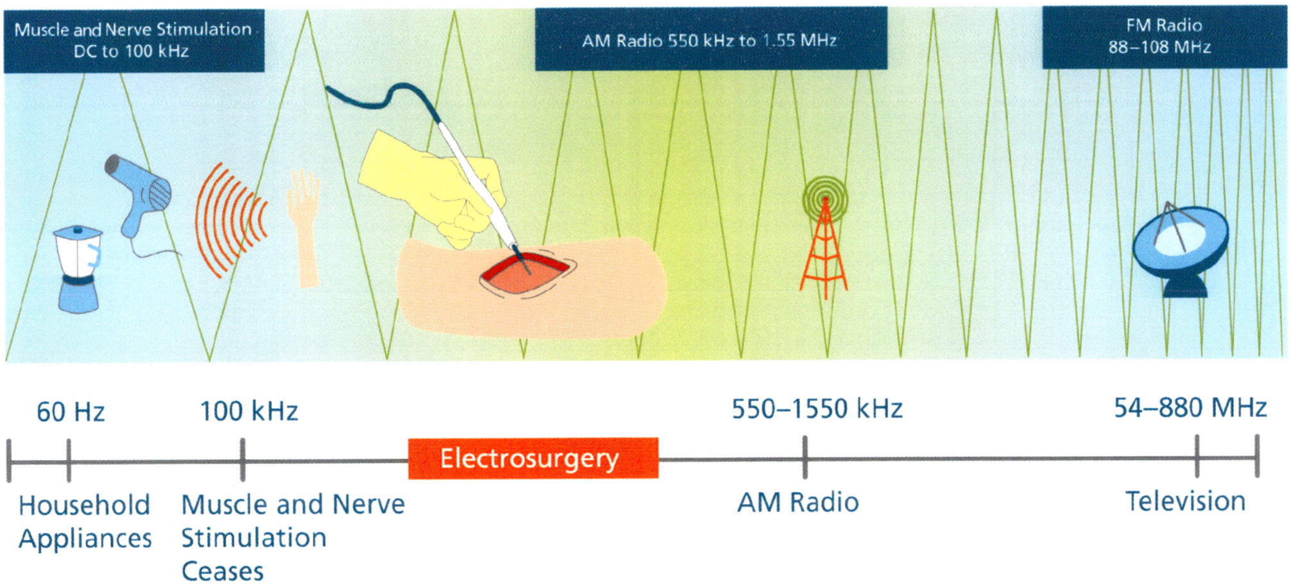

Figure 2 Electrosurgery uses high frequency alternating current that is in the radiofrequency range.

of light, these electrons produce heat as they overcome the opposition or resistance to conduction by tissue constituents—termed "impedance" in the case of AC. Resultant thermodynamic phenomena during the intervening tissue conduction ultimately increase tissue temperature, causing a variety of phenomena and tissue effects described as cutting (vaporization), fulguration, coagulation, or desiccation (8). Hence, high-frequency AC is conducted through an insulated surgical instrument–electrode assembly and then into living tissue. Since electricity will always seek an electron reservoir such as the ground (i.e., the earth) by following the pathways of least resistance, there must be a complete electrical circuit during electrosurgery so the current can return to ground.

During monopolar electrosurgery, the complete electrical circuit includes the electrosurgical generator unit, the active electrode, and patient's tissues (9). Once electrical current is applied to the tissue target, it is conducted from the surgical site via a myriad of pathways through the patient to be distributed over a much larger area via the dispersive (aka grounding) electrode. The larger surface area and substantially lower current density at the dispersive electrode site precludes tissue heating sufficient to burn (Fig. 3). On the other hand, during bipolar electrosurgery, both the active and dispersive electrodes are isolated to the small amount of tissue at the surgical site and thermal effects are evenly distributed between the surfaces of each electrode.

Electricity is a form of electromagnetic energy. At its root are the particles that orbit atoms: negatively charged electrons, positively charged protons, and neutrons. Electrons flow from one atom to another, and this flow of electrons is termed electricity.

Electrical current (I), a term that is often used interchangeably with electricity, is defined as the amount of electricity moving through an area or conductor over a specific amount of time. Given a significant difference in electrical potential, electrons are set in motion in a particular direction within a conductor to carry an electrical current that is measured in amperes (A) and represents the rate of flow of electrical charge. The electromotive force that pushes the current through the conductor is referred to as voltage (V) (8,10). Resistance (termed impedance with high-frequency AC), is measured in Ohms and represents the property of a conductor that opposes the flow of the current (Fig. 4).

Electricity is governed by Ohm's law:

$$V\text{ (voltage)} = I\text{ (current)} \times R\text{ (resistance/impedance)}$$

Current (I) is directly proportional to voltage (V) and inversely proportional to resistance (R). Greater resistance therefore requires greater voltage (11). If the resistance is a fixed variable, greater voltage will create greater current (Fig. 4). On the other hand, power (the numerical designation that a surgeon keys into the electrosurgical generator) quantifies the rate of work

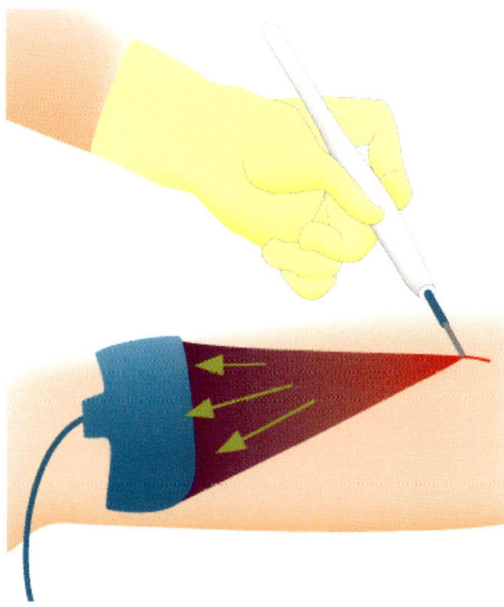

Figure 3 High-current concentration occurs where the tip of the hand-held pencil electrode is placed next to the skin. As the current travels through the body to the dispersive electrode, it is distributed over a substantially larger surface area and is less concentrated, precluding any thermal tissue effects.

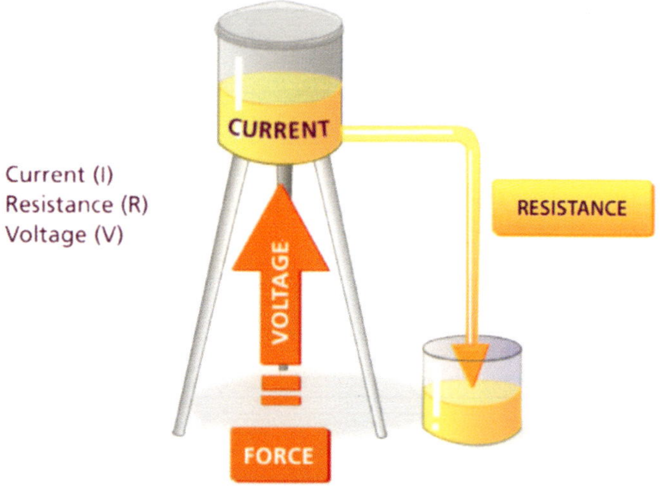

Figure 4 The fundamental elements of electricity—current, resistance, and voltage—and their relationships are depicted by a water tower. Just as it takes pressure to fill the reservoir, voltage is the electromotive force that drives current across an electrical circuit. As more fluid or a smaller diameter outlet would require greater pressure, greater current or increasing resistance requires higher voltage. (Ohm's law: $V = I \times R$.)

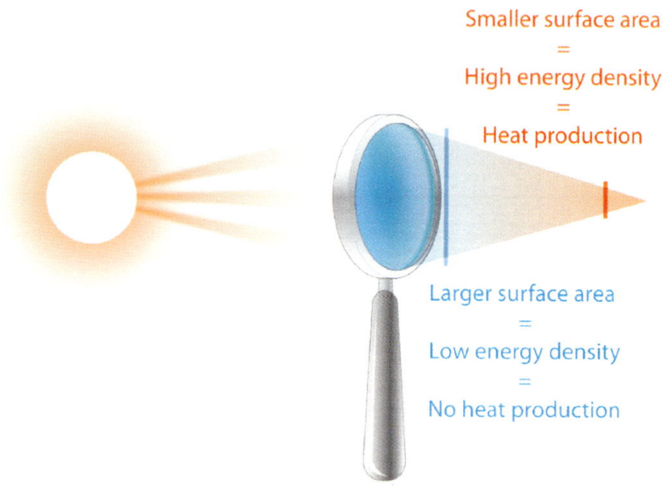

Figure 5 Energy density: Just as the sun can be variably focused with a magnifying glass to produce heat, the generation of thermal effects during electrosurgery is dependent upon the amount of current concentration, or current density.

being done and is expressed in watts (W). This is expressed by the following equation:

$$W = I \times V, \text{ or alternatively as } W = I^2 \times R \text{ and } W = V^2 R$$

Three important concepts can be derived from these relationships:

1. When an electrode is applied to tissues with higher impedance (e.g., fat), the electrosurgical generator correspondingly outputs greater voltage (V) provided the power setting (W) remains the same.
2. Similarly, output voltage (V) will be greater whenever current (R) is conducted via the high impedance pathways of carbonized tissue products that inevitably encrust electrode surfaces.
3. Since voltage (V) is electromotive force that drives the transit of charged particles across a potential difference, *greater voltage has the propensity to produce greater lateral and deeper thermal necrosis.*

A "pathway" or completed circuit must exist for electrons to flow. Since energy can be neither created nor destroyed, heat is produced as the moving electrons encounter resistance, so-called resistive heating. *This ability of electricity to produce work in the form of heat in living tissue is central to the mechanism of electrosurgery.* The surgeon's goal during electrosurgery is to attain anatomic dissection with hemostasis while causing the least amount of collateral damage and subsequent scar tissue formation.

The term electrocautery is often used—albeit incorrectly—to describe electrosurgery. Electrocautery is the intentional burning of tissue with a hot surgical instrument, such as a wire-looped hyfrecator, that is heated by using DC. During electrocautery, the patient is not a part of any electrical circuit and there is no ability to objectively moderate or precisely control the thermal effects on tissue (11). In contrast, during electrosurgery, the patient's tissues are part of a complete electrical circuit (12) and variable thermal effects can be achieved and precisely controlled. *Electrocautery is not electrosurgery.*

The rate of heat production from the conduction of current in living tissue ultimately determines whether cutting or coagulation of the target occurs; this fundamentally depends on the applied current concentration, known as current density. Practically speaking, manipulating electrode surface area (i.e., current density) will determine whether coagulation or cutting predominates (Fig. 5). This means coagulation will occur whenever a larger electrode surface area is used, causing tissue dehydration, vessel wall shrinkage, and coagulation of blood constituents by slow tissue heating; on the other hand, a small electrode surface area will result in tissue cutting or vaporization by delivering a much higher density of electrical energy that rapidly superheats intracellular water. In both instances, the output current (i.e., *cut, blend, and coag*) or power settings (W) on the electrosurgical generator have little bearing on the desired electrosurgical endpoint. In essence, the more concentrated the current, the more rapidly heat is produced. Consequently, higher energy concentration or density is more effective and produces more heat per unit time (Fig. 6). This explains why heat is concentrated at the active electrode and not at the substantially larger dispersive electrode during monopolar electrosurgery.

BIPOLAR AND MONOPOLAR ELECTROSURGERY

Bipolar Electrosurgery

Electrosurgery is traditionally described as either in bipolar or monopolar mode. In fact, all electrosurgery is intrinsically bipolar because of the use of AC (13). With the conventional bipolar mode, the patient is in essence not part of the circuit; the current does not enter the patient's body beyond the immediate surgical site (Fig. 7). Rather than coursing through the body, the flow of AC is symmetrically distributed, reversing direction every 1/2 cycle, and is conducted from the electrosurgical generator (ESU) to one electrode (of a two-poled surgical instrument), through the tissue being grasped or contacted, to the second electrode, and back to the generator. In the bipolar mode, the energy is delivered and returned at the same site with no need for a larger dispersive electrode. Since the distance between the active electrodes is so small, power requirements are substantially less than they are during

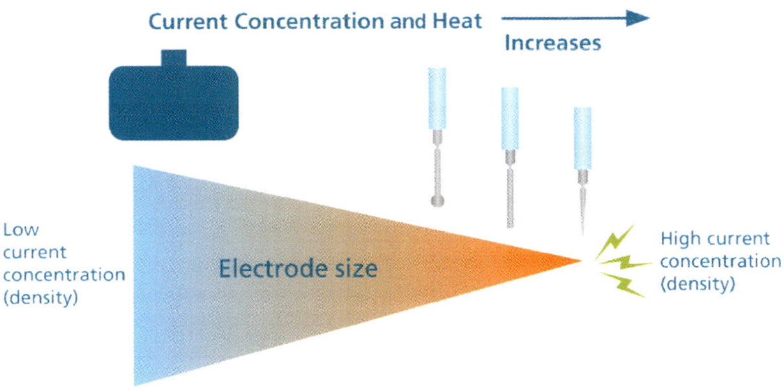

Figure 6 Since the production of heat during electrosurgery depends upon the current density, it is moderated by the electrode surface area.

monopolar electrosurgery. This intrinsically limits the use of conventional bipolar electrosurgery to desiccation and coagulation of tissue (10).

Intuitively then, bipolar electrosurgery has some advantages over monopolar electrosurgery. It is a reliable method of occluding and sealing blood vessels, and it can limit the amount of effected tissue. It also has a more limited area of thermal spread and produces less smoke. Because the two electrodes are in close proximity, it can work well under saline or nonelectrolyte solutions in the surgical field. In addition, it potentially alleviates cross-interference with implanted electrical devices such as cardiac pacemakers (7).

Despite the isolation of tissue between the bipolar electrodes, thermal damage may occur well beyond their confines. Desiccation of tissue percolates heated intracellular water into adjacent tissues. The unabated application of current after attaining this endpoint can propagate a secondary thermal bloom that disruptively bubbles steam throughout the surrounding parenchyma. Further application of current using older electrosurgical generators may heat enough to carbonize and cause a sticky tissue amalgam. These adverse phenomena are best prevented by terminating current on tissue whitening and when water vapor can no longer be seen to percolate

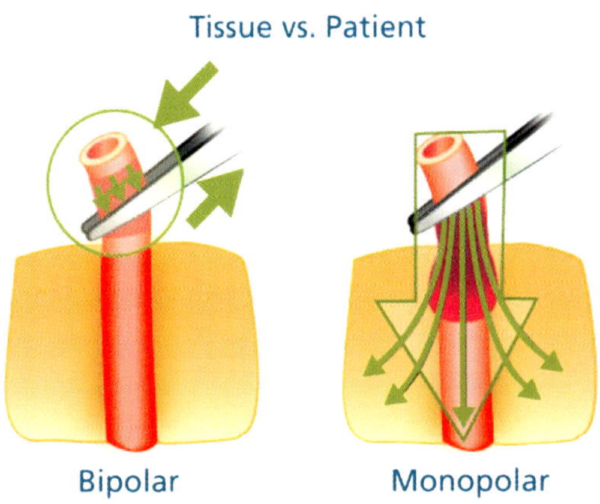

Figure 7 In bipolar electrosurgery, the current flows from the electrosurgical generator into a two-poled instrument, through the intervening tissue, and then back to the generator without entering the rest of the body. Since all thermal effects occur in the tissue contacted by the instrument, a dispersive electrode is not required to complete the circuit.

from the heated tissue. Despite its propriety for determining the endpoint for bipolar tubal sterilization, the use of an in-line ammeter, which meters the flow of current between the tissue and the jaws of the bipolar grasper, does not prevent this problem. Rather, it tends to promote over-desiccation of tissue. Since larger coapted tissue pedicles generate greater heat, unwanted thermal damage can also be minimized by selectively utilizing the sides or tips of a slightly open bipolar device to directly tamponade and then desiccate with the episodic application of current. Rather than subjecting a desiccated pedicle to mechanical trauma, an electrosurgically frozen pedicle can usually be dislodged by activating the active electrodes while immersed in a conductive irrigant (14).

New Bipolar Ligating-Cutting Devices

The latest advances in bipolar electrosurgery arise from the evolution and development of instant feedback technology that delivers either pulsed or continuous electrical output with constant voltage by only moderating the output current. This new breed of electrosurgical generators is paired with a variety of novel ligating-cutting devices, which are manufactured to provide continuous feedback about tissue impedance (resistance) at the treatment site. By near instantaneous response to incremental changes in tissue resistance, total energy delivery using these newer devices is dramatically less than it is with conventional bipolar systems. Once tonal feedback from the electrosurgical generator signals complete desiccation of the tissue bundle, the pedicle is typically cut by advancing a centrally set mechanical blade. These devices should logically reduce tissue carbonization, sticking, plume, and lateral thermal damage. As a general rule, low-voltage bipolar desiccation of coapted vessels is more effective under reduced tissue tension. All are able to adequately seal blood vessels up to 7 mm in diameter.

To date, there are three innovative bipolar platforms that utilize low constant voltage and impedance feedback along with paired ligating-cutting devices. Having established that vessel wall fusion can be achieved using electrical energy to denature collagen and elastin in vessel walls to reform into a permanent seal, the LigaSure® Vessel Sealing Device (Covidien, Boulder, Colorado) applies a high coaptive pressure to the tissue bundle during the generation of tissue temperatures under 100°C; hydrogen cross-links are first ruptured and then renatured, resulting in a vascular seal that has high tensile strength. Similarly, the EnSeal® Laparoscopic Vessel Fusion System (Ethicon Endo-Surgery, Inc.) desiccates by utilizing a set of thermoelastic plastic jaws embedded with nanometer-sized spheres of carbon that conduct a locally regulated current and cuts by the advancing of a mechanical blade, which squeezes the tissue bundle under very high pressure to create a coaptive seal and rapidly express tissue water. A third device, the Plasmakinetics® Cutting Forceps (Gyrus ACMI, a division of Olympus Corporation), delivers pulsed energy with continuous feedback control using conventional tissue grasping.

Monopolar Electrosurgery

During monopolar electrosurgery, the entire patient is potentially part of the circuit (Fig. 8). The electrical current oscillates from the electrosurgical generator to a single-poled surgical instrument or electrode, to the surgical site, through the patient's body, into a dispersive (return) electrode, and back to the generator. While the electrical current does travel some distance in the patient's body, the tissue effect is confined to the immediate area of the active electrode, where the current is highly concentrated.

Compared to bipolar electrosurgery, monopolar electrosurgery requires substantially higher voltage (*V*) to propel the current (*I*) along the myriad of tissue conductors between the active and dispersive electrode to complete the significantly longer electrical circuit. While this provides a greater range of available tissue effects, it also poses increased potential for undesired effects such as burns at the dispersive electrode site and the consequences of stray electrical currents.

Electrosurgical Waveforms: Cut, Blend, and Coag

The AC used for electrosurgery is a sinusoidal waveform (constantly changing directions). The typical output settings labeled *cut*, *blend*, and *coag* on the face of conventional electrosurgical generators are simply variations of current and voltage in relation to time called waveforms (Fig. 9). Despite the common presumption that the labels *cut*, *blend*, and *coag* on a typical electrosurgical generator are necessarily related to specific tissue effects, they are not required for any particular electrosurgical tissue endpoint.

A pure *cut* waveform (also referred to as continuous, unmodulated, or undamped) is an uninterrupted sine wave of low voltage. Compared to the other outputs, the average current is the highest (uninterrupted) and the peak voltage is lowest. Because the current concentration between the closely placed electrodes with bipolar electrosurgery is extremely high, the low voltage *cut* waveform is automatically delivered as the default output for this modality.

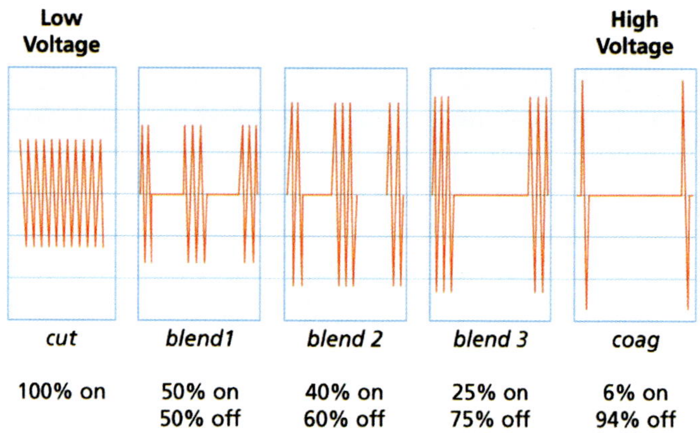

Figure 9 Waveforms produced by an electrosurgical generator range from the continuous low-voltage *cut* output to the discontinuous high-voltage *coag* output, providing outputs of varying current and voltage.

The *blend* output should not be misconstrued as being some mixture or blend of other types of waveforms. The term "blend" refers to a blend of the net surgical effects of tissue cutting and coagulation, not a literal blend of different types of electrosurgical current outputs. Correctly speaking, electrosurgical generator settings in this mode (i.e., *blend 1*, *blend 2*, etc.) simply produce progressive drops in average current by inserting current interruption of greater duration (i.e., *blend 1* is "on" 50% of the time, *blend 2* 40%, and *blend 3* 25%, respectively). As current progressively drops with higher blend settings, the output voltage must progressively increase to conserve energy (recall that $V = I \times R$).

The pure *coag* waveform (also referred to as noncontinuous, modulated, or damped) is a highly interrupted current with frequent and prolonged gaps. Switched to this mode, significantly higher voltage is delivered, but the current is "on" (the duty cycle) only 6% of the time. Comparatively, the pure cut mode is "on" 100% of the time. In order to maintain the same power output (*W*), the significantly lower average current (*I*) of the *coag* output is automatically balanced by the generation of a higher output voltage (recall that $W = I \times V$).

To achieve numerous tissue effects, the surgeon can use the electrosurgery waveforms in combination with many other factors: power settings (*W*), the electrode dwell time (the length of exposure or velocity), the volume of tissue treated, the proximity of the tissue to the active electrode, and the current density (electrode surface area). Tissue impedance (resistance), which primarily depends on water content, will also affect the electrosurgical outcome. Power requirements will be higher whenever an electrode is applied to an area of higher impedance. Impedance is high in desiccated tissues, moderate in adipose tissues, and very low in vascular tissues. The impedance of tissue is dynamic during electrosurgery. For example, as tissue coagulates and water evaporates, impedance rises—at times to the point that the current is inhibited from flowing through the tissue. If the surgeon reflexively increases the power setting (*W*) and consequently the output voltage (*V*), the current (*I*) is more likely to seek an alternate pathway via the least resistance to the ground, which

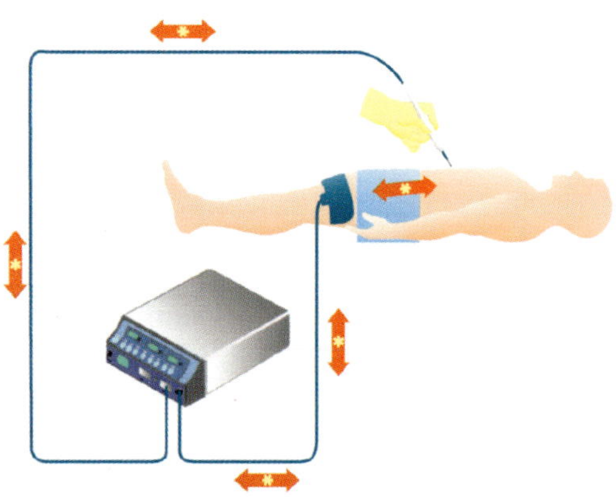

Figure 8 In monopolar electrosurgery, current flows from the electrosurgical generator (ESU) to an electrode, where it is used to achieve tissue effects. The current then moves beyond the point of the tissue effects, through the body, and to the dispersive electrode, where it is returned to the generator.

may lead to thermal injury. Therefore, it is always advisable to use the lowest power setting to achieve the desired tissue effect. Moreover, the power (W) needed to accomplish a particular electrosurgical effect may vary from one patient to another. Lean, muscular patients are better overall conductors of electricity. Obese or emaciated patients may provide more tissue impedance to the electrical current, and so may require more applied power to achieve the same effect.

ELECTROSURGICAL TISSUE ENDPOINTS

The three fundamental types of electrosurgical tissue phenomena—cutting, fulguration, and coagulation—may be further differentiated as being contact or noncontact in nature (Fig. 10).

Noncontact Phenomena: Cutting and Fulguration

Cutting/Vaporization

The capacity to electrosurgically cut (vaporize) living tissue is dependent upon the ability to deliver output current of sufficient current density. Electrosurgical sparking, the active ionization of the air gap between the active electrode and the target tissue, confines the current to a small strike zone and requires at least 200 V of electromotive force. Since the *cut*, *blend*, and *coag* waveforms all satisfy this requirement, electrosurgical cutting can be accomplished using any of these output settings (Fig. 11).

Using conventional electrosurgical generators, thermal damage at the margins of a cut is governed by the amount of voltage used. Decreases in current from progressive current interruption—*cut* to *blend* to *coag*—lead to greater output voltage ($V = I \times R$). With conventional electrosurgical generators, the higher voltages of *blend* and *coag* waveforms create progressively wider zones of thermal damage (Fig. 12) at the margins of the incision. These effects are amplified by using broad surface electrodes and lower cutting velocity. Using *blend* or *coag* waveforms to cut in order to provide wider hemostasis can be helpful during myomectomy, when operating down the broad ligament and along the vaginal fornices during hysterectomy, or across vascular adhesions. Higher voltage outputs also facilitate incision of tissues with greater impedance, such as fatty

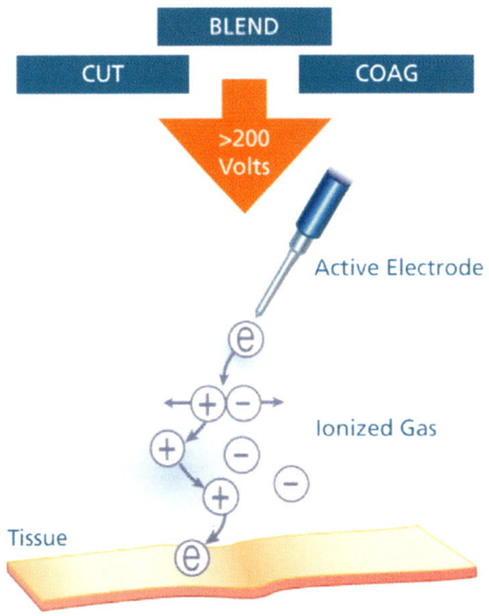

Figure 11 Since all electrosurgical waveforms provide sufficient voltage to generate a spark between the electrode and tissue surface, vaporization or tissue cutting can be accomplished using any output setting on the electrosurgical generator in a noncontact mode.

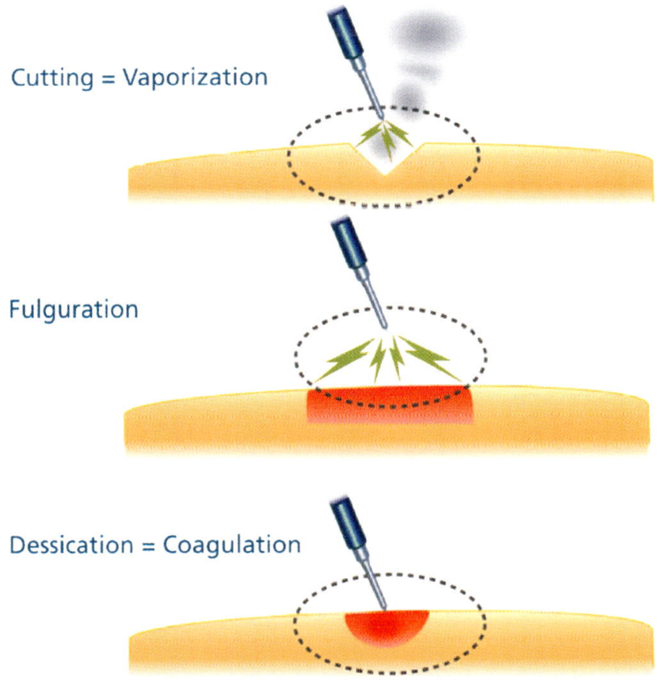

Figure 10 Vaporization, fulguration, and coagulation are the primary tissue phenomena achievable with electrosurgery.

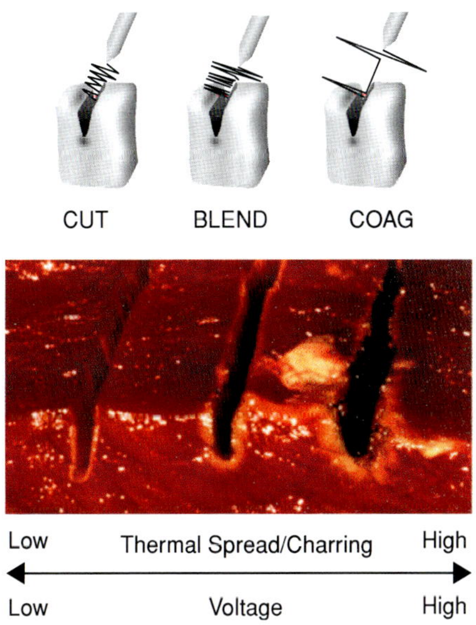

Figure 12 Cutting can be accomplished using any of waveform, but the higher voltages of *blend* and *coag* create wider zones of thermal damage. Less coagulation effect occurs based on the shape and speed at which the electrode passes through tissue.

or desiccated pedicles and adhesions. It is advisable to use the *cut* waveform via the edge of an electrode whenever lateral thermal spread may pose liability to adjacent tissues (15).

While the relative zone of lateral thermal necrosis of the cut margins is progressively greater when using the higher voltage outputs (i.e., *blend* and *coag*) of conventional electrosurgical generators, newer units that employ impedance feedback provide more constant thermal margins regardless of the chosen waveform. The faster an electrode passes over or through tissue, the less thermal effects occur, and newer automatic ESU technology that integrates feedback from the active electrode can deliver constant voltage to achieve the depth of coagulation, independent of the cutting rate (16). The active electrode can continuously monitor changes in the tissue impedance up to 4000 times per second and can adjust output voltage, current, and power every 300 microseconds. For instance, if 40-W power output is selected, that output is delivered regardless of impedance change. This newer type of closed-loop controlled technology maintains the selected power setting despite variable tissue impedance by increasing the current output, *not the voltage*. This allows physicians to use lower power settings and to cause less thermal spread. Consequently, electrosurgical performance is markedly enhanced and the tissue product is more uniform and predictable (13).

Fulguration

Fulguration (aka superficial coagulation or spray coagulation) uses high-voltage sparking produced by the *coag* output to coagulate a broad surface with open vessels on end where coaption is not feasible or desirable. As opposed to the continuous arcing produced by the *cut* output, the highly interrupted *coag* output causes the arcs to strike the tissue surface in a widely dispersed and random fashion. With fulguration, sparks jump from one area to another randomly, "sprayed" rather than concentrated. High-voltage sparking results in high temperature tissue changes, including carbonization; this technique leads to more rapid thermal change, creating a zone of superficial coagulation for fast control of bleeding across a wide area, such as oozing capillary beds or venous bleeding. Fulguration can be effective to control small bleeders up to 2 mm cut on end, such as along the undersurface of the ovarian cortex during cystectomy, and atop the myometrial bed during myomectomy (16). Despite the high-voltage output involved, fulguration is ineffective in a wet, conductive surgical field due to the widespread diffusion of current in blood. Some electrosurgical generators use argon, an inert and noncombustible gas, as part of the current delivery system. At the active electrode, the emitted current is surrounded by argon gas. The current ionizes the gas; it becomes more conductive than air and provides an efficient pathway to the tissue. By definition, this technology is argon-enhanced fulguration. Because the beam concentrates the electrosurgical current, a smoother, more pliable eschar is produced. At the same time, the gas disperses the blood, ostensibly improving visualization. Because the heavier argon displaces some of the oxygen at the surgical site, less smoke is produced (8,17).

Contact Phenomena: Desiccation and Coagulation

Coagulation is a general term that includes both fulguration and desiccation (also called deep coagulation). Touching tissue with the surface of any active electrode, regardless of the selected waveform, obliterates any ionizable gap and leads to the diffusion of current with substantially lower current density. Consequently, the tissue is heated more slowly, causing cellular dehydration by gradual percolation, rather than by the volumetric explosion by superheated steam that is produced with higher current densities. Desiccation and coagulation can occur whenever an activated electrode comes into direct contact with tissue for a sufficient amount of time. Desiccation occurs as cells become dehydrated but still preserve their form. When intracellular temperature reaches 70°C to 80°C, protein denaturation occurs and a white coagulum forms. At 90°C, there is just enough heat to destroy tissue without carbonizing it, causing an effect between hyperemia and carbonization. Further heating leads to development of eschar—carbonized blood and tissue—that occurs when tissue is hyperheated. Because of its low conductivity, eschar buildup on an electrode induces higher resistance (impedance) levels. A higher voltage may then be needed to overcome the resistance in order to complete the circuit (recall that $W = I \times V$) (7). Correspondingly, clean electrodes require less power, are more efficient, and produce more predictable thermal tissue effects.

Compared to noncontact electrosurgical cutting and fulguration, which consume energy to ionize the air gap for sparking, contact desiccation heats tissue more efficiently. Since there is more available energy to heat tissue, thermal damage is predictably deeper and more widespread during contact electrosurgical phenomena. When using *coag* waveform, the peak voltage is very high, so contact coagulation using this waveform is generally limited to superficial layers. The high-voltage tissue strikes limit conduction in deeper layers by accelerating the buildup of tissue impedance from rapid desiccation and carbonization at the surface (Fig. 13). Conversely, when using the lower voltage *cut* waveform, electrode contact heats tissue more gradually, leading to deeper and more effective penetration. Thus, both contact as well as coaptive coagulation using electrosurgery are predictably more effective using the *cut* waveform. For example, these precepts can help determine the best waveform to electrosurgically ablate endometriosis. Since superficial-appearing implants may extend deeply into the retroperitoneal tissues, these types of lesions are best ablated using a broad surface electrode in contact with the *cut* waveform. In contrast, superficial implants on the ovarian cortex may be more prudently treated using a smaller surface electrode in contact with the *coag* waveform to help minimize thermal injury to adjacent follicular tissue.

Coaptive vessel sealing with electrosurgery using any type of current may be ineffective if the blood flow remains uninterrupted. Unless a vessel is sufficiently squeezed before electricity is applied, the current density is significantly reduced by conduction in blood, and luminal temperatures undergo little change as any heat is dissipated by convection from the flow of blood. Directed by the appearance of a

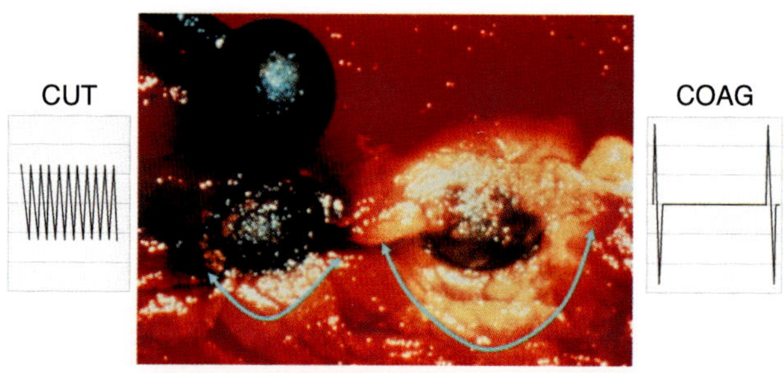

Figure 13 Unlike the corresponding appearance of thermal effects on the tissue surface, desiccation-coagulation is deeper and more effective with the lower voltage, *cut* waveform and most superficial with the higher voltage, *coag* waveform during contact electrosurgery.

well-coagulated tissue pedicle, a fully pulsatile vascular core can be an unwelcome discovery at the time of surgical incision.

REDUCING RISK DURING CONVENTIONAL AND LAPAROSCOPIC ELECTROSURGERY

Electrosurgical Burns

The most commonly reported complication during electrosurgery is a dispersive electrode burn resulting from improper application of this electrode. Indeed, such burns account for two-thirds of electrosurgical accidents. Alternate site burns, such as to cardiac monitor leads, result from improper grounding and the application of high power and voltage levels.

Given that electricity seeks the path of least resistance, potentially unintended current pathways to the ground include the operating room table, metal stirrups, EKG leads, and the surgeon. Furthermore, if the current return to the dispersive electrode is not spread over a sufficiently large area or if the dispersive electrode becomes partially detached, the current could be concentrated enough to cause a third-degree burn to the skin and deeper tissues. Even with a dispersive electrode monitoring system, thermal injuries can still occur. The localization of current during bipolar electrosurgery removes the propensity of current to seek alternate current pathways to ground (13).

The ideal dispersive electrode safely collects and then removes current during monopolar electrosurgery. Early dispersive electrodes were metal plates placed under the patient; a conductive gel ensured tissue–electrode contact. Today, water based gel foam pads and adhesive pads are applied to the tissue. Complete contact between skin and dispersive electrode is essential to eliminate burns at the return site. A complicating factor in laparoscopic procedures is that most of the conductors, including part of the active electrode, are commonly out of the surgeon's field of view. Consequently, some injuries, such as burns to the bowel, may not be recognized immediately.

Because it is possible to misdiagnose or be unaware of electrosurgical burns, the prevalence of complications resulting from laparoscopic monopolar electrosurgery specifically is likely underreported and underestimated. Prevention of these complications is of paramount importance, requiring the surgeon to remain vigilant when utilizing all electrosurgical instrumentation or techniques.

Three types of stray current injuries are possible, especially during laparoscopic electrosurgery: direct coupling, capacitive coupling, and insulation failure. All of these phenomena are more likely to occur with the use of high-voltage *coag* waveform. Using the lowest possible power settings (*W*) and the lower voltage *cut* waveform may help reduce such risks (18).

Direct Coupling

Direct coupling occurs when the user accidentally activates the electrosurgical generator (ESU) while the active electrode is near another metal instrument (Fig. 14). The secondary instrument becomes energized, and the energy seeks a pathway to complete the circuit to the dispersive electrode. Electrical sparks or arcing may be seen. If the pathway is via the viscera, and is of sufficient current density, unrecognized thermal injury may occur.

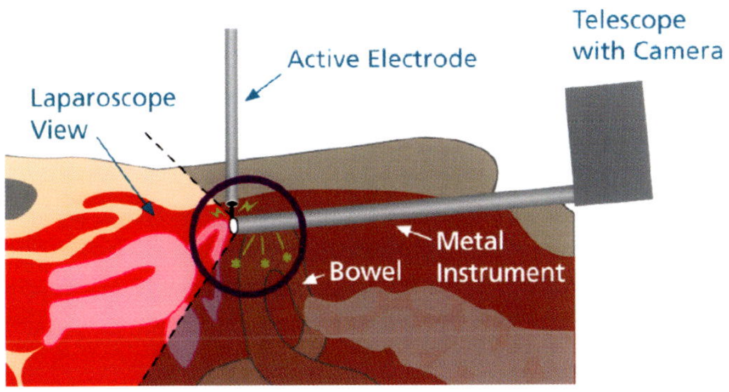

Figure 14 Significant thermal injury may occur if the electrosurgical generator is activated while the active electrode is located near another metal instrument that contacts the viscera along a small surface area.

Capacitance

Capacitance is the property of an electrical circuit to store energy. A capacitor exists whenever two conductors with different potentials are separated by an insulator. A difference of potential or voltage will exist between two conductors that have differing numbers of free electrons (an overall negative charge on the conductor with excess, and a positive charge on the electron-deficient conductor). Although separation by an insulator prevents the flow of electrons between these conductors, the potential difference nevertheless creates an attraction or electrostatic force between them. This force results in an electric field and creates a reservoir of stored energy. When an AC flows through a circuit, the applied voltage and flow of current periodically changes direction. With each reversal of current flow, the energy of the stored electric field is discharged. Although no actual current flows through the capacitor, the charged current from capacitance completes the circuit and in essence conducts the AC. The amount of capacitance is directly proportional to the voltage (i.e., lowest with the *cut* and highest with the *coag* waveforms, respectively).

Capacitive Coupling

Capacitive coupling occurs when energy from an active electrode is transferred across the insulator surrounding it to another conductor (7), such as to an outer trocar sheath of an electrosurgical instrument. Although there is an insulator between the electrode and the trocar sheath, an electrostatic field between the two bodies induces the current to flow through the insulation, momentarily moving current from the active electrode to the trocar sheath (Fig. 15). The localization of current during bipolar electrosurgery eliminates the risk of capacitive coupling during laparoscopic surgery and the propensity of current to seek alternate current pathways to ground (13).

If the trocar sheath is in direct contact with the abdominal wall, the induced charge is released by ready conduction to the dispersive electrode. However, if the sheath is isolated by a plastic collar or other insulated material, the charge remains isolated to the outer cannula as long as the electrosurgical generator is on. If isolated, and if the current density is of sufficient magnitude, contact between the sheath and adjacent tissue such as the bowel can result in thermal injury—often outside of the surgeon's field of view (Fig. 16).

Even if an all-plastic system is used, there is still a risk for capacitive coupling, as the patient's tissues can act as the second conductor. For example, if a patient's bowel is draped over a plastic trocar sheath, energy could travel by that pathway to body structures. The risk of capacitive coupling increases with longer instruments, thinner electrode insulation, narrow cannulas, and again, higher voltage waveforms (7).

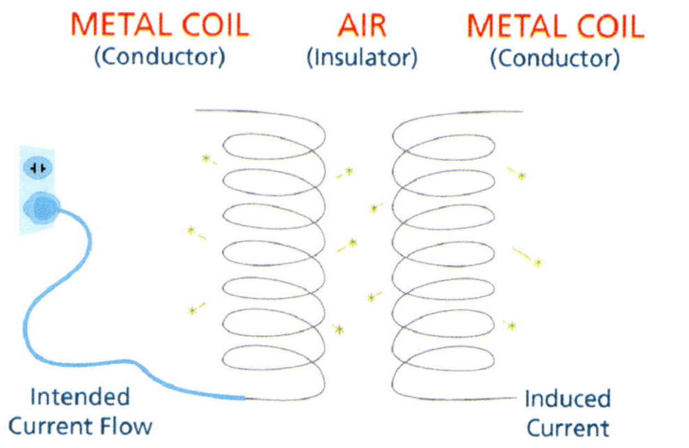

Figure 15 Capacitive coupling: An electrostatic field between the two bodies induces the current to flow through the insulation, momentarily moving current from the active to passive conductor.

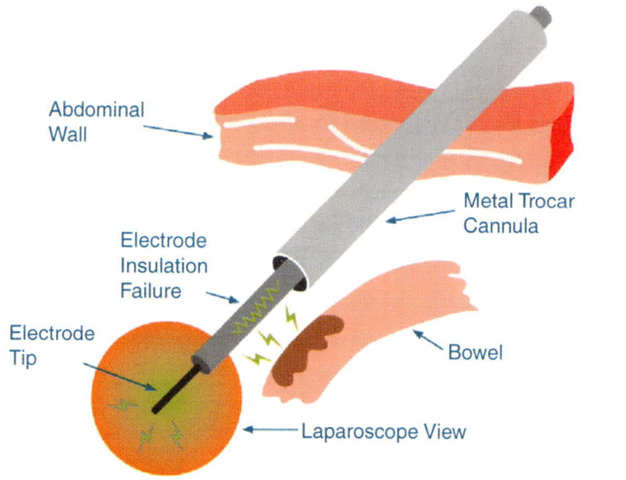

Figure 17 Insulation failure causing thermal injury to the bowel out of the laparoscopic view.

All surgeons have experienced an unexpected shock across their gloved fingers while stabilizing a clamp in contact with a monopolar electrode. Although many such burns occur from the direct conduction of concentrated current through the hydrated rubber or a hole in the surgeon's glove, these phenomena can also result from capacitive coupling. In the latter case, the electrified clamp and the surgeon's fingers are conductors with significantly different potentials. Activating the electrode, especially prior to contacting the clamp (generating higher voltage), induces a coupled current on the surgeon's fingers. If the area of contact between the fingers and the clamp is small, the current density will be high enough to generate a burn. Capacitance-induced burns across surgical gloves can be eliminated by avoiding open circuit (noncontact) activation and cradling the surgical clamp with a large surface area.

Insulation Failure

Insulation failure potentially produces an alternate current pathway (Fig. 17). The often-undetectable smaller insulation breaks are more dangerous than larger breaks because of current concentration. Failure may occur as a result of normal wear and tear, microscopic imperfections, routine use of the higher voltage *coag* waveform, and repeated electrode insertion into a trocar. To reduce the risk of insulation failure, electrodes should undergo periodic assessment for excess wear and minimizing the use of high-voltage levels associated with the *coag* and higher *blend* waveforms.

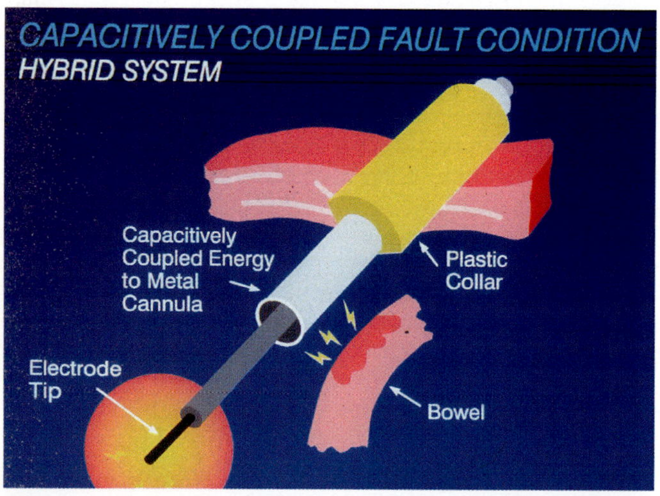

Figure 16 If the trocar is isolated by a plastic collar during electrosurgery, the charge is coupled to the metallic sheath. If the current density is of sufficient magnitude, contact between the sheath and the bowel can result in a significant burn.

Alternate Current Pathways

Early electrosurgery units used current directly from wall outlets and were "ground-referenced." The current passed from the electrosurgical generator to the active electrode, to the surgical site, to the dispersive electrode, back to the generator, and to the ground. However, if the dispersive electrode was compromised, or if it did not present the path of least resistance, the current could exit the body at another site (e.g., a finger in contact with metal, an electrocardiograph lead, a stirrup). The current could also split and follow two routes (known as current division), exiting the body at the dispersive electrode and at the second site, causing a burn at the latter.

The 1960s saw the introduction of "isolated" electrosurgical generators, which use wall outlet current to produce a second isolated current that recognizes only the generator as ground. In the absence of a return pathway to the electrosurgical generator, the unit ceases function. This technology has virtually eliminated alternate burn sites.

Dispersive Electrode Site Placement

Dispersive electrodes used with monitoring systems (or interrogation circuits) have become standard electrosurgical components. Contact quality monitoring uses a split pad design, which, although more expensive, incorporates an "interrogation circuit" and thereby prevents injury. The circuit is part of a system that actively monitors the impedance at the patient/electrode interface and, in the event of dangerously high impedance, is designed to deactivate the electrosurgical generator (19). Peeling of the electrode disrupts the current and automatically terminates current deliver. This technologic advance has eliminated the risk for burns from an unpeeled dispersive electrode.

To maintain an optimal dispersive electrode site, the surgeon should select well-vascularized muscle mass and avoid sites that can increase impedance such as irregular body contours, bony prominences, scar tissue, adipose tissue, and areas with excessive hair (6). Impedance can also be increased by fluid invasion (6). Choosing a site close to the surgical field will ensure a short current pathway and lower power settings. Maintaining full contact between the dispersive electrode and the tissue will help to preclude current concentration and potential burns.

Body Jewelry

If the surface area of contact between the patient and the capacitively coupled object is small, the density of leakage current may be high enough to create thermal damage (20). If body jewelry cannot be removed prior to surgery, it should be covered with gauze and taped in place to increase the contact area and to reduce the risk of current concentration, which can cause an inadvertent burn. If jewelry were in a direct line between the active and dispersive electrodes, the electrode would need to be repositioned.

Implanted Electronic Devices

Implanted electronic devices may malfunction during electrosurgery due to electromagnetic interference (energy transmission from one device to another). Among common implanted electronic devices are pacemakers, deep-brain stimulators to treat Parkinson's disease, spinal cord stimulators to treat pain or incontinence, cochlear implants, and infusion pumps. If monopolar electrosurgery is used, the dispersive electrode should be placed as close as possible to the surgical site, and far from the electronic device. In addition, it is important to avoid electrode placement over a metal prosthesis, since scar tissue can impede current return and potentially cause tissue burn. An implantable cardioverter defibrillator (ICD) should be inactivated beforehand since electrosurgery could cause the device to deliver a shock to the patient (21).

Surgical Smoke and Fire

Smoke produced during electrosurgery can not only impede the visual field but it can contain toxic substances such as formaldehyde, benzene, carbon monoxide, and hydrogen cyanide. If no smoke evacuation system is available during laparoscopic surgery, smoke should be intermittently evacuated through one of the laparoscopic port sites.

To prevent fire in the operating room, an electrode should be activated only when it is visible and deactivated before removing it from the surgical site. Avoiding or minimizing the use of enriched oxygen and nitrous oxide at the surgical site, ensuring that flammable vapors and gases do not accumulate (such as in the bowel or under surgical drapes), and avoiding eschar buildup on electrode tips can help further prevent fires.

CONCLUSIONS

Science becomes art and art becomes function when fundamental principles are utilized to dictate surgical practice. Most importantly, the risk for inadvertent thermal injury during electrosurgery can be minimized by a sound comprehension of the predictable behaviors of electricity in living tissue.

Guided by the Hippocratic charge to "primum non nocere," the ultimate aim of energy-assisted surgery is the attainment of anatomical dissection and hemostasis with the least amount of collateral damage and subsequent scar tissue formation. Ideally, the surgeon's final view of the operative field should accurately approximate the topography discoverable after postoperative healing. Despite the continued innovation of products borne to reduce thermal damage and then marketed as being comparatively safer, it is the hands and mind of the surgeon that serve to preserve tissue integrity by reducing the burden of delayed thermal necrosis and taking steps to prevent excessive devitalization of tissue. Regardless of the chosen modality, the inseparable and exponentially linked elements of time and the quantity of delivered energy must be integrated while purposefully moderating to attain the desired tissue effect. Ultimately, the reduction of unwanted thermal injury is inherently linked to good surgical judgment and technique, a sound comprehension of the applied energy modality, and the surgeon's ability to recognize anatomical structures within the field of surgical dissection as well as those within the zone of significant thermal change.

During the use of any energy-based device for hemostasis, out of sight must never mean out of mind. If the bowel, bladder, or ureter is in close proximity to a bleeder, they should be sufficiently mobilized before applying energy. Thermal energy should always be withheld until an orderly sequence of anatomical triage is carried out. Whenever a vital structure cannot be adequately mobilized, hemorrhage is preferentially controlled by using mechanical tamponade or suture ligature.

REFERENCES

1. Wicker P. Electrosurgery – part 1: The history of diathermy. Br J Theater Nurs 1990; 27(8):6–7.
2. Kelly HA, Ward GE. History. Electrosurgery. Philadelphia, PA: W B Saunders, 1932:1–9.
3. Pearce J. Early experiments with high frequency current. Electrosurgery. London: Chapman and Hall, 1986:2–7.
4. Geddes, LA, Roeder, RA. Deforest and the first electrosurgical unit [abstract]. IEEE Eng Med Biol Mag 2003; 22(1):84–87. http://ieeexplore.ieee.org/xpl/freeabs_all.jsp?tp=&arnumber=1191454&isnumber=26703. Last accessed 3/16/09.
5. O'Connor JL, Bloom DA, William T. Bovie and electrosurgery [abstract]. Surgery 1996; 119(4):390–396. http://cat.inist.fr/?aModele=afficheN&cpsidt=3038632. Accessed 16 March, 2009.
6. ValleyLab. Clinical Information Hotline Electrosurgery News. 10(2). http://www.valleylab.com/education/hotline/pdfs/hotline_0303.pdf. Accessed 16 March, 2009.
7. Harrell AG. Energy Sources in Laparoscopy [abstract]. Semin Laparosc Surg 2004; 11(3)201–209. http://sri.sagepub.com/cgi/content/abstract/11/3/201. Accessed 16 March, 2009.
8. Brill AI. Energy Systems for Operative Laparoscopy: It's not the wand, it's the magician. J Am Assoc Gynecol Laparosc 1998; 5(4):335–349.
9. Brill AI, Feste JR, Hamilton TL, et al. Patient safety during laparoscopic monopolar electrosurgery-principles and guidelines. JSLS 1998;2:221–225.
10. Soderstrom R, Brill AI. Principles of electrosurgery as applied to gynecology. In: Rock JA, Jones HW, eds, Te Linde's Operative Gynecology. 10th ed. Philadelphia, PA: Lippincott-Raven Publishers, 2008:280–297.
11. Brill AI. Bipolar electrosurgery: Convention and innovation. Clin Obstet Gynecol 2008; 51(1):153–158.
12. Wu MP, et al. Complications and recommended practices for electrosurgery in laparoscopy [abstract]. Am J Surg 2000; 179: 67–73. http://cat.inist.fr/?aModele=afficheN&cpsidt=1288652. Accessed 16 March, 2009.
13. Brill A. Principles & Practice: Electrosurgery and Ultrasonics. As presented at AAGL 2007. http://www.obgyn.net/AAGL-Online-Endoupdate/electrosurgery/transcript_brill.pdf. Accessed 16 March, 2009.

14. Brill AI. The use of contemporary energy modalities during operative laparoscopy. In: Peter Joseph O'Donovan, Charles E. Miller, eds, Modern Management of Abnormal Uterine Bleeding. Section III. Informa Health Care, 2008:98. ISBN 0415454794, 9780415454797. http://books.google.com/books?id=X21Iwxw DYPgC&printsec=frontcover&dq=Modern+Management+of+ Abnormal+Uterine+Bleeding#PPR5,M1.
15. Brill A. Energy-based techniques to ensure hemostasis and limit damage during laparoscopy. OBGMgmt 2003; 15(5):23–27. http://www.obgmanagement.com/article_pages.asp?AID= 3125&UID. Accessed 16 March, 2009.
16. Tucker RD. Applied electrophysics in endometrial ablation. In: Eric J. Bieber, Franklin D Loffer, eds. Hysteroscopy, Resectoscopy & Endometrial Ablation. Cambridge, MA: Informa Health Care, 2003:133. ISBNs 1842141171, 9781842141175. http://www.shrunkin.com/18212. Accessed 16 March, 2009.
17. Rothrock JC. The RN First Assistant. 3rd ed. Philadelphia, PA: Lippincott, 1999:327–323. http://www.tycohealth-ece.com /files/d0000/ty_ihtmnu.pdf. Accessed 16 March, 2009.
18. Brill AI. Energy systems in laparoscopy. In: A Practical Manual of Laparoscopy & Minimally Invasive Gynecology. UK: Informa Healthcare/CRC Press, 2007:86–89. http://www.shrunkin.com /18216. Accessed 16 March, 2009.
19. Odell RC. Electrosurgery in laparoscopy. Infertil Reprod Med Clin North Am 1993;4:289–304.
20. AORN Recommended Practices Committee. Recommended Practices for Electrosurgery. AORN J 2005; 81(3):616–642. Available online at http://findarticles.com/p/articles/mi_m0FSL /is_3_81/ai_n13471132. Accessed 16 March, 2009.
21. ValleyLab. Clinical Information Hotline Electrosurgery News. 7(3). http://www.valleylab.com/education/hotline/pdfs/hot line_0211.pdf. Accessed 15 March, 2009.

4

Principles for laparoscopic peritoneal access

Andrew I. Brill

The art of laparoscopic surgery is inextricably linked to how well the strategic needs for any anticipated surgical procedure are established. Moreover, patient safety and technical efficacy are closely linked to preoperative assessments, including an assiduous review of all relevant prior surgical records.

Surgical access to the peritoneal cavity may be by laparotomy or mini-laparotomy (open access), by laparoscopy, or by vaginal approach. Determining the most prudent technique for peritoneal access depends on the ergonomic and technical needs of the intended surgical procedure(s), the abdominal habitus, any prior laparotomic or laparoscopic surgeries, the spatial configuration of any underlying pelvic or abdominal pathology, and the experience of the surgeon. Since no particular technique is universally applicable or foolproof, it is the duty of every surgeon to be knowledgeable about alternative procedures for entry into the peritoneal cavity. This chapter will be confined to laparoscopic access.

Without question, the most life-threatening surgical accidents during laparoscopic surgery are apt to occur during peritoneal access, including injury to the underlying intestinal viscera and retroperitoneal vessels. One group in Switzerland prospectively followed 14,243 patients over two years and found 22 trocar and 4 Veress needle injuries (0.18%), including 19 injuries to large and small bowel and 7 to retroperitoneal vessels (1). With these detailed concerns in mind, the surgeon addresses the challenge of Veress needle and trocar entry in every case. Planning, knowledge of relevant anatomy, and carefully controlled maneuvers are the best insurance against complications from peritoneal access.

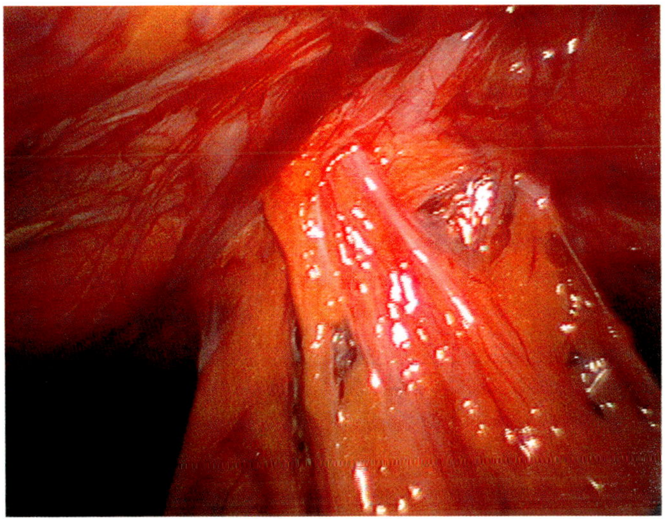

Figure 1 Intra-abdominal adhesions below the umbilicus from prior postpartum tubal ligation as viewed from the left upper quadrant.

METHODS TO REDUCE RISK

Since the overall safety of inserting a Veress needle or a trocar into the peritoneal cavity is critically dependent on mobility of the underlying viscera, every effort should be made to anticipate the probability of intraabdominal adhesions between underlying the bowel and the anterior abdominal wall. Prior operative reports and hospital discharge summaries should be carefully reviewed for the likelihood of intraabdominal adhesions. Any history of postoperative peritonitis and abdominal surgical scars should be especially suspect for the presence of intraabdominal adhesions. Adhesions between the bowel and anterior abdominal wall are the enemy of every laparoscopist (Fig. 1). Whenever these are suspected, alternative techniques for insufflation and/or access to the peritoneal cavity are necessary. Given the propensity of the intestine and its fatty appendages to adhere to fresh edges of any peritoneal incision beneath the anterior abdominal wall, all abdominal incisions must be treated as potentially harboring immobile bowel below. In 362 women undergoing operative laparoscopy after laparotomy, adhesions were present between the anterior abdominal wall and underlying omentum or bowel in 27% after Pfannenstiel incisions, in 55% after midline incisions below the umbilicus, and in 67% after midline incisions above the umbilicus (2). Even patients with one previous laparoscopic procedure should be approached with a measure of caution, as both omentum and bowel may be adherent beneath the umbilicus from Valsalva on extubation or accidental suturing during closure of the umbilical defect.

Furthermore, the preoperative examination should include a detailed assessment of the umbilical anatomy and the abdominal wall including the distribution of any scars and adiposity. Extremes of body weight may pose technical difficulty and greater risk. Overweight women especially those with centripetal obesity can present a strategic challenge for uneventful insufflation and trocar entry (3). Additionally, the very slender women, especially those with an android-type pelvis and prominent sacral promontory, present specific hazards as the depth of the umbilicus may lie just 1 to 2 cm above the anterior surface of the aorta (4).

After final supine positioning under general anesthesia, the depth of subcutaneous fat and degree of laxity of the abdominal wall can be judged by elevation between the thumb and index finger. Any palpable mass can be outlined using a sterile pen and should be carefully assessed for mobility, shape, and size. The spatial orientation and relative position of the aortic bifurcation can be estimated by transabdominal palpation for aortic pulsations and by ascertaining the fixed reference points of the anterosuperior iliac spines and summit of the iliac crest. In most women, the aortic bifurcation rests between the fourth and fifth lumbar vertebrae and within

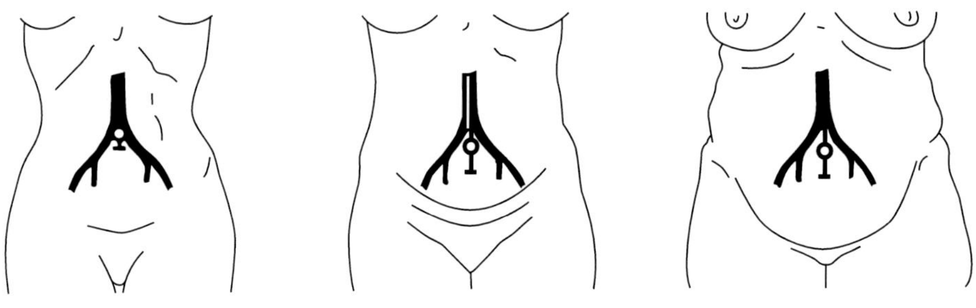

Figure 2 Relationship of the umbilicus to increasing BMI.

1.25 cm above or below the highest points of the iliac crests (5). Since the position of the umbilicus in relation to the bifurcation is quite variable, it should not be used to define its location. The position of the umbilicus relative to the aortic bifurcation has been shown to be negatively correlated with body mass index (BMI) (6) (Fig. 2). However, the risk of vascular injury below the bifurcation still remains; one group reported that the space between the common iliac arteries was always at least partially occupied by the left common iliac vein and was completely filled by this vessel in 19 (28%) of 97 cases studied (7).

Logically then, the most dependable safeguard for the underlying retroperitoneal vessels is to limit the depth of insertion of the Veress needle or primary trocar by minimizing thrust force and perception of the moment of peritoneal entry. This includes measures such as using slow progressive movements with sharp instruments, maintaining secure control of the abdominal wall, using slow screw-like turns with blunt instruments, ensuring adequate incision to prevent soft tissue dystocia, and gripping the Veress needle or primary trocar in a way that controls the tip and may serve as a brake. Moreover, maximal pneumoperitoneal distention is helpful by making it easier to perceive the moment of entry as is lowering the height of the operating table to the level of the surgeon's waist or below. Virtually, every technical maneuver during laparoscopic surgery can be affected by table height. It should ideally be at the level of the surgeon's waist or lower. As the table rises above the waist, critical elements of control and finesse diminish incrementally as any proprioceptive feedback and motor control shift from the surgeon's hand and wrist to the larger and less-sensitive elbow, upper arm, and shoulder girdle.

As a general rule, the Veress needle and/or primary trocar should ideally be inserted while the patient is maintained in an unaltered supine position. Changing the patient's position can adversely affect the surgical perspective regarding both the midline by premature lateral rotation and the sacral promontory by head-down positioning. Without altering the angle of insertion, Trendelenburg position may align the position of the retroperitoneal vessels more directly in target with a 45-degree transumbilical insertion angle (Fig. 3). In one study, the aortic bifurcation was located caudal to the umbilicus in only 11% of women undergoing laparoscopy when supine compared to 33% women in Trendelenburg position (7).

Sharp entry is best done directly through the base of the umbilicus, which is the thinnest portion of the anterior abdominal wall. The retracted umbilical fossa represents the region of abdominal skin where it is fused to underlying linea alba. Union of peritoneum to the postnatal umbilical plate prevents stretching at this site during sharp entry (Fig. 4). Inspection of the umbilical fossa usually reveals a sunburst of folds that run vertically. When the umbilicus is narrow, a dominant vertical fold should be chosen for the site of incision.

Since the topographic alignment of collagen bundles and lines of tension run in a parallel direction, this type of incision leads to the best cosmetic result with the least amount of bleeding (8). If the navel is naturally wide, everted, or flat with the abdominal wall, the surgeon's best choice is to make a transverse incision carefully fashioned to the skin fold defined by the inferior rim. In most cases, the inferior margin may be grasped and lifted with the surgeon's nondominant hand by

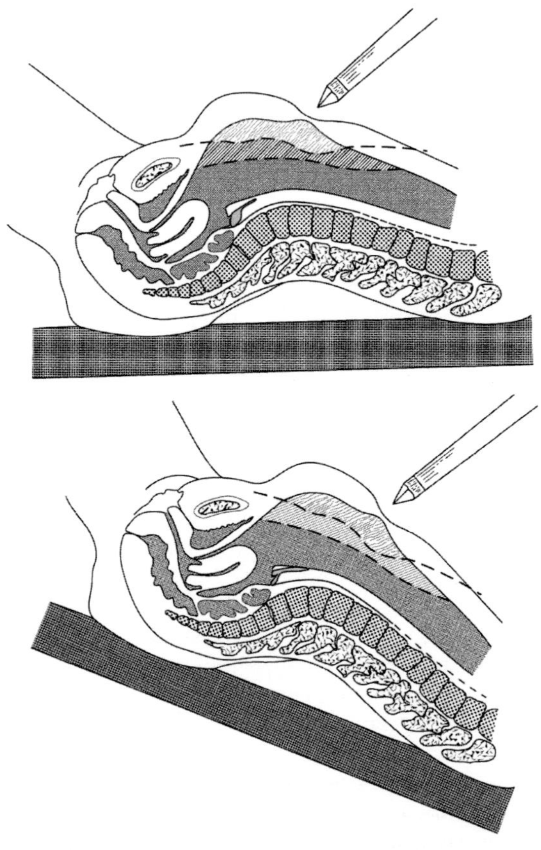

Figure 3 The propensity of Trendelenburg position to align the retroperitoneal vessels with the axis of entry.

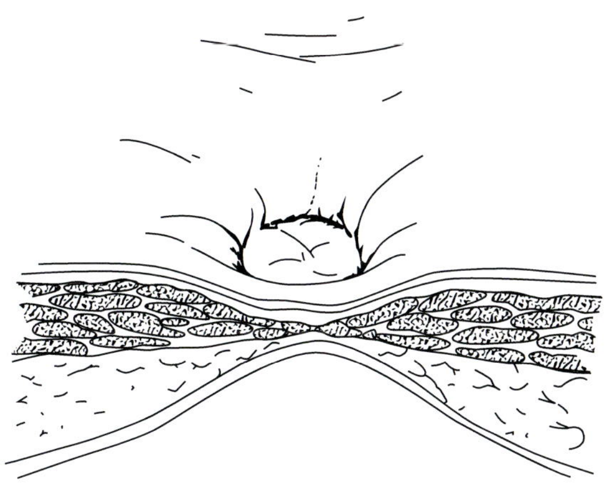

Figure 4 Fusion of the abdominal wall layers at the umbilical plate.

using an Allis clamp and rolled outward and upward at a 45-degree angle. The assistant then uses a Kelly clamp to spread open the umbilicus to expose the base of the fossa and delineate skin folds. Using a no. 11 blade, a superficial vertical or horizontal incision is completed to escape the fossa up to the Allis clamp. The Kelly clamp is used to dissect the umbilical ring bluntly free of tissue investments, first in parallel and then at 90-degrees to the incision, to develop sufficient girth for the primary trocar. The Allis clamp is removed after the size of the incision is checked with the back of the scalpel holder (about 1 cm in width), the surgeon's small finger, or the trocar sheath.

If a Veress needle will be used to establish the pneumoperitoneum, it should be inspected to ensure that the spring is properly loaded, and reassembled to confirm that the inner and outer sheath are properly mated. The stopcock and holding screw should be tightly fastened. The blunt tip of the needle should be pushed against something flat to confirm that it retracts easily and springs forward smoothly and rapidly. Finally, flushing with saline checks the patency of the needle.

ABDOMINAL WALL AND PERITONEAL ENTRY TECHNIQUES

No particular method for abdominal wall elevation is singularly superior. Regardless of technique, it should be comfortable for the surgeon. The abdominal wall must be securely grasped to provide controlled countertension, and the amount and angle of abdominal wall elevation should naturally accommodate the safest and most logical approach to the peritoneal cavity. Two approaches are most commonly used for elevating the abdominal wall before placement of the Veress needle or primary trocar. In the first, the skin and subcutaneous tissue on either side of the umbilicus are grasped either manually or with towel clips (taking great care to grasp only subcutaneous tissue) and the abdominal wall is elevated at a 90-degree angle, assumedly increasing the distance between it and underlying vital intraabdominal structures (9). Overzealous grasping with towel clips, especially in thin patients, risks inadvertent entrapment of underlying omentum and even bowel. In the second approach, skin and fat of the abdominal wall are manually grasped midway between the mons pubis and umbilicus and elevated caudally at a 45-degree angle, assumedly stretching peritoneum below the umbilicus and making penetration of the needle much easier. Whether elevation of the umbilicus either manually or with towel clips actually elevates the peritoneum has been a subject of debate; since the fascia is tightly applied to underlying muscle, abdominal wall elevation may only in fact be elevating underlying subcutaneous tissue per se. Using a suprapubic port, the efficacy of manual elevation below the umbilicus was compared with towel clips placed within and 2 cm from the umbilicus (10). Only towel clips provided significant elevation of the fascia with peritoneum that was maintained during the force of primary trocar insertion. With or without abdominal wall elevation, the Veress needle must be inserted under maximum control. Entry should be within the base of the umbilicus to minimize the chance for preperitoneal insufflation. Keeping the valve open during insertion may help prevent bowel injury by capitalizing on negative intraperitoneal pressure on entry. While the outside of the surgeon's hand rests on the patient's abdominal wall, the needle is grasped midway along the shaft like a dart to maximally translate resistance at the tip, gently passed into the infraumbilical incision, and angled at 45 to 90 degrees depending on the thickness of the abdominal panniculus. As the needle is passed through the abdominal wall, two consecutive layers of resistance followed by give will be felt as it meets and traverses fascia and then peritoneum. A distinct click can often be heard as the blunt tip portion of the Veress needle finally springs forward into the peritoneal cavity. The needle is then aimed in the midline toward the uterus, away from pelvic blood vessels, and toward the hollow of the sacrum. Once the surgeon perceives peritoneal entry, no further thrusting is continued (Fig. 5). Intraperitoneal location may be confined by conducting an orderly series of tests. A 10-mL syringe is filled with 5 mL saline and the plunger removed is connected to the Veress needle. Free flow of saline into the peritoneal cavity signals peritoneal entry. With the plunger in place, it is aspirated to assess whether blood or bowel contents enter the barrel of the syringe. Saline is then instilled and flow should proceed without resistance. On aspiration, no saline should return; otherwise preperitoneal placement is indicated. The stopcock is left open and the syringe is disconnected. Several drops of saline are instilled into the hub of the

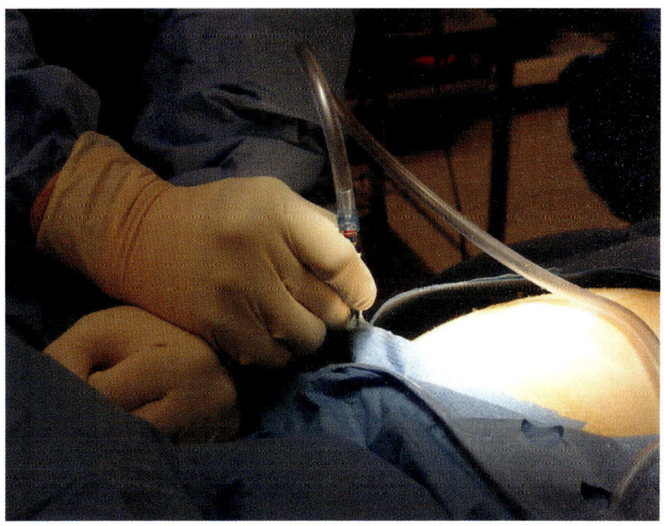

Figure 5 While the outside of the surgeon's hand rests on the patient's abdominal wall, the Veress needle is grasped midway along the shaft like a dart to maximally translate resistance at the tip.

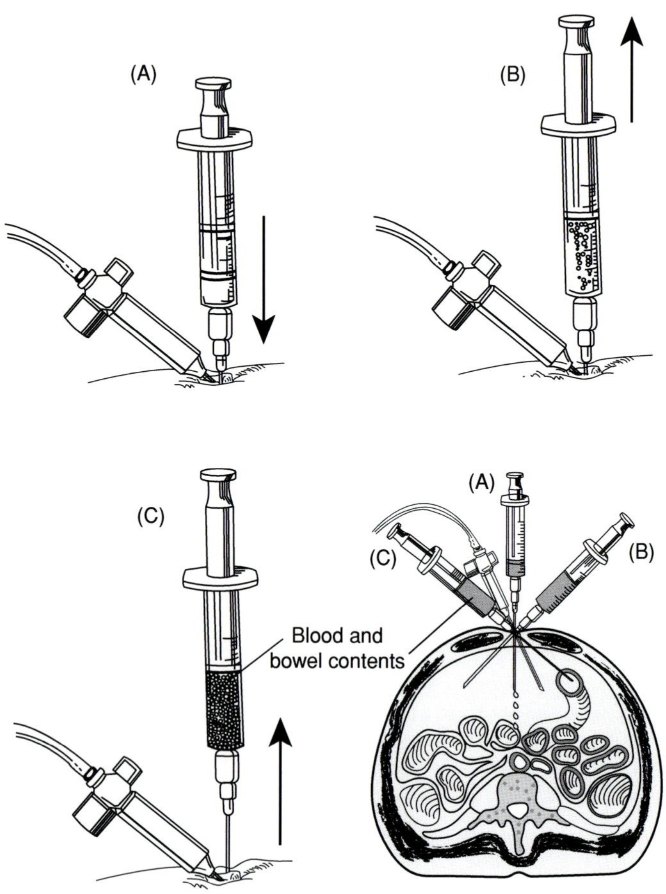

Figure 6 Peritoneal mapping after Veress insufflation using a spinal needle to aspirate with a partially filled syringe.

needle that should rapidly fall into the abdominal cavity on elevation of the abdominal wall. Alternatively, proper placement can be ascertained using a saline-filled 10-mL syringe directly attached to the needle with the valve open. Under these circumstances, room air pressure coupled with negative pressure within the abdominal cavity during respiration will produce a rapid flow of saline by gravity alone, giving a good visual end point (Fig. 6). While all of these techniques maximize safe peritoneal entry, none is foolproof. Once the surgeon is certain that the tip of the needle lies within the peritoneal cavity, the insufflation line can be connected. The flow of carbon dioxide should be turned to 1 L/minute, and the indicator on the machine for total carbon dioxide infused should be reset to zero. Pressure in the abdomen during initial insufflation should register less than 8 mm Hg regardless of body mass and typically less than 5 mm Hg. If insufflation pressure is high or there is no flow, the needle should be rotated to assess whether the opening in the shaft is resting on the abdominal wall, omentum, or bowel (the inflow hole is always on the same side of the needle as the stopcock). High pressure may also be secondary to a small piece of tissue blocking the needle opening, which is easily dislodged by flushing with 2 to 3 mL of saline. Movements that swing the Veress needle to and fro should be avoided to reduce the risk of making a laceration larger. Insufflation should not be continued if the surgeon is uncertain about the location of the tip of the Veress needle. When the needle is correctly placed, peritoneum should effectively seal it off; if carbon dioxide bubbles out along the shaft, one must suspect that the needle tip has migrated into a preperitoneal locale. Unresolved high insufflation pressures should always signal misplacement, mandating removal and reinsertion or consideration of an alternative site for peritoneal access. Any preperitoneal gas pocket should be evacuated before reinsertion is attempted. If a second or even third attempt is successful, it is advisable to temporarily inflate the abdominal cavity beyond 25 mm to distend the peritoneum against the abdominal wall in preparation for trocar insertion. If the needle cannot be comfortably and successfully inserted an alternative method for insufflation should be used. The first definitive sign that the Veress needle lies in the abdominal cavity is loss of dullness to percussion over the liver during early insufflation at 500 to 700 mL of gas. The abdominal wall should continue to expand symmetrically with loss of the sharp contour of costal margins. Downward pressure in an upper quadrant should easily create symmetric elevation of the contralateral lower quadrant.

As with the Veress needle, insertion of the primary trocar is blind and may be associated with significant complications. Safety is maximized by understanding the construction and function of each type of cannula and by rigorously adhering to logical methodology. The spring-loaded mechanism of a disposable-shielded trocar is never considered to be fail-safe and does not always prevent injury to underlying viscera. As a significant number of complications occurred with shielded systems, the Food and Drug Administration directed all trocar manufacturers in August 1996 to remove the term "safety trocar" from their product labeling.

The signature of controlled entry into the peritoneal cavity is reduced thrust force to minimize the depth of entry. Undoubtedly, the type of trocar tip affects entry force. Although it is generally presumed that force required is greater for conical than for pyramidal tips, this is not necessarily the case with 5-mm devices (11). Furthermore, conical tips theoretically reduce the risk of injury to blood vessels within the abdominal wall. When using sharp pyramidal trocars, the potential for soft tissue trauma is minimized by directly advancing the instrument in a continuous fashion. While blunt conical systems require significantly greater force than pyramidal or cutting-dilating (linear-bladed) systems, radially expanding trocars require the greatest force because of the need for progressive dilatation of the polymeric sheath with a blunt obturator. A screw-in (turning) technique must be considered when using any blunt trocar.

In the virgin abdomen, the primary trocar is best directed into the vertical or horizontal skin defect at the inferior base of the umbilicus. Placing the distal assembly into the defect while the abdominal wall is not retracted assesses adequacy of the incision. Meeting excessive resistance signifies a mismatch that can be easily remedied by stretching or extending the incision. If the incision is of insufficient size, a cannula shield can hang up at the skin and fail to spring back into position once the sharp tip has entered the abdominal cavity. Increasing pneumoperitoneal pressure to at least 20 mm Hg before trocar insertion further reduces risk by increasing volume, providing firmer countertraction, and pushing peritoneum more firmly against the abdominal wall. The trocar is held in the palm of the surgeon's dominant hand, and the index or middle finger is extended down the shaft of the sheath to act as a brake to prevent sudden or deep advancement [Fig. 7(A)]. For the small-handed surgeon unable to enwrap the proximal trocar assembly, the nondominant forearm can be laid across the patient's upper abdomen and used as a fulcrum to control the force and depth of insertion. Alternatively, encircling

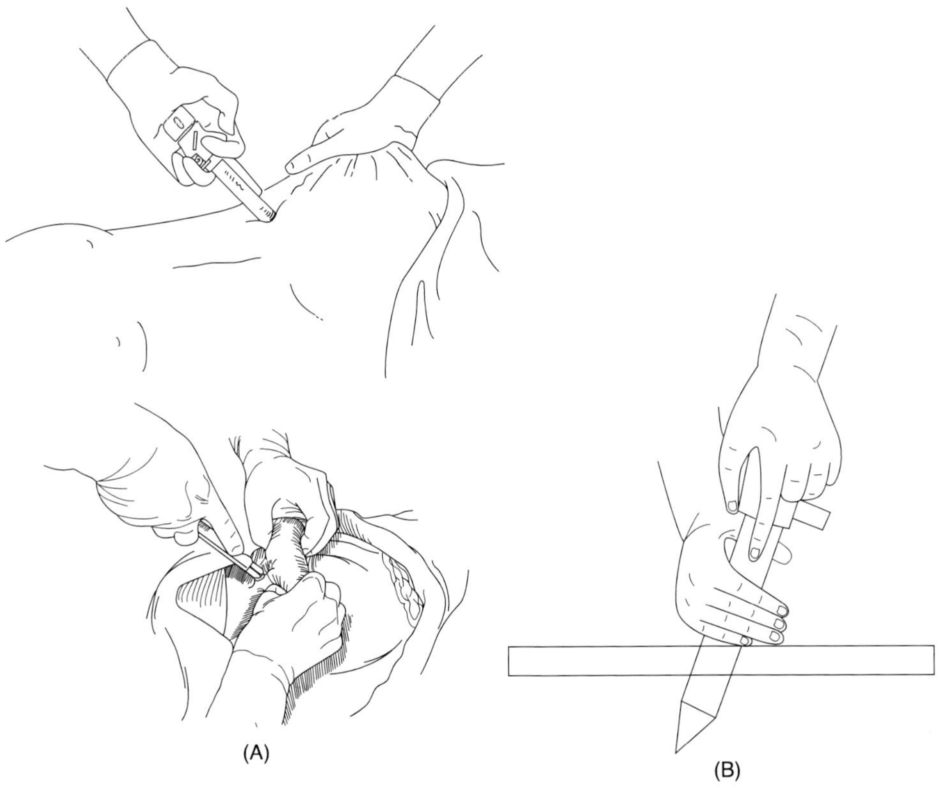

Figure 7 (A) One-handed braking during insertion of the primary umbilical cannula. (B) Two-handed braking during insertion of a cannula.

two to three fingers around the sheath may limit the depth of penetration. In the presence of a tense pneumoperitoneum, further elevation of the abdominal wall is usually unnecessary in most patients [Fig. 7(B)]. In very obese women, towel clips or intraumbilical Kelly forceps can be retained on either side of the umbilicus to elevate and immobilize the umbilicus, thereby facilitating initial trocar insertion at a perpendicular angle. An assistant placing pressure against the patient's abdomen above the umbilicus can provide additional abdominal elevation and countertraction. Using slow, steady force (rotational for pyramidal or conical, vertical for linear-bladed cannulas), the trocar is initially inserted perpendicularly to penetrate the skin and subcutaneous fat. In the nonobese patient, it is then tilted downward at a 60- to 70-degree angle, directing the tip into the abdominal cavity by aiming midway between the sacral promontory and bladder. If the patient is obese, trocar insertion should be completely perpendicular but with controlled minimal entry to ensure the shortest route into the abdominal cavity.

For a reusable trocar, inadvertent withdrawal from the peritoneal cavity, the sheath should be gently advanced as the obturator is withdrawn. For a disposable trocar, the surgeon should appreciate an audible click as the safety shield is engaged as the peritoneal cavity is entered. Despite these steps, the ability to perceive the moment of entry into the peritoneal cavity may be more difficult than presumed, even with visual entry trocars.

Several innovations in trocar design have evolved in an attempt to offset the inherent risk of blind peritoneal entry with a sharp tip. Two trocar-cannula systems are equipped with blunt conical tips: the TroGard™ (ConMed Corp., Utica, New York) and the Step™ (Covidien, Norwalk, Connecticut), a radially expanding device. Conical devices penetrate layers of the abdominal wall primarily by dilating rather than cutting. The Step™ device requires a 1.9 mm diameter Veress needle to insert a radially expanding sheath that is subsequently expanded from 3 to 12 mm with a blunt dilator for cannula insertion.

An optical trocar is a visually directed assembly equipped with either a transparent blunt conical tip with plastic tissue separators (EXCEL™, Ethicon Endosurgery, Cincinnati, Ohio) or a fine, laterally separating blade (VISIPORT™, Covidien, Norwalk, Connecticut) that provides a sequential view of tissues penetrated during insertion as yellow fat, white fascia, red muscle, and transparent peritoneum. Despite the presumed advantages, using medical device–reporting databases, 79 serious complications were identified with optical-access trocars, with 37 major vascular injuries, 18 bowel perforations, and 20 cases of severe bleeding including liver and stomach perforation (12).

Irrespective of the primary trocar/cannula used, it is introduced with the patient in supine position. The obturator is removed and the laparoscope inserted through the cannula to inspect the underlying bowel and mesentery before tilting the patient into Trendelenburg position.

A more recently introduced laparoscopic access cannula (EndoTIP, Karl Storz Endoscopy America, Culver City, California) virtually eliminates the need for axial penetration force during insertion. This cannula has a single thread winding around its outer distal surface, ending in a blunt tip. Rather than directing force internally, the device is rotated clockwise, thereby causing layers of the abdominal wall to be spread radially and lifted in an Archimedean fashion, under laparoscopic visualization, until the peritoneum is transilluminated.

DIRECT TROCAR INSERTION

The theoretical benefits of trocar insertion without a pneumoperitoneum are shortened operating time and elimination of the risks associated with the Veress needle, such as pelvic vessel laceration, gas embolism, failed pneumoperitoneum, and preperitoneal insufflation. It can be further argued that a flaccid abdomen permits higher elevation of the abdominal wall, less force to achieve trocar insertion, and easier perception of each layer during insertion. When 252 women were randomly assigned to compare these two techniques, no major complications were found to have occurred in either group; however, preperitoneal insufflations, failed entry, and multiple insertions were more frequent with the Veress needle. In the 113 women who underwent sterilization procedures, mean laparoscope insertion time was significantly less using direct insertion (2.2 vs. 5.9 min) (13). Moreover, no major complications were reported with direct insertion with a 12-mm disposable cannula through the left upper quadrant, 2 to 3 cm below the costal margin, in 23 women having undergone pelvic surgery (14). Critically, the security of this approach is predicated on elevation of the abdominal wall, sharp instruments, controlled entry, and firm knowledge of anatomy. Since the safety of this technique is vitally dependent on mobility of underlying bowel and control of the abdominal wall, it should be performed with caution in women who have had previous abdominal surgery and in very thin or obese women. Vascular laceration with a large trocar is far less forgiving than that which may occur with a Veress needle.

After a vertical intraumbilical incision is made, the trocar is directly inserted into the abdominal cavity while the abdomen is held upward using hands on both sides of the abdomen, midway between the umbilicus and pubic symphysis. It must be carefully aimed toward the pelvic hollow and slowly inserted while perceiving each layer on penetration. On removal of the obturator, the abdominal wall is elevated and the laparoscope is inserted in parallel to confirm the presence of bowel in the visual field. The peritoneal cavity is then insufflated and underlying bowel, mesentery, and vessels are carefully checked for injury. A complication of this technique is perforation of omentum as it adheres to the peritoneum. When this occurs, the pneumoperitoneum will elevate omentum partially off underlying bowel, and a curtain of omentum will appear before the laparoscope as an abdomen seemingly filled with adhesions. To correct this, the tip of the laparoscope is withdrawn back into the sleeve, the sleeve is brought perpendicular to the abdomen, and omentum will slide off the trocar onto the bowel.

PRIOR SURGERY

In women having undergone laparoscopy either through the umbilical fossa or left upper quadrant, a 20-gauge spinal needle attached to a syringe partly filled with saline can be used once pneumoperitoneum is established with a Verres needle through the umbilical fossa to estimate the clarity of the anticipated cannula insertion tract by exploring for adhesions, omentum, and bowel beneath the incision. With the Veress needle in situ, the spinal needle is sequentially inserted while aspirated to outline the circumference of the incision up to 5 cm caudad. Absence of significant adhesions and bowel are presumed by aspiration of carbon dioxide bubbles; negative aspiration is interpreted as abutment with adhesions or insertion into bowel wall (Fig. 6). Although aspiration of stool is disturbing even to the most experienced surgeon, a potentially catastrophic bowel injury from the subsequent thrust of a trocar is averted at the price of little, if any, morbidity. In the presence of significant adhesions, this technique may help delineate a free pathway for trocar insertion. Failure to satisfy these criteria mandates trocar insertion at either the left upper quadrant or by open laparoscopy.

NONUMBILICAL ENTRY TECHNIQUES

The left upper quadrant is arguably the safest alternative insertion site for peritoneal access in women having undergone earlier laparotomies. Despite its unorthodox location, this site can be used as an operative port if the umbilicus is used for the laparoscope. Extremely versatile, this approach is contraindicated only in women who have had splenic or gastric surgery, or who suffer from significant hepatosplenomegaly. Nevertheless, a sine qua non is that gastric contents must be emptied by nasogastric or oral gastric suction before beginning this method, as is routine with all laparoscopies. The first skin incision should be made with a scalpel below the left costal margin between the left midclavicular and anterior axillary lines in order to minimize the risk injuring the superior epigastric artery. Choosing a site closer to the costal margin exploits the adherence of the peritoneum to the last rib to resist downward placement of the anterior abdominal wall. The abdominal wall is both stabilized and lifted caudal to the skin incision with the assistant's grip or a towel clip. To target an insertion path for the Veress needle in the left upper quadrant, the abdominal wall is stabilized while the needle is advanced on an angle midway between the umbilicus medially and exit of the external iliac vessels laterally. Initially, the needle is perpendicularly inserted by holding it between the index finger and thumb with the wrist stabilized on the patient's abdominal wall to maximize proprioception, and then cautiously aimed following an axis that avoids both midline retroperitoneal and ipsilateral iliac vessels. Differing from the two "pops" classically perceived while traversing the fused layers of the umbilical plate, passage through the left upper quadrant is perceived as three pops; due to the relative flexibility of the peritoneum underlying this area, the third pop is easily perceived as resistance of stretched peritoneum is finally overcome. After sufficient insufflation, a 5-mm trocar is inserted taking great care at first to direct it perpendicular to the anterior abdominal wall. A 5-mm telescope is then inserted to confirm safe entry and peruse the subumbilical area for anatomic freedom. To minimize potential scarring and bleeding from a 5-mm trocar, insufflation may be accomplished in a similar fashion, using a larger Veress needle outfitted to accommodate a microlaparoscope (15). Alternatively, the left upper quadrant can be used by inserting the Veress needle directly through the eighth or ninth intercostal space. The initial skin incision is made at the anterior axillary line along the superior surface of the lower rib to avoid injuring the underlying neurovascular bundle. Due to strict adherence of peritoneum to the ribs in this area, passage into the peritoneal cavity is perceived as two pops. As the Veress needle is inserted perpendicularly and then slowly advanced, thick intercostal cartilage is immediately perceived, after which sudden release of resistance by strictly adherent peritoneum heralds peritoneal entry. The dramatic difference between resistance of intercostal tissue and peritoneal cavity enables the surgeon predictably to insert the needle only several millimeters into the peritoneal cavity. However, caudal apices of the pleura may in rare instances extend to this

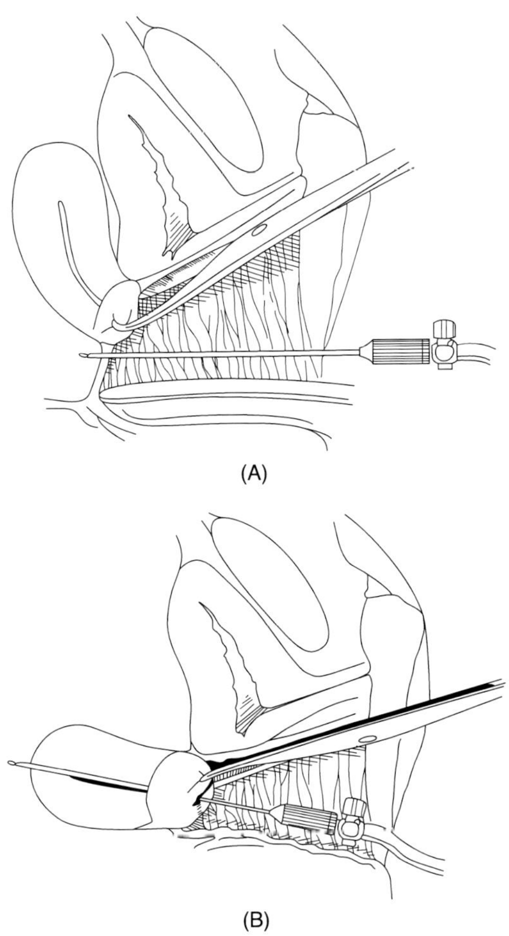

Figure 8 (A) Utilizing the cul-de-sac as an alternative method for peritoneal insufflation. (B) Utilizing transfundal passage as an alternative method for peritoneal insufflation.

level of the thoracic wall, and iatrogenic pneumothorax from insufflation directly into the pleural cavity may occur with this method.

In difficult cases, pneumoperitoneum can be safely and effectively introduced through the cul-de-sac. With the patient in Trendelenburg position, a single-tooth tenaculum is used to grasp and place the posterior cervix on anterior traction to tauten the posterior vaginal fornix. The tip of a long Veress needle (17 cm) is placed precisely in the midline, nearly 2 cm below the junction of the rugae of the vaginal vault and smooth epithelium of the cervical lip, and slowly advanced no more than 3 cm [(Fig. 8(A)]. After attaining adequate pneumoperitoneum, the needle is removed only under direct laparoscopic vision. This technique should not be performed in the presence of a cul-de-sac mass, rectovaginal endometriosis with cul-de-sac obliteration, or fixed uterine retroversion, or whenever the patient had prior vaginal vault surgery.

Insufflation may also be accomplished by transuterine insertion of the Veress needle. With the patient in Trendelenburg position, the anterior lip of the cervix is grasped with a single-tooth tenaculum and placed on traction to straighten any flexion. The position of the uterus and the length and direction of the uterine cavity are confirmed by inserting a uterine sound. A long Veress needle is inserted into the uterine cavity in midline and used to antevert the uterus away from the sacral hollow, rectosigmoid, and large retroperitoneal vessels to avoid the risks of visceral or vascular insult and gas embolism. Directing this step under intraoperative sonographic guidance may be safer. While holding the collar of the Veress needle, the fundus is penetrated and intraperitoneal location presumed by the spring release of the needle on entry [(Fig. 8(B)]. The needle is removed under direct laparoscopic vision as the uterus and adjacent structures are inspected for bleeding or injury. If chromopertubation is an essential part of the procedure, this technique should not be performed in women with multiple leiomyomata, extensive pelvic inflammatory disease, or prior uterine suspension, or whenever a risk of postsurgical adhesions between bowel and fundus exists, such as after myomectomy or hysterotomy.

OPEN LAPAROSCOPY

With open laparoscopy, the abdomen is first entered through a small umbilical incision under direct vision. Its use is indicated in the presence of a gravid uterus and can be used to facilitate the removal of larger pelvic masses. This technique reduces the risk of sharp trauma to retroperitoneal vessels and minimizes but does not completely obviate the risk of entering the lumen of adherent bowel. However, to exercise the same degree of caution used during laparotomy, visual access must remain unimpeded and underlying anatomic relationships should be predictable. In some patients, limiting the initial incision and subsequent dissection of this region of the abdominal wall can be difficult due to anatomic variation of the umbilicus itself, a large abdominal panniculus, and scarring or retraction secondary to a prior midline laparotomy. Previous laparotomy in the vicinity of the umbilicus can dramatically alter usual subumbilical anatomic relationships between the linea alba, rectus muscles, preperitoneal adipose tissue, and peritoneum. Tissue planes can be unrecognizable secondary to fusion of peritoneum and overlying fascia by scar formation, attenuation of the fascial plane, and fixation of the rectus muscles. Occasionally, especially when a previous abdominal incision has been extended lateral and superior to the umbilicus, the bowel is attached directly to the abdominal wall below the umbilical fossa, fixed to fascia without a discernible layer of peritoneum. In this situation, injury to the bowel will not necessarily be avoided by maintaining awareness of the depth of incision of fascial layers. Categorically, then, entering the lumen of the bowel on incision of fascia during open laparoscopy remains one of the rare but predictable complications of this technique.

The skin of the lower umbilical fold is held under tension by two Allis clamps and incised vertically for a distance of 1 to 3 cm, beginning inside the umbilicus and extending it inferiorly. Allis clamps are repositioned on skin edges, which are retracted laterally with S-shaped retractors. The cleavage plane is enlarged and deep fascia cleaned by inserting closed scissors and bluntly dissecting as they are separated using a spreading maneuver. Grasped with two small Kocher clamps, fascia is raised, incised transversely, and bluntly enlarged. With the S-shaped retractor below each fascial edge, a suture of sufficient tensile strength is passed through each edge and tagged. If the peritoneal cavity has not been inadvertently entered, it is exposed with the S-shaped retractors and gently entered by spreading with a hemostat. After affixing the cone sleeve to the shaft appropriate for the thickness of the abdominal wall, the blunt cannula is inserted into the peritoneal defect. Insufflation is begun. Tagged sutures are pulled upward and threaded into the cannula to anchor the fascia firmly against the cone, providing an airtight seal. The blunt obturator is removed and the laparoscope inserted. When the procedure is completed, the cannula is withdrawn after desufflation and fascia is approximated with previously tagged sutures. A retrospective review of the literature coupled with one group's experience culled data on 489,335 patients with the Veress technique and 12,444 with open laparoscopy (16). Rates of visceral and vascular injury were 0.083% and 0.075% after closed laparoscopy, and 0.048% and zero after open laparoscopy. Vascular injury occurred significantly more frequently in patients having closed laparoscopy. No study to date has reported a direct comparison between open and closed techniques in a randomized, controlled fashion.

INSERTION OF ACCESSORY TROCARS

The site and size of accessory trocars depend on the anatomic configuration of pelvic viscera and any associated pathology, instruments required for the planned procedure, and the type of surgery to be performed. Trocars must be arrayed so that they are not too close to each other to prevent interference between the tops of the sheaths and striking one another within the surgical field. Similarly, an accessory port placed too close to the plane of the primary trocar will inhibit simultaneous access to the surgical field. Ideally, accessory trocars should be inserted at 90-degree angles to each other, forming an equilateral triangle or diamond matrix around the operative site. Each point of entry should be chosen to aid the surgical procedure as much as possible. The risk of injury to vessels of the abdominal wall is substantially greater whenever an accessory trocar is placed lateral to midline.

Immediately above the pubic symphysis, both superficial and inferior epigastric arteries are at their most lateral locations. Each vessel has a specific origin and anatomic distribution. The superficial epigastric artery arises from femoral vessels to branch superiorly to supply skin and subcutaneous tissues of the abdominal wall; the inferior epigastric artery arises from external iliac vessels and courses around the inguinal ligament to ascend the posterior surface of the rectus abdominus muscle to become the primary supply to lower abdominal segments (Fig. 9). Superficial epigastric vessels can usually be identified by transillumination. This is not always possible, however, in obese and dark-skinned patients or in the presence of a dense surgical scar. To the contrary, the subrectus locale of inferior epigastric arteries usually precludes visualization by transillumination. Location of these arteries should be identified laparoscopically by integrating their known anatomic distribution. Under normal conditions, these vessels can be visually mapped to course along the parietal peritoneum between the medial umbilical ligament and exit of the round ligament into the internal ring. Two companion veins, railroad-track in appearance, can often be seen running parallel below the surface of the pulsatile artery (Fig. 10). When inferior epigastric vessels cannot be identified, inserting the trocar medial to the medial umbilical ligament or lateral to the exit of the round ligament can reduce the risk of injury. Using computed tomographic images of 21 reproductive-age women, the mean location of the inferior epigastric vessel immediately above the symphysis was found only 5.6 cm from midline, and thus this suggested that the lateral trocar must be placed 4 cm or less from midline to avoid this vessel consistently (17,18). Because the lateral margin of the rectus abdominus muscle is the least vascular area, the site least likely to cause vascular injury would be at its margins or approximately 8 cm from midline in women of normal weight and somewhat more lateral in overweight patients. This same concept substantiates the recommendation to target at or lateral to the midclavicular line during peritoneal access in the left upper quadrant. Neither directive is absolute.

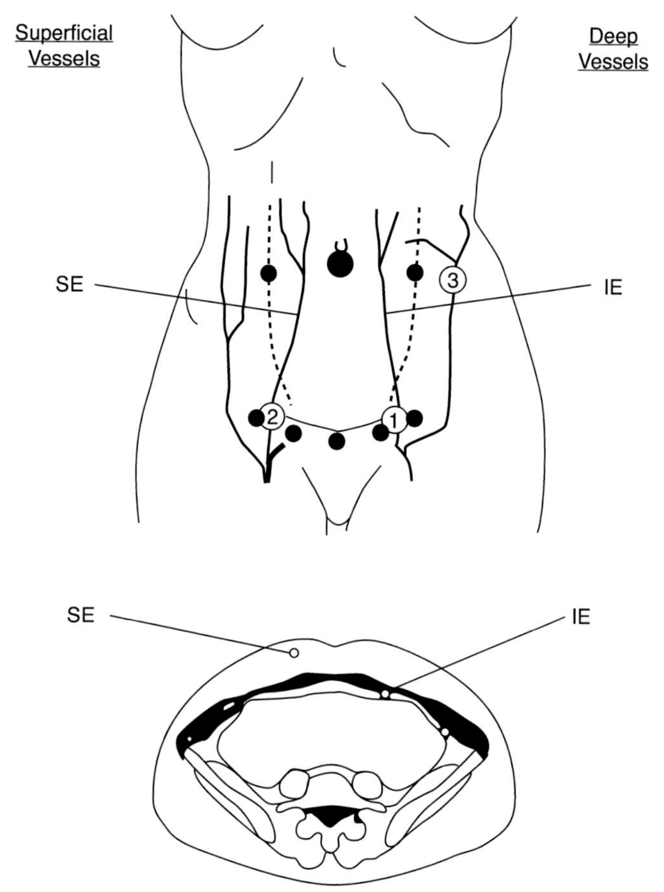

Figure 9 The anatomical distribution of the superficial (SE) and inferior epigastric (IE) vessels.

Since large cannulas are more likely to encounter a blood vessel than small ones, the smallest trocars possible are preferentially placed at lateral sites. While a conical tip is theoretically less likely to lacerate a vessel than a multiblade pyramidal tip, its utility must be weighed against the extra force required for insertion. Once the sites are chosen, the skin is incised superficially with a no. 11 blade in a somewhat curvilinear fashion, just enough to accommodate the diameter of the trocar. A Kelly clamp is inserted into the subcutaneous defect and the incision is widened enough to allow dissection down to the fascia. The point of the closed clamp should be visualized laparoscopically, as it tents fascia and peritoneum. The trocar is held so the index or middle finger extends down the sheath to act as a brake. For the small-handed surgeon, the nondominant forearm can be laid across the patient's lower trunk and used as a fulcrum to control the force and depth of trocar insertion. The assistant should push on the patient's upper abdomen or the contralateral abdominal wall to further elevate the insertion site. Under continuous laparoscopic monitoring, the trocar is inserted using a slow motion (side-to-side for pyramidal, twisting for conical, linear for linear cutting) initially in a perpendicular fashion until it superficially penetrates the fascia. After fascial engagement, the direction of the sheath is directly altered in line with the pelvic hollow and

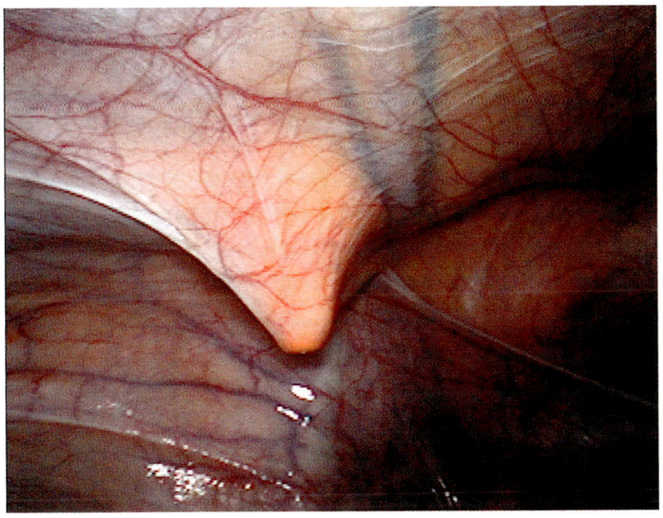

Figure 10 Inferior epigastric vessels including paired veins along the undersurface of the abdominal wall during insertion of accessory trocar.

away from any pelvic mass. The trocar tip must be visualized continuously during all phases of peritoneal entry. Failure to engage fascia before angulation into the pelvis risks injury to abdominal wall vessels caused by sliding and then penetrating in a "Z" fashion. If the sheath is not properly redirected to the surgical field, particularly in obese patients, the surgeon will have to put significant pressure on the sheath each time an instrument is inserted in order to redirect it to the surgical field.

Although incisional herniations may occur at both umbilical and extraumbilical sites, they are most likely to occur at port sites of 10 cm or larger, especially when placed lateral to the rectus sheath (19). This risk appears to be magnified whenever self-retaining fascial screws are used and after longer procedures with excessive manipulation of the port site. One multicenter report of 3560 operative laparoscopies found the risk of herniation through a 12-mm trocar site to be 13-fold greater than that for a 10-mm site (20). Therefore, when larger extraumbilical ports (≥10 mm) are placed lateral to midline, the fascial defect should be closed transmurally to include fascial and peritoneal components; adequate closure of the fascial defect alone does not preclude occurrence of a Richter's hernia, which may occur lateral to the rectus abdominus muscle. Closing the entire defect is best achieved with laparoscopic closure devices that can be directed by the intraperitoneal view. General preventive recommendations to reduce herniation of bowel into peritoneal and fascial defects include deflating the abdomen before trocars are removed and postoperatively instructing the patient to avoid straining and heavy lifting for a month after surgery.

SUMMARY

By virtue of the strategic importance and potential operative morbidities, placement of primary and secondary cannulas during peritoneal access remains the gynecologic surgeon's most important concern during a laparoscopic surgery. Success and safety are closely predicated on knowledge of underlying visceral and vascular anatomy as well as any space-occupying pelvic pathology. While a variety of techniques can serve to avert injury to underlying structures, control of entry force and limiting the depth of insertion are the foremost sentinels during blind entry into the abdominal cavity. The final locations of secondary cannulas depend upon body habitus, the topography of any underlying pelvic pathology, and the technical needs of the planned surgical procedure. Since no singular technique for primary peritoneal entry is applicable for all patients, the laparoscopic surgeon must be able to utilize alternative methods for access to the abdominal cavity.

REFERENCES

1. Schafer M, Lauper M, Krahenbuhl L. Trocar and Veress needle injuries during laparoscopy. Surg Endosc 2001; 15:275–280.
2. Brill A, Nezhat F, Nezhat C, et al. The incidence of adhesions after prior laparotomy: A laparoscopic appraisal. Obstet Gynecol 1995; 85:269–272.
3. Loffer FD, Pent D. Laparoscopy in the obese patient. Am J Obstet Gynecol 1976; 125:104–107.
4. Hulka JF. Major vessel injury during laparoscopy. Am J Obstet Gynecol 1980; 138:590.
5. Goss GM, eds. Gray's Anatomy of the Human Body. 28th ed. Philadelphia, PA: Lea & Febiger; 1966:646–647.
6. Hurd WW, Bude RO, DeLancey JO, et al. The relationship of the umbilicus to the aortic bifurcation: Implications for laparoscopic technique. Obstet Gynecol 1992; 80:48–51.
7. Nezhat F, Brill AI, Nezhat CH, et al. Laparoscopic appraisal of the anatomic relationship of the umbilicus to the aortic bifurcation. J Am Assoc Gynecol Laparosc 1998; 5:135–140.
8. Toth A, Graf M. The center of umbilicus as the Veress needle's entry site for laparoscopy. J Reprod Med 1984; 29:126–128.
9. Loffer FD, Pent D. An alternate technique in penetrating the abdomen for laparoscopy. J Reprod Med 1974; 13:37–40.
10. Roy GM, Bazzurini L, Solima E, et al. Safe technique for laparoscopic entry into the abdominal cavity. J Am Assoc Gynecol Laparosc 2001; 8:399–401.
11. Hurd WW, Wang L, Schemmel MT. A comparison of the relative risk of vessel injury with conical versus pyramidal laparoscopic trocars in a rabbit model. Am J Obstet Gynecol 1995; 173:1731–1733.
12. Sharp HT, Dodson MK, Draper ML, et al. Complications associated with optical-access laparoscopic trocars. Obstet Gynecol 2002; 99:553–555.
13. Nezhat FR, Silfen SL, Evans D, et al. Comparison of direct insertion of disposable and standard reusable laparoscopic trocars and pervious pneumoperitoneum with Veress needle. Obstet Gynecol 1991; 78:148–150.
14. Howard FM, El-Minawi AM, DeLoach VE. Direct laparoscopic cannula insertion at the left upper quadrant. J Am Assoc Gynecol Laparosc 1997; 4:595–600.
15. Audebert AJM, Gomel V. Role of microlaparoscopy in the diagnosis of peritoneal and visceral adhesions and in the prevention of bowel injury associated with blind trocar insertion. Fertil Steril 2000; 73: 631–635.
16. Bonjer JJ, Hazebroek EJ, Kazemier G, et al. Open versus closed establishment of pneumoperitoneum in laparoscopic surgery. Br J Surg 1997; 84:599–602.
17. Hurd WW, Bude RO, DeLancey JO, et al. The location of abdominal wall blood vessels in relationship to abdominal landmarks apparent at laparoscopy. Am J Obstet Gynecol 1994; 171:642–646.
18. Hurd WW, Pearl ML, DeLancey JO, et al. Laparoscopic injury of abdominal wall blood vessels: A report of three cases. Obstet Gynecol 1993; 82:673–676.
19. Boike GM, Miller CE, Spirtos NM, et al. Incisional bowel herniations after operative laparoscopy: A series of nineteen cases and review of the literature. Am J Obstet Gynecol 1995; 172:1726–1731.
20. Kadar N, Reich H, Liu CY, et al. Incisional hernias after major laparoscopic gynecologic procedures. Am J Obstet Gynecol. 1993; 168:1493–1495.

5

Surgical dissection and anatomy of the female pelvis for the gynecologic surgeon

Robert M. Rogers, Jr. and Richard H. Taylor

The anatomy used by gynecologic surgeons is the anatomy relevant to surgical dissection in specific areas of the female pelvis. The bridge between the knowledge of pelvic anatomy and an efficient surgical practice is the mastery of the several techniques of surgical dissection. This chapter discusses the three fundamentals that are essential for a gynecologic surgeon to be successful—techniques of tissue dissection, the dynamics of surgical teamwork, and a working knowledge of surgical anatomy. Proper tissue dissection concerns both lysis of adhesions within the pelvic cavity itself and exploration of many areas of the pelvic retroperitoneum. Collaboration is essential to perform a successful surgery. Teamwork involves leadership skills to coordinate the roles of the several team members in order to achieve a "synergy of purpose." Anatomically, areas that are to be discussed include the presacral space, the pelvic brim, the pelvic sidewall, the base of the broad ligament/cardinal ligament, the paravesical space, the retropubic space, the vesicovaginal space, the pararectal space, and the rectovaginal space.

SURGICAL DISSECTION—THEORY AND DISCUSSION OF TECHNIQUES

The purpose of deliberate surgical dissection is not to do any harm to the patient, while safeguarding vital anatomic structures and blood vessels. The goal is to perform the dissection in order to avoid injuring the viscera, ureter, and somatic nerves and to limit blood loss. Most surgeons read, study, and strive to master the knowledge of surgical anatomy. However, they assume that skilled dissection techniques will soon follow. Not so!—tissue dissection techniques must be learned, understood, and practiced as rigorously and consistently as any other surgical skill, such as laparoscopic suturing or use of new surgical products. Correct knowledge and focused practice gradually result in safe and efficient dissection techniques. Importantly, the surgeon must acknowledge that he/she cannot operate alone and must have assistants to aid him/her in the surgical procedure. The surgeon is only one part of a surgical team that can accomplish any surgery when working in an environment of experience and mutual respect.

The purpose of surgical dissection is to thin out adhesions, scar tissue, and/or visceral connective tissues, in order to visualize the anatomic structures contained therein or situated nearby. In the pelvic cavity itself, adhesions can be fine and filmy to denser and shorter and, then, to very thick, nodular, and hard. Some cases require minor surgical lysis. In other more challenging cases, the denser and harder scarring can result in the dangers of surgical dissections in a "frozen pelvis." Adhesions can and do adhere from the female organs to the bladder peritoneum, to the serosa of the colon and intestines, and to the parietal peritoneum of the cul-de-sac and sidewall. In the retroperitoneal areas and spaces, both normal visceral connective tissues and scar tissue can coexist, to challenge the dissectional skills of the surgeon. Dissections in both the pelvic cavity and the retroperitoneum use the same techniques.

In the retroperitoneum, the visceral connective tissues serve two important purposes (1). One is to envelope and mechanically support the visceral blood vessels, nerves, and lymph nodes and channels that service the viscera. The other is to follow these visceral structures to their viscera for the purposes of mechanical suspension of these organs, such as the bladder, cervix and vagina, and the rectum. The visceral connective tissues anchor the pelvic viscera to the parietal fascia of the back wall and sidewall of the pelvis. For example, the cardinal ligament/uterosacral ligament complex of visceral connective tissue envelopes the internal iliac artery and vein and is led to the pericervical ring by the uterine artery. The cardinal ligaments and uterosacral ligaments are anchored to the back wall and sidewall of the pelvis. They suspend the cervix and upper vagina over the tendinous levator plate. The levator plate is the dynamic backstop that functions to help prevent uterine and vaginal prolapse during the episodes of increased intrapelvic (Valsalva) pressure.

The first and most important principle of surgical dissection is the exposure of anatomic structures. Ideally, the surgeon should not cut into tissues that he/she does not understand and cannot see with his/her own eyes. Therefore, sharp and blunt dissections must literally proceed "millimeter by millimeter." The dissection carefully spreads out and thins the adhesion, the scar, or the visceral connective tissues so that the operator can visualize the structures enveloped within. Surgical dissection must reveal structures, not obscure or confuse them. Therefore, knowledge of the structures contained in the area to be dissected and anatomic orientation during the dissection are essential to meticulous and safe dissection techniques. This also requires the operator to think spatially in three dimensions. Additionally, the surgeon must learn the palpable "feel" of the dissection. Remember, the operator only employs two of the five senses when performing a surgical procedure—sight and palpation. These two senses are equally important. These senses must be consciously developed, practiced, and improved by repetition and experience.

By dissecting "millimeter by millimeter," the surgeon achieves four goals. First is the maintenance of correct anatomic orientation and direction of dissection. Second is the allowance for re-evaluation of dissection techniques and use of instrumentation. The surgeon has time to think the dissection technique step by step and change techniques, approach, or instrumentation, if needed. Flexibility, ingenuity, and experience are essential characteristics of an accomplished surgeon. Third is proceeding in small steps under direct visualization, in order to safely reveal the vital anatomic structures to be safeguarded. Fourth is limitation of any injury to an anatomic structure by 1 mm or less. By dissecting deliberately and slowly, in most cases, the operator can readily control any bleeding encountered or see an unavoidable injury to a viscus or an anatomic structure. Therefore, major bleeding or gross visceral injury should be minimized.

There are several techniques that the operator must master. These techniques of surgical dissection are the same in any area of the pelvis irrespective of the route of entry to that anatomic area, whether by laparotomy, laparoscopy, or per vaginum. The techniques are grasp and tent, "mm" incisions under clear visual control, push and spread, traction and countertraction, rotation and counterrotation of the grasped tissue, and gentle wiping of tissue by judicious blunt dissection. Some of these techniques can be facilitated by the technique of hydrodissection. Hydrodissection is the injection of sterile fluid into the tissues to be dissected, in order to tent and thin these tissues. Again, these dissection techniques must be performed slowly and deliberately in small 1-mm increments.

By *grasping and tenting* the adhesion, scar, peritoneum, or visceral connective tissue, the operator, in most cases, elevates or moves the grasped tissue away from a viscus or vital anatomic structure, even if that distance is only a millimeter or two. Grasping and tenting also help to thin out the grasped tissue so that an edge of bowel serosa may be seen, a ureter can be seen peristalsing, or an artery can be seen pulsating. With tenting and with anatomic knowledge and orientation, the surgeon can then *incise* the grasped tissue by 1 mm with a knife, scissors, or laser. The incision should be placed on the side away from any vital anatomic structure or organ. For example, adhesions from the uterus to the bowel should be incised on the uterine serosa and not toward the bowel serosa. The techniques of tenting and traction countertraction would be useful in this case.

With re-evaluation of the incision, the surgeon can then carefully use a *push and spread* technique "millimeter by millimeter" to further expose the contents of the adhesion, scar, or visceral connective tissue. The tissue is further spread out and thinned by grasping the edges of the dissected tissues and gently pulling them apart by using *traction and countertraction*. Obviously, there is a "feel" to these maneuvers.

In some situations, gentle *rotation of the grasped tissue* will further thin the tissues and may reveal the underlying structures. *Rotation and counterrotation* can further fracture scars and adhesions to thin them out. In dense adhesions or scar tissue, sharp dissection with the knife or scissors or with laser "millimeter by millimeter" can be augmented with gentle localized *wiping* "millimeter by millimeter" as a form of traction and countertraction. This technique is also known as "teasing the tissues." Broad, blunt strokes of the *wiping* technique should not be used. Such quick, sweeping moves do not allow for controlled dissection. This is an uncontrolled, "blind" method of dissection that can tear into blood vessels, bladder, or bowel. Another technique is the directed injection of sterile saline or other physiologic fluid into the dissection field. This technique, *hydrodissection*, further spreads, thins, and tents the tissues in a gentle manner. Hydrodissection can and does facilitate vaginal dissections in the vesicovaginal, paravaginal, rectovaginal, and paravaginal spaces.

YOU CANNOT OPERATE WITHOUT A TEAM

No matter how skilled and experienced you are as a surgeon, you cannot operate safely, efficiently, and effectively without an experienced team in the operating room. This team consists of you, your surgical assistant, scrub nurse, nurse circulator, and, of course, your anesthesiologist. You cannot operate without a properly anesthetized, comfortable patient who has adequate muscle relaxation and does not move. You would waste your time if you had to take the time to gather your own instruments, sterilize them, and set them up on a sterile table. You would not be able to prep and drape your patient yourself and then insert cords into the machines surrounding the operating table without breaking scrub. In many cases, you cannot assist yourself during the surgical dissections. In more challenging surgical cases, you will require additional personnel for retraction. You are the leader of a team that allows you to perform your best surgical techniques and procedures. You are a clumsy, grossly inefficient surgeon without the team. The team allows you to shine forth. Better surgical results are achieved when there is a "synergy of purpose" with the members of the team working together to achieve a common purpose of safety and efficiency.

When the individual members of a team work independently or at odds with one another, the loss of cohesive respect fractures the quality and efficiency of the working environment. A tense, uncomfortable atmosphere in the operating room does not allow the optimal surgical result. First, do no harm. Professionals care about their behavior and performance. The entire team must be dedicated to patient safety and procedural efficiency.

Learn to be an appreciative leader. Your surgery will become smoother and better in a pleasant professional environment. Accept suggestions and compromise in order to improve surgical safety and procedural flow. Be mindful of the comfort of the team members, especially those who assist and retract. Appreciate team input during your surgeries. Your team members may give you information or reminders that you may not have noticed or remembered. You cannot observe everything that is going on in the operating room when you are focused on a small field of dissection. Your assistant may see something around the dissection field that you may not have seen. You may have been distracted when manipulating an instrument or performing a dissection.

Remember, there is no "I" in a team, unless you can say, "I am proud of our team." You have spent years in learning and developing your knowledge and skills in surgical anatomy, dissections, accepted procedures, and judgment and management of complications. However, you must remember that you did very little of this development on your own. You had teachers, mentors, and experienced operating personnel to guide and encourage you. Therefore, in return, you must develop an attitude of appreciation and respect for them, your "team" members of past, present and future. Positive motivation should come willingly from within the individuals of the surgical team, not by fear of embarrassment or verbal punishment. The more you give to others in courtesy and respect, the more those others will give you in facilitating your surgeries. The atmosphere in the operating room will become respectful and comfortable. The members of the surgical team are your colleagues. Respect them, teach them, listen to them, and complement them. Everyone involved in a surgery responds positively when he/she is a part of a respected and successful team that brings the best care to each patient.

AREAS OF ANATOMIC DISSECTION IN THE FEMALE PELVIS

The areas of dissection in the female pelvis relevant to the gynecologic surgeon are the presacral space, the pelvic brim, the pelvic sidewall, the base of the broad ligament or the cardinal ligament, the paravesical space, the retropubic space, the vesicovaginal space, the pararectal space, and the rectovaginal space. The paravesical (paravaginal), vesicovaginal, and rectovaginal spaces are discussed from both the intrapelvic and the intravaginal routes. Mention of surgical dissections in each of these areas refers to the dissection techniques already discussed. The reader should actively review and learn them.

The Presacral Space

The *presacral space* is the area of surgical dissection and performance of the "presacral neurectomy" for women with "central" chronic pelvic pain, severe dysmenorrhea, and proven endometriosis (2,3). However, heated controversy and continuing debates exist, concerning the real use of this procedure in the gynecologist's armamentarium of operations for patients with pelvic pain issues (4).

This space is actually the prelumbar space, since it lies over the anterior longitudinal ligament on the fourth and fifth lumbar vertebrae (Fig. 1). This potential space is bordered superiorly by the bifurcation of the aorta at the level of the fourth lumbar vertebra, and inferiorly by the promontory of the first sacral vertebra. Laterally to the right travels the right common iliac artery and right ureter, while on the left courses the left common iliac vein and left ureter. Anteriorly, covering the presacral space is the peritoneum. Posteriorly, the middle sacral artery (from the aorta!) and a plexus of fragile veins on the anterior longitudinal ligament are found.

Between the peritoneum and the posterior border of the presacral space are found several fused sheets of visceral connective tissue enveloping the multiple visceral nerves coursing through this area. These nerves emanate from preaortic ganglia and, eventually, enter into the right and left hypogastric nerves, which then travel in the pelvic sidewalls to feed into the respective inferior hypogastric plexuses, also known as the pelvic plexuses of visceral nerves. These presacral nerves, or visceral nerves of the superior hypogastric plexus, are very fine or invisible to the naked eye. They are enveloped in and obscured by the fatty areolar tissue within the sheets of visceral connective tissue. The presacral plexus forms a geometric

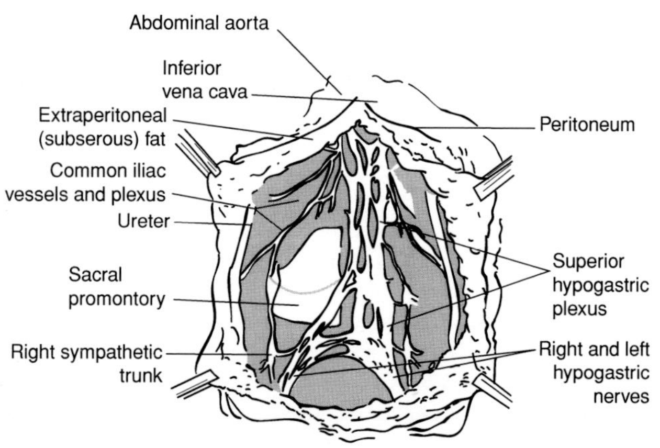

Figure 1 Presacral space.

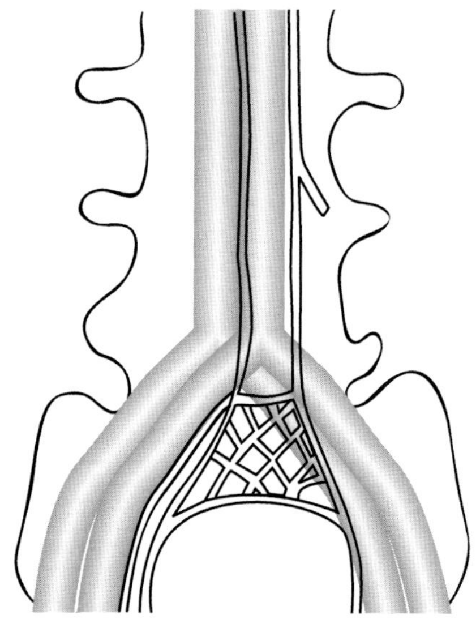

Figure 2 Presacral nerves.

webbing that is quite variable in location, formation, and size. This webbing of unseen nerves can even be found overlying the left common iliac vein and artery, lateral and away from the presacral space (Fig. 2) (5).

Dissection must use the tenting of tissues, and gentle traction and countertraction to thin out the several layers of visceral connective tissues, in order to see the larger structures bordering this space, while lifting the visceral connective tissues away from very vascular posterior border. The operator then removes these visceral connective tissues, which contain the visceral nerves of the presacral plexus. Remember, these fine nerves can only be seen if some of the nerves have physically coalesced together. Even then, some or many nerves may not be removed since the bulk of the plexus may pass laterally to the left, as noted. Tissues should not be excised from this space unless the operator has positively seen all the bordering anatomic structures. If this rule is not followed, the potential for massive hemorrhage or injury to the ureters is very real.

The Pelvic Brim

This is the area most likely to be unaltered by endometriosis, an ovarian remnant pelvic, infection, and subsequent scarring or adhesion formation. Therefore, this is the area most ideally suited to begin a retroperitoneal sidewall dissection in order to find the ureter and major blood vessels entering into the pelvis. This is especially so on the patient's right side. On the left side, the mesentery of the sigmoid colon adds more layers of areolar tissue that must be dissected in order to expose the anatomic structures (Fig. 3). The structures of the pelvic brim enter into the pelvis, one over another, in a vertical orientation and then rotate 90° to form the three surgical layers of the pelvic sidewall. These anatomic structures are the *parietal peritoneum* covering the *ovarian vessels* in the *infundibulopelvic ligament*, coursing over the *ureter*, which passes over the *bifurcation of the common iliac artery*, located at the pelvic brim overlying the sacroiliac joint. Between the bifurcation of the common iliac artery and sacroiliac joint are found the *common iliac vein*, the medial edge of the psoas muscle, and the *obturator nerve* overlying the parietal fascia over the capsule of the sacroiliac

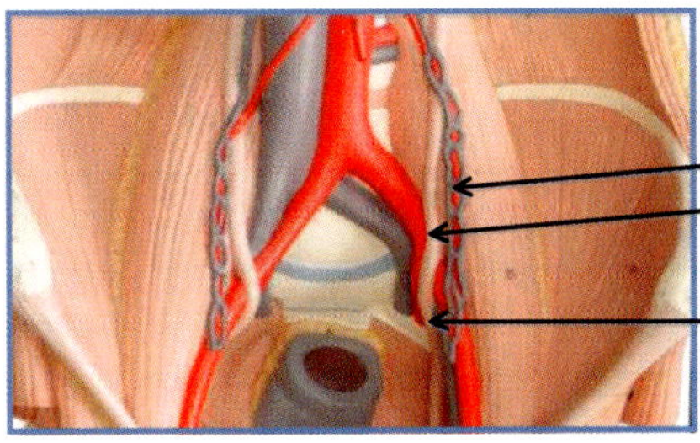

Figure 3 Key structures at the pelvic brim.

joint. The common iliac artery bifurcates into the internal iliac artery (hypogastric artery) and the external iliac artery, which courses on the medial portion of the anterior surface of the psoas muscle. The external iliac vein courses on the medial edge of the psoas muscle, just medial and posterior to the external iliac artery.

When performing oophorectomy, ureteral injury or occlusion can occur in this area during ligation or coagulation of the infundibulopelvic ligament. All the discussed dissection techniques are safely used in this area to the surgeon's great advantage to see and isolate the ureter, great vessels, and obturator nerve. These same techniques are essential for sampling and excision of the lymph nodes along the common, external, and internal iliac vessels.

The Pelvic Sidewall

The *pelvic sidewall* is that area of the pelvic retroperitoneum that starts at the pelvic brim and extends to the base of the broad ligament where the ureter courses just posterior to the uterine blood vessels. It is bordered medially by the parietal peritoneum and laterally by the parietal fascia of the obturator internus muscle. Sandwiched in between are the multiple, fused sheets of visceral connective tissues that envelope the visceral vessels, nerves and lymph nodes, and channels that service the bladder, uterus, cervix and vagina, and the lower rectum. From a surgical need to dissect in avascular planes, the pelvic sidewall structures are found in three layers. These three layers are separated by two avascular dissection planes (Fig. 4).

The first layer, or the ureteral layer, is the ureter and its surrounding visceral connective tissue sheath attached to the parietal peritoneum. The second layer, or the visceral layer, is the internal iliac artery and vein ensheathed by the multiple sheets of the visceral connective tissue of the cardinal ligament. The third layer, or the parietal layer, is the external iliac artery and vein on the medial aspect of the psoas muscle, and the obturator nerve and the obturator artery and vein, found coursing along the anterior aspect of the obturator internus muscle. The avascular dissection planes are found between each of these three layers, unless there is significant scarring from prior disease processes or former sidewall dissections. Here, the goal of dissections is to identify the ureter and the parietal structures of the third layer. Then, because of the rich vascular collateral circulation in the pelvis, the visceral blood vessels in the second layer can be clamped, sutured, and coagulated safely without injuring other pelvic structures.

Also found in the second surgical layer of the pelvic sidewall are the visceral branches of the internal iliac artery and vein (Fig. 5)—the uterine, superior vesical leading to the obliterated umbilical, the inferior vesical, the vaginal, the middle rectal, and the inferior gluteal. The operator must be aware that these vessels may originate from surrounding parietal vessels but may still be safely clamped, tied, and coagulated. Another way to find the internal iliac artery (hypogastric artery) is to identify the obliterated umbilical artery and follow and dissect it back, underneath the round ligament, in the broad ligament, to the superior vesical artery, and, then, to the terminus of the internal iliac artery. At this same terminus, the operator finds the medial arterial offshoot, which is the beginning of the uterine artery, which may be followed to course anterior to the ureter. This is a safe area in which to ligate or coagulate the uterine artery, with the ureter in view.

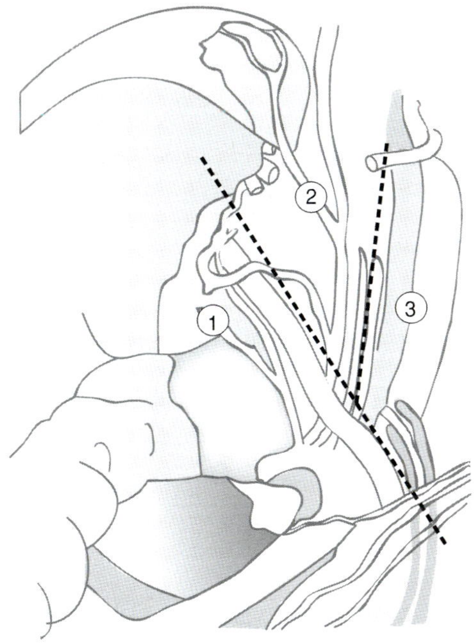

1. FIRST LAYER OF PELVIC SIDEWALL
   Parietal peritoneum and ureter
2. SECOND LAYER OF PELVIC SIDEWALL
   Internal iliac vessels and their tributaries: uterine, superior and inferior vesical, vaginal, internal pudendal, and inferior gluteal vessels
3. THIRD LAYER OF PELVIC SIDEWALL
   Obturator internus muscle
   Obutrator nerve, artery and vein
   External iliac artery and vein

Figure 4 Three layers of pelvic sidewall.

At the time of laparotomy or laparoscopy, the operator can see many of these structures through the thin peritoneal covering, especially on the right side. Anteriorly and laterally situated are the external iliac artery and vein on the medial portion of the psoas muscle. Just lateral to the external iliac vein is the bony ridge of the arcuate line of the ilium, which cannot be seen. More posteriorly through the parietal peritoneum of the pelvic sidewall are the ureter, occasionally demonstrating peristalsis, and the internal iliac artery, demonstrating regular pulsations. The other structures of the third layer cannot be visualized without opening the peritoneum and dissecting laterally and inferiorly.

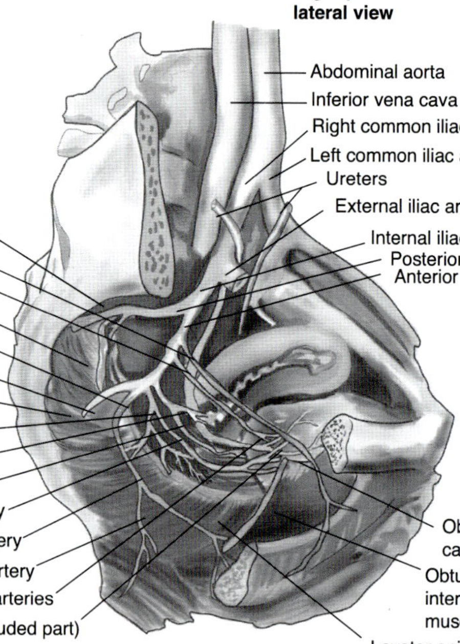

Figure 5 Visceral branches of internal iliac artery.

Base of the Broad Ligament/Cardinal Ligament—Protect the Ureter

Dissection of the pelvic sidewall inferiorly toward the uterine and superior vesical arteries leads the operator to the *base of the broad ligament*, which is also the *base of the cardinal ligament*, where the oblique crossing of the ureter is found underneath the uterine artery and vein in most cases. This anatomic landmark allows the surgeon to proceed anteriorly and laterally into the *paravesical space*, or posteriorly and laterally into the *pararectal space*, or posteriorly and medially into the *rectovaginal space* (Fig. 6). The paravesical space is simply the lateral compartment of the *retropubic space (of Retzius)*, which is easily entered by dissection toward the pubic bone medially.

The intersection of the uterine artery and ureter occurs surgically close to the side of the lower uterine segment and cervix. The distance is within 1 to 2 cm in the natural state, without traction on the uterus. This area is also just lateral to the insertion of the uterosacral ligament to the posterolateral aspect of the cervix.

The obvious challenge in hysterectomy or uterine artery ablation is to ligate or coagulate the uterine vessels without damaging the ureter. Ideally, the ureter and uterine vessels are successfully dissected for clear visualization by the surgeon, and then the uterine vessels are occluded under direct visualization, with the ureter being clearly seen safely away. There are two main routes to achieve this visualization. These

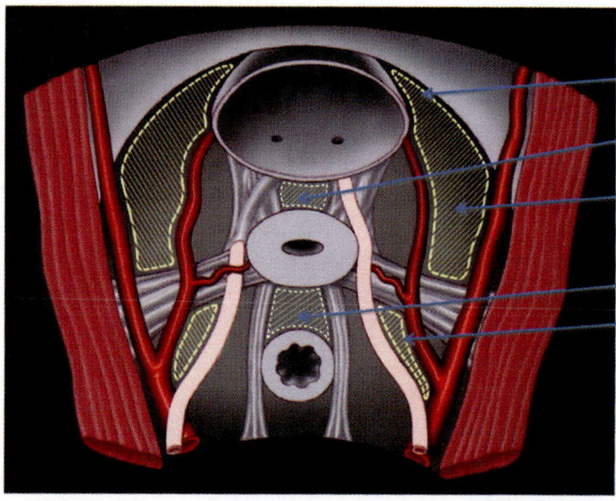

Figure 6 Key retroperitoneal spaces in the pelvis.

must be used in cases of significant scarring in the base of this area by endometriosis, infection, or tumor. First, the ureter can be dissected carefully from the pelvic brim in the pelvic sidewall until the uterine artery is seen coursing medially from the terminus of the internal iliac artery, where the superior vesical artery continues anteriorly into the broad ligament and underneath the round ligament to become the obliterated umbilical artery. Second, the operator can open the round ligament, pull on the obliterated umbilical artery, which is responsible for the medial umbilical fold of peritoneum, and follow this anatomic cord posteriorly to the base of the internal iliac artery, where the uterine artery is the medial branch. Note that the median umbilical fold of peritoneum is formed by the urachus, while the lateral umbilical fold of peritoneum is formed by the inferior epigastric artery and vein. These inferior epigastric vessels are located just medial to the exit of the round ligament through the internal inguinal ring.

However, in most cases of hysterectomy, the operator does not, nor is required by present standard of care, to visually identify the junction of the ureter crossing underneath the uterine vessels (Fig. 3). Therefore, the surgeon must follow two important surgical principles. First, the uterus must be mechanically manipulated, with the direction depending upon the route of hysterectomy. If the hysterectomy is being performed through the abdominal/pelvic route via laparotomy or laparoscopy, the operator must push, with an intrauterine manipulator, or pull, with a tenaculum on the fundus, the uterus superiorly and medially away from the ureter, to be protected from clamping or coagulation. This maneuver significantly elevates and pulls the uterine artery and vein away from the ureter. If the hysterectomy is being pursued through the vaginal route, the operator must pull the cervix and uterus inferiorly toward the vaginal introitus to achieve anatomic separation between the ureter and the uterine vessels.

Second, once the appropriate traction has been placed on the uterus, as described, the gynecologic surgeon must clamp or coagulate immediately adjacent to the palpable, lateral edge of the uterus and cervix. Unless the ureter can be seen, any clamping or coagulating more laterally into the parametrium will increase the risk of ureteral injury or obstruction. The parametrium is the anatomic area of vascular and visceral connective tissues lateral to the lower uterine segment and cervix. With proper mechanical traction on the uterus, the lateral border of the lower uterine segment and the cervix will be easily felt by the clamp or coagulating forceps. Any cutting and ligating must occur between the clamp and the side of the uterus/cervix. In order to significantly decrease "back bleeding," the surgeon should clamp or coagulate both the right and the left sides of the lower uterine segment and cervix before cutting these uterine artery pedicles. If any question of ureteral function arises, a simple intraoperative cystoscopy can easily be performed with or without intravenous indigo carmine dye.

Paravesical/Obturator Space

The *paravesical space* is an avascular potential space that is bordered by the uterine artery posteriorly, the pubic bone anteriorly, the edge of the bladder medially, and the obturator internus muscle and fascia laterally (Fig. 6). The lateral border extends to the external iliac vein on the anterior edge of the obturator internus muscle. The space is covered by the peritoneum superiorly. Its floor is the pubocervical fascia, which is the fibromuscular visceral connective tissue coating surrounding the vaginal epithelium. The pubocervical fascia extends laterally to the arcus tendineus fasciae pelvis. Note that the ureter courses just posterior to the uterine artery, and then, courses anteriorly and medially across the pubocervical fascia. The ureter is only 2 to 3 cm superior and medial to the ischial spine, where it passes by the uterine artery. The ureter then continues across the pubocervical fascia for 2 cm to enter the bladder, approximately at the junction of the middle third and upper third of the vagina.

Within the paravesical space are situated the superior vesical artery, coursing anteriorly toward the obliterated umbilical artery, and the obturator nerve and vessels, coursing inferiorly toward the obturator notch. The obturator notch is the groove on the posterior side of the superior pubic ramus and leads to the adductor muscles in the upper, medial thigh. The obturator notch is located approximately 4 cm lateral to the pubic symphysis. With the patient in the supine or dorsal lithotomy position, the ischial spine can be found in the paravesical space, approximately 5 to 6 cm directly posterior to the obturator notch. Remember, the paravesical space is the lateral compartment of the retropubic space of Retzius.

Within the paravesical space is the *obturator space*. The obturator space has the same boundaries as the paravesical space, except that the medial border is the superior vesical artery. The obturator lymph nodes are harvested in this space—laterally to the obturator internus fascia, anterior to the obturator nerve, and just posterior to the external iliac vein. Within this space is found the obturator nerve, a somatic nerve. This nerve is surrounded by loose areolar tissue and is easily visualized by gently wiping this tissue down along the nerve to the obturator notch. The standard dissection techniques allow the experienced surgeon to open this area in an avascular manner. In addition to the excision of lymph nodes contained in the areolar tissues found here, the surgeon also performs paravaginal defect repairs and retropubic colposuspensions in the paravesical space.

The Retropubic Space

The *space of Retzius* is the anatomic *retropubic space*. It is a potential space consisting of an anterior compartment and two lateral compartments. The lateral compartments have been discussed already and are the right and left paravesical spaces (Fig. 7). The anterior compartment is bordered anteriorly by the pubic bones and posteriorly by the visceral fascial capsules that surround the bladder and the urethra. The anterior portion of the visceral connective tissue capsule of the bladder continues laterally and anteriorly, just underneath the peritoneum, to drape over the external iliac artery and vein, and superiorly to the umbilicus between the peritoneum and the parietal transversalis fascia. The superior extension of this visceral connective tissue is named the *vesicoumbilical sheet*. When entering the retropubic space through the pelvic cavity, the vesicoumbilical sheet of visceral fascia is found just deep to the superficial incision through the peritoneum incised between the bladder and the pubic bone. The vesicoumbilical sheet is what keeps the round ligament out of the retropubic space.

The bladder rests on the pubocervical fascia of the anterior vaginal wall of the upper two-thirds of the vagina. Laterally in the paravesical space, the pubocervical fascia is the floor of the lateral compartment of the retropubic space. Running longitudinally, parallel to the long axis of the vagina in the pubocervical fascia, are arterioles and veins, making dissection potentially bloody here. In addition, the visceral connective tissue capsules of the bladder and urethra contain

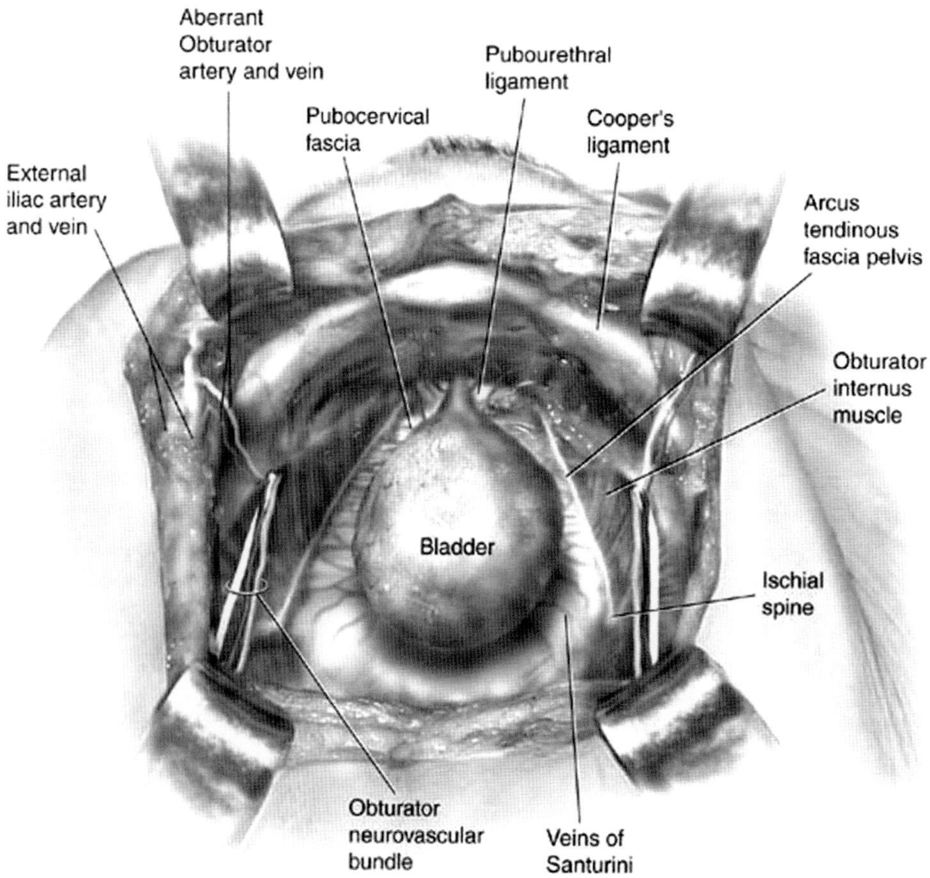

Figure 7 Retropubic space with anatomical boundaries and structures.

a rich network of perivesical venous sinuses within deposits of areolar fat. Centrally over the urethra, running underneath the pubic arch, is the deep dorsal vein of the clitoris, feeding these venous channels. This vast venous plexus of Santorini drains into the uncharted internal iliac venous system. The retropubic space is a potential space with very vascular borders. The external iliac artery and vein are found laterally, coursing on the anterior edge of the superior pubic ramus, while the obturator artery and vein, and obturator nerve, travel in the lateral compartment on the underside (posterior edge) of the superior pubic bone.

Fortunately, dissection in the retropubic space is usually bloodless, especially when performed via the laparoscope with a pneumoperitoneum. The pneumoperitoneum gently opens the space for gentle blunt dissection, while compressing some of the smaller venous sinuses. The space is filled with loose areolar fatty tissues. Dissection begins sharply, anterior to the bladder, centrally through the peritoneum and the vesicoumbilical sheet to enter into the fatty retropubic space. The dissection proceeds gently and bluntly toward the back of the pubic bone, laterally to the obturator internus muscle, and posteriorly to the floor, formed by the pubocervical fascia, where it attaches laterally to the arcus tendineus fasciae pelvis. Again, in these areas, the operator performs paravaginal defect repairs for anterior vaginal wall prolapse and retropubic colposuspensions for patients with stress urinary incontinence and a hypermobile urethra.

The Vesicovaginal/Vesicocervical Space

The vesicovaginal/vesicocervical space is a potential space between the anterior surface of the vagina/cervix and the posterior aspect of the bladder (Fig. 6). This space is bordered laterally by the bladder "pillars" that are conduits for the ureters, inferior vesical vessels, and visceral nerves to the bladder. These structures pass just lateral to the lower uterine segment and cervix, and course medially on the pubocervical fascia of the anterolateral fornix of the upper third of the vagina.

When performing a hysterectomy in the pelvic cavity via laparotomy or laparoscopy, the surgeon sharply incises the uterovesical peritoneum and dissects centrally on the pubocervical fascia of the cervix and upper vagina. This includes incising the supravaginal septum, which is the visceral connective tissue reflected from the bladder capsule to the pubocervical fascia of the cervix. The dissection proceeds sharply and centrally for 1 to 2 cm, depending on how much of the upper vagina is to be removed with the cervix. Aggressive lateral dissection with blunt pushing with a sponge is not necessary, especially since it brings the dissection closer to the ureter and vesical artery and vein in the more lateral bladder "pillar." Remember that the trigone begins at the junction of the middle third and upper third of the vagina. This is also the approximate juncture where the ureters enter the bladder, approximately 5 cm apart from one another.

This space can also be surgically entered and developed through the vaginal route via an anterior vaginal wall colpotomy incision or by transversely incising the anterior vaginal wall overlying the anterior portion of the cervix. The anterior colpotomy incision should begin 1 to 2 cm proximal to the urethrovesical junction, in the midline, and proceed toward the vaginal apex. A full thickness of the vaginal wall must be incised, allowing the pubocervical fascia, also known as the fibromuscular coat, to remain on the vaginal epithelium. The dissection then proceeds with careful sharp and blunt dissection in the avascular space in a lateral direction toward the fascia of the obturator internus muscle. Because of the lateral fusion of visceral connective tissues in this area, sharp or blunt dissection laterally is necessary to truly enter the paravaginal (paravesical) space and touch the obturator internus fascia.

When performing a vaginal hysterectomy, the operator transversely incises the vaginal epithelium and sharply dissects centrally on the cervix to incise the supracervical septum and then the vesicouterine peritoneum in order to enter the anterior cul-de-sac. Here, the dissection needs not be too lateral, as mentioned before. Care must be taken to direct the dissection superiorly, and not posteriorly into the cervix or anteriorly into the bladder. This requires a palpable "feel" for the dissection plane. Any entry into the bladder during this dissection will be 1 to 2 cm above the trigone in the center of the bladder. A two-layer closure with absorbable suture, followed by cystoscopic confirmation of bilateral ureteral function, is required, along with catheter drainage of the bladder for a week. Some surgeons also recommend a retrograde cystogram one week postop to confirm satisfactory healing before the catheter is removed from the bladder.

The Pararectal Space

The *pararectal space* is still another potential, avascular space. It is located posterior to the crossing of the ureter with the uterine artery (Fig. 6). The medial border is the ureter on the rectum and the lateral border is the internal iliac artery. The space also contains the uterosacral ligament passing laterally and posteriorly toward the sacrum. The ischial spines and sacrospinous ligaments can also be approached through this space. Here, dissections are done for endometriosis or tumors when performed by laparotomy or by laparoscopy. The pararectal space is commonly dissected bluntly with the finger when approached by the vaginal route through the rectovaginal space.

The Rectovaginal Space

The *rectovaginal space* is anterior and medial to the pararectal space. It is bounded posteriorly by the cul-de-sac peritoneum and the uterosacral ligaments, laterally by the iliococcygeus muscles, inferiorly by the rectum, and superiorly by the visceral connective tissue surrounding the vagina (Fig. 6). The rectum may be easily and bluntly dissected away from the vagina in developing the rectovaginal space. The dissection may safely be carried laterally in the pararectal spaces to the iliococcygeus muscles and down to the level of the ischial spines and the sacrospinous ligaments. Within this space is situated the rectovaginal fascia, which loosely adheres to the vaginal visceral capsule. The rectovaginal fascia is a separate sheet of fibroelastic connective tissue between the visceral connective tissue capsules of the vagina and the rectum (6).

The rectovaginal space is safely dissected through the pelvic cavity by laparotomy or laparoscopy. Much more commonly, this space is entered and dissected by the vaginal route by a vertical posterior colpotomy incision or, even, by a transverse vaginal incision at the junction of the lower third and middle third of the posterior vagina. Again, this dissection proceeds using careful sharp and blunt dissection in the avascular plane. This requires a full-thickness incision through the posterior vaginal wall, allowing the visceral connective tissue to remain on the vaginal epithelium.

REFERENCES

1. Retzky SS, Rogers RM, Richardson AC. Anatomy of female pelvic support. In: Brubaker LT, Saclarides TJ, eds. The Female Pelvic Floor: Disorders of Function and Support. Philadelphia, PA: FA Davis, 1996:3–21.
2. Zullo F, Palomba S, Zupi E, et al. Effectiveness of presacral neurectomy in women with severe dysmenorrhea caused by endometriosis who were treated with laparoscopic conservative surgery: A 1-year prospective randomized double-blind controlled trial. Am J Obstet Gynecol 2003; 189:5–10.
3. Zullo F, Palomba S, Zupi E, et al. Long-term effectiveness of presacral neurectomy for the treatment of severe dysmenorrhea due to endometriosis. J Am Assoc Gynecol Laparosc 2004; 11(1):23–28.
4. Rogers RM. Pelvic denervation surgery. In: Sharp H, guest ed. Clinical Obstetrics and Gynecology, Vol. 46, No. 4. Philadelphia, PA: Lippincott, Williams & Wilkins, 2003:767–772.
5. Curtis AH, Anson BJ, Ashley FL, et al. The anatomy of the pelvic autonomic nerves in relation to gynecology. Surg Gynecol Obstet 1942; 75:743–750.
6. Uhlenhuth E, Wolfe W, Smith E, et al. The rectogenital septum. Surg Gynecol Obstet 1948; 86:148–163.

Note: There are few references in this chapter since most of this chapter is based on extensive personal observations and surgical experiences of both Robert Rogers and Richard Taylor.

6

Uterine anomalies

Barry Sanders

The primary function of the uterus is to allow the growth and development of a pregnancy. It follows, therefore, that a variety of congenital and acquired abnormalities of the mullerian system can interfere with uterine structure or function, thus contributing toward infertility, pregnancy loss, or preterm delivery.

The congenital abnormalities include those resulting from abnormal differentiation of the mullerian system in utero. Most cases are sporadic, although familial and teratogen-associated cases have been reported. While present at birth, most congenital mullerian anomalies remain asymptomatic and undetected until puberty, or until investigations are initiated for infertility or pregnancy losses. The acquired abnormalities include conditions such as intrauterine adhesions (IUAs) (Asherman's syndrome), uterine myomas (see chaps. 7 and 19), and endometrial polyps. They, too, are often detected during investigations for infertility or pregnancy loss and disorders of menstruation.

This chapter will review the established relationships of abnormalities of the uterus to infertility and pregnancy loss. The evidence, or lack thereof, for these associations will be discussed. Treatment recommendations are often controversial, but the evidence for standard treatment options will be presented.

EMBRYOLOGY OF THE UTERUS

The mullerian ducts derive from invagination of the coelomic epithelium on the lateral surface of the paired urogenital ridges in the fifth week of embryonic life. The mullerian ducts migrate caudally and medially as they enter the pelvis. By the eighth week of embryonic life, the mullerian ducts fuse in the midline to form a single structure, the origin of the urogenital canal (Fig. 1A). By the 10th week, the intervening septum has degenerated to form a single endometrial cavity (Fig. 1B). Smooth muscle appears in the walls of the genital canal between 18 and 20 weeks, and by 24 weeks the uterine muscular wall is well developed (Fig. 1C). Cervical glands appear by 15 weeks and endometrial glands by 19 weeks, although the endometrium remains poorly developed until puberty (1).

CONGENITAL UTERINE ABNORMALITIES

Development: Congenital uterine abnormalities result from aberrant differentiation of the mullerian system. Understanding the underlying pathophysiology is a key prerequisite to evaluating the patient and assessing the potential for a successful surgical repair. Various anomalies can be categorized into defects in development, canalization, or midline fusion of the ducts, or in the resorption of the midline septum (Fig. 1 and Table 1).

Mullerian malformations may be associated with renal and skeletal abnormalities. However, ovarian function, secondary sexual characteristics, and external genitalia are usually normal.

Classification: Uniform descriptive criteria are critical for evaluating the frequency of various abnormalities, their natural history, and their response to surgical interventions.

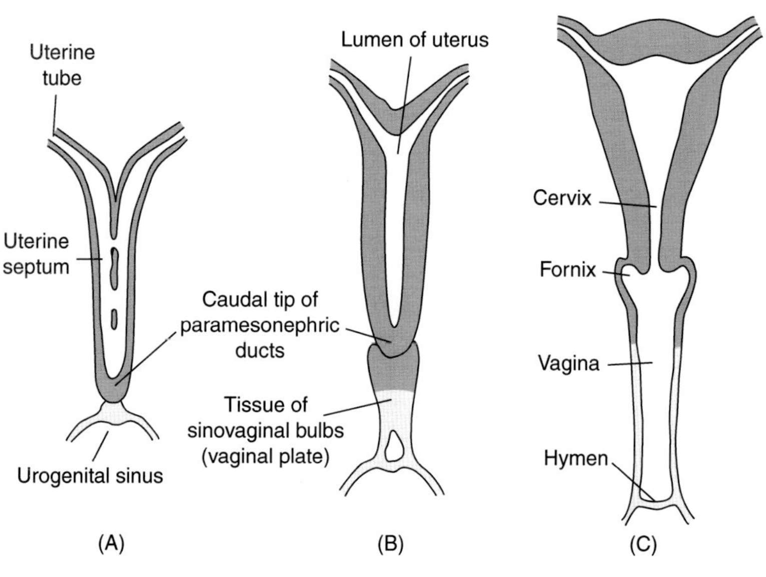

Figure 1 Embryologic development of the human uterus and vagina. **(A)** Fusion of the mullerian ducts in the midline. **(B)** Resorption of the midline septum and early development of the uterine muscular walls. **(C)** Well-developed uterine muscular walls and canalization of the cervix and vagina.

Table 1 Disturbances in Mullerian Development Affecting the Uterus

Defect	Extent	Example
Failure of development of one or both mullerian ducts	Complete bilateral	Rokitansky–Kuster–Hauser syndrome
	Complete unilateral	Unicornuate
	Partial	Rudimentary horn
Failure of canalization	Complete	Rudimentary horn without functioning endometrium
	Partial	Cervical atresia
Failure of midline fusion	Complete	Uterine didelphys
	Partial	Bicornuate uterus
Failure of resorption of the midline septum	Complete	Septate
	Partial	Arcuate

The American Fertility Society (2) classification of congenital uterine abnormalities is the most commonly used system (Fig. 2). It allows standardized intraoperative descriptions and uniform reporting. Unfortunately, however, considerable variability still exists in the literature with regard to the use of different diagnostic methods and classification criteria, making meaningful comparisons difficult.

Incidence: The precise incidence of congenital mullerian abnormalities is difficult to determine, as these are likely over-reported among women with infertility or recurrent pregnancy loss and under-reported among healthy fertile women. In a review article encompassing 9 publications and 1392 cases, Grimbizis and colleagues reported that approximately 4.3% of women in the general population have congenital uterine anomalies (Table 2) (3). Taken together, septate and arcuate uteri are the most common, comprising more than half of the cases (Table 2). All of the congenital uterine abnormalities, to varying degrees, may be associated with a reduction in successful reproduction (Table 3) (4).

Mullerian Agenesis

Complete bilateral mullerian atresia is the rarest of the anomalies, affecting about 0.10% of the general population and comprising 2.9% of all congenital uterine abnormalities (Table 2). Complete aplasia is not amenable to surgical restoration, although fertility can still be achieved using the woman's oocytes and a gestational carrier. However, cases of focal aplasia or hypoplasia involving the cervix, lower uterine segment, or endocervical canal may be amenable to surgical correction. While cervical patency and menstrual function may be restored, fertility is unlikely, aside from sporadic case reports (5,6).

Unicornuate Uterus

A unicornuate uterus arises from arrested or defective development of one of the mullerian ducts. It affects 0.41% of the general population and comprises nearly 10% of all congenital uterine anomalies (Table 2). As with other mullerian anomalies, the unicornuate uterus appears to have an increased incidence of pregnancy loss and preterm delivery (Table 3). Some authors suggest that the unicornuate uterus is associated with the poorest reproductive outcome (4), although not all agree (3).

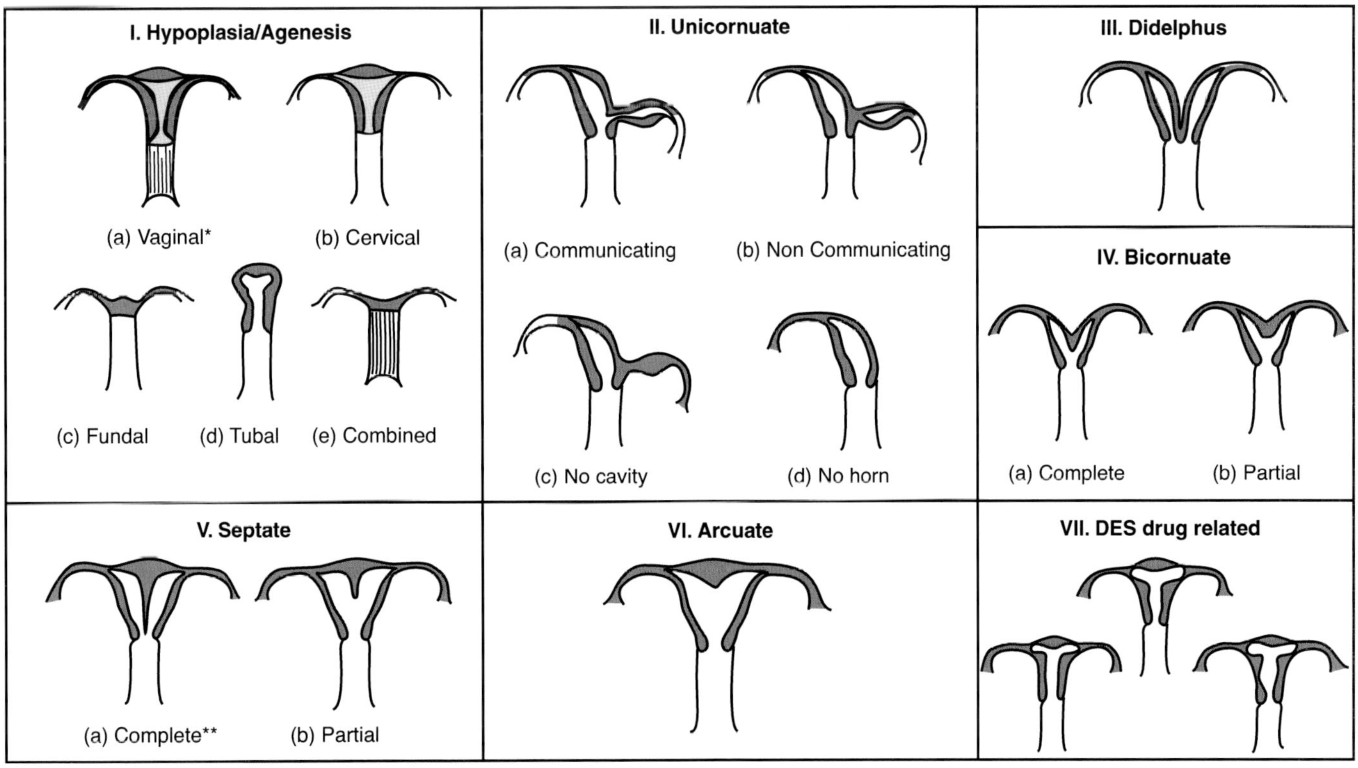

*Uterus may be normal or take a variety of abnormal forms.
**May have two distinct cervices

Figure 2 American Fertility Society (1988) classification of mullerian anomalies.

Table 2 Incidence of Various Uterine Malformations

	All cases	Arcuate	Septate	Bicornuate	Unicornuate	Didelphys	Agenesis
Total	1392	255	486	362	134	114	40
% all anomalies	-	18.3	34.9	26.0	9.6	8.2	2.9
Incidence in population	4.3	0.77	1.5	1.1	0.41	0.35	0.10

Source: Adapted from Ref. 3.

Table 3 Pregnancy Outcome with Untreated Congenital Uterine Anomalies

	Pregnancies	SAB (*n*)	Preterm deliveries (*n*)	Live births (*n*)
Population-based comparisons[a]	–	10–15%	9–12%	82%
Unicornuate uterus	393	34% (135)	43% (170)	54% (213)
Didelphys uterus	86	21% (18)	24% (21)	69% (59)
Bicornuate uterus	56	25% (14)	25% (14)	63% (35)
Septate uterus	1459	76% (1105/1459)	10% (146/1459)	58% (90/155)
Arcuate uterus	283	20% (57/283)	5% (10/195)	66% (129/195)

[a]Derived from U.S. National Vital Statistics database, 1976–2001.
Source: Adapted from Ref. 4.

Approximately 65% of unicornuate uteri have an associated rudimentary horn (Fig. 2). As many as 40% of these may have associated urinary tract abnormalities, especially in the presence of a noncommunicating rudimentary horn (7,8). Approximately one-third of the rudimentary horns contain endometrial tissue and about one-half of these communicate with the main endometrial cavity (9).

HSG will reveal the characteristic unicornuate cavity (Fig. 3), but MRI or precise transvaginal sonographic examination will be needed to detect the rudimentary horn and the presence of functioning endometrium (Fig. 4). It is prudent to document associated renal abnormalities by renal ultrasound, IVP, or MRI.

The presence of a rudimentary horn does not alter the reproductive potential associated with a unicornuate uterus; rather, the primary risk is that of a rudimentary horn pregnancy. This may occur when a communication exists with the main uterine cavity or following transmigration of sperm. The primary indication for surgery in this group is the presence of *functioning* endometrium in the rudimentary horn. Removal of an externally separated functioning rudimentary horn eliminates the risk of catastrophic pregnancy rupture in the horn and can alleviate cyclic pain from a localized hematometra in a noncommunicating horn. However, if the functioning rudimentary horn is contained within the main uterine body, then a communication between the main uterine cavity and the rudimentary horn cavity may be established hysteroscopically (5). An asymptomatic nonfunctioning rudimentary horn does not require to be removed.

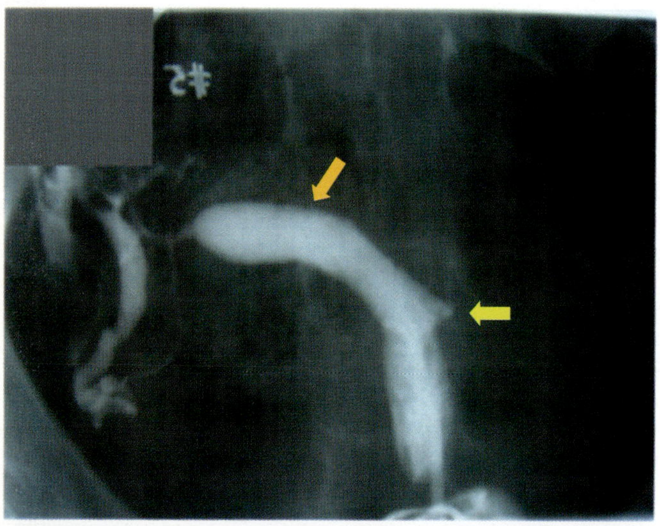

Figure 3 Hysterosalpingogram of a unicornuate uterus (*orange arrow*) with a hypoplastic rudimentary communicating horn (*yellow arrow*).

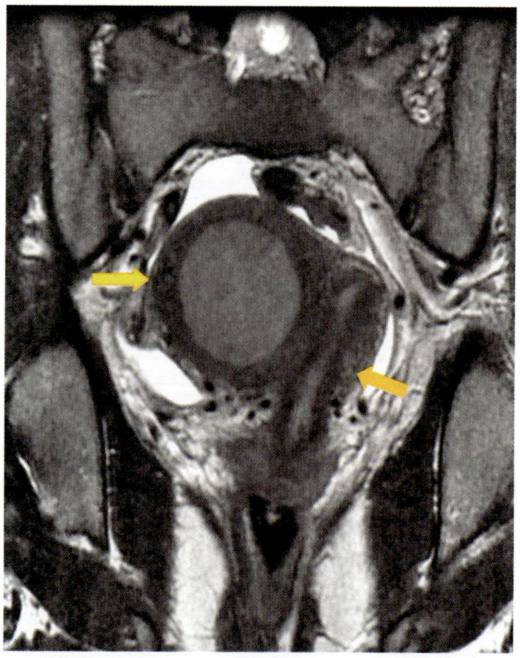

Figure 4 This MRI demonstrates a unicornuate (*orange arrow*) uterus with a noncommunicating obstructed rudimentary horn with functioning endometrium (*yellow arrow*). The patient had severe dysmenorrhea.

Uterus Didelphus

Failure of midline fusion of the mullerian ducts results in uterus didelphus (Figs. 1 and 2). This anomaly is associated with two endometrial cavities and two cervices that are fused in the lower uterine segment, often accompanied by a longitudinal vaginal septum. The incidence in the general population is about 0.35%. It is thought to comprise 8.2% of all congenital uterine abnormalities but may be difficult to distinguish from a complete bicornuate (IV-a) or a complete septate (V-a) uterus (Fig. 2), depending on the degree of extension of the midline septum into the cervix. Renal anomalies, particularly renal agenesis, are common, occurring in approximately 20% of this group (10). The diagnosis may be apparent on physical examination, with the documentation of two vaginas or a longitudinal vaginal septum leading to two cervices. Confirmation can be obtained with transvaginal ultrasound, MRI, or HSG (Fig. 5). Renal ultrasound, IVP, or MRI can be used to document associated renal abnormalities.

Uterus didelphus has the best prognosis of all the major uterine malformations (Table 3). The only potential corrective surgical procedure is the Strassman metroplasty. However, it is technically difficult to perform and the results are frequently disappointing, so it is infrequently indicated.

Bicornuate Uterus

A bicornuate uterus results from incomplete mullerian duct fusion. This results in two separate but communicating endometrial cavities with external fundal indentation and a single cervix (Fig. 6), the key features distinguishing it from septate and didelphic uteri (Fig. 2). Failure of fusion may range from partial to more extensive. Bicornuate uteri occur in about 1% of the general population and make up about one-fourth of all congenital uterine anomalies (Table 2).

The reproductive outcome associated with bicornuate uteri predominantly involves pregnancy loss or preterm delivery (Table 3) rather than infertility (11). Traditional surgical correction of the bicornuate uterus involved a Strassman procedure for uterine unification. However, initial experience with the procedure pre-dated the use of the AFS classification system and may have inadvertently included patients with a septate uterus. Indeed, a recent study of 35 patients with recurrent pregnancy loss in the presence of a divided uterine cavity

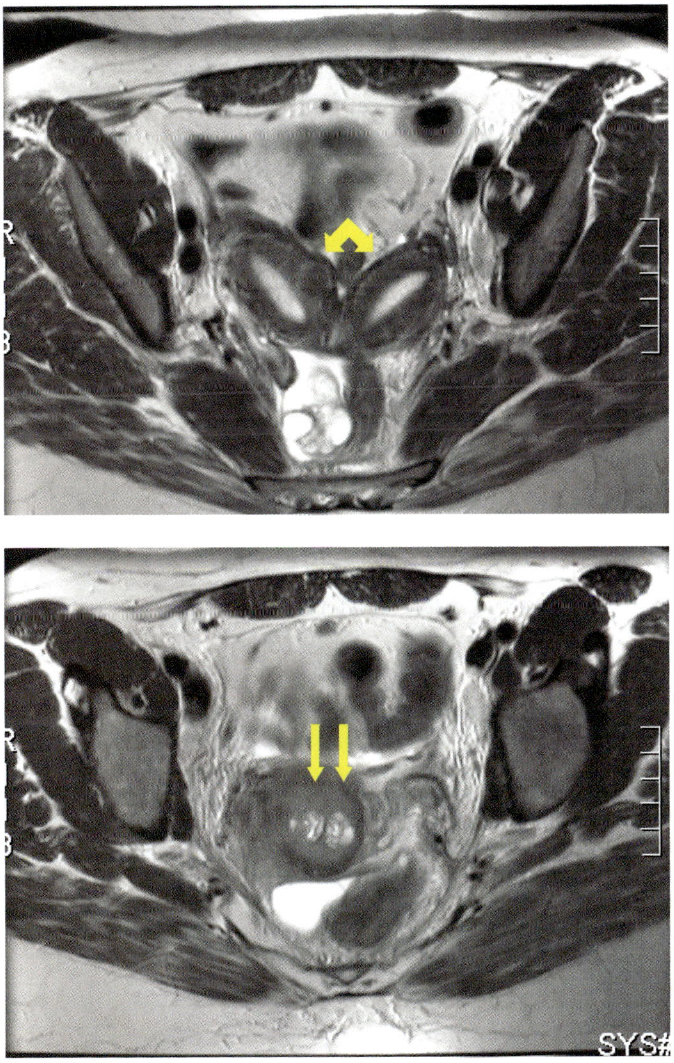

Figure 5 MRI showing uterus didelphys. The upper image shows the duplex uterine corpus and the lower image shows the duplex cervix.

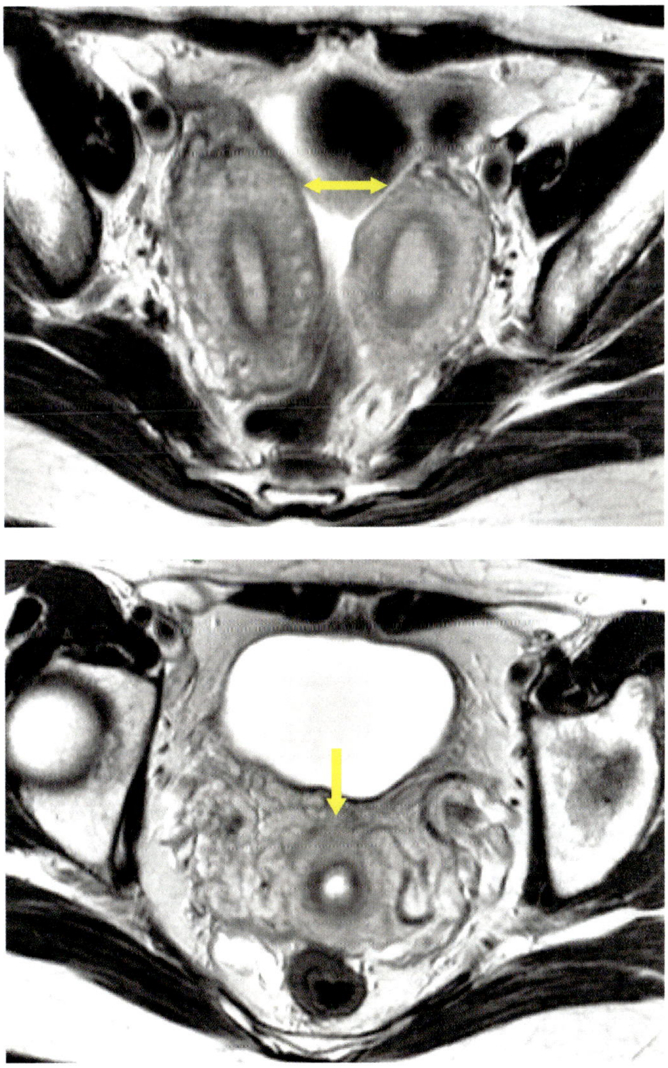

Figure 6 MRI of a bicornuate uterus. The upper image demonstrates duplication of both internal and external contours of the uterine corpus. The lower image shows the single cervix.

Table 4 Reduction in the Spontaneous Abortion Rate after Hysteroscopic Metroplasty

		Before metroplasty		After metroplasty	
Author	No. of patients	No. of pregnancies	No. of spontaneous abortions (%)	No. of pregnancies	No. of spontaneous abortions (%)
March and Israel (15)	57	240	212 (88)	56	8 (14)
Daley et al. (16)	55	150	130 (87)	75	15 (20)
Fedele et al. (17)	71	>139	>139	65	10 (16)
Carrach et al. (18)	62	176	160 (91)	41	12 (29)
Pabuccu et al. (19)	49	108	96 (89)	44	2 (4.5)
Valle (20)	115	299	258 (86.3)	103	12 (12)
Venturoli et al. (21)	72	171	171 (100)	52	13 (25)
Total	481	>1283	>1166 (91)	436	72 (17)

revealed that all the abnormalities were septate and not bicornuate (12).

One recent series reported 19 live births in 22 women following a Strassman procedure (13). However, similar improvements have also been reported following the less complex procedure of cervical cerclage (9). At least one series indicated that reproductive outcome in untreated women improved with successive pregnancies, suggesting a beneficial effect of repeated distention on uterine capacity (11). It, therefore, appears that the Strassman procedure for bicornuate unification should be reserved for highly selected patients with otherwise unexplained recurrent pregnancy losses.

Septate Uterus

A uterine septum results from the failure of resorption of the fibromuscular midline septum between the fused mullerian ducts. The degree of impairment of resorption varies. The separation of cavities may be limited or may extend through the entire uterus, cervix, and vagina.

A septate uterus is the most common (34.9%) of congenital uterine abnormalities, occurring in about 1.5% of the general population. It is associated with some of the poorest reproductive outcomes (14), especially spontaneous abortions (Table 3). It is estimated that 15 % to 25% of all spontaneous abortions occur in women with uterine septa. While the mechanism for pregnancy loss is unknown, impaired vascular development of the endometrium at the implantation site is commonly implicated in causation.

The reproductive outcome of women with an untreated septate uterus (Table 3) appears better than that quoted in series of patients undergoing hysteroscopic metroplasty (Table 4) (22). Likely the patients undergoing hysteroscopic metroplasty represent a highly selective group of patients with a particularly poor reproductive outcome. However, the reproductive outcome of untreated septate uterus is significantly impaired in both circumstances, thus justifying hysteroscopic metroplasty for both prophylactic reasons as well as for those with a past history of pregnancy loss.

Clearly, the reported rates of pregnancy loss before and after hysteroscopic metroplasty provide the strongest evidence of surgical benefit for the treatment of women with a septate uterus (Table 4).

Unfortunately, there are only a few studies in the literature (23,24) that compare patients with a uterine septum who undergo surgical treatment and to those who do not. While these studies do suggest improved outcomes in surgically treated patients, their small sample sizes and methodology hamper conclusive results.

Table 5 The Pregnancy Rate After Hysteroscopic Metroplasty in Patients with Primary Infertility That Was Otherwise Unexplained

Author	No. of patients	Crude pregnancy rate (%)
Daley et al. (16)	15	47
Marabini et al. (25)	14	44
Pabuccu and Gomel (26)	61	41
Colacurci et al. (27)	21	29
Venturoli et al. (21)	69	52
Total	180	43

It is generally accepted that a septate uterus does not cause infertility. The incidence of septate uterus is similar in both the fertile and the infertile populations (3). Septoplasty is often undertaken in the infertility setting, but largely with the hope of reducing subsequent pregnancy wastage. While the crude pregnancy rate after hysteroscopic metroplasty in patients with primary infertility suggests surgical benefit (Table 5) (22), these data are inherently biased by the use of the same infertile patients as their own controls.

The diagnosis of a uterine septum requires that the internal contour of the uterus is duplex (Fig. 7) while the external contour is singular. If both the endometrial cavity and the external contour of the uterus are duplex, then the abnormality is a bicornuate uterus (Fig. 8). Accurate differentiation

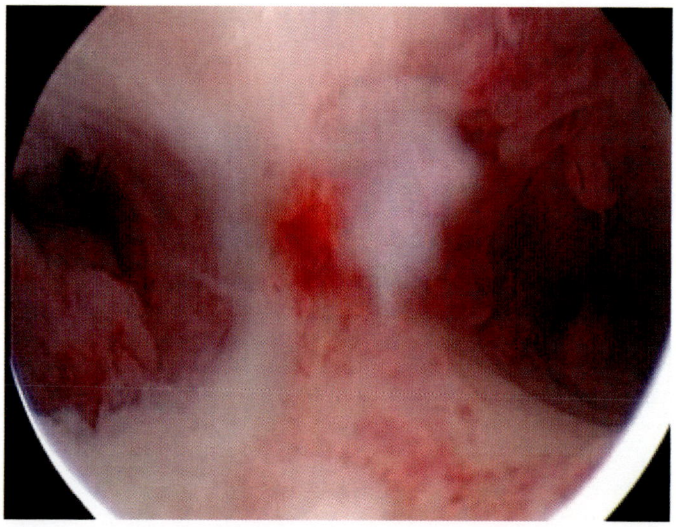

Figure 7 This hysteroscopic picture of a septate uterus demonstrates a typical duplex endometrial cavity immediately prior to septum incision.

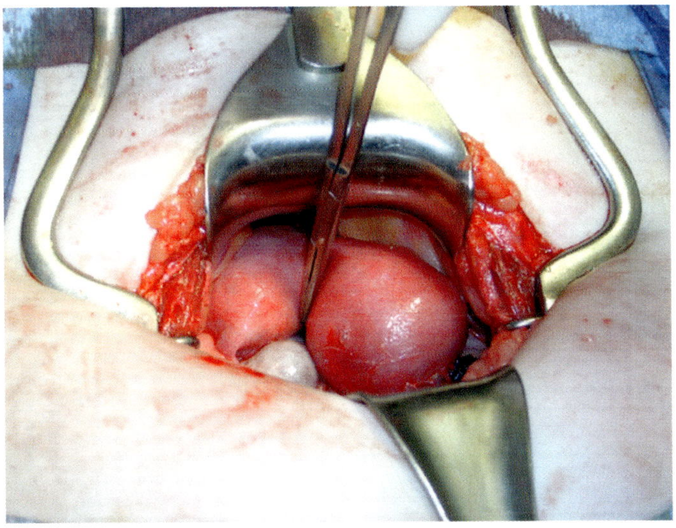

Figure 8 Bicornuate uterus prior to Strassman procedure.

between septate and bicornuate uteri is essential prior to the treatment. This requires imaging or direct visual assessment of both the internal and the external anatomy of the uterus. Combined hysteroscopy and laparoscopy is considered the gold standard. However, internal duplication may be identified by hysterosalpingography, and ultrasound or magnetic resonance imaging may provide the diagnosis (Fig. 9).

Surgical Procedure

Surgical correction is usually undertaken by hysteroscopic incision of the septum. Similar to the treatment of synechiae, the septum may be divided by scissors and electro- or laser vaporization. This author's preference is to use a continuous-flow resectoscope with a right-angle electrode for electrovaporization of the septum. A major advantage to the use of a resectoscope is that it provides a wider and larger field of view than a standard operating hysteroscope. This allows one

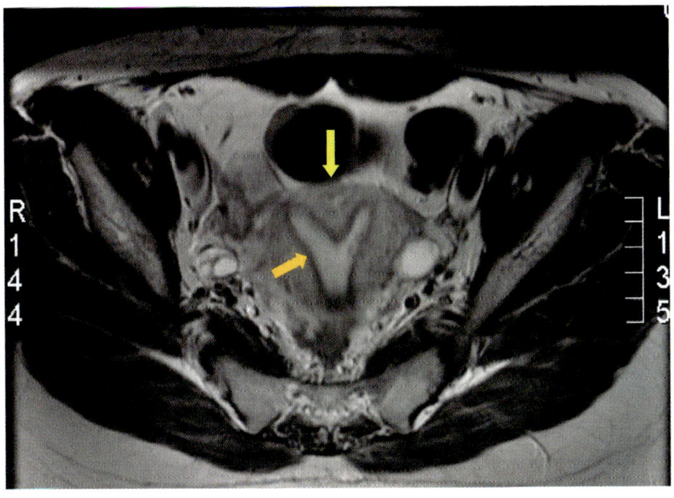

Figure 9 MRI demonstrating a septate uterus in a woman with recurrent pregnancy losses. There is a duplex endometrial cavity (*orange arrow*), but the external contour of the uterine fundus is single (*yellow arrow*).

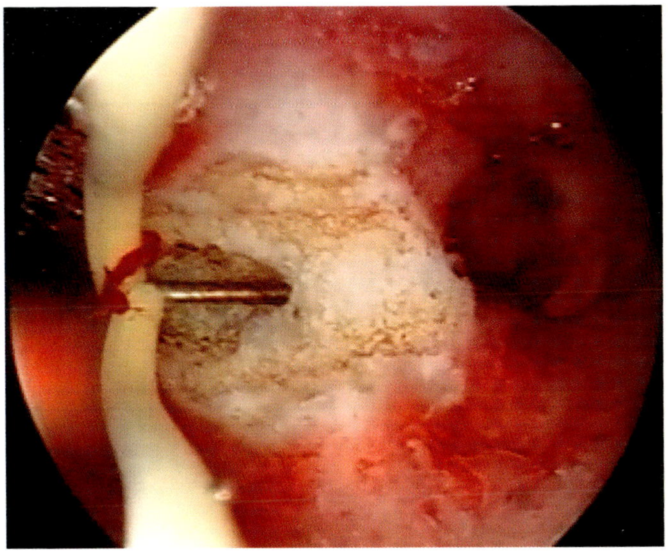

Figure 10 This hysteroscopic picture shows a right-angle electrode incising a uterine septum in a plane equidistant between anterior and posterior uterine walls.

to keep not only the septum but also both uterine horns in view. A disadvantage is the potential restriction of surgical space due to the use of a large instrument in a cavity already narrowed by the presence of a septum.

With the right-angle electrode being extended into one uterine horn, incision of the septum begins at the caudal tip, at a point that is equidistant from the anterior and the posterior walls of the uterus (Fig. 10). The right-angle electrode is positioned perpendicular to the septum, and the incision is made horizontally from one uterine horn to the other. As the incision progresses toward the fundus, care should be taken to ensure that the site of the incision remains on plane with the natural curvature of the uterus. Otherwise, the incision may encroach upon either the anterior or the posterior walls. The electrical current may be nonmodulated, since there is little vascularity in the septum, and minimal thermal vascular injury is desired. The incision is complete when there is only a minimal convex curvature to the fundus of the uterus and the resectoscope or extended electrode can be moved easily from one cornual recess to the other. Laparoscopy, which is not usually required if the diagnosis has previously been confirmed, occasionally may be used to assist in determining the depth of dissection.

Adjuvant preoperative preparation of the endometrium with gonadotropin-releasing hormone (GnRH) analogs and postoperative treatments with antibiotics, hormonal therapy, and uterine balloon catheter are controversial and not evidence based, but are sometimes used empirically (14). This author's preference is to perform the procedure early in the proliferative phase of the menstrual cycle under perioperative prophylactic antibiotic coverage. A postoperative balloon catheter is not usually employed, except perhaps with difficult dissections, multiple coexisting anomalies, or repeat procedures. Their use may justify continued antibiotic coverage.

While the results of hysteroscopic septum division are similar to those performed via laparotomy, the endoscopic approach is much simpler and less intrusive, requires minimal hospitalization and recovery, and allows for safe subsequent

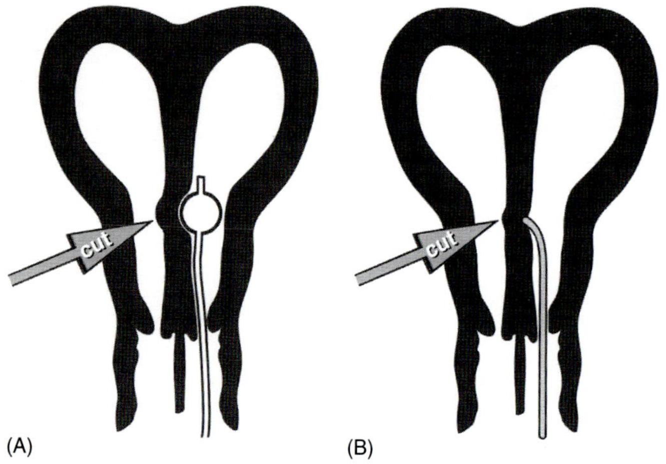

Figure 11 Placement of either a pediatric Foley catheter (**A**) or a curved uterine dilator (**B**) in the contralateral uterine horn from the location of the hysteroscope. The visible bulge in the septum defines the site to initiate hysteroscopic incision of a complete uterine septum.

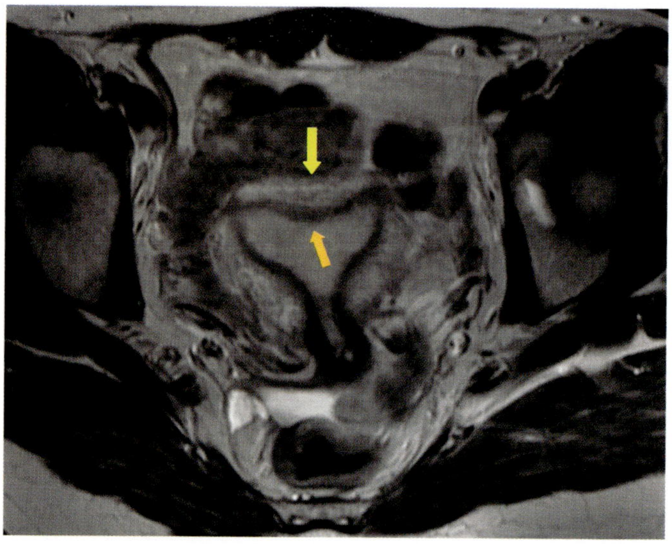

Figure 12 MRI of an arcuate uterus shows the small convex indentation of the endometrial cavity (*orange arrow*) and the singular external contour of the uterine fundus (*yellow arrow*).

vaginal delivery. However, case reports of uterine rupture have been published (28–30).

Controversy exists regarding the effects a residual septal remnant (<1 cm) on subsequent reproductive outcome. Fedele and colleagues reported no significant effect on conception or delivery rates (31), while Kormanyos et al. reported an increased chance of successful pregnancy when the septum was completely removed, either at the primary or at a subsequent procedure (32).

A complete uterine septum with duplex cervix and longitudinal vaginal septum does not appear to be associated with infertility, but there is debate whether it may be associated with pregnancy loss. In a series of 51 such cases, Heinonen observed a live birth rate of 72% without treatment and concluded that metroplasty is only indicated for selected patients demonstrating recurrent pregnancy loss (33). In contrast, Patton et al. reported an apparent improvement in miscarriage and delivery rates in nine women following hysteroscopic unification of the uterine corpus (Fig. 11) (34).

In a randomized controlled trial of 28 women with the same abnormality, Parsanezhad et al. reported that concomitant resection of the cervical septum made the procedure easier and safer, without adversely influencing reproductive outcome (35).

Arcuate Uterus

An arcuate uterus occurs in about 0.77% of the general population and represents about 18.3% of all congenital uterine malformations. It involves a minor convex change to the fundal contour of the uterine cavity, with no change to the external contour of the uterus (Fig. 12). The arcuate uterus is often considered a variation of the normal uterus, with few reproductive consequences (36).

Unfortunately, there are no widely accepted criteria for differentiating a minimal arcuate configuration from a more clinically important septate uterus. Although there is no uniformity of definition, most authors appear to characterize an arcuate uterus as one with less than 10 to 15 mm of protrusion into the cavity, with the term septate reserved for deeper indentations.

It appears that arcuate and septate uteri are variations along the same continuum of midline resorption defects, albeit with very different reproductive outcomes. The difficulty in differentiating an arcuate uterus from a septate uterus has led to the wide variations in reproductive outcome associated with this anomaly.

ACQUIRED UTERINE ABNORMALITIES

Intrauterine Adhesions

In 1894, Fritsch (37) first reported adhesions in the uterine cavity. In 1948, Asherman (38) further described the condition that is now associated with his name. Asherman's syndrome refers to partial or complete obliteration of the endometrial cavity due to IUAs.

The exact mechanism by which IUAs develop is not known. However, it is generally believed that IUAs may develop after trauma to the basal layer of the endometrium. Vigorous curettage of the recently pregnant uterus is the most common clinical precedent. The basal layer of the endometrium is most susceptible to injury in the first 2 to 4 weeks postpartum. Curettage at this time is most likely to result in IUAs. Estrogen-deficient states are also more likely to expose the basal layer of the endometrium to trauma.

While infection is commonly thought to play a role in causation, most patients who develop IUAs have not had evidence of clinical infection. Furthermore, any endometrial injury, such as that occurs with cesarean section, myomectomy, or endometrial tuberculosis, may result in IUAs. Despite common belief that IUAs are infrequent, their incidence was found to be 16% after one, 14% after two, and 32% after three D&Cs (39).

The adhesions may be avascular and composed of thin filmy strands of fibrous tissue, or vascular with dense bands of inactive endometrium and/or myometrium. In an attempt to unify reporting, the American Fertility Society developed a classification system in 1988 that has since become the standard (Table 6) (2).

Table 6 The American Fertility Society Classification System for Intrauterine Adhesions

Extent of cavity involved	<1/3	1/3–2/3	>2/3
	1	2	4
Type of adhesions	Filmy	Filmy and dense	Dense
	1	2	4
Menstrual pattern	Normal	Hypomenorrhea	Amenorrhea
	0	2	4

The score for extent, type, and menstrual pattern is added together for a cumulative score.
Stage I (mild) score = 1–4; stage II (moderate) score = 5–8; stage III (severe) score = 9–12.

IUAs may result in a variety of menstrual bleeding abnormalities, but most common is a reduction of bleeding. Infertility and spontaneous pregnancy loss are also potential sequelae of IUAs. While the correlation is not perfect, in general the more extensive the adhesions, the greater are the reduction in bleeding and the potential for successful fertility. If adhesions completely obliterate the endometrial cavity or block access to the fallopian tubes, spontaneous fertilization may not be possible. In less extensive cases, fertilization may occur, but adhesions may hinder successful implantation or placentation.

IUAs may be suspected in patients with reduced menstrual bleeding, infertility, or previous pregnancy loss, who demonstrate filling defects in the endometrial cavity by hysterosalpingography or sonohysterography. Confirmation of the diagnosis is made by direct visualization with hysteroscopy.

Surgical Procedure

Treatment by hysteroscopic-directed division of the adhesions is indicated for relief of menstrual abnormalities or to improve fertility. The modality chosen is operator dependent but may include scissor dissection, electrosurgery, or laser vaporization. This author's preference is to use a continuous-flow operating hysteroscope with a semiflexible scissors advanced through the operating channel to incise the adhesions (Fig. 13). An endometrial cavity with significant IUA is often markedly reduced in volume with few visual reference landmarks, thus compromising both surgical orientation and the surgical field. The smaller operating hysteroscope is usually preferable, as the contracted surgical field may not allow insertion or adequate visualization and surgical dissection required for a resectoscope.

Small stepwise incisions are made to recreate a normal cavity. Continual reorientation to any available reference landmarks helps to prevent myometrial trauma and perforation. Bleeding is infrequent if the incisions are limited to the adhesions, so electrosurgery is generally not required. In fact, if excessive bleeding is encountered, one should suspect that the myometrium has been incised. Concurrent laparoscopy or ultrasound may be undertaken to assist in the dissection and to help prevent uterine perforation, but it is not a required adjunct. In selected circumstances, concurrent tubal cannulation may also be undertaken to ensure access to the fallopian tubes and patency of the tubal ostia (Fig. 14) (5).

Focal or segmental adhesions are easier to treat and afford higher degrees of successful resolution than more extensive adhesions (Figs. 15 and 16). If the adhesions are extensive, several procedures may be required. Capella-Allouc et al. reported restoration of normal anatomy in 31 patients with severe adhesions after one ($n = 16$), two ($n = 7$), three ($n = 7$), and four ($n = 1$) surgical procedures (40). Even with multiple procedures, restoration of normal anatomy and function may not always be possible. Although the literature contains only limited observational studies, the term pregnancy rate, after hysteroscopic treatment of IUAs, appears to correlate inversely with the severity of adhesions (Table 7) (22).

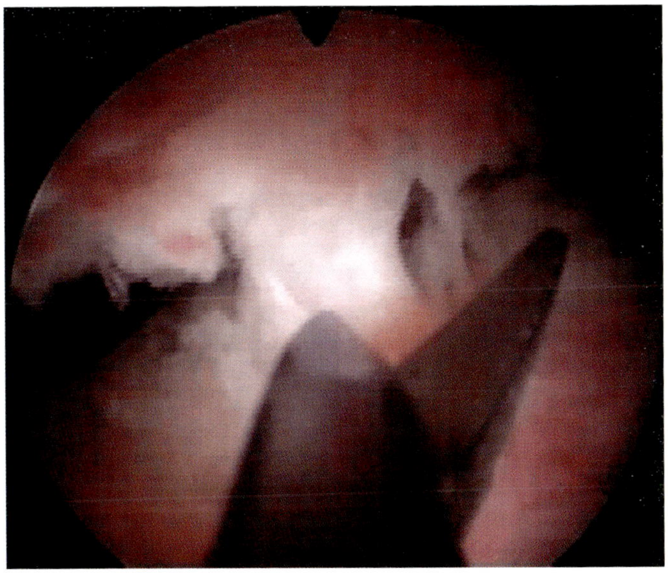

Figure 13 Small scissors may be introduced through the operating channel of a hysteroscope for precise incision of IUAs.

Traditionally, a large-loop intrauterine contraceptive device (IUD) was placed into the uterine cavity and left in place for two months, postoperatively. Copper-bearing and progestin IUDs were considered too small to prevent adhesion formation and the copper IUDs could induce a counterproductive inflammatory reaction. This practice was thought to separate the raw dissected surfaces during the initial healing phase and reduce the chance of re-adherence.

Currently, many surgeons empirically leave a balloon catheter in the endometrial cavity at the conclusion of the procedure for the same purpose (Cook Balloon Uterine Stent®

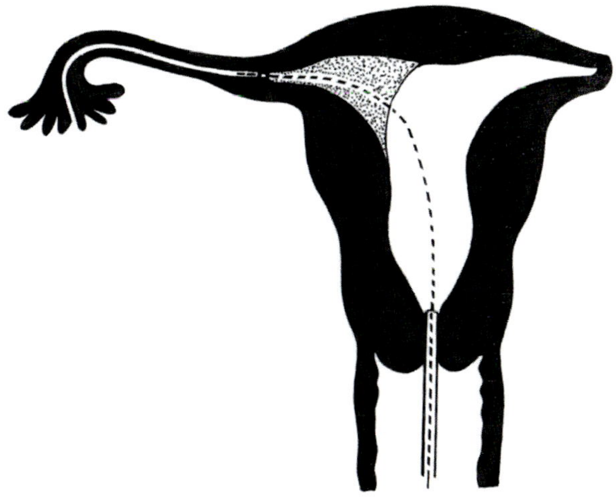

Figure 14 Tubal cannulation prior to hysteroscopic lysis of IUA to ensure access and patency of the tubal ostium.

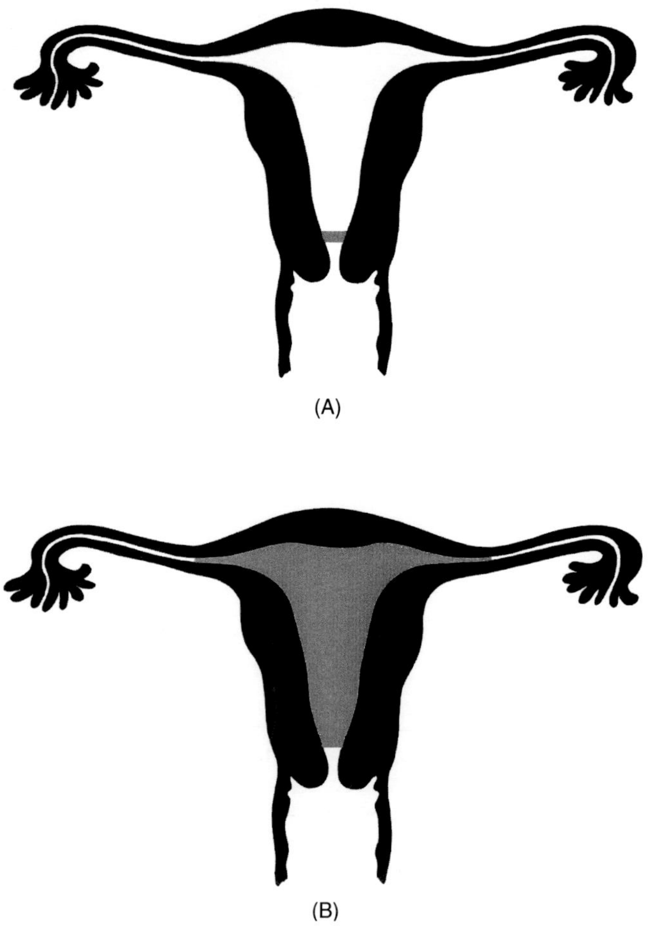

Figure 15 (**A** and **B**). Segmental versus extensive IUAs. The initial hysteroscopic appearance of both segmental cervical IUA (**A**) and extensive intrauterine IUA (**B**) is the same. However, the surgical procedure is considerably easier and expected outcomes are better for the former than for the latter.

or pediatric Foley catheter). The catheter is left in place for approximately one week. Postoperative antibiotics and estrogen are empiric adjuvant agents that are thought to help prevent infection and to aid in rapid proliferation of endometrium at the operative site.

To date, there has been little systematic evaluation of the postoperative adjuvant therapies. Orhue et al. compared the postadhesiolysis clinical outcome in 51 patients using a IUD for three months with 59 patients treated for 10 days with a pediatric Foley catheter. Restoration of normal menses and a higher conception rate occurred in the Foley catheter group (43).

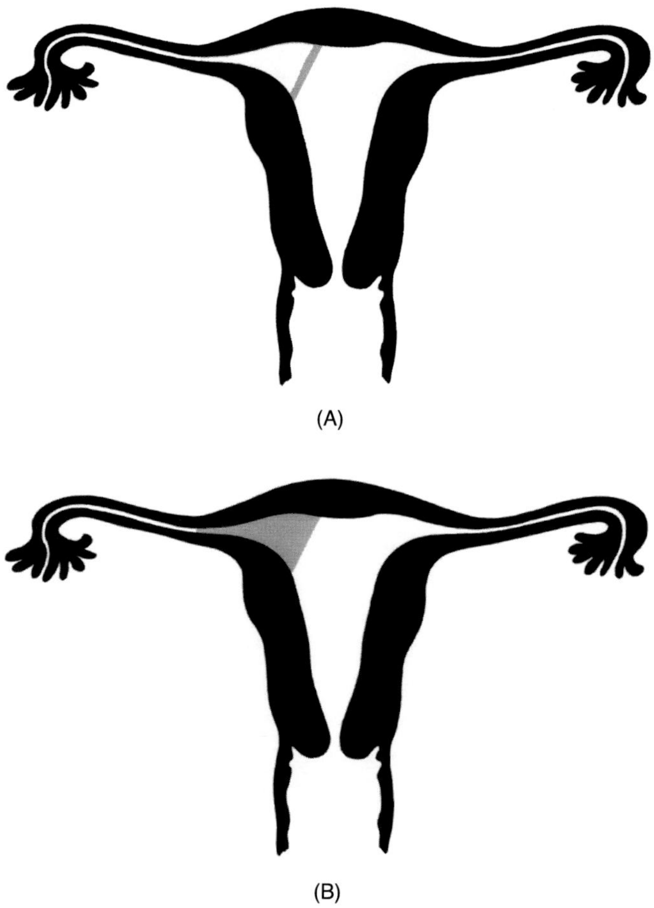

Figure 16 (**A** and **B**). Segmental cornual adhesions versus extensive cornual adhesions. The initial hysteroscopic appearance for both segmental cornual adhesions (**A**) and extensive cornual adhesions resembles that of a unicornuate uterus. The former is easier to treat and is associated with higher successful resolution than the latter.

Table 7 Term Pregnancy Rates After Hysteroscopic Division of Mild, Moderate, and Severe Intrauterine Adhesions

	Term pregnancy rate					
	Mild IUA		Moderate IUA		Severe IUA	
	%	*n*	%	*n*	%	*n*
Valle and Sciarra (41)	87.5	43	84.2	97	55.6	47
Pabuccu et al. (42)					57.5	40
Capella-Allouc et al. (40)					32.1	28

Endometrial Polyps

Endometrial polyps are a common cause of abnormal uterine bleeding (AUB), but their role in infertility and spontaneous abortion is uncertain. Endometrial polyps are often found in patients with infertility and recurrent pregnancy loss. However, this association does not imply causation, although recent trials have attempted to address this issue.

Implantation is the biologic transition of a free-floating blastocyst in the endometrial cavity attaching to the endometrium, invading the underlying stroma and establishing a trophoblast. The processes that govern implantation largely remain unexplained. Polyps may adversely affect fertility by bleeding, presenting an abnormal site for implantation, or by influencing some of the factors that affect fertilization and implantation.

Glycodelin is a glycoprotein secreted by the endometrial epithelial cells into the uterine cavity. Its levels are lowest in the follicular phase; they rise with increasing ovarian progesterone secretion and peak by postovulatory day 12. Elevated levels in the periovulatory period may impair fertilization, implantation, and sperm–oocyte binding. Richlin et al. demonstrated elevated periovulatory plasma and uterine cavitary concentrations of glycodelin among patients with endometrial polyps. They speculated that endometrial polyps may

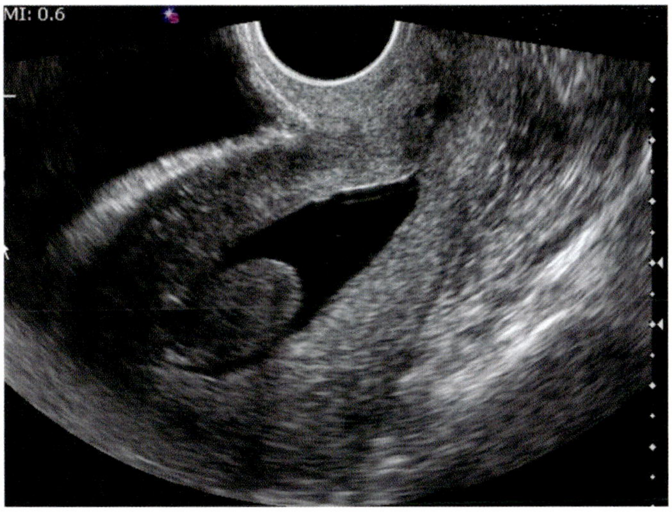

Figure 17 Saline-infused sonography clearly demonstrates a fundal endometrial polyp in this woman with intermenstrual spotting.

impair fertilization and endometrial receptivity via increased glycodelin levels (44).

Endometrial polyps may be identified by transvaginal sonography, sonohysterography, or hysterosalpingography (Fig. 17). Confirmation is usually by direct visualization and histology, i.e., hysteroscopy with directed biopsy, extraction, and/or resection. The typical hysteroscopic appearance is that of a fleshy polypoid lesion, with similar coloring to the surrounding endometrium and a stalk of variable thickness (Fig. 18). Sonographically, a feeding vessel may be identified in the stalk. Submucous myomas, in contrast, are often paler than the surrounding endometrium, with more obvious surface vasculature. While myomas may have a stalk, they more commonly have a degree of myometrial extension. Ultimately, histologic differentiation may be required.

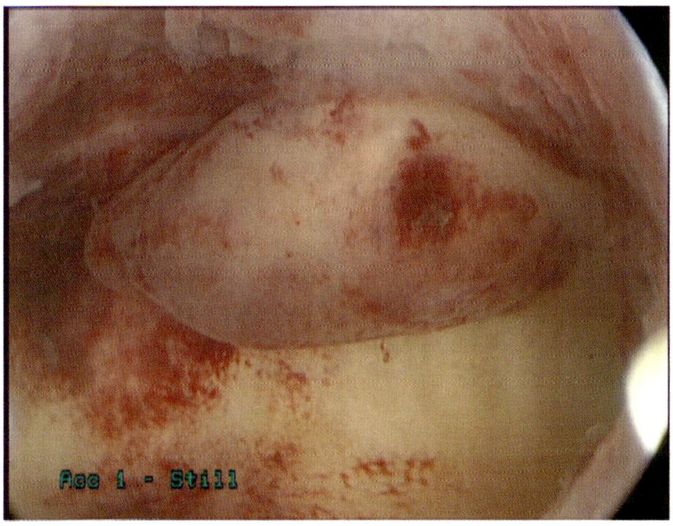

Figure 18 This picture was obtained immediately prior to hysteroscopic resection of this benign endometrial polyp in a patient planning IVF.

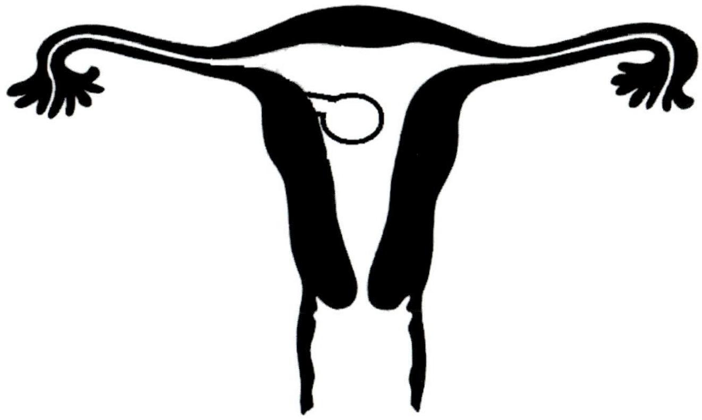

Figure 19 Endometrial polyp. An endometrial polyp arises from the endometrium and remains attached to it. It does not attach to the underlying myometrium.

Surgical Procedure

Larger polyps are commonly removed by electrosurgical resection with a continuous-flow resectoscope. The polyp may need to be morcellated to be removed through the cervix. Serial sections may be made with the cutting loop electrode, but only activating the electrode when the loop is moved from far to near field. The pedicle should be transected last.

Smaller polyps may be resected similarly or extracted with an operating hysteroscope using grasping forceps and/or scissors inserted through the operating channel. Both techniques enable the polyp to be removed completely, under direct visual guidance. Unlike myomas that may have a degree of myometrial extension, polyps are always surface abnormalities. Therefore, the basal layer of the endometrium can usually be preserved and the risk of subsequent synechiae should be minimal (Fig. 19). There is no need for the use of any adjuvant agents; however, some commonly employ empiric perioperative antibiotic prophylaxis.

If endometrial polyps have the potential to contribute to infertility or pregnancy loss, it follows that their removal should result in improved pregnancy and miscarriage rates. To date, only one randomized controlled trial has addressed this issue, involving 215 patients with endometrial polyps undergoing intrauterine insemination for infertility. Perez-Medina et al. reported that polypectomy was associated with a higher incidence of pregnancy (RR 2.1, 95% CI 1.5–2.9) and a shorter time to conception. The effect was apparent despite stratification for polyp size from <5 to >20 mm. This study provides the strongest evidence supporting polypectomy in infertile women (45).

Supportive findings are also available from two other retrospective studies. Varasteh et al. reported higher pregnancy and live birth rates and a shorter time to conception following hysteroscopic polypectomy compared to infertile controls with a normal hysteroscopic examination (46). Lass and colleagues reported that small endometrial polyps did not appear to decrease pregnancy rates but tended to increase pregnancy loss rates during IVF-ET. Hysteroscopic polypectomy appeared to reverse this trend (47).

Uterine Fibroids

Fibroids are benign monoclonal smooth muscle tumors that arise in the myometrium. They are the most common solid pelvic tumors found in women. Their occurrence increases with age, until menopause. It is estimated that 20% to 80% of women older than 30 years may have uterine fibroids. Fibroids may be solitary or multiple, and their size may vary widely. Subserosal fibroids are located on the outside of the uterus, intramural fibroids are positioned within the myometrium, and submucosal fibroids protrude into the endometrial cavity. Studies have shown that fibroids frequently contain chromosomal aberrations. A large number of genes may be involved in their tumorigenesis (48). It is thought that fibroids develop initially by the transformation of normal myocytes into abnormal myocytes that subsequently grow into clinically apparent tumors. The etiology of this neoplastic transformation is unknown. Each fibroid is derived from the mutation of a single myometrial cell. Subsequent growth occurs via clonal expansion. Furthermore, since each fibroid arises from a single monoclonal cell line, each fibroid is genetically different and may behave differently. However, in general fibroids tend to respond by hypertrophy in the presence of estrogen and tend to shrink in its absence. There is an increasing evidence that progesterone may also be implicated in their growth, and this knowledge is a focus of investigation for alternative medical methods of therapy.

Leiomyomas are continually undergoing degeneration. The most common type of degeneration is fibrosis; thus, they are commonly referred to as fibroids. Cystic, calcific, and red degenerations are uncommon, while malignant transformation is controversial. Genetic differences between fibroids and leiomyosarcomas suggest that leiomyosarcomas do not result from malignant transformation of a fibroid. Leiomyosarcoma is reported to occur in 0.29% to 1% of women with fibroids. The incidence of leiomyosarcoma is estimated to be 0.23% in premenopausal women and peaks to <2% in postmenopausal women (49). However, it remains uncertain whether leiomyosarcoma is a de novo disorder or a result of malignant transformation. Rapid growth is commonly thought to be a sign of malignant change, although there is no evidence to support this. Furthermore, since there are no norms for the rate of growth, rapid growth is subjective.

Fibroids may be symptomatic or asymptomatic. Clinical symptoms have been shown to occur in up to 50% of women with uterine fibroids (49). The most common symptom experienced is AUB. Fibroids that distort the endometrial cavity are most commonly associated with menstrual bleeding abnormalities (Fig. 20). Submucosal fibroids are most commonly implicated, but intramural fibroids that impinge on the endometrial cavity may also be associated with abnormal bleeding. As fibroids grow they may compress other adjacent structures, resulting in symptoms such as pain, bloating, abdominal distension, urinary frequency, and constipation. These bulk-related symptoms are more common with subserosal and intramural fibroids.

The most common indication for the treatment of fibroids is for AUB. Medical management may be effective in improving bleeding in some cases, although this beneficial effect may be achieved without any direct influence on the fibroids. Radiologic-guided treatment with vascular embolization and therapeutic ultrasound has also been developed recently, primarily for symptom control. Surgery is commonly recommended as the primary treatment, but even when other modalities are chosen first, surgery is frequently required for circumstances of other treatment modality failure.

To date, there has not been a meta-analysis of hysteroscopic myomectomy for women with submucous fibroids and AUB. The available data include many observational trials, demonstrating a range of successful resolution of AUB from 65% to 90% (Table 8). Since the first report of hysteroscopic myomectomy by Neuwirth and Amin (55) in 1976, it has increasingly been incorporated into clinical practice worldwide and is currently considered a safe and effective standard surgical procedure.

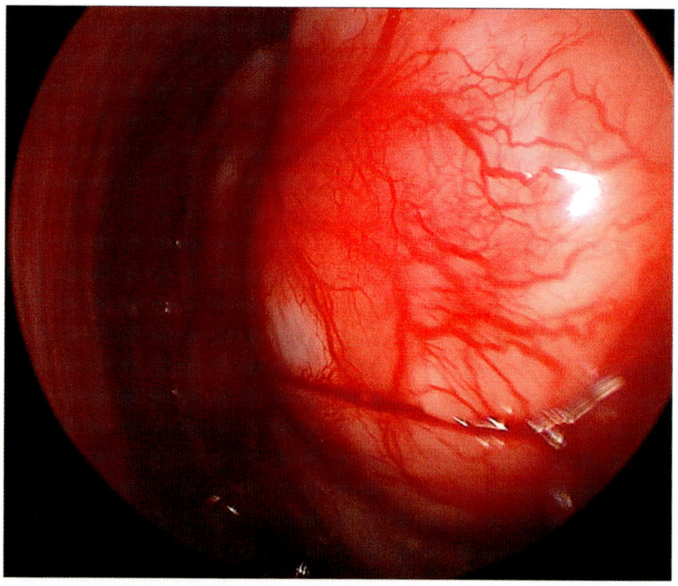

Figure 20 This hysteroscopic picture demonstrates a 5-cm submucous myoma that fills the endometrial cavity in a patient with secondary infertility.

Long-term success of hysteroscopic myomectomy seems to relate to complete resection of the submucous fibroid(s), the subsequent growth of other fibroids at other sites, and other potential causes for AUB that may pre-exist or subsequently develop.

The role of fibroids in reproduction remains a subject of considerable controversy. While they have been commonly implicated in infertility and pregnancy loss, there are no current randomized controlled trials to support this. The available evidence for support and regarding treatment of fibroids for this indication is found in chapter 19.

Surgical Procedure

Hysteroscopic myomectomy is a minimally invasive surgical procedure for excision of submucous or intramural fibroids with an intracavitary component. Submucous fibroids are commonly classified according to the degree of myometrial penetration (Table 9). The classification system of the European Society of Hysteroscopy is commonly used worldwide (56).

Hysteroscopic myomectomy is made more difficult when a greater proportion of the fibroid is intramural than intracavitary. The deeper the required dissection into the myometrium, the greater the risk of excessive bleeding, intravasation of distension media, and perforation of the

Table 8 Results of Hysteroscopic Myomectomy for Abnormal Uterine Bleeding

Author	Year	Cases (*n*)	Follow-up (yr)	Success (%)
Derman et al. (50)	1991	94	9	84
Hart et al. (51)	1999	113	2.3	86
Vercellini et al. (52)	1999	101	3.4	70
Campo et al. (53)	2005	63	2	68
Loffer (54)	2005	104	-	81

Table 9 The European Society of Hysteroscopy Classification of Submucous Fibroids

	Intramural extension (%)	Intracavitary portion (%)
Type 0 (T0)	0	100
Type I (TI)	<50	>50
Type II (TII)	>50	<50

uterus. Knowledge of the thickness of the myometrium between the outer edge of the fibroid and the serosal surface of the uterus would be ideal both prior to surgery and real time during surgery, but frequently this information is not available (Fig. 21). Preoperatively, transvaginal ultrasound, with or without saline infusion, may be able to provide a reasonable estimate of the thickness of this outer layer of myometrium (Fig. 22). However, this can best be determined by MRI (Fig. 23), although not as commonly performed due to cost. It is commonly recommended that the thickness of the myometrium between the fibroid and the serosa should be at least 1 cm, in order to attempt complete hysteroscopic fibroid resection. In expert hands, if the myometrium is only 5-mm thick over a relatively small surface area, then complete resection may be planned. Size, specific location within the endometrial cavity, and vascularity are additional factors that influence ease and success of surgery. Fibroids greater than 4 cm in diameter, those deep in the cornu, and TII fibroids are probably best reserved for experienced hysteroscopic surgeons.

Once the decision has been made to proceed with hysteroscopic myomectomy, preoperative administration of GnRH agonist may be considered. GnRH agonists have been shown to reduce preoperative anemia, size of submucous fibroids (57,58), surgical time, intraoperative bleeding, and the volume of distension fluid required, though conflicting results have been reported (53,59). Practically, their use also assists in surgical booking by removing the restriction to the early proliferative phase of the menstrual cycle. Conversely, some disadvantages to the use of GnRH agonists prior to surgery are their high cost, frequency of unpleasant side effects, and tendency to reduce to size of endometrial cavity and elasticity of the cervix. The latter problem may be countered by preoperative intravaginal misoprostol, which promotes cervical softening and dilation and reduces the risk of cervical lacerations.

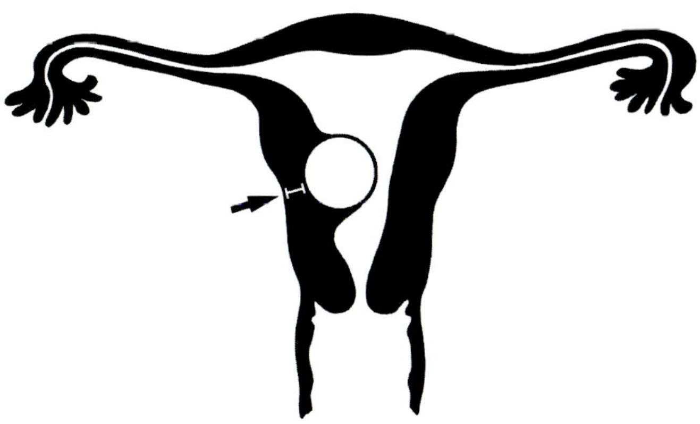

Figure 21 Myometrial thickness between the uterine serosal surface and outer edge of a fibroid.

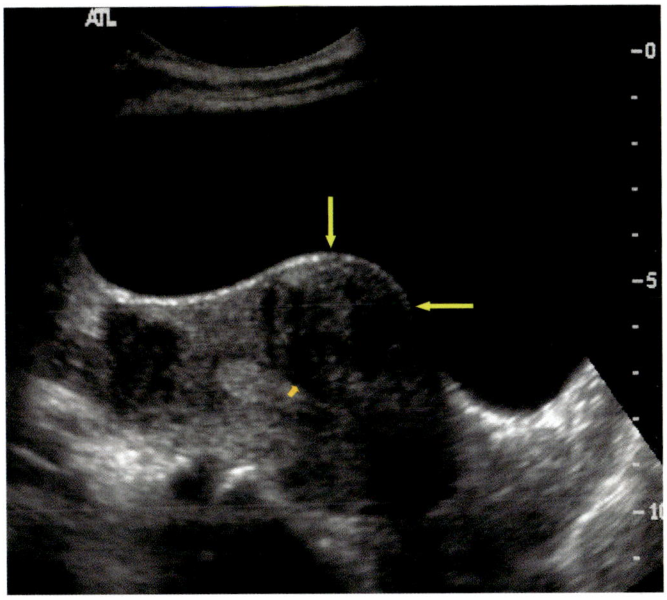

Figure 22 Transvaginal ultrasound demonstrates a 3-cm intramural myoma. While the myoma is surgically accessible via the anterior wall of the endometrial cavity (*orange arrow*), there is no safe margin of myometrium between the myoma and the uterine serosa (*yellow arrows*). Hysteroscopic myoma resection was not deemed appropriate.

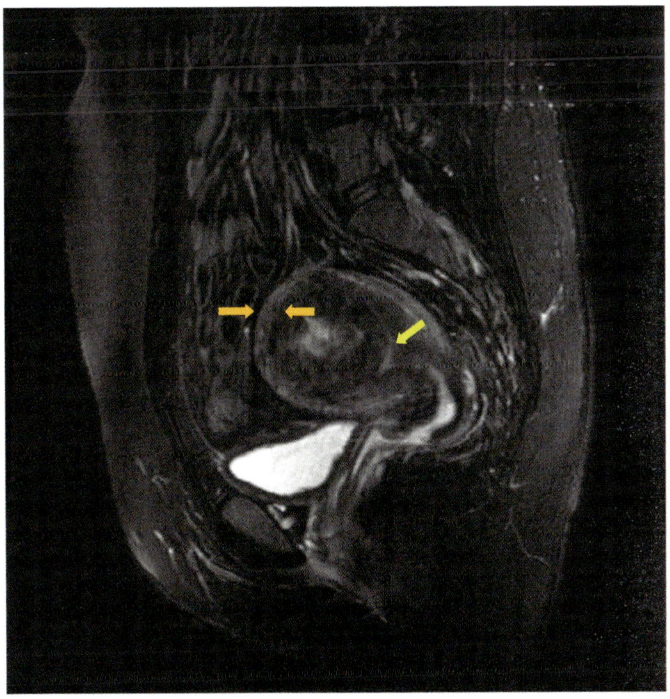

Figure 23 This MRI demonstrates a 2-cm margin of myometrium between the outer edge of this submucous myoma and the uterine serosa (*orange arrows*). The myoma compresses the superior aspect of the endometrial cavity (*yellow arrow*). Total hysteroscopic myoma resection was deemed safe.

Hysteroscopic myomectomy is typically performed under general or regional anesthesia with a continuous-flow resectoscope. The resectoscope should be assembled first. The continuous flow of distention fluid provides a clear visual field for the entire procedure.

Traditionally, hysteroscopic resection is performed with monopolar electrosurgery. With monopolar electrosurgery, it is necessary to use a distention fluid that is electrolyte free, such as low-viscosity 1.5% glycine, 2.7% sorbitol with 0.54% mannitol, 3% sorbitol, or 5% mannitol. The recent development of bipolar hysteroscopic systems allows surgery to be performed in an electrolyte-rich media such as normal saline. The advantage of this is that if there is a problem with fluid overload, it is not further compromised by hyponatremia. However, one should recognize that even with isotonic solutions severe fluid overload with patient compromise has occurred.

Surgery with a monopolar resectoscope requires the return electrode to be placed at a distant site such as the patient's thigh. Electrical current is conducted from the active electrode, through the path of least resistance in the patient's body to the return electrode on the thigh, then back to the generator. In contrast, with a bipolar resectoscope, the return electrode is located on the distal portion of the resectoscope itself, near the active electrode. This virtually eliminates the likelihood of stray electrical current finding an unintended alternate pathway, such as with capacitive coupling. Furthermore, bipolar technology minimizes the amount of unwanted tissue damage as the exposed current is constrained to only the small volume of tissue between the active and return electrode. Also, bipolar electrosurgery requires less generator power output to accomplish equivalent results at the target tissue. In spite of the safety advantages of bipolar electrosurgery, most resectoscopic surgery is performed with monopolar systems with a low incidence of complications.

Methods to try to reduce the risk of intravasation include the following:

1. Maintain the intrauterine pressure below the woman's mean arterial pressure.
2. Monitor inflow and outflow of fluid closely during the operation. In many facilities, the use of a fluid management system has become the standard of care. These systems provide a real-time accurate measurement of fluid balance, by weight. General guidelines for fluid overload are as follows:
   (a) Volume >1000 cc—stop, assess clinical status, obtain serum electrolytes, only proceed if patient is stable, but aim for quick completion.
   (b) Volume >1500 cc—stop completely, assess clinical status, obtain serum electrolytes, and transfer to PAR for ongoing management.
3. Use a GnRH agonist preoperatively.

The cervix must be dilated sufficiently to accommodate the resectoscope. Most commonly a 26-French resectoscope is used; therefore, the cervix must be dilated to ≥9 mm. It is generally preferable to slightly overdilate the cervix to enable easier insertion of the linear resectoscope through the curvilinear cervical canal. In addition, slight overdilation of the cervix should help to reduce the risk of air embolism that may occur with a piston-type action of a blunt instrument forcing air into a potentially open vascular space. Furthermore, reduced intrauterine pressure should help to reduce the risk of fluid intravasation. The resectoscope may be inserted visually or blindly with an obturator. Dilute Pitressin solution (20 mL of 0.05 U/mL), injected into the cervical wall, has been shown to decrease intraoperative blood loss, decrease distension fluid absorption, and facilitate cervical dilatation (60).

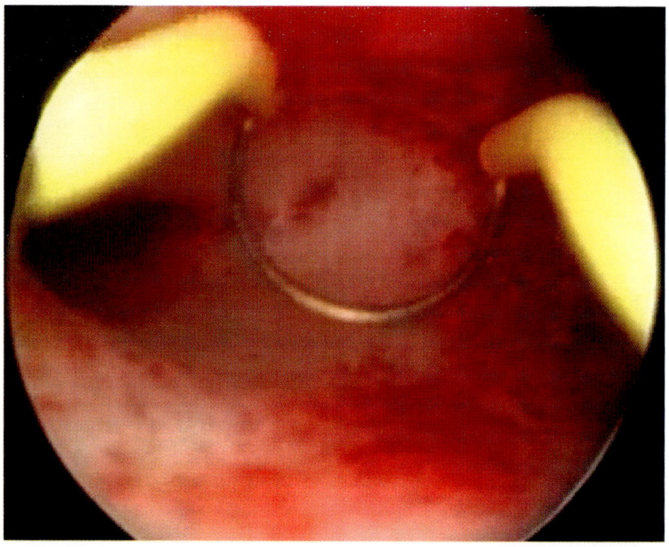

Figure 24 The cutting loop electrode inside the endometrial cavity.

The resection is performed using a wire monopolar or bipolar cutting loop (Fig. 24). The loop electrode is passed cephalad to the fibroid to be resected, and, as it is retracted toward the insulated sheath of the resectoscope, the electrosurgical generator is activated. Only the cutting mode of the generator is activated; this provides a nonmodulated electrical current. The current should only be activated when the electrode is moving from the far to the near field of view. Care should always be taken to ensure that the electrode is only in contact with the fibroid, when the current is activated, to prevent injury to the surrounding endometrium. This may be aided by continually directing the base of the loop electrode toward the center of the fibroid and resecting from lateral to central.

When resecting a T0 fibroid, the progressive resection should be continued until the fibroid is morcellated to a size that can be removed through the dilated cervix. Then the pedicle may be transected and, if there is bleeding from the resection base, the open vessels should be visualized and coagulated with the "coag mode" that gives a modulated current. The strips of tissue may be removed as the case proceeds or at the end of the procedure. The procedure is finalized when a close visual inspection demonstrates that the endometrial cavity has been normalized.

TI and TII fibroids require a slightly different approach. The technique preferred by this author is to start the resection at one of the lateral margins of the myoma near the site where it protrudes from the uterine wall. The base of the electrode should point toward the center of the myoma. The first resection trough should be level to that of the surrounding normal endometrial cavity (Fig. 25A). This approach will demarcate the margin of the intracavitary portion of the fibroid from the intramural portion of the fibroid. This will assist, when resecting the intramural portion later. Serial resection should continue to remove this lateral intracavitary quarter of the fibroid (Fig. 25B). Resection should occur from the lateral aspect toward the center of the myoma, to protect against inadvertent injury to normal tissue. Resected tissue

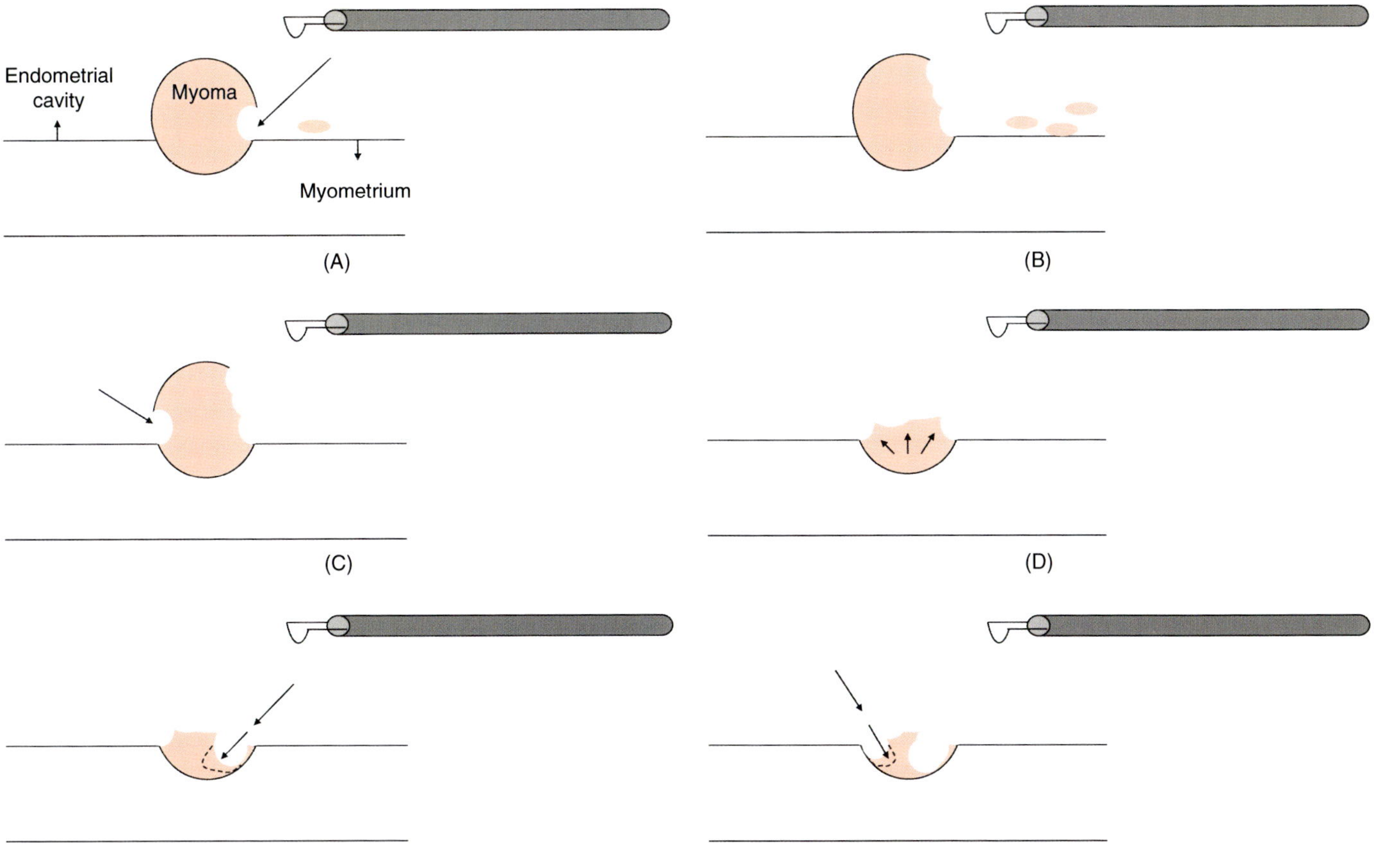

Figure 25 (A) The initial incision into a submucous myoma with the cutting loop electrode should start at the margin between the intracavitary and the intramural portions of the fibroid. (B) The lateral side of the intracavitary myoma is sequentially resected. (C) The margin between the intracavitary and intramural portions of the fibroid on the opposite side should then be identified and resected. (D) Once the intracavitary portion of the myoma has been resected, the intramural portion of the myoma will begin to extrude into the endometrial cavity. (E) Careful resection of the intramural portion should begin at one lateral margin of the fibroid, preserving normal myometrium and following the border of the fibroid. (F) Next, the opposite lateral margin should be carefully resected. This will help to extrude the remaining central component of the intramural portion.

should be removed, from the uterine cavity, whenever vision is impaired. The opposite quarter of the intracavitary portion should now be resected in the same manner, working from lateral to central (Fig. 25C). When this has been completed, all of the remaining myoma is its intramural portion. It will tend to extrude into the endometrial cavity, with a convex contour (Fig. 25D). This may be promoted by reducing the pressure in the cavity.

Resection of the intramural portion may continue with the loop electrode. Serial sections should be obtained while keeping the base of the electrode pointed toward the deeper portion of the fibroid. Resection should proceed starting at one lateral aspect of the myoma, attempting to dissect out the fibroid from the surrounding normal myometrium (Fig. 25E). Once the dissection plane is well established on one side of the fibroid, the operator should move to the contralateral side of the fibroid and dissect out the tissue plane there (Fig. 25F). This will promote protrusion of the central portion of the fibroid into the uterine cavity. If the intramural portion is relatively small, then this technique will allow one to fashion a pedicle. As the remaining portion of the fibroid is protruded into the cavity, resection may continue to remove the deeper portion of the fibroid.

Ideally, resection would continue until the intramural portion is completely removed, which would be evident by the visual distinction between the tissue of a fibroid and that of normal myometrium. In addition, when the fibroid has been completely removed, the resection base will have a concave contour, not convex. However, the operator must always guard against perforation of the uterus. Perforation with an activated electrode risks injury not only to the uterus but also to other surrounding intra-abdominal organs. The deeper the resection, the greater the risk of perforation. The operator must exercise judgment and may decide to leave a small portion of fibroid at the resection base. In some cases, a second procedure may be booked, within a few weeks, in order to remove the retained portion of the myoma. Often, with time the surrounding myometrium will force further protrusion of the remnant portion, making resection safer. The second procedure should be booked within a month prior to any significant regeneration of the fibroid.

Alternative methods for hysteroscopic myomectomy include the use of a vaporizing electrode to vaporize rather than resect tissue and the use of a "cold loop" to bluntly dissect the intramural extension of the fibroid from the uterine wall. Vaporization is performed with a monopolar resectoscope using either a spherical or a cylindrical electrode. The electrode is rolled over the surface of the fibroid, from far to near field, using high-power "cut" current delivering a non-modulated waveform. The advantage is the absence of tissue strips requiring removal from the surgical field. However, this is also a disadvantage since the tissue is not available for histologic review.

"Cold loops" may be used to bluntly dissect out the tissue plane between the fibroid and the uterine wall after the intracavitary portion of a TI or TII fibroid has been removed. The advantage is that there is no electrical energy used in the deeper aspect of the uterine wall.

Complications Associated with Hysteroscopic Surgery

Complications of hysteroscopy include uterine perforation, fluid overload, hemorrhage, cervical laceration, infection, air or gas embolism, and rarely death. Complications are more common with operative hysteroscopy than with diagnostic hysteroscopy. While complication rates with hysteroscopic surgery range from 1% to 12% in the literature, the rate of 4% is commonly quoted. The Scottish audit of hysteroscopic surgery for menorrhagia registered 978 cases. Of these, 732 women were followed for a minimum of 6 months and 554 for 12 months. Thus, both immediate and delayed complications were identified and followed. Furthermore, this method of evaluation represents the results of everyday practice rather than being limited to that of the most experienced surgeons. Fluid overload between 1 and 2 L occurred in about 5% of cases, and >2 L in about 1%. However, there were no cases of pulmonary edema. Uterine perforation occurred in about 1% of cases and excessive bleeding in about 3%, and there was one death presumed to be from toxic shock syndrome (61). In another study that analyzed the factors influencing fluid loss during transcervical resection of submucous fibroids, only intramural extension of the myoma and operating time were identified by multiple linear regression to be positively related (62). A more recent review of complications of hysteroscopic surgery in 2007 recognized that two-thirds of their complications were uterine entry related. The authors conclude that strict fluid monitoring and terminating of procedures when fluid balance exceeds 1000 mL contributed to their low incidence of media-related complications (63). The MISTLETOE study included 10,686 women in the United Kingdom and Wales who had endometrial ablation (by a variety of techniques) by 690 doctors. They documented a 4% complication rate, of which about one-half of their complications were hemorrhage. The presence of fibroids significantly increased their documented rate of hemorrhage (64).

Factors that increase the probability of complication with hysteroscopic myomectomy include

1. greater degree of myometrial extension,
2. multiple fibroids,
3. larger fibroids,
4. length of operating time, and
5. inexperienced surgeon.

Some methods to reduce the risk of fluid intravasation, perforation, and air embolism have previously been discussed. Hemorrhage is often secondary to deep myometrial dissection and may most commonly be managed with electrocoagulation. If persistent, temporary tamponade with a 30 cc intrauterine Foley catheter is usually effective. While infection is uncommon, some employ empiric prophylactic antibiotics.

SUMMARY

The uterus is an integral organ in human fertility. Some of the anatomic anomalies that may interfere with successful reproduction may be amenable to surgical correction. One of the great advances in gynecologic endoscopy over the past two decades has been the development of hysteroscopic procedures to surgically correct anomalies involving the endometrial cavity. The current methods of imaging and visual assessment allow for very accurate diagnosis. The surgical instruments and techniques that have been developed facilitate precise restoration of normal anatomy and function, in many cases. There is considerable medical evidence that supports the use of hysteroscopic surgery for the treatment of women with uterine anomalies and disorders of menstruation. However, at the present time, there are some limitations to the medical evidence that confirms the role of hysteroscopic surgery for uterine anomalies to enhance fertility. Further investigation that focuses on surgical methodology, along with medical adjuvant therapy, and patient outcomes is required to optimize counseling and treatment of patients with uterine anomalies.

ACKNOWLEDGMENTS

Thanks to Drs. T.M. Chandler and L.S. Machan for HSG and MR images shown in Figs. 3 to 6, 9, and 12.

REFERENCES

1. Robboy SJ, Bentley RC, Russell P. Embryology of the female genital tract and disorders of abnormal sexual development. In: Kurman RJ, ed. Blaustein's Pathology of the Female Reproductive Tract. New York, NY: Springer, 2002:3–36.
2. The American Fertility Society. Classifications of adnexal adhesions, distal tubal occlusion, tubal occlusion secondary to tubal ligation, tubal pregnancies, Mullerian anomalies and intrauterine adhesions. Fertil Steril 1988; 49(6):944–955.
3. Grimbizis GF, Camus M, Tarlatzis BC, et al. Clinical implications of uterine malformations and hysteroscopic treatment results. Hum Reprod Update 2001; 7(1):161–174.
4. Lin PC. Reproductive outcomes in women with uterine anomalies. J Womens Health 2004; 13(1):33–39.
5. Sanders BH, Machan LS, Gomel V. Complex uterine surgery: A cooperative role for interventional radiology with hysteroscopic surgery. Fertil Steril 1998; 70(5):952–955.
6. Fluker MR, Bebbington MW, Munro MG. Successful pregnancy following zygote intrafallopian transfer for congenital cervical hypoplasia. Obstet Gynecol 1994; 84(4 Pt 2):659–661.
7. Rock JA, Schlaff WD. The obstetric consequences of uterovaginal anomalies. Fertil Steril 1985; 43(5):681–692.
8. Rollen AC, Choquette AJ. Rudimentary uterine horn: Obstetric and gynecologic implications. Obstet Gynecol 1966; 27:806–813.
9. Patton PE. Anatomic uterine defects. Clinical Obstet Gynecol 1994; 37(3):705–721.
10. Golan A, Langer R, Bukovsky I, et al. Congenital anomalies of the mullerian system. Fertil Steril 1989; 51(5):747–755.
11. Maneschi F, Marana R, Muzii L, et al. Reproductive performance in women with bicornuate uterus. Acta Eur Fertil 1993; 24(3):117–120.
12. Procter JA, Haney AF. Recurrent first trimester pregnancy loss is associated with uterine septum but not with bicornuate uterus. Fertil Steril 2003; 80(5):1212–1215.
13. Lolis DE, Paschopoulos M, Makrydimas G, et al. Reproductive outcome after Strassman metroplasty in women with a bicornuate uterus. J Reprod Med 2005; 50(5):297–301.
14. Homer HA, Li TC, Cooke ID. The septate uterus: A review of management and reproductive outcome. Fertil Steril 2000; 73(1):1–14.
15. March CM, Israel R. Hysteroscopic management of recurrent abortion caused by septate uterus. Am J Obstet Gynecol 1987; 156:834–842.

16. Daley DC, Walters CA, Soto-Albors CE, et al. Hysteroscopic metroplasty: Six years' experience. Obstet Gynecol 1989; 73:201–205.
17. Fedele L, Arcaini L, Parazzini F, et al. Reproductive prognosis after hysteroscopic metroplasty in 102 women: Life-table analysis. Fertil Steril 1993; 59:768–772.
18. Carrach M, Penella J, Ubeda A, et al. Hysteroscopic incision of the septate uterus: Scissors versus resectoscope. Hum Reprod 1994; 9:87–97.
19. Pabuccu R, Atay V, Urman, B, et al. Hysteroscopic treatment of septate uterus. Gynaecol Endosc 1995; 4:213–215.
20. Valle RF. Hysteroscopic treatment of partial and complete uterine septum. Int J Fertil Menopausal Stud 1996; 41:310–315.
21. Venturoli S, Colombo FM, Vianello F, et al. A study of hysteroscopic metroplasty in 141 women with a septate uterus. Arch Gynecol Obstet 2002; 266:157–159.
22. Sanders B. Uterine factors and infertility. J Reprod Med 2006; 51(3):169–176.
23. Heinonen PK. Reproductive performance of women with uterine anomalies after abdominal or hysteroscopic metroplasty or with no surgical treatment. J Am Assoc Gynecol Laparosc 1997; 4(3):311–317.
24. Valli E, Vaguero E, Lazzarin N, et al. Hysteroscopic metroplasty improves gestational outcome in women with recurrent spontaneous abortion. J Am Assoc Gynecol Laparosc 2004; 11(2):240–244.
25. Marabini A, Gubbini G, Stagnozzi R, et al. Hysteroscopic metroplasty. Ann N Y Acad Sci 1994; 734:488–492.
26. Pabuccu R, Gomel V. Reproductive outcome after hysteroscopic metroplasty in women with septate uterus and otherwise unexplained infertility. Fertil Steril 2004; 81(6):1675–1678.
27. Colacurci N, De Placido G, Mollo A, et al. Reproductive outcome after hysteroscopic metroplasty. Eur J Obstet Gynecol Reprod Biol 1996; 66:147–150.
28. Mencaglia L, Tantini C. Hysteroscopic treatment of septate and arcuate uterus. Gynaecol Endosc 1996; 5:151–154.
29. Nisolle M, Donnez J. Endoscopic treatment of uterine malformations. Gynaecol Endosc 1996; 5:155–160.
30. Lobaugh ML, Bammel BM, Duke D, et al. Uterine rupture during pregnancy in a patient with a history of uterine metroplasty. Obstet Gynecol 1994; 83:838–840.
31. Fedele L, Bianchi S, Marchini M, et al. Residual uterine septum of less than 1 cm after hysteroscopic metroplasty does not impair reproductive outcome. Hum Reprod 1996; 11:727–729.
32. Kormanyos Z, Molnar BG, Pal A. Removal of a residual portion of a uterine septum in women of advanced reproductive age: Obstetric outcome. Hum Reprod 2006; 4:1047–1051.
33. Heinonen PK. Complete septate uterus with longitudinal vaginal septum. Fertil Steril 2006; 85(3):700–705.
34. Patton PE, Novy MJ, Lee DM, et al. The diagnosis and reproductive outcome after surgical treatment of the complete septate uterus, duplicated cervix and vaginal septum. Am J Obstet Gynecol 2004; 190:1669–1678.
35. Parsanezhad ME, Alborzi S, Zarei A, et al. Hysteroscopic metroplasty of the complete uterine septum, duplicate cervix, and vaginal septum. Fertil Steril 2006; 85(5):1473–1477.
36. Raga F, Bausel C, Remohi J, et al. Reproductive impact of congenital Mullerian anomalies. Hum Reprod 1997; 12(10):2277–2281.
37. Fritsch H. Ein Fall von volligen Schund der gebarmutter Hohle nach Auskratzung. Contralbl F Gynak 1894; 18:1337–1339.
38. Asherman JG. Amenorrhea traumatica (atretica). J Obstet Gynaecol Br Empire 1948; 55:23–30.
39. Friedler S, Margalioth EJ, Kafka I, et al. Incidence of post-abortion intra-uterine adhesions evaluated by hysteroscopy—a prospective study. Hum Reprod 1993; 8:442–444.
40. Capella-Allouc S, Morsad F, Rongieres-Bertrand C, et al. Hysteroscopic treatment of severe Asherman's syndrome and subsequent fertility. Hum Reprod 1999; 14(5):1230–1233.
41. Valle R, Sciarra JJ. Intrauterine adhesions: Hysteroscopic diagnosis, classification, treatment, and reproductive outcome. Am J Obstet Gynecol 1988; 158(6):1459–1470.
42. Pabuccu R, Atay V, Orhon E, et al. Hysteroscopic treatment of intrauterine adhesions is safe and effective in the restoration of normal menstruation and fertility. Fertil Steril 1997; 68(6):1141–1143.
43. Orhue AA, Aziken ME, Igbefoh JO. A comparison of two adjunctive treatments for intrauterine adhesions following lysis. Int J Gynaecol Obstet 2003; 82(1):49–56.
44. Richlin SS, Ramachandran S, Shanti A, et al. Glycodelin levels in uterine flushings and in plasma of patients with leiomyomas and polyps: Implications for implantation. Hum Reprod 2002; 17(10):2742–2747.
45. Perez-Medina T, Bajo-Arenas J, Salazar F, et al. Endometrial polyps and their implication in the pregnancy rates of patients undergoing intrauterine insemination: A prospective, randomized study. Hum Reprod 2005; 20(6):1632–1635.
46. Varasteh NN, Neuwirth RS, Levin B, et al. Pregnancy rates after hysteroscopic polypectomy and myomectomy in infertile women. Obstet Gynecol 1999; 94(2):168–171.
47. Lass A, Williams G, Abusheikha N, et al. The effect of endometrial polyps on outcomes of in vitro fertilization (IVF) cycles. J Assist Reprod Genet 1999; 16(8):410–415.
48. Wang H, Mahadevappa M, Yamamoto K, et al. Distinctive proliferative phase differences in gene expression in human myometrium and leiomyomata. Fertil Steril 2003; 80(2): 266–276.
49. Guarnaccia MM, Rein, MS. Traditional surgical approaches to uterine fibroids: Abdominal myomectomy and hysterectomy. Clin Obstet Gynecol 2001; 44(2):385–400.
50. Derman SG, Rehnstrom J, Neuwirth RS. The long-term effectiveness of hysteroscopic treatment of menorrhagia and leiofibroids. Obstet Gynecol 1991; 77:591–594.
51. Hart R, Molnar BG, Magos A. Long term follow up of hysteroscopic myomectomy assessed by survival analysis. Br J Obstet Gynecol 1999; 106:700–705.
52. Vercellini P, Zaina B, Yaylayan L, et al. Hysteroscopic myomectomy: Long-term effects on menstrual pattern and fertility. Obstet Gynecol 1999; 94:341–347.
53. Campo S, Campo V, Gambadauro P. Short-term and long-term results of resectoscopic myomectomy with and without pretreatment with GnRH analogs in premenopausal women. Acta Obstet Gynecol Scand 2005; 84:756–760.
54. Loffer FD. Improving results of hysteroscopic submucosal myomectomy for menorrhagia by concomitant endometrial ablation. J Minim Invasive Gynecol 2005; 12:254–260.
55. Neuwirth RS, Amin HK. Excision of submucous fibroids with hysteroscopic control. Am J Obstet Gynecol 1976; 126:95–99.
56. Cohen LS, Valle RF. Role of vaginal sonography and hysterosonography in the endoscopic treatment of uterine myomas. Fertil Steril 2000; 73:197–204.
57. Mencaglia L, Tantini C. GnRH analogs and hysteroscopic resection of myomas. Int J Gynaecol Obstet 1993; 43:285–288.
58. Donnez J, Schrurs B, Gillerot S, et al. Treatment of uterine fibroids with implants of gonadotropin-releasing hormone agonist: Assessment by hysterography. Fertil Steril 1989; 51: 947–950.
59. Perino A, Chianchiano N, Petronio M, et al. Role of leuprolide acetate depot in hysteroscopic surgery: A controlled study. Fertil Steril 1993; 59:507–510.
60. Corson SL, Brooks PG, Serden SP, et al. Effects of vasopressin administration during hysteroscopic surgery. J Reprod Med 1994; 39(6):419–423.
61. Scottish Hysteroscopy Audit Group. A Scottish audit of hysteroscopic surgery for menorrhagia: Complications and follow up. Br J Obstet Gynaecol 1995; 102:249–254.
62. Emanuel MH, Hart A, Wamsteker K, et al. An analysis of fluid loss during transcervical resection of submucous myomas. Fertil Steril 1997; 68(5):881–886.
63. Shveiky D, Rojansky N, Revel A, et al. Complications of hysteroscopic surgery: "Beyond the learning curve." J Minim Invasive Gynecol 2007; 14:218–222.
64. Overton C, Hargreaves J, Maresh M. A national survey of the complications of endometrial destruction for menstrual disorders, the MISTLETOE study. Minimally invasive surgical techniques—laser, endothermal or endoresection. Br J Obstet Gynecol 1997; 104:1351–1359.

7

Treatment of leiomyoma

Jean-Bernard Dubuisson and William H. Parker

SYMPTOMS RELATED TO MYOMAS THAT MAY REQUIRE TREATMENT

Careful evaluation should be undertaken to ensure that the presence of symptoms is related to the presence of myomas. Associated symptoms may include abnormal uterine bleeding, dyspareunia, bloating, infertility, pelvic pain or pressure, and urinary symptoms. Some women with myomas may have menorrhagia, and etiologic theories include venous ectasia resulting from mechanical compression of veins by myomas, or storage of vasoactive growth factors produced by myomas (1,2). The presence of myomas does not necessarily lead to menorrhagia, and other possible etiologies should be considered, including coagulopathies such as von Willebrandt's disease (3).

Studies of non–care-seeking women evaluated by abdominal and transvaginal sonography found that the presence of myomas was not necessarily related to prolonged or heavy menstrual flow (4). Another study (5) found that gushing blood and length of periods were related to the size of myomas, but not to the presence of submucous myomas or multiple myomas. A population-based study (6) found that women with myomas were only slightly more likely to report moderate or severe dyspareunia or noncyclic pelvic pain and had no higher incidence of moderate or severe dysmenorrhea than women without myomas. Following uterine artery embolization (UAE) and a 35% reduction in uterine volume, frequency and urgency were improved in 68% of women, slightly improved in 18%, and unchanged or worse in only 14%, suggesting that increased uterine volume associated with myomas is related to urinary symptoms (7).

DIAGNOSIS

Uterine size, as assessed by bimanual examination, correlates well with uterine size and weight at pathological examination, even in overweight women (BMI > 30) (8). Sonography, saline-infusion sonography, hysteroscopy, and magnetic resonance imaging (MRI) may help select patients for surgical treatment by accurately assessing the size, number, and position of myomas.

Sonography, the most readily available and least costly technique, may be inadequate for determining the precise number and position of myomas (9). Saline-infusion sonography better defines submucous myomas, polyps, or other endometrial pathology. MRI, although expensive, is an excellent method for evaluating the size, position, and number of myomas; submucous myoma penetration into the myometrium; and differentiation of adenomyosis from myomas (10,11). In a study of women scheduled for hysterectomy (10), preoperative transvaginal sonography, saline-infusion sonography, hysteroscopy, and pelvic MRI were all performed. Submucous myomas were best identified with MRI (100% sensitivity and 91% specificity) and less accurately with transvaginal sonography (83% sensitivity and 90% specificity), saline-infusion sonography (90% sensitivity and 89% specificity), and hysteroscopy (82% sensitivity and 87% specificity).

Myomas and Fertility

The literature relating myomas and fertility is unfortunately limited by a lack of prospective, randomized, controlled studies. Most studies are observational and lack the statistical power to make valid conclusions. Many studies omit evaluation of the uterine cavity with hysteroscopy or saline-infusion sonography or do not report the size and number of myomas, patient ages, or type of fertility treatment. A meta-analysis found that only submucous myomas decreased and removal of myomas increased fertility to baseline rates (12). Neither intramural nor subserosal myomas appeared to affect fertility rates, and their removal was not found to increase fertility (12). The risks of myomectomy include operative and anesthetic risks, infection, postoperative adhesions, incrementally greater risk of uterine rupture, increased incidence of cesarean section, and the direct and indirect expenses of the procedure and recovery from surgery. Therefore, removal of intramural myomas to increase fertility should be carefully considered as addressed in chapter 13. (See chap. 19 on myomas and fertility.)

Influence of Myomas on Pregnancy

Large groups of pregnant women examined with routine second trimester sonography, with follow-up and delivery at the same institution, have been reported in two studies. In one (13) study, there were no significant differences in women with and without myomas (similar clinical management) regarding the incidence of preterm delivery, premature rupture of membranes, fetal growth restriction, placenta previa, placental abruption, postpartum hemorrhage, or retained placenta. Only cesarean section was more common among women with myomas. Another study (14) found no increased risk of premature rupture of membranes, operative vaginal delivery, chorioamnionitis, or endomyometritis; however, there was an increased risk of preterm delivery (19.2% vs. 12.7%), placenta previa (3.5% vs. 1.8%), and postpartum hemorrhage (8.3% vs. 2.9%) and cesarean section. Pregnancy outcomes following myomectomy have not been compared with women having untreated myomas.

TREATMENT OF SYMPTOMATIC UTERINE MYOMAS

Watchful Waiting

There is no evidence that failure to treat myomas results in harm, except for women with severe anemia from myoma-related menorrhagia or significant hydronephrosis due to obstruction of the ureter(s) from an enlarged myomatous uterus. A nonrandomized study (15) of women with uterine size eight weeks or greater, choosing hysterectomy or "watchful waiting," found that more than three-quarters of women choosing observation had no significant changes in the degree of bothersome symptoms, mental health, general health, or activity indexes at the end of one year. However, one quarter of the women decided on hysterectomy during the course of the year.

For women wishing to preserve fertility, myomectomy is presently the gold standard for the treatment of symptomatic leiomyomas. The abdominal approach remains the most frequent procedure, since patients may often consult the surgeon late in the evolution of the symptoms, with big leiomyomas (16). Myomectomy may be performed by laparoscopy in selected cases, particularly in subserous and intramural leiomyomas (17–20).

PREOPERATIVE EVALUATION

Careful preoperative detection and evaluation of the leiomyomas are important. This preoperative workup should include transvaginal (and often abdominal) ultrasonography and measurement of hemoglobin levels. Serum ferritin should be measured, particularly in patients with abnormal uterine bleeding. Examination of the uterine cavity is performed by diagnostic hysteroscopy, saline-infusion sonography, or MRI if submucous leiomyomas are suspected. Sonographic evaluation should include measurement of the entire uterus, number of leiomyomas, and type (intramural, subserous, or pedunculated), size, and location (anterior, posterior, fundus, broad ligament, or isthmus) of the dominant leiomyomas. Measurement of the distance between the endometrium and the leiomyoma, and the serosa and the myoma should be noted (21). It is also important to include a systematic search for adenomyosis, as this may modify the operative approach (22,23).

The blood supply of the dominant leiomyoma can be evaluated using Doppler sonography. This examination can provide important information concerning the origin of the vessels associated with the dominant leiomyoma: right or left uterine artery, both uterine arteries, or ovarian artery. Experience shows that a left-side leiomyoma is vascularized by the left uterine artery (or both uterine arteries) and a right-side leiomyoma by the right uterine artery (or both); a fundal leiomyoma may be vascularized by the uterine arteries as well as the ovarian arteries.

MRI is helpful when the ultrasound examination is difficult to analyze. Saline-infusion sonography might be useful for evaluating relationships between the leiomyomas and the uterine cavity (24). In infertile patients, a full infertility evaluation should be performed before surgery. If other fertility factors, including male factors are abnormal, the overall benefit on fertility may be substantially reduced. This should be assiduously discussed preoperatively (25).

PREOPERATIVE TREATMENT

Correction of iron deficiency anemia is essential in order to reduce the risk of blood transfusion. It may be necessary to postpone myomectomy until the blood count has been normalized. Oral iron may be given, although correction of anemia may take several months. Erythropoietin alpha and epoietin, given weekly for three weeks prior to elective surgery, has been shown to significantly increase hemoglobin concentrations (by 1.6 g/dL) and decrease transfusion rates when compared to controls (26,27). No side effects have been noted in these studies.

Gonadotropin-releasing hormone-a (GnRH-a) may be used preoperatively to stop abnormal uterine bleeding. A study (28) of women with myomas and initial mean hemoglobin concentrations of 10.2 g randomized the women to GnRH-a plus oral iron and placebo plus oral iron. After three months, three-quarters of the women treated with GnRH-a and iron had hemoglobin levels greater than 12 g as compared to less than half of the women receiving iron alone. GnRH agonists may also be used preoperatively to decrease uterine and myoma volumes. Maximal reduction is achieved by 12 weeks of therapy, with no further change observed after 24 weeks of treatment (29). Matta and colleagues observed that GnRH agonists also reduce uterine blood flow (30).

In patients undergoing laparoscopic myomectomy, preoperative treatment with GnRH agonists is controversial. A reduction in blood loss during both abdominal and laparoscopic myomectomy has been demonstrated; however, no difference in transfusion rates have been shown (31–33). The author (JBD) and others have found that preoperative treatment with GnRH agonists (whatever the duration of the treatment) increases the risk of conversion to laparotomy because of increased difficulties in identifying and dissecting the cleavage plane between the leiomyoma and its pseudocapsule (34–36). In addition, small intramural myomas may be more difficult to detect during surgery, which may increase the risk of persistence of leiomyomata (37).

Abdominal myomectomy can be considered for a woman with large uterine myomas who wishes to retain her uterus. A study of 90 women with uterine size larger than 16 weeks (range of 16–36 weeks) reported no conversions into hysterectomy (16). Complications included one bowel injury, one bladder injury, and one reoperation for incarcerated bowel (3%). The cell saver was used prophylactically in 70 women, and only 7 required homologous blood transfusion (38).

INDICATIONS FOR OPERATIVE LAPAROSCOPY

Laparoscopic Myomectomy

Currently available instruments make laparoscopic myomectomy feasible, although its use may be limited by the size and number of myomas reasonably removed, and the technical difficulty of myoma dissection and laparoscopic suturing (39). Preoperative evaluation is particularly important because it is impossible to palpate the myometrium thoroughly.

Case series (without controls) show the feasibility of laparoscopic surgery in women with large myomas. Of 144 women with a mean myoma diameter of 7.8 cm (largest myoma 18 cm), only 2 (1.4%) required conversion into laparotomy (40). Another study of 332 consecutive women undergoing laparoscopic myomectomy for myomas smaller than 15 cm, only 3 (0.9%) women required conversion into laparotomy (41).

The main published series of laparoscopic myomectomy show that this approach is mostly used for medium-sized myomas (about 5 cm) that are relatively few in number (one or two per patient) (42). In Dubuisson's opinion this procedure should not be attempted when more than two or three leiomyomas are present at ultrasound investigation for several reasons. First, the conversion rate increases with the number of leiomyomas (43). Second, operative time and difficulties increase with the number of leiomyomas, leading to strain on the surgeon. Third, when myomas are numerous, ultrasound investigation might underestimate the true number of leiomyomas. One of the authors (Parker) routinely performs MRI on all women for whom laparoscopic myomectomy is considered in order to better define position and sizes of the myomas and, ultimately, procedure feasibility.

Subserous and intramural leiomyomas are an indication for elective operative laparoscopic removal. Several studies suggest that laparoscopic myomectomy should only been performed for leiomyomas not exceeding 10 cm (42–45). Leiomyomas situated in the broad ligament or at the uterine isthmus can also be treated by operative laparoscopy, taking care not to damage the ureters and the uterine vessels. Although other physicians have far higher limits (up to 15 cm), difficulties may arise with increasing leiomyoma size for a number of reasons: the largest leiomyomas will have highly distended vessels due to compression by the leiomyoma; growth of certain leiomyomas results in reorganization of the myomatous tissues and neighboring myometrium, making the attachments of the myomas difficult to sever; the time required for laparoscopic myomectomy increases with size; and large leiomyomas can cause a lack of operating space (42,46–49). The upper size limit may also depend on other characteristics including the location and depth of penetration of the leiomyomas, the BMI of the patient, or the presence of pelvic adhesions (21).

Although removal of a entirely intracavitary leiomyoma must be performed by operative hysteroscopy when its diameter is less than 4–5 cm, cases with deep intramural leiomyoma with a submucosal component are difficult to treat by this method and may require repeat procedures (50,51). Cases of medium-sized (4–7 cm) leiomyomas involving the uterine cavity appear to be easy to treat by the laparoscopic approach, thus providing an interesting alternative to hysteroscopic resection (21). On the other hand, in cases where an entire submucous leiomyoma of small diameter (2–3 cm) is associated with other subserous or intramural leiomyomas, the submucous myoma is treated first by operative hysteroscopy. Since operative hysteroscopy distends the uterus, it may cause bleeding when performing hysterotomy and myoma enucleation.

An anterior location of the dominant leiomyoma may increase the technical difficulty and conversion rate (21,44). This may be explained by the fact that the anterior wall of the uterus is less accessible to the operating trocars when the leiomyoma is large. This is particularly evident for hemostasis and suturing. Compared to a midline or oblique incision, an anterior transverse uterine incision is easier to close with laparoscopic suturing.

Ideally, a curved needle should penetrate and traverse the myometrium perpendicularly to ensure accurate approximation, obliteration of dead space, and hemostasis.

OPERATIVE TECHNIQUE OF LAPAROSCOPIC MYOMECTOMY

The main complications of laparoscopic myomectomy, as with myomectomy by laparotomy, are the risks of perioperative bleeding and postoperative adhesion formation. The use of laparoscopic access to perform myomectomy heightens certain issues: hemostatic enucleation of the leiomyomas is absolutely essential to retain a clear view of the operative field to continue the procedure. As by laparotomy, a perfect suture should be achieved to obtain a good-quality scar. Therefore, the use of the technique of laparoscopic myomectomy is based on several basic principles:

1. The principles of atraumatic surgery and microsurgery must be applied to laparoscopic myomectomy to avoid adhesion formation as well as injury to other pelvic organs (e.g., ovary, tube, and bowel).
2. To help avoid intraoperative hemorrhage during enucleation and suturing of the hysterotomy, especially with hypervascularized leiomyomas, preventive vascular occlusion can be accomplished using a vascular clip applied to the uterine artery in the paravesical space. One or two uterine arteries may be providing the vascular supply to the myoma, according to the preoperative Doppler examination (52).
3. With laparoscopic myomectomy, it may not be possible to use the same incision to remove all the myomas as by laparotomy. Indeed, a long anterior sagittal hysterotomy may cause excessive bleeding and take too long to suture by laparoscopy.
4. Dissection must take place along the cleavage plane, separating the leiomyoma from the adjacent myometrium. This cleavage plane is bound by a pseudocapsule made up of compressed muscular fibers and diverted uterine vessels (34,49). This allows healthy adjacent myometrium to be preserved, and helps prevent damage to the perimyomatous vessels, which are often distended due to compression by the leiomyoma (48) and can be the origin of considerable bleeding.
5. Electrocoagulation must be used as sparingly as possible to achieve hemostasis at the edges of the uterine incision. Certain cases of uterine rupture during pregnancy have been reported after laparoscopic myomectomy (53–56) and after myolysis (57). Both suggest that the use of excess electrosurgery may induce significant thermal necrosis of the myometrium, resulting in a postoperative fistula or in a low-quality scar.
6. Suture of the myoma bed should always follow the same time-honored principles employed during laparotomy. Indeed, any technical deficiency when carrying this out may result in uterine rupture during a subsequent pregnancy (54). Other than for pedunculated myomas, myomectomy sites should always be sutured; case reports when no suturing was performed demonstrated that uterine scars were thin or noted to be dehiscing (20,47). One, two, or three layered-closure should be used to close all dead space and provide good hemostasis and to avoid hematoma formation (58–60). An intramyometrial hematoma can cause weakness in the scar and even a uterine-peritoneal fistula (47). To achieve these goals, consideration may be given to performing laparoscopic-assisted myomectomy (LAM). Laparoscopy is used to expose the myoma and begin or achieve enucleation, and then a mini-laparotomy is performed to suture the uterine defect(s) and remove the leiomyoma(s) (61,62).

Instrumentation

Certain instruments may be helpful for performing laparoscopic myomectomy. A monopolar needle or harmonic scalpel enables incision of the myometrium. Curved scissors can enable dissection between the leiomyoma and the myometrium. Needle holders, atraumatic forceps, and a knot-pusher are useful when intra- or extracorporeal suturing is performed. A strong grasping 10-mm tenaculum or claw forceps is useful for efficient traction during enucleation.

Ideally, an electric morcellation device (Steiner or the Rotocut, Karl Storz, Germany, or X-tract, Gynecare) allows large leiomyomas to be removed via a 12- or 15-mm port. Morcellators are easy to use after a learning phase and greatly reduce operative times (63).

Preparation

The patient lies with thighs spread, with abduction providing access to the vagina and buttocks protruding generously over the edge of the table in order to be able to manipulate the uterus with an intrauterine cannula. The main surgeon stands to the patient's side (left or right), with the first assistant opposite and the second assistant, if present, between the patient's legs.

In infertile patients with no previous tubal investigation, the injection of diluted methylene blue into the uterine cavity is useful to confirm tubal patency and enable the endometrium to be identified if entered during surgery. A uterine manipulator is placed, allowing uterine anteversion, retroversion, and also rotation during the operation.

Description of the Operative Technique: Laparoscopic Myomectomy

The technique of laparoscopic myomectomy comprises four main phases: uterine incision and visualization of the pseudocapsule of the leiomyoma, enucleation, hemostasis and suturing of the myomectomy site, and extraction of the leiomyoma (52,64,65). Surgical technique may vary among surgeons.

Laparoscopy can be performed transumbilically, supraumbilically, or via the left upper quadrant, depending on the uterine size. Two 5-mm lateral trocars and one 12-mm midline trocar are inserted in the suprapubic position. Alternatively, two trocars may be placed laterally, the first just medial to the iliac crest and the second about 4 cm cephalad to the first (WHP). This allows an ergonomic approach to laparoscopic suturing (53). Generally, the two lateral trocars should be placed high and outside the epigastric vessels so that good access is provided for leiomyomas in various locations and it is ensured that the surgeon has sufficient operating space for movement when performing enucleation or suturing.

Uterine Incision

The uterine incision is lined up over the leiomyoma in the case of a posterior leiomyoma, some surgeons use a sagittal uterine incision and, in the case of an anterior myoma, may utilize oblique and transverse uterine incisions because these are easier to suture. Ultimately, the direction of the uterine incision depends on the available access to the myoma. Transverse incisions run parallel to the arcuate vessels and may decrease blood loss. The myometrium is incised with a laparoscopic needle using unmodulated monopolar current in cut mode or a harmonic scalpel in order to safeguard the myometrium as far as possible (Fig. 1). Hemostasis is carried out as needed using bipolar forceps. The leiomyoma is easy to recognize by its smooth appearance and pearly white color, which contrasts with the adjacent myometrium. It is important to incise the myometrium, often into the myoma, to identify the pseudocapsule, as dissection in the proper avascular plane decreases blood loss.

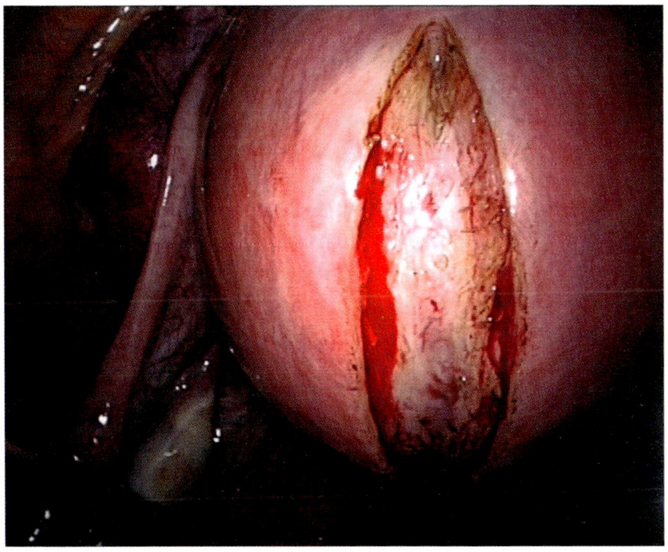

Figure 1 Uterine incision performed with a monopolar laparoscopic needle.

Enucleation

Dissection of the leiomyoma should continue within the avascular plane. Identification of this avascular plane is assisted by the magnifying effect of the laparoscopic images (Figs. 2–4). The leiomyoma is grasped with a strong 10-mm claw or tenaculum, and traction is applied as needed toward the anterior abdominal wall or cephalad, while the surgeon or the assistant exerts countertraction with the uterine manipulator or with an instrument applied to the myometrial edges. Dissection proceeds from the superficial areas inward under visual control in order to identify the tissue adhering to the leiomyoma. The tip of a blunt instrument may be used to press against the leiomyoma. Tissues adhering to the leiomyoma are desiccated and then divided. The bed of the myomectomy is often free from hemorrhage if care has been taken to follow the avascular cleavage plane (Fig. 5). Bipolar desiccation may be used, if necessary (Fig. 6).

Suturing the Uterine Defect

Delayed absorbable sutures, 00 or 0 gauge, mounted on a curved needle with an atraumatic tip (Vicryl, Polyglactine 910, Ethicon®) are placed in one, two, or three layers, as needed, adhering to surgical technique during laparotomy.

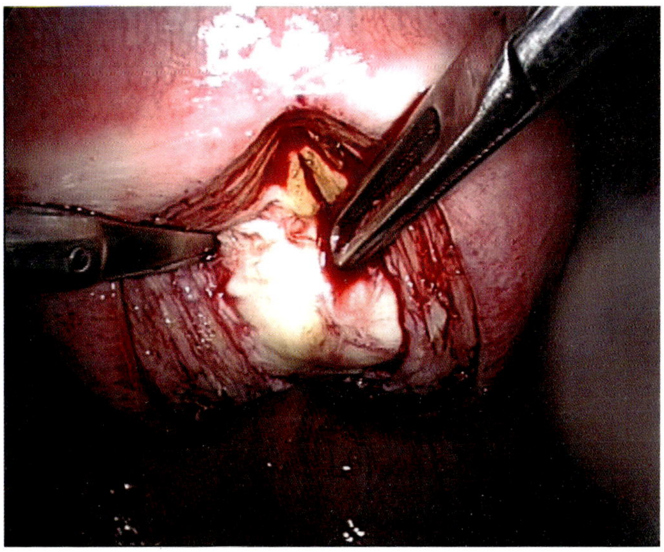

Figure 2 Laparoscopic uterine incision to expose the leiomyoma.

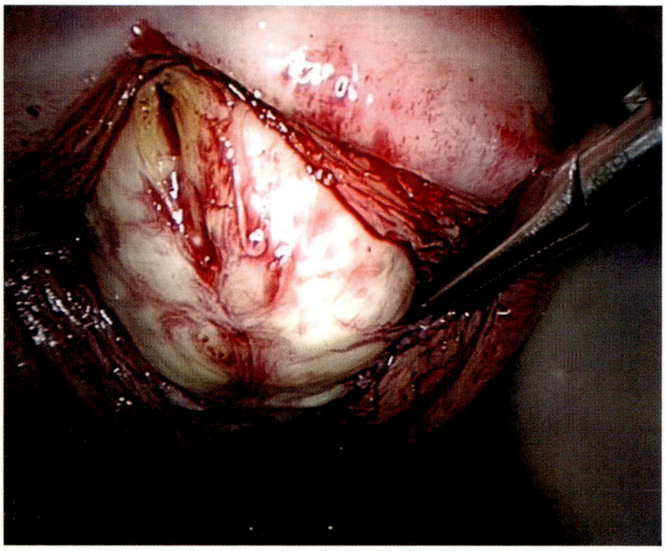

Figure 3 Enucleation of the leiomyoma during laparoscopy.

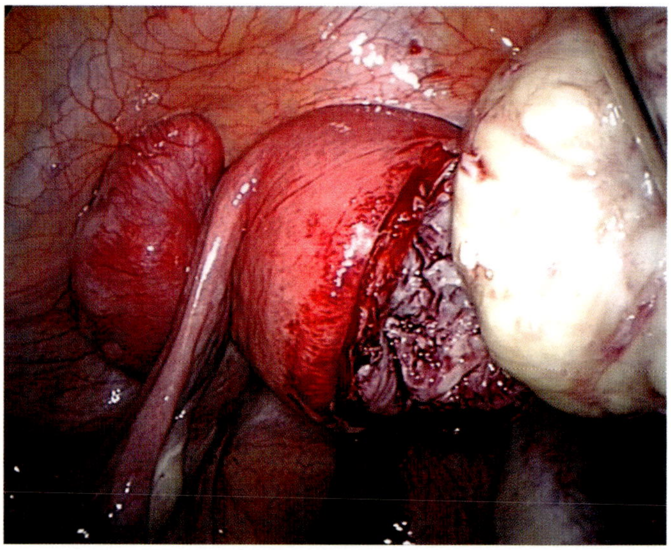

Figure 5 Precise dissection avoids opening the uterine cavity.

For subserosal leiomyomas, a one-layered closure of interrupted sutures tied with intracorporeal knots, placed through the whole thickness of the myometrium and serosa, may be used. Sutures should be placed sufficiently close for the edges to be approximated completely, yet far enough apart to avoid weakening the myometrium.

When the incision is deep into the myometrium, or the uterine cavity has been entered, the defect should be closed in two or three layers (Figs. 7 and 8). The serosal layer may be closed using either a running or an interrupted suture. When suturing the deep plane, it may sometimes be difficult to pass the needle through the thickness of the defect. In this case, it can be an advantage to use Vicryl-1 with a large curved needle and to perform a U-shaped transfixing stitch, running through the uterine serosa and the whole thickness of the edges of the incision (42). One or two of these stitches are sufficient to ensure that all the deep part of the hysterotomy is brought into contact. When the uterine suture proves difficult to carry out, as may be the case with large anterior or deep intramural leiomyomas, mini-laparotomy can be considered.

Extraction of the Leiomyomas

Various methods are available for the extraction of myomas, including direct abdominal extraction, extraction via posterior colpotomy, or electromechanical morcellation.

Direct extraction of small leiomyomas may be performed through an ancillary incision (suprapubic), which may be enlarged if needed. Alternatively, morcellation may be carried out by bringing the leiomyoma up to the incision, holding it against the peritoneum to prevent loss of CO_2 and then fragmenting it with a small blade under laparoscopic control.

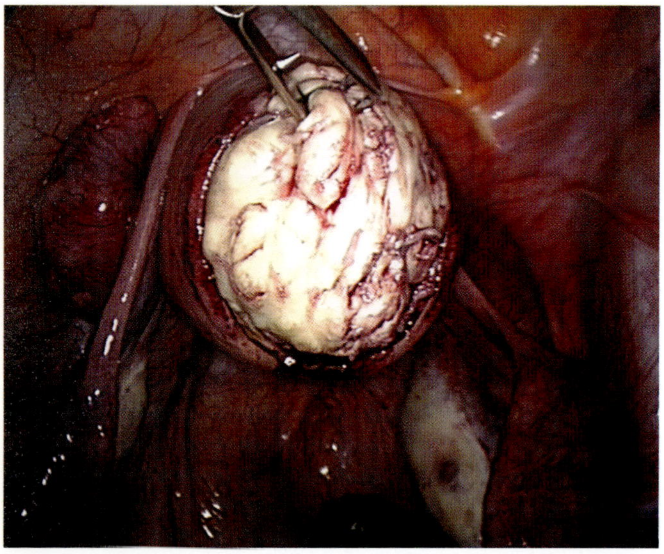

Figure 4 End of enucleation of the leiomyoma using a strong 10 mm tenaculum.

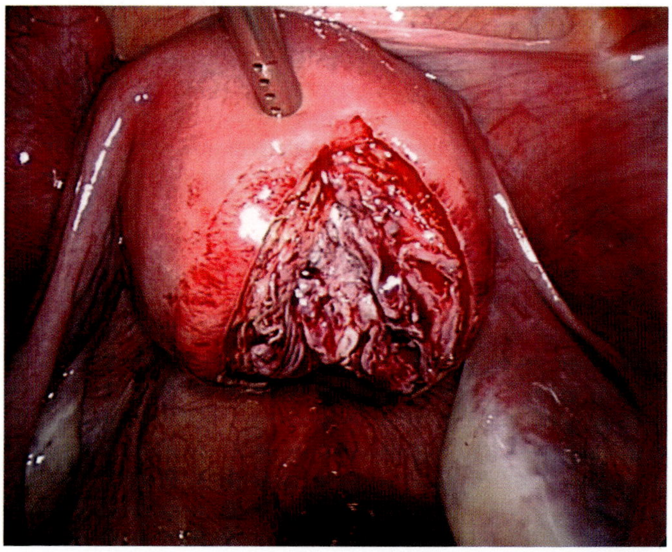

Figure 6 Hemostasis of uterine bed and incision.

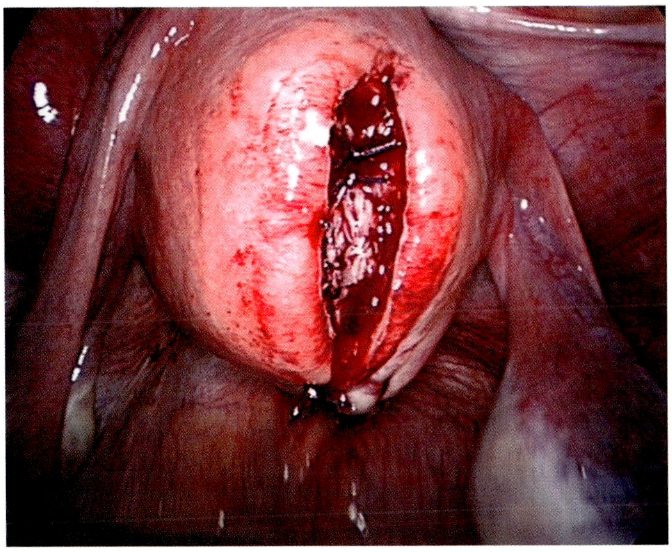

Figure 7 Laparoscopic closure of the myometrium (first layer).

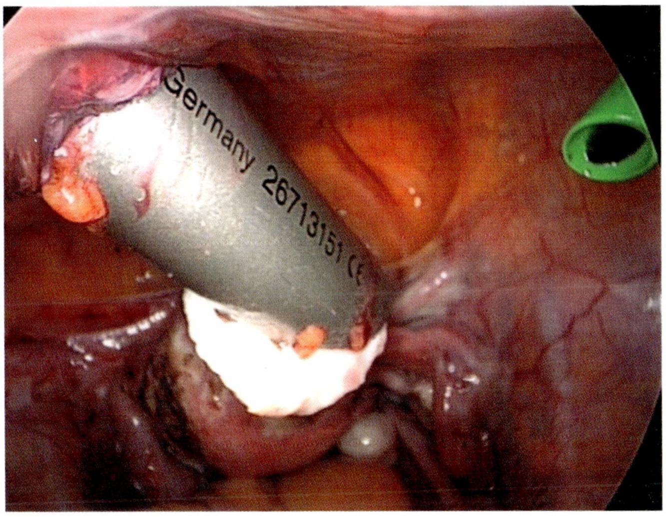

Figure 9 Electricomechanical morcellation of leiomyoma.

Posterior colpotomy also allows large leiomyomas to be extracted (63). The colpotomy incision may be performed laparoscopically or through the vagina. The leiomyoma is grasped through the colpotomy under laparoscopic control and extracted directly or after morcellation. In the case of large or numerous myomas, the C.C.L. Vaginal Extractor (Karl Storz, Germany) is useful to prevent leakage of gas.

Electromechanical morcellation is carried out using a rotating cylindrical blade introduced via a 12- or 15-mm port (Fig. 9). A 10-mm forceps or tenaculum is inserted through the morcellator channel to grasp the leiomyoma and pull it into the rotating blade, which will morcellate it like peeling an orange. The position of the rotating blade must be carefully controlled in order to avoid any risk of damaging any neighboring organs. Morcellation is best accomplished in the anterior midpelvis. The rotating blade should always be in view to avoid inadvertent injury to nearby structures.

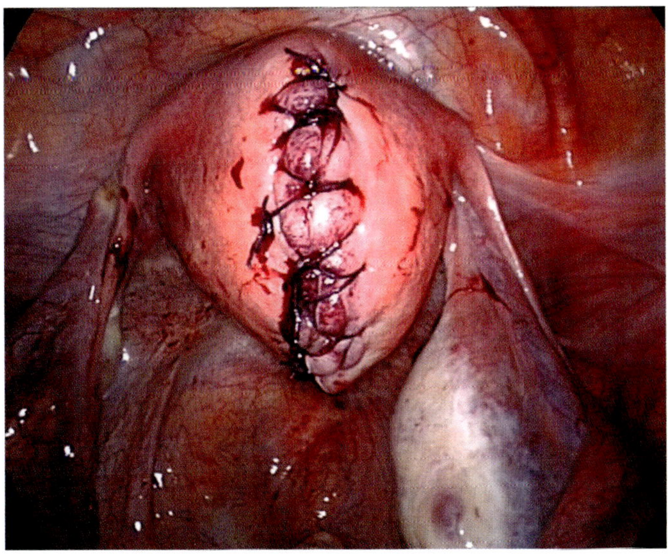

Figure 8 Closure of the myometrium (superficial layer).

Preventive Uterine Artery Occlusion Combined with Laparoscopic Myomectomy

In highly vascular leiomyomas, it is important to limit blood loss during leiomyoma enucleation and myometrium suture. Before 2001, in some cases of excessive bleeding during laparoscopic myomectomy, occlusion of one or two uterine arteries during the procedure was one of the only methods to prophylactically prevent uterine bleeding. A comparative study was completed in order to demonstrate the advantages of this adjunctive procedure (52). Typically, the uterine artery occlusion is performed at the beginning of laparoscopy (on one or both sides) if a highly vascular leiomyoma of more than 6 cm is suspected by Doppler ultrasonography. This procedure is not indicated when the leiomyoma is poorly vascularized or has a typical aspect of degeneration at ultrasonography, MRI, or laparoscopy. Furthermore, it is not helpful when the leiomyoma is exclusively vascularized by the ovarian vessels. Moreover, this procedure is not feasible when the leiomyoma is very large and fixed, preventing access to the uterine arteries before the myomectomy. Uterine artery occlusion is performed using the following technique:

1. Broad ligament access of the uterine artery: Before myomectomy, a 3-cm incision along the peritoneum, with scissors, on the upper part of the broad ligament, behind the round ligament. The umbilical artery is then dissected free within the perivesical space and followed to the origin of the uterine artery. The origin of the uterine artery is then dissected from the uterine veins. Medial to the artery, the ureter is also visualized, adherent to the peritoneum. To occlude the artery, one or two nonabsorbable clips (titanium Ligaclip, Karl Storz) placed at its origin. Hemostasis of small vessels is performed as necessary. A few minutes after the occlusion, the leiomyoma turns white, before the uterus itself. At the end of the laparoscopic myomectomy, the peritoneum of the broad ligament is closed using a 00-Vicryl running suture. The same procedure is performed on the other broad ligament if necessary. Then the uterine incision is performed.

2. Posterior access of the uterine artery: The occlusion of the uterine artery may be performed using a posterior access. The uterus is pulled hard toward the anterior abdominal wall using the intrauterine cannula. On the chosen side, the uterine artery is visualized under the peritoneum at the inferior area of the posterior leaf of the broad ligament, close to the uterus, just above the origin of the ipsilateral uterosacral ligament. The ureter is also visualized under the pulsating artery. A 1-cm incision of the peritoneum gives immediate access to the uterine artery. One or two clips are then placed, away from the ureter. This second procedure is quick and easy to perform if this access is possible. The peritoneum is then closed with a 00-Vicryl single suture.

ROBOTICALLY-ASSISTED MYOMECTOMY

More recently, robot-assisted technology has been integrated into minimally invasive gynecologic surgery. Much of this experience revolves around the da Vinci surgical system, which was approved by the Food and Drug Administration for gynecologic applications in April 2005. Putative advantages of the robotic approach are the improved dexterity and precision of the instruments coupled with three-dimensional imaging. Limitations include the absence of haptic (tactile) feedback, bulkiness of the system, lack of vaginal access, and cost (66). Using a retrospective case-matched analysis of 58 patients, Advincula et al. compared the surgical outcomes of myomectomy by robot-assisted laparoscopy with those performed by more traditional laparotomy including financial impact (67). Patients with robot-assisted laparoscopic myomectomy had decreased estimated blood loss and length of stay when compared with the laparotomy group. Operative times were significantly longer in the robotic group whereas complication rates were higher in the laparotomy group. Professional and hospital charges were statistically higher for the robotic group. Nezhat et al. similarly compared 15 consecutive laparoscopic robotic-assisted myomectomy to a matched control group of 35 having undergone standard laparoscopic myomectomy. Whereas surgical time was longer for the robotic-assisted group, blood loss, hospitalization time, and postoperative complications were not significantly different. These authors concluded that in the hands of a skilled laparoscopic surgeon, robotic-assisted laparoscopic myomectomy does not offer any major advantage (68).

OPERATIVE TECHNIQUE OF ABDOMINAL MYOMECTOMY FOR LARGE MYOMAS

A Pfannenstiel incision can be used in all patients, and the linea alba should be dissected to the umbilicus to allow adequate exposure and delivery of the uterine fundus. If the uterus cannot be delivered, accessible lower uterine segment myomas should be removed first, which will allow access to fundal myomas (38). A small amount of dilute Pitressin (20 U/60 to 100 mL normal saline) is injected deep into each myoma using an 18-gauge spinal or laparoscopic needle. Approximately 5 mL of Pitressin is injected slowly while the patient is observed for evidence of bradycardia and hypertension. If no change in blood pressure or pulse is observed, additional Pitressin can be injected by always aspirating for blood before injection.

Uterine incisions are made transversely in order to avoid the arcuate vessels and are carried through the uterine serosa, myometrium, and entire pseudocapsule using a needle-point electrode. The myoma is grasped with a tenaculum, and the overlying myometrium and pseudocapsule are bluntly wiped down and off of the myoma. Only myomas near each incision are removed, and tunneling through the myometrium is avoided to provide good hemostasis and full repair of the defect. Each uterine incision is promptly closed in multiple layers of running 0-Vicryl suture. Heparin 5000 U in 1000 mL normal saline can be used as an irrigating solution to help prevent blood clotting and allow red blood cell salvage for processing by the cell saver (Haemmetics, Braintree, Massachusetts) if this is used. The serosa can be covered with an adhesion barrier such as Seprafilm (Genzyme, Cambridge, Massachusetts). The results of this technique have been reported to be excellent (16).

RESULTS

Conversion Rates and Operative Time for Laparoscopic Myomectomy

The percentage of conversions into laparotomy reported in retrospective studies varies from 0% to 41% (40,42). Case series without controls show the feasibility of laparoscopic surgery in women with large myomas. In a series of 144 women with the largest myoma up to 18 cm (mean = 7.8 cm.), only two (1.4%) required conversion into laparotomy (40). Of 332 consecutive women undergoing laparoscopic myomectomy for symptomatic myomas smaller than 15 cm, only 3 (0.9%) women required conversion into laparotomy (41).

In one group's experience with 426 laparoscopic myomectomies, the rate of conversion into an open procedure (either laparotomy or LAM) was 11.3%. Several independent factors were found to increase the risk of conversion: size of the dominant leiomyoma at ultrasonography, anterior location, intramural type, or preoperative use of GnRH agonists (21). The difficulties associated with identifying the cleavage plane after GnRH use, which can cause degeneration of the myoma, and/or the presence of an adenomyoma or associated adenomyosis makes laparoscopic myomectomy more difficult (44). In one study (43), where the use of laparoscopic myomectomy was not restricted to cases with a low number of leiomyomas, the conversion rate was found to increase with the number of leiomyomas. Some women may require conversion into laparotomy due to the presence of severe pelvic adhesions and/or severe undiagnosed adenomyosis (45).

The mean operative time is about two hours for the main series published (42). Two controlled studies comparing laparoscopic myomectomy with myomectomy by laparotomy found an increase in the operative time when the procedure was carried out by the laparoscopic route (69,70). The size and depth of penetration in the myometrium of the dominant leiomyoma are the most important parameters to consider. In the case of large and deeply infiltrating leiomyomas, the operating time will increase with enucleation, suturing, and morcellation. The surgeon must also take into account his/her own experience. The initial occlusion of one or two uterine arteries before the uterine incision, in the case of a highly vascularized leiomyoma, may limit the risk of conversion.

Risk of Hemorrhage

Myomectomy has the reputation of being associated with operative blood loss. However, in two randomized controlled studies, laparoscopic myomectomy was associated with a significant reduction in the drop of the hemoglobin level compared to those who had a myomectomy by laparotomy (69,71). The laparoscopic route presents two theoretical advantages over laparotomy: the pressure of the pneumoperitoneum may decrease blood extravasation from the intramyometrial capillaries and veins and the magnification provided by the laparoscope helps to identify the cleavage plane more precisely and enables selective coagulation of the small vessels feeding the leiomyoma.

Meticulous, preventive coagulation of the tissue connecting the leiomyoma to the adjacent myometrium must be carried out (44). One author (60) has proposed a technique for temporary hemostasis that can be used with laparoscopy (compression of the uterine pedicles at the isthmus, using a broad, single strand suture). Infiltration of the myometrium adjacent to the myoma with appropriately diluted vasoconstrictive agents (vasopressin derivatives) is very useful for limiting the bleeding (72). These agents may be used in the smallest effective dose after approval of the anesthesiologist.

Postoperative Course

Two randomized clinical trials have demonstrated that laparoscopic myomectomy has proven advantages compared to abdominal approach in terms of postoperative course. Laparoscopic approach may offer the benefits of lower postoperative pain and shorter recovery time in comparison with laparotomy (71). It also reduces hospital stay and transient episode of febrile morbidity (69).

Complication rates, in experienced hands, are not higher with laparoscopic myomectomy. Among 40 women randomized to abdominal and laparoscopic myomectomy for subserosal and intramural myomas smaller than 6 cm, estimated blood loss and surgical times were similar and there were no major complications in either group (71). A study (69) of 131 women randomized to abdominal and laparoscopic myomectomy for nonpedunculated myomas larger than 5 cm (mean = 7 cm) found significantly higher postoperative hemoglobin, lower incidence of postoperative fever, and shorter hospital stays with laparoscopic myomectomy.

Postoperative Adhesions

There are several arguments suggesting that the laparoscopic approach reduces the risk of postoperative adhesions after myomectomy. Laparoscopic surgery can be performed respecting the principles of microsurgery including atraumatic manipulation, fine instruments, and thorough irrigation. In a nonrandomized cohort study, Bulletti and colleagues (73) found a statistically significant decrease in the degree of postoperative adhesions and the proportion of patients with adhesions associated with the use of the laparoscopic route. Furthermore, in the retrospective studies with a systematic laparoscopic second look after myomectomy, the percentages of patients presenting adhesions after laparoscopic myomectomy are 51.1% and 89.6% after laparotomy. The proportions of patients presenting adnexal adhesions connected to the myomectomy are 30.5% after laparoscopic myomectomy and 68.9% after laparotomy (42).

Adhesion barriers may also be considered to decrease the rate of adhesion formation. A Cochrane review found that Interceed® (Ethicon) reduced the incidence of adhesion formation, both de novo and re-formation, at both laparoscopy and laparotomy. However, there were insufficient data to support its use to improve pregnancy rates (74). In one study, Interceed was placed following laparoscopic myomectomy in 25 women, and at second-look laparoscopy, 60% of the women had no adhesions found, compared to 25 women who did not have Interceed placed, and only 12% were adhesion free (75). In a recent study (76), 63 women having an abdominal myomectomy were randomized to intraoperative use of Seprafilm, Dextran, factor 13 with fibrinogen, and a control group. At second-look laparoscopy one week later, uterine adhesions were found in 14% of women treated with Seprafilm, 70% treated with Dextran, 75% treated with factor13/fibrinogen, and 69% in the control group.

Second-look laparoscopy, two or three months after laparoscopic myomectomy, may be considered for patients desiring pregnancy and who have sutured uterine scars, in order to remove adhesions after myomectomy and to assess the appearance of the uterine scar using a methylene blue test (77–79). Systematic use of second-look laparoscopy could reduce adhesions after myomectomy and possibly enhance fertility (80,81).

Obstetric Quality of Laparoscopic Myomectomy Scars

There is considerable debate concerning the strength of uterine scars after laparoscopic myomectomy (82). To date, 11 reports of uterine rupture following laparoscopic myomectomy have been published (54–56,83,84). All these cases of rupture occurred after small (3–5 cm), single myomas were removed, and quite remarkably they took place before labor actually began. However, it is difficult to draw any definite conclusions from these cases because it is not known how frequently this accident occurs; the cases are reported in isolation, without any indication of the number of normal pregnancies and deliveries occurring after laparoscopic myomectomy.

Between 1989 and 1996, the risk of uterine rupture, specifically due to laparoscopic myomectomy, was reported as 1.0% (95% CI: 0.0–5.5) among 100 deliveries after laparoscopic myomectomy (79). Recently, a spontaneous uterine rupture occurred at 33 weeks subsequent to previous superficial laparoscopic myomectomy (85). This publication confirms that it is difficult to evaluate the risk of uterine risk of rupture. To date, seven other teams have reported on pregnancies after laparoscopic myomectomy and none has observed any uterine rupture (19,57,86–89). It is difficult to say whether this risk is greater than that after myomectomy by laparotomy.

Uterine rupture during pregnancy or delivery as a consequence of abdominal myomectomy appears to be extremely rare. A report of 98,872 deliveries over 30 years found 76 cases of uterine rupture in the third trimester, but only one of these cases of rupture followed myomectomy, while 16 of the women had no prior uterine incisions (90). Another study of 137,582 pregnancies found 133 cases of uterine rupture after the 28th week of pregnancy, of which 3 followed abdominal myomectomies (91). In these two studies, the number of women who had a previous myomectomy is not known, so the incidence of rupture cannot be calculated.

However, the largest series are old and the rate of cases lost to follow-up is not specified. Furthermore, observations of uterine ruptures after laparotomy have been reported regularly in the literature (91,92). Finally, in a retrospective study made in the Trinidad maternity hospital, the rate of rupture observed during labor after myomectomy by laparotomy was 4.4% (95% CI: 0.5–14.8) (93). All these elements suggest, in fact, that the risk of rupture after myomectomy by laparotomy is underestimated. In the randomized clinical trial of Seracchioli and colleagues (69), 27 women in the laparotomic group and 20 women in the laparoscopic myomectomy group had deliveries after myomectomy. There was no uterine rupture in either group. However, comparative studies covering a larger number of cases are still needed to see if the risk of rupture differs according to the approach.

At present, we consider that this risk is low and that it should not prevent laparoscopic approach being used when the myomectomy is needed. However, when performing laparoscopic myomectomy, particular care must be given to proper uterine closure (see Suturing the Uterine Defect). Indeed, proper closure requires experience in laparoscopic suturing and laparoscopic surgical techniques.

Uterine Artery Occlusion and Pregnancy

The combined procedure of uterine artery occlusion and laparoscopic myomectomy influences the vascularization of the myometrium. In a study using a contrast-enhanced MR scan, Katsumori et al. have shown that myometrial perfusion was normal at one, two, three, four, and six months and a year after uterine artery embolization (UAE) (94). In a recent paper, Holub et al. published 15 pregnancies with normal infant weights after UAE (95). These publications confirm our preliminary results concerning patients treated with laparoscopic myomectomy and bilateral uterine artery occlusion: normal postoperative Doppler color of the uterus and normal infant weights at delivery (Dubuisson JB, 2003, unpublished data).

Persistence or New Appearance of Myomas

Myomas detected after myomectomy, often referred to as recurrence, either are the result of persistence of myomas left at the time of surgery or are newly developed myomas. Although new myomas may grow following myomectomy, most women will not require additional treatment. A study of 125 women followed after abdominal myomectomy reported that a second surgery was required during the follow-up period (average 7.6 years; range = 5–10 years) for 11.1% of women who had one myoma removed initially and for 26.3% of women who had multiple myomas removed (96). Crude rates of hysterectomy after myomectomy vary from 4.3% to 16.8% over five years (97,98).

Only one study has been devoted specifically to the risk of recurrence after laparoscopic myomectomy (99). The cumulative rate at five years (51%) is higher than those observed in the series of myomectomy by laparotomy and the time lapse before recurrence is shorter (35,100,101). However, 81 women randomized to either laparoscopic or abdominal myomectomy were followed with transvaginal sonography every 6 months for at least 40 months (102). Myomas larger than 1 cm were found in 27% of women following laparoscopic myomectomy compared to 23% in the abdominal myomectomy group. However, no woman in either group required reoperation or other intervention.

With the laparoscopic route, it is impossible to palpate the myometrium thoroughly and small intramural nuclei that do not deform the uterine serosa can be overlooked, resulting in incomplete removal more often than with laparotomy. If these results are confirmed, then considerable caution should be exercised before using the laparoscopic route for multiple leiomyomas. MRI is an excellent method of detecting even small myomas prior to the planned laparoscopic myomectomy and may help determine the feasibility of removing all myomas.

Laparoscopic myomectomy is a safe technique that has several advantages, including lower postoperative pain, shorter recovery time, and a lower rate of postoperative adhesions in comparison with laparotomy. However, it is a difficult operation and the surgeon requires to be well experienced in laparoscopic surgery. Because of increasing difficulties during laparoscopic myomectomy, it is essential to respect limits. We recommend the following:

1. Preoperative evaluation of the leiomyomas should be meticulous and requires ultrasound and hysteroscopic examination. MRI should be considered if the evaluation is unsatisfactory despite the preceding examinations.
2. The preoperative blood count should be assessed, and sideropenic anemia should be corrected.
3. High-frequency electrosurgical generators and monopolar needles or harmonic scalpels should be used to limit destruction of normal myometrium.
4. Particular care must be taken when suturing the uterus to prevent bleeding and weakening of the myometrium;
5. An electric morcellator should be employed for the extraction of large leiomyomas.

Hysterectomy

Women with severe symptoms who have not been helped by other treatments may benefit from hysterectomy. Following hysterectomy, the Maine Women's Health Study reported that 72% of women felt "much better" and another 16% felt a "little better" than they did before surgery (15).

Alternative modes of surgical therapy such as endometrial ablation; hysteroscopic, laparoscopic, or abdominal myomectomy; UAE; or focused ultrasound were not used in this study. As these procedures become more available to women, the need for hysterectomy should decrease.

Laparoscopic Hysterectomy

Total or supracervical laparoscopic hysterectomy is often feasible for women with uterine myomas. However, if a vaginal hysterectomy is technically feasible for a patient, there is no benefit to laparoscopic hysterectomy. A prospective, randomized study of women with a mobile uterus less than 16 weeks size compared outpatient laparoscopy-assisted vaginal hysterectomy with vaginal hysterectomy (103). Although laparoscopy-assisted vaginal hysterectomy took approximately 55 minutes longer, the outcomes of the two groups were otherwise comparable. Other studies have confirmed these findings (104).

A prospective, randomized study of 80 women with uterine size between 280 and 700 g concluded that laparoscopic-assisted hysterectomy offered the benefits of less invasive surgery without increased risk (105). Laparoscopy-assisted vaginal hysterectomies were compared with abdominal hysterectomies. Estimated blood loss, postoperative day 1 hemoglobin, postoperative pain, and postoperative hospital stay were all significantly better for the laparoscopy-assisted hysterectomy group. Seven complications occurred in the abdominal hysterectomy group including a cuff hematoma, delayed bleeding requiring reoperation, and five women with fever compared with fever in two women in the laparoscopic group.

In experienced hands, the benefits of laparoscopic hysterectomy may also be extended to women who have large myomas. Outcomes of laparoscopic hysterectomy for 34 women with uterine weights greater than 500 g (range = 500–1230 g) were compared with 68 women with uterine weights less than 300 g (106). No difference in complications rates, blood loss, hospital stay, or postoperative recovery was found, but operating times were shorter in women with smaller uteri. No woman required conversion into laparotomy.

UTERINE ARTERY EMBOLIZATION

While the effects of UAE on premature ovarian failure, fertility, and pregnancy are unclear, UAE is an effective treatment for some women with uterine myomas.

Percutaneous cannulation of the femoral artery is performed and gelatin sponges, polyvinyl alcohol particles, or tris-acryl gelatin microspheres are injected to embolize the uterine artery.

Women usually spend one night in the hospital for pain management and take nonsteroidal anti-inflammatory medications for one to two weeks, although about 10% of women have pain for longer time. Postembolization syndrome occurs in about 10% of women. Symptoms include diffuse abdominal pain, nausea, vomiting, low-grade fever, malaise, anorexia, and leukocytosis, and these women require readmission to the hospital. Persistent fever should be managed with antibiotics. Failure to respond to antibiotics may indicate sepsis and should be managed with hysterectomy.

The largest prospective study of UAE included 555 women, aged 18 to 59 years, and found that menorrhagia improved in 83%, dysmenorrhea improved in 77%, and urinary frequency in 86% of women (7). Volume reduction of the largest fibroid was 33% at three months, but improvement in menorrhagia was not related to preprocedural uterine volume. Eight women required hysterectomy: two for infection, four for persistent postembolization pain, one for a prolapsed myoma, and one for continued vaginal bleeding. Also, 41% of women older than 50 years had amenorrhea, although only 3% percent of women younger than 40 years had amenorrhea.

Potential fertility following UAE is uncertain, since an analysis of women actively attempting and achieving pregnancy following UAE has not been performed. Nor have fertility rates following UAE been compared with rates following myomectomy or with that in untreated women with similar myomas. Nevertheless, pregnancies have been reported following UAE. Of 34 pregnancies subsequent to UAE, 32% of women had a spontaneous abortion (107). In a report of 164 women desiring future fertility prior to UAE, 21 women achieved pregnancy, 4 (19%) had a spontaneous abortion, 2 had elective terminations, and 18 had live births during 24 months of follow-up (108). For women achieving pregnancy, one study reported that 6% had postpartum hemorrhage, 16% had premature delivery, and 11% had malpresentation (7,108). Another study reported eight term and six preterm deliveries, but two women had placenta previa and one woman had a membranous placenta.

Uterine Artery Occlusion

Alternatives methods of uterine artery occlusion have been developed, both more and less invasive than UAE, including laparoscopic uterine artery occlusion and nonincisional transvaginal uterine artery occlusion. Laparoscopic occlusion has similar short-term results as UAE but requires general anesthesia, is invasive, and requires a skilled laparoscopic surgeon. Transvaginal occlusion is performed by placing a specially designed clamp in the vaginal fornices and, guided by Doppler ultrasound auditory signals, is positioned to occlude the uterine arteries. The clamp is left in place for six hours and then removed. Results are preliminary, but this technique may develop into an alternative, noninvasive method to decrease myoma size (109).

Considerations for Management of Uterine Myomas

Treatment options will depend on the primary symptoms, wishes regarding future fertility, and wishes of the patient. Multiple treatment options often exist, and the following points might be considered.

Asymptomatic Women

For asymptomatic women who desire future fertility, evaluation of the uterine cavity with saline-infusion sonography, hysteroscopy, or MRI provides useful information regarding the possible impact of myomas on fertility. If the cavity is not deformed, myomas need not be treated and conception may be attempted. If the cavity is deformed, myomectomy (hysteroscopic or abdominal) can be considered. Laparoscopic myomectomy may be offered by experienced laparoscopic surgeons with the ability to perform multilayered myometrial closures.

For an asymptomatic woman who does not desire future fertility, observation (watchful waiting) should be considered. If there is concern that the uterus may be near the ureter(s) at the pelvic sidewall, renal ultrasound or IVP should be considered to rule out significant hydronephrosis.

Bleeding as the Primary Symptom

For women who have heavy uterine bleeding and desire future fertility, evaluation of the uterine cavity with saline-infusion sonography, hysteroscopy, or MRI can help determine the appropriate treatment. In submucous fibroids are present, hysteroscopic excision should be carried out. If the cavity is deformed, myomectomy (hysteroscopic or abdominal) should be considered. Laparoscopic myomectomy may be offered by experienced laparoscopic surgeons.

For women with heavy bleeding not desiring future fertility, a levonorgestrel-IUS or hysteroscopic myomectomy and/or endometrial ablation may be appropriate. Hysterectomy (vaginal, laparoscopic, or abdominal) or UAE can be considered. Women choosing hysterectomy and who are not at high risk of ovarian cancer should consider ovarian conservation (110).

Pain or Pressure as Primary Symptom

If the symptoms of pain or pressure (bulk symptoms) are bothersome and future fertility is desired, abdominal myomectomy should be considered. Laparoscopic myomectomy may be offered by experienced laparoscopic surgeons.

For women who do not desire future fertility, observation (watchful waiting) can be considered if no treatment is desired at the time. Perimenopausal women may wish observation until menopause when symptoms usually diminish. If treatment is desired, myomectomy, hysterectomy, UAE, or focused ultrasound (presently limited by size and number of myomas) may be considered. Symptoms suggestive of uterine sarcoma (irregular bleeding, pelvic pain, and uterine growth) can be evaluated with MRI-Gd and LDH (111).

REFERENCES

1. Farrer-Brown G, Beilby JO, Tarbit MH, et al. The vascular patterns in myomatous uteri. J Obstet Gynaecol Br Commonw 1970; 77(11):967–975.
2. Farrer-Brown G, Beilby JO, Tarbit MH, et al. Venous changes in the endometrium of myomatous uteri. Obstet Gynecol 1971, 38(5):743–751.

3. Munro MG, Lukes AS. Abnormal uterine bleeding and underlying hemostatic disorders: Report of a consensus process. Fertil Steril 2005; 84(5):1335–1337.
4. Marino JL, Eskenazi B, Warner M, et al. Uterine leiomyoma and menstrual cycle characteristics in a population-based cohort study. Hum Reprod 2004; 19:2350–2355.
5. Wegienka G, Baird DD, Hertz-Picciotto I, et al. Self-reported heavy bleeding associated with uterine leiomyomata. Obstet Gynecol 2003; 101:431–437.
6. Lippman SA, Warner M, Samuels S, et al. Uterine fibroids and gynecologic pain symptoms in a population-based study. Fertil Steril 2003; 80:1488–1494.
7. Pron G, Bennett J, Common A, et al. The Ontario uterine fibroid embolization trial. Part 2. Uterine fibroid reduction and symptom relief after uterine artery embolization for fibroids. Fertil Steril 2003; 79:120–127.
8. Cantuaria GH, Angioli R, Frost L, et al. Comparison of bimanual examination with ultrasound examination before hysterectomy for uterine leiomyoma. Obstet Gynecol 1998; 92:109–112.
9. Dueholm M, Lundorf E, Hansen ES, et al. Accuracy of magnetic resonance imaging and transvaginal ultrasonography in the diagnosis, mapping, and measurement of uterine myomas. Am J Obstet Gynecol 2002; 188:409–415.
10. Dueholm M, Lundorf E, Hansen ES, et al. Evaluation of the uterine cavity with magnetic resonance imaging, transvaginal sonography, hysterosonographic examination, and diagnostic hysteroscopy. Fertil Steril 2001; 76:350–357.
11. Dueholm M, Lundorf E, Hansen ES, et al. Magnetic resonance imaging and transvaginal ultrasonography for the diagnosis of adenomyosis. Fertil Steril 2001; 76:588–594.
12. Pritts EA. Fibroids and infertility: A systematic review of the evidence. Obstet Gynecol Surv 2001; 56:483–491.
13. Vergani P, Ghidini A, Strobelt N, et al. Do uterine leiomyomas influence pregnancy outcome? Am J Perinatol 1994; 11:356–358.
14. Qidwai GI, Caughey AB, Jacoby AF. Obstetric outcomes in women with sonographically identified uterine leiomyomata. Obstet Gynecol 2006; 107:376–382.
15. Carlson KJ, Miller BA, Fowler FJ Jr. The Maine Women's Health Study: II. Outcomes of nonsurgical management of leiomyomas, abnormal bleeding, and chronic pelvic pain. Obstet Gynecol 1994; 83:566–572.
16. Davids A. Myomectomy: Surgical technique and results in series of 1150 cases. Am J Obstet Gynecol 1952; 63:592–604.
17. Daniell JF, Gurley LD. Laparoscopic treatment of clinically significant symptomatic uterine fibroids. J Gynecol Surg 1991; 7:37–39.
18. Dubuisson JB, Lecuru F, Foulot H, et al. Myomectomy by laparoscopy: A preliminary report of 43 cases. Fertil Steril 1991; 56:827–830.
19. Hasson HM, Rotman C, Rana N, et al. Laparoscopic myomectomy. Obstet Gynecol 1992; 80:884–888.
20. Nezhat C, Nezhat F, Silfen SL, et al. Laparoscopic myomectomy. Int J Fertil 1991; 36:275–280.
21. Dubuisson JB, Fauconnier A, Fourchotte V, et al. Laparoscopic myomectomy: Predicting the risk of conversion to an open procedure. Hum Reprod 2001; 16:1726–1731.
22. Atri M, Reinhold C, Mehio AR, et al. Adenomyosis: US features with histologic correlation in an in-vitro study. Radiology 2000; 215:783–790.
23. Chiang CH, Chang MY, Hsu JJ, et al. Tumor vascular pattern and blood flow impedance in the differential diagnosis of leiomyoma and adenomyosis by color Doppler sonography. J Assist Reprod Genet 1999; 16:268–275.
24. Cohen LS, Valle RF. Role of vaginal sonography and hysterosonography in the endoscopic treatment of uterine myomas. Fertil Steril 2000; 73:197–204.
25. Fauconnier A, Dubuisson JB, Ancel PY, et al. Prognostic factors of reproductive outcome after myomectomy in infertile patients. Hum Reprod 2000; 15:1751–1757.
26. Wurnig C, Schatz K, Noske H, et al. Subcutaneous low-dose epoietin beta for the avoidance of transfusion in patients scheduled for elective surgery not eligible for autologous blood donation. Eur Surg Res 2001; 33(5–6):303–310.
27. Sesti F, Ticconi C, Bonifacio S, et al. Preoperative administration of recombinant human erythropoietin in patients undergoing gynaecologic surgery. Gynecol Obstet Invest 2002; 54(1):1–5.
28. Friedman AJ, Harrison-Atlas D, Barbieri RL, et al. A randomized, placebo-controlled, double-blind study evaluating the efficacy of leuprolide acetate depot in the treatment of uterine leiomyomata. Fertil Steril 1989; 51:251–256.
29. Lumsden MA, West CP, Baird DT. Goserelin therapy before surgery for uterine fibroids. Lancet 1987; 1:36–37.
30. Matta WH, Stabile I, Shaw RW, et al. Doppler assessment of uterine blood flow changes in patients with fibroids receiving the gonadotropin-releasing hormone agonist Buserelin. Fertil Steril 1988; 49:1083–1085.
31. Friedman AJ, Rein MS, Harrison-Atlas D, et al. A randomized, placebo-controlled, double-blind study evaluating leuprolide acetate depot treatment before myomectomy. Fertil Steril 1989; 52:728–733.
32. Campo S, Garcea N. Laparoscopic myomectomy in premenopausal women with and without preoperative treatment using gonadotrophin-releasing hormone analogues. Hum Reprod 1999; 14:44–48.
33. Zullo F, Pellicano M, De Stefano R, et al. A prospective randomized study to evaluate leuprolide acetate treatment before laparoscopic myomectomy: Efficacy and ultrasonographic predictors. Am J Obstet Gynecol 1998; 178:108–112.
34. Acien P, Quereda, F. Abdominal myomectomy: Results of a simple operative technique. Fertil Steril 1996; 65:41–51.
35. Beyth Y. Gonadotropin-releasing hormone analog treatment should not precede conservative myomectomy [letter]. Fertil Steril 1990; 53:187–188.
36. Reich H, Thompson KA, Nataupsky LG, et al. Laparoscopic myomectomy: An alternative to laparotomy or hysterectomy? Gynaecol Endosc 1997; 6:7–12.
37. Fedele L, Vercellini P, Bianchi S, et al. Treatment with GnRH agonists before myomectomy and the risk of short-term myoma recurrence. Br J Obstet Gynaecol 1990; 97:393–396.
38. West S, Ruiz R, Parker WH. Abdominal myomectomy in women with very large uterine size. Fertil Steril 2006; 85:36–39.
39. Parker WH, Rodi IA. Patient selection for laparoscopic myomectomy. J Am Assoc Gynecol Laparosc 1994; 2(1):23–26.
40. Malzoni M, Rotond M, Perone C, et al. Fertility after laparoscopic myomectomy of large uterine myomas: Operative technique and preliminary results. Eur J Gynecol Oncol 2003; 24: 79–82.
41. Andrei B, Crovini, Rosi A. Uterine myomas: Pelviscopic treatment. Clin Exp Obstet Gynecol 1999; 26:44–46.
42. Dubuisson JB, Fauconnier A, Babaki-Fard K, et al. Laparoscopic myomectomy: A current view. Hum Reprod Update 2000; 6:558–594.
43. Daraï E, Deval B, Darles C, et al. Myomectomie: Coelioscopie ou laparotomie. Contracept Fertil Sex 1996; 24:751–756.
44. Dubuisson JB, Chapron C, Lévy L. Difficulties and complications of laparoscopic myomectomy. J Gynecol Surg 1996; 12:159–165.
45. Benhaim Y, Ducarme G, Madelenat P, et al. Les limites de la myomectomie coelioscopique. Gynécol Obstét Fertil 2005; 33:44–49.
46. Adamian LV, Kulakov VI, Kiselev SI, et al. Laparoscopic myomectomy in treatment of large myomas. J Am Assoc Gynecol Laparosc 1996; 3:S1.
47. Hasson HM. Laparoscopic myomectomy. Infertil Reprod Med Clin North Am 1996; 7:143–159.
48. Farrer-Brown G, Beilby J, Tarbit MH. Venous changes in the endometrium of myomatous uteri. Obstet Gynecol 1971; 38:743–751.
49. Vollenhoven BJ, Lawrence AS, Healy DL. Uterine fibroids: A clinical review. Br J Obstet Gynaecol 1990; 97:285–298.
50. Donnez J, Polet R, Smets M, et al. Hysteroscopic myomectomy. Curr Opin Obstet Gynecol 1995; 7:311–316.

51. Wamsteker K, Emanuel MH, Kruitt JH. Transcervical hysteroscopic resection of submucous fibroids for abnormal uterine bleeding: Results regarding the degree of intramural extension. Obstet Gynecol 1993; 82:736–740.
52. Dubuisson JB, Malartic C, Jacob S, et al. Preventive uterine artery occlusion combined with laparoscopic myomectomy: A valid procedure to prevent bleeding. J Gynecol Surg 2004; 20:105–112.
53. Koh C, Janik G. Laparoscopic myomectomy: The current status. Curr Opin Obstet Gynecol 2003; 15:295–301.
54. Dubuisson JB, Chavet X, Chapron C, et al. Uterine rupture during pregnancy after laparoscopic myomectomy. Hum Reprod 1995; 10:1475–1477.
55. Harris WJ. Uterine dehiscence following laparoscopic myomectomy. Obstet Gynecol 1992; 80:545–546.
56. Pelosi M, Pelosi MA. Spontaneous uterine rupture at thirty-three weeks subsequent to previous superficial laparoscopic myomectomy. Am J Obstet Gynecol 1997; 177:1547–1549.
57. Vilos GA, Daly LJ. Tse BM. Pregnancy outcome after laparoscopic electromyolysis. J Am Assoc Gynecol Laparosc 1998; 5:289–292.
58. Miller CE, Johnston M, Rundell M. Laparoscopic myomectomy in the infertile woman. J Am Assoc Gynecol Laparosc 1996; 3:525–532.
59. Dubuisson JB, Chapron C, Chavet X, et al. Traitement coeliochirurgical des volumineux fibromes utérins. Technique opératoire et résultats. J Gynecol Obstet Biol Reprod 1995; 24:705–710.
60. Ostrzenski A. A new laparoscopic myomectomy technique for intramural fibroids penetrating the uterine cavity. Eur J Obstet Gynecol Reprod Biol 1997; 74:189–193.
61. Nezhat C, Nezhat F, Bess O, et al. Laparoscopically assisted myomectomy: A report of a new technique in 57 cases. Int J Fertil Menopausal Stud 1994; 39:39–44.
62. Tulandi T, Youseff H. Laparoscopy assisted myomectomy of large uterine myomas. Gynaecol Endosc 1997; 6:105–108.
63. Carter JE, McCarus SD. Laparoscopic myomectomy. Time and cost analysis of power vs. manual morcellation. J Reprod Med 1997; 42:383–388.
64. Dubuisson JB, Chapron C, Fauconnier A, et al. Laparoscopic myomectomy and myolysis. Curr Opin Obstet Gynecol 1997; 9:233–238.
65. Pritts EA, Parker WH. Predictive value of myomectomy. Fertil Steril 2006; 85:c5.
66. Advincula AP, Song A. The role of robotic surgery in gynecology. Curr Opin Obstet Gynecol 2007; 19(4):331–336.
67. Advincula AP, Xu X, Goudeau S 4th, et al. Robot-assisted laparoscopic myomectomy versus abdominal myomectomy: A comparison of short-term surgical outcomes and immediate costs. J Minim Invasive Gynecol 2007; 14(6):698–705.
68. Nezhat C, Lavie O, Hsu S, et al. Robotic-assisted laparoscopic myomectomy compared with standard laparoscopic myomectomy—a retrospective matched control study. Fertil Steril 2009; 91(2):556–559.
69. Seracchioli R, Rossi S, Govoni F, et al. Fertility and obstetric outcome after laparoscopic myomectomy of large myomata: A randomized comparison with abdominal myomectomy. Hum Reprod 2000; 15:2663–2668.
70. Stringer NH, Walker JC, Meyer PM. Comparison of 49 laparoscopic myomectomies with 49 open myomectomies. J Am Assoc Gynecol Laparosc 1997; 4:457–464.
71. Mais V, Ajossa S, Guerriero S, et al. Laparoscopic versus abdominal myomectomy: A prospective, randomized trial to evaluate benefits in early outcome. Am J Obstet Gynecol 1996; 174:654–658.
72. Ginsburg E, Benson C, Garfield J, et al. The effect of operative technique and uterine size on blood loss during myomectomy: A prospective randomised study. Fertil Steril 1993; 60:956–962.
73. Bulletti C, Polli V, Negrini V, et al. Adhesion formation after laparoscopic myomectomy. J Am Assoc Gynecol Laparosc 1996; 3:533–536.
74. Farquhar C, Vandekerckhove P, Watson A, et al. Barrier agents for preventing adhesions after surgery for subfertility. Cochrane Database Syst Rev 2000:CD000475.
75. Mais V, Ajossa S, Iras B, et al. Prevention of de-novo adhesion formation after laparoscopic myomectomy: A randomized trial to evaluate the effectiveness of an oxidized regenerated cellulose absorbable barrier. Hum Reprod 1995; 10:3133–3135.
76. Tsuji S, Takahashi K, Yomo H, et al. Effectiveness of antiadhesion barriers in preventing adhesion after myomectomy in patients with uterine leiomyoma. Eur J Obstet Gynecol Reprod Biol 2005; 123:244–248.
77. Dubuisson JB, Fauconnier A, Chapron C, et al. Second look after laparoscopic myomectomy. Hum Reprod 1998; 13:2102–2106.
78. Dubuisson JB, Fauconnier A, Chapron C, et al. Reproductive outcome after laparoscopic myomectomy in infertile women. J Reprod Med 2000; 45:23–31.
79. Dubuisson JB, Fauconnier A, Deffarges JV, et al. Pregnancy outcome and deliveries following laparoscopic myomectomy. Hum Reprod 2000; 15:869–873.
80. Tulandi T, Murray C, Guralnick M. Adhesion formation and reproductive outcome after myomectomy and second look laparoscopy. Obstet Gynecol 1993; 82:213–215.
81. Ugur M, Turan C, Mungan T, et al. Laparoscopy for adhesion prevention following myomectomy. Int J Gynecol Obstet 1996; 53:145–149.
82. Nezhat C. The "cons" of laparoscopic myomectomy in women who may reproduce in the future. Int J Fertil Menopausal Stud 1996; 41:280–283.
83. Friedmann W, Maier RF, Luttkus A, et al. Uterine rupture after laparoscopic myomectomy. Acta Obstet Gynecol Scand 1996; 75:683–684.
84. Mecke H, Wallas F, Brocker A, et al. Pelviskopische Myomenukleation: Technik, Grenzen, Komplicationen. Geburtshlife Frauenheilkd 1995; 55:374–379.
85. Soriano D, Dessolle L, Poncelet C, et al. Pregnancy outcome after laparoscopic and laparoconverted myomectomy. Eur J Obstet Gynecol Reprod Biol 2003; 108:194–198.
86. Daraï E, Dechaud H, Benifla JL, et al. Fertility after laparoscopic myomectomy: Preliminary results. Hum Reprod 1997; 12:1931–1934.
87. Nezhat CH, Nezhat F, Roemisch M, et al. Pregnancy following laparoscopic myomectomy: Preliminary results. Hum Reprod 1999; 14:1219–1221.
88. Reich H. Laparoscopic myomectomy. Obstet Gynecol Clin North Am 1995; 22:757–780.
89. Ribeiro SC, Reich H, Rosenberg J, et al. Laparoscopic myomectomy and pregnancy outcome in infertile patients. Fertil Steril 1999; 71:571–574.
90. Palerme GR, Friedman EA. Rupture of the gravid uterus in the third trimester. Am J Obstet Gynecol 1966; 94:571–576.
91. Garnet JD. Uterine rupture during pregnancy. An analysis of 133 patients. Obstet Gynecol 1964; 23:898–905.
92. Quakernack K, Bordt J, Nienhaus H. Placenta percreta and rupture of the uterus. Geburtshlife Frauenheilkd 1980; 40: 520–523.
93. Roopnarinesingh S, Suratsingh J, Roopnarinesingh A. The obstetric outcome of patients with previous myomectomy or hysterotomy. West Indian Med J 1985; 34:59–62.
94. Katsumori T, Nakajima K, Tokuhiro M. Gadolinium-enhanced MR imaging in the evaluation of uterine fibroids treated with uterine artery embolization. Am J Roentgenol 2001; 177:303–307.
95. Holub Z, Eim J, Jabor A, et al. Complications and myoma recurrence after laparoscopic uterine artery occlusion for symptomatic myomas. J Obstet Gynaecol Res 2006; 32:55–62.
96. Malone L. Myomectomy: Recurrence after removal of solitary and multiple myomas. Obstet Gynecol 1969; 34:200–203.
97. Vavala V, Lanzone A, Monaco A, et al. Postoperative GnRH analog treatment for the prevention of recurrences of uterine myomas after myomectomy. A pilot study. Gynecol Obstet Invest 1997; 43:251–254.

98. Dadak C, Feiks A. Organ-sparing surgery of leiomyomas of the uterus in young females. Zentralbl Gynakol 1988; 110:102–106.
99. Doridot V, Dubuisson JB, Chapron C, et al. Recurrence of leiomyomata after laparoscopic myomectomy. J Am Assoc Gynecol Laparosc 2001; 8:495–500.
100. Finn WF, Muller PF. Abdominal myomectomy: Special reference to subsequent pregnancy and to the reappearance of fibromyomas of the uterus. Am J Obstet Gynecol 1950; 60: 109–114.
101. Candiani GB, Fedele L, Parazzini F, et al. Risk of recurrence after myomectomy. Br J Obstet Gynaecol 1991; 98:385–389.
102. Rossetti A, Sizzi O, Soranna L, et al. Long-term results of laparoscopic myomectomy: Recurrence rate in comparison with abdominal myomectomy. Hum Reprod 2001; 16:770–774.
103. Summitt RL Jr, Stovall TG, Lipscomb GH, et al. Randomized comparison of laparoscopy-assisted vaginal hysterectomy with standard vaginal hysterectomy in an outpatient setting. Obstet Gynecol 1992; 80:895–901.
104. Garry R, Fountain J, Mason S, et al. The eVALuate study: Two parallel randomised trials, one comparing laparoscopic with abdominal hysterectomy, the other comparing laparoscopic with vaginal hysterectomy. BMJ 2004; 328:129.
105. Marana R, Busacca M, Zupi E, et al. Laparoscopically assisted vaginal hysterectomy versus total abdominal hysterectomy: A prospective, randomized, multicenter study. Am J Obstet Gynecol 1999; 180:270–275.
106. Wattiez A, Soriano D, Fiaccavento A, et al. Total laparoscopic hysterectomy for very enlarged uteri. J Am Assoc Gynecol Laparosc 2002; 9:125–130.
107. Goldberg J, Pereira L, Berghella V, et al. Pregnancy outcomes after treatment for fibromyomata: Uterine artery embolization versus laparoscopic myomectomy. Am J Obstet Gynecol 2004; 191:18–21.
108. Pron G, Mocarski E, Bennett J, et al. Pregnancy after uterine artery embolization for leiomyomata: The Ontario multicenter trial. Obstet Gynecol 2005; 105:67–76.
109. Vilos GA, Vilos EC, Romano W, et al. Temporary uterine artery occlusion for treatment of menorrhagia and uterine fibroids using an incisionless Doppler-guided transvaginal clamp: Case report. Hum Reprod 2006; 21:269–271.
110. Parker WH, Broder MS, Liu Z, et al. Ovarian conservation at the time of hysterectomy for benign disease. Obstet Gynecol 2005; 106:219–226.
111. Goto A, Takeuchi S, Sugimura K, et al. Usefulness of Gd-DTPA contrast-enhanced dynamic MRI and serum determination of LDH and its isozymes in the differential diagnosis of leiomyosarcoma from degenerated leiomyoma of the uterus. Int J Gynecol Cancer 2002; 12:354–361.

8

Laparoscopic evaluation of adnexal malignancies

Denis Querleu, Gwenael Ferron, Arash Rafii, and Eva Jouve

Adnexal malignancies encompass ovarian and tubal cancer. Fallopian tube cancer is much less common than ovarian cancer and is diagnosed and managed in a similar way.

Laparotomy has for long been the mainstay of surgical management of these conditions, even though laparoscopy has been routinely used in the diagnosis of adnexal masses. The need for routine midline laparotomy was the result of requirement for hysterectomy, omentectomy, comprehensive lymph node dissections, biopsies in any part of the abdomen, and appendectomy even in the case of early adnexal malignancy.

With the development of advanced laparoscopic techniques, the technical limits have gradually been pushed, and at this time the only absolute limitation of laparoscopic surgery is the presence of large tumor masses. The laparoscope may thus presently be used as a diagnostic tool at any stage of the disease, any step of the management, and any time during the natural history of the disease.

This chapter will present an overview of the technical aspects of laparoscopic surgery in the field of adnexal malignancies. The chapter concludes with recommendations to the general gynecologist and a brief summary of the role and indications of laparoscopy in adnexal neoplasms.

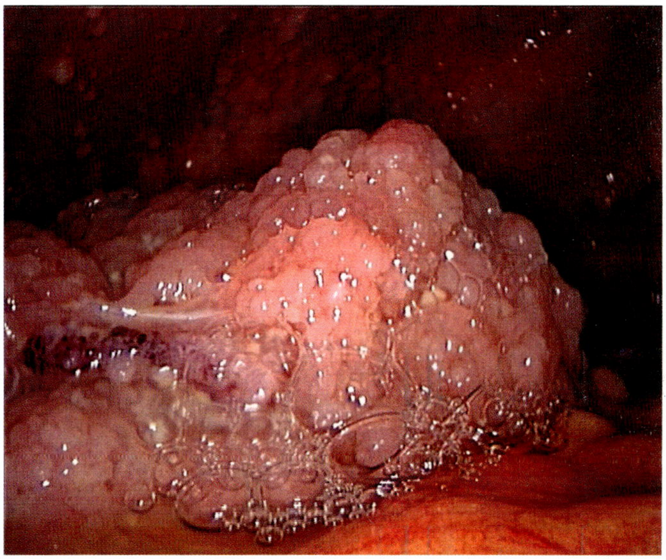

Figure 1 The presence of papillary growth suggests malignancy.

LAPAROSCOPIC DIAGNOSIS OF OVARIAN CANCER

A comprehensive workup including a pelvic ultrasonography and, in menopausal patients, plasma Ca-125 levels is required to reduce the rate of unexpectedly finding ovarian malignancies. However, even after careful preoperative workup, unrecognized malignancies may be encountered at the time of laparoscopy. Moreover, apparently benign masses may turn out to be malignant at definitive pathological examination. Thus, the general gynecologist must be aware of a few essential diagnostic criteria and guidelines for the management of previously unsuspected malignancy and adnexal masses in general.

The presence of extracapsular papillary or solid growth, peritoneal deposits, and ascites strongly suggests malignant disease (Figs. 1–4). However, the gynecologist must be aware that not all ascites, not all solid masses, and not all exophytic tumors require radical surgery. This is crucial in the case of young patients, knowing that young age is associated with a higher incidence of germ cell tumors and borderline tumors that can almost invariably be managed with preservation of fertility. Rather than rushing to open the patient, care must be taken to describe the intraperitoneal lesions, and take photographs and biopsies in order to refer the patient to a tertiary oncological center with a maximum of relevant information.

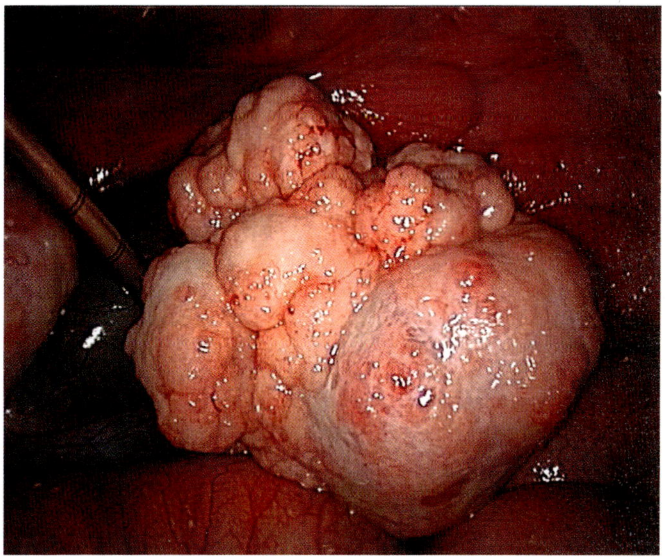

Figure 2 The association of solid growth suggests malignancy.

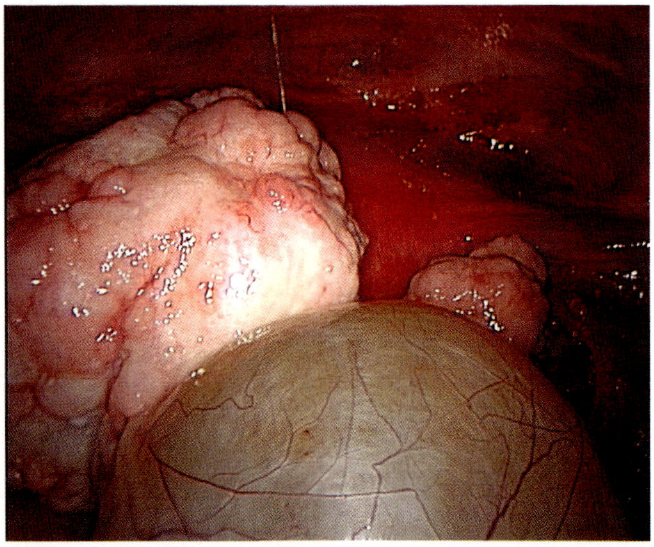

Figure 3 The association of solid and papillary growth suggests malignancy.

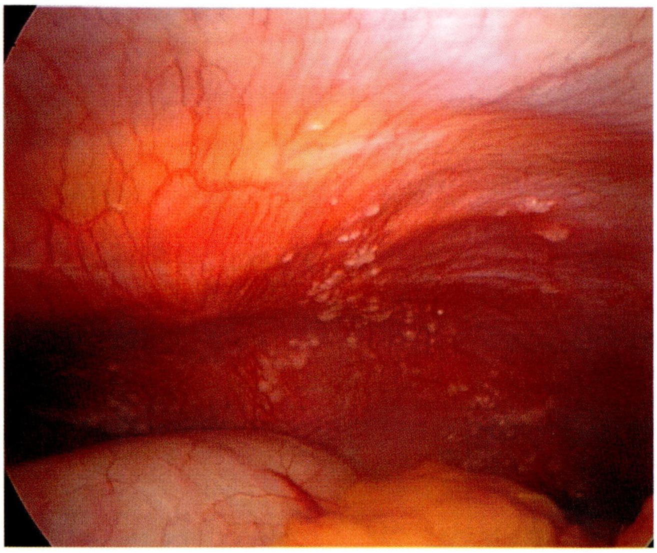

Figure 5 Minute peritoneal papillary lesions.

LAPAROSCOPIC EVALUATION OF THE PERITONEAL CAVITY

The rationale for the use of laparoscopy for the evaluation of the peritoneal cavity in patients presenting with suspicious or malignant adnexal masses is based on a conjunction of several points. Laparoscopy is an invaluable tool to explore the entire peritoneal cavity while avoiding a midline laparotomy. A number of peritoneal growths related to adnexal malignancies are too small to be identified by modern imaging techniques including computerized tomography scan, magnetic resonance imaging, and positron emission tomography. In addition, adnexal malignancies may metastasize to any point of the peritoneal cavity.

However, the pattern of malignant peritoneal growth has never been extensively described. In this chapter, the appearance of the diseased peritoneum will be systematically described using a terminology similar to the one used by colposcopists. As a matter of fact, many of the peritoneal lesions feature "atypical transformation" quite similar to cervical lesions familiar to the colposcopist. The resulting concept may be deemed as "peritoneal colposcopy," emphasizing the need to examine carefully the peritoneal surface, taking the advantage of the magnification provided by the laparoscope. Elementary images then various anatomical locations will be described.

Elementary Lesions of the Diseased Peritoneum

In this chapter, we describe papillary lesions (type 1), white lesions (type 2), nodules (type 3), vascular anomalies (type 4), and, finally, invisible lesions defined only after optical manipulation.

Type 1: Papillary Lesions

Peritoneal papillary lesions ("condyloma like") may be minute in size (Fig. 5) or large and sometimes confluent (Fig. 6).

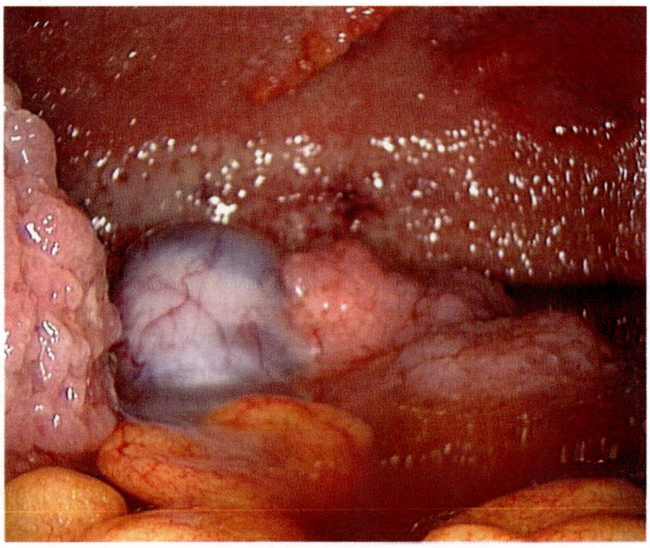

Figure 4 The additional presence of ascites further suggests malignancy.

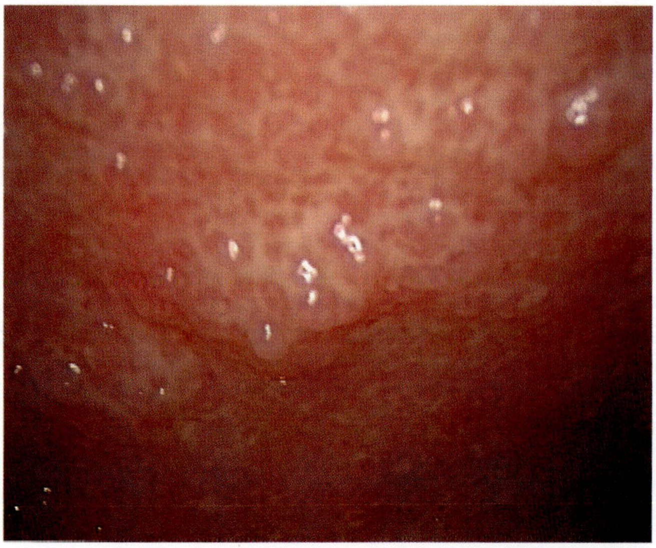

Figure 6 Confluent peritoneal papillary lesions.

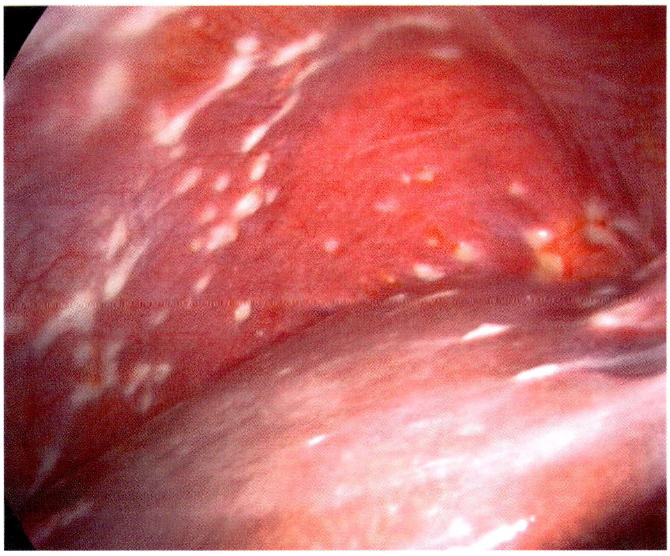

Figure 7 Small nonconfluent lesions.

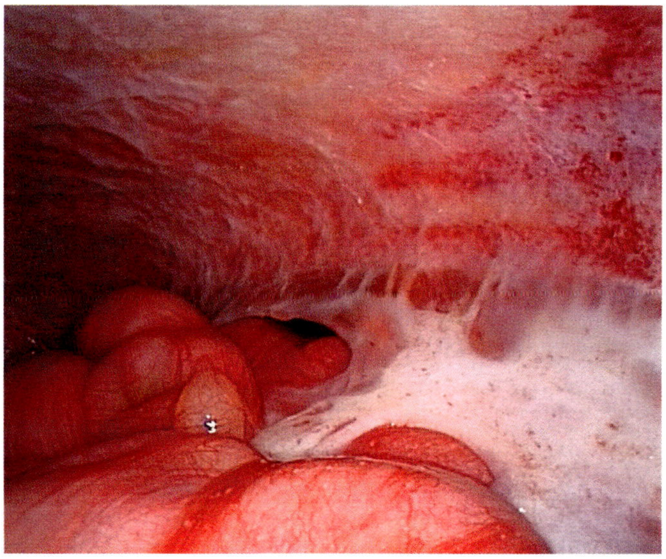

Figure 9 Thick confluent white lesions.

Type 2: White Lesions

Malignant peritoneal disease may feature a white color related to the thickening of the peritoneum. Small, nonconfluent lesions look like wax spots (Fig. 7). White lesions can also be confluent (Fig. 8). Thick and confluent white lesions are described as "plaques" (Fig. 9). White spots may be associated with exophytic lesions with a combination of various features including plaques (Fig. 10). A rare but characteristic feature is the "white web" (Fig. 11) that covers the visceral and parietal peritoneum without forming plaques.

Type 3: Nodules

Nodules can be small or large. Small or micro nodules are often disseminated in the peritoneal cavity, forming the so-called miliary (Fig. 12). Large nodules are not different from large white lesions.

Type 4: Vascular Anomalies

The normal appearance of peritoneal vasculature is regular and made of a few thin vessels. The diseased peritoneum may feature irregular vessels, of different diameters, with multiple anastomoses (Fig. 13; see also Fig. 8).

Type 5: Nonvisible Lesions

Microscopic lesions may not be visible. New fluorescence techniques may reveal peritoneal grafts. Drugs injected in the blood are concentrated in tumor cells and elicit fluorescent light when submitted to stimulating wavelengths. Currently,

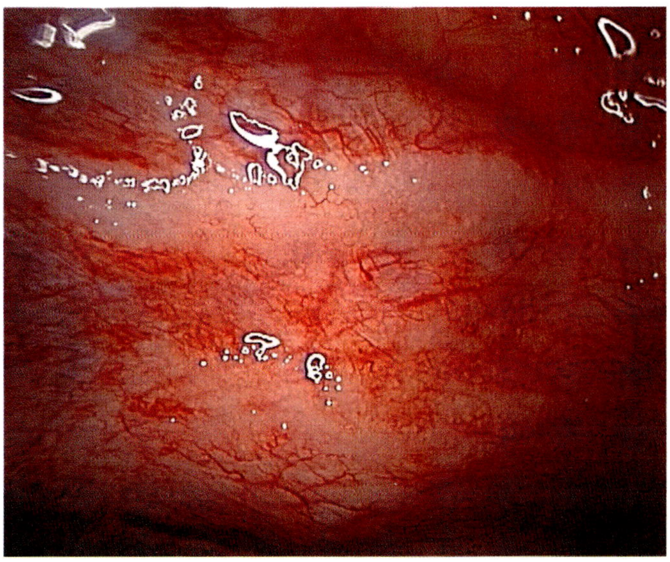

Figure 8 Confluent white lesions.

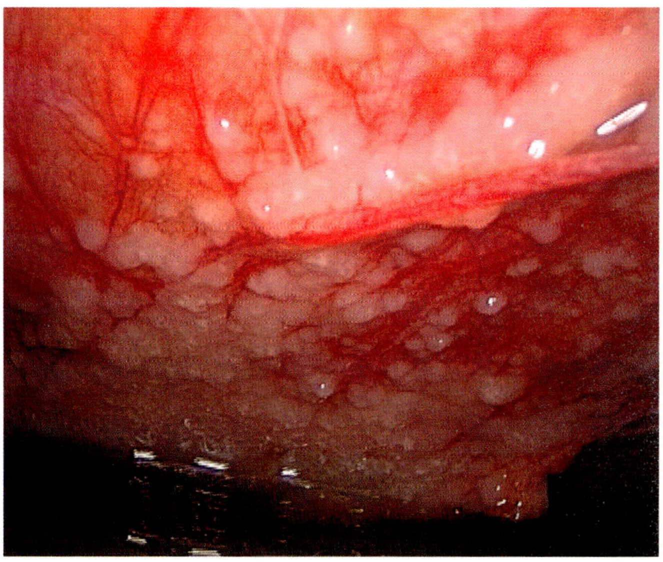

Figure 10 White spots associated with exophytic lesions.

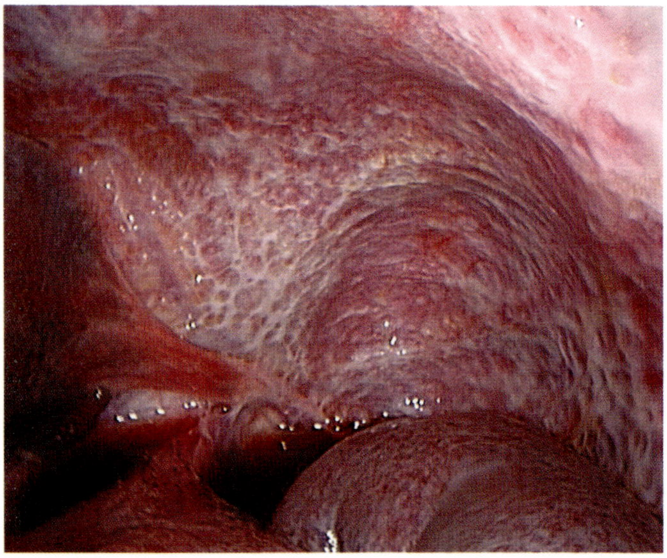

Figure 11 A "white web" covering the peritoneum.

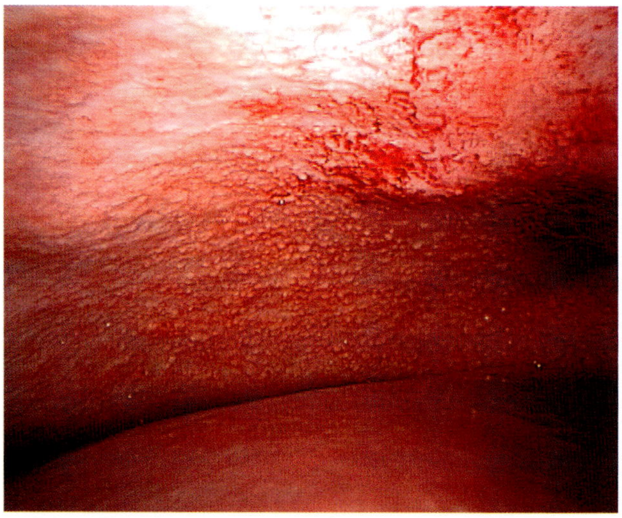

Figure 12 Micromodules in the peritoneal cavity.

the most used compound is the aminolevulinic acid and esters (Figs. 14 and 15).

Anatomical Extension of Disease

Every intraperitoneal organ may be involved. Thorough and methodic exploration is then mandatory to make sure that even small and isolated deposits are diagnosed. A complete mapping of the peritoneum is possible.

Pelvis

The pouch of Douglas, the vesicouterine fold, and the posterior leaf to broad ligaments must be examined (Fig. 16), and the rectal and sigmoid colon serosa (Fig. 17) as well.

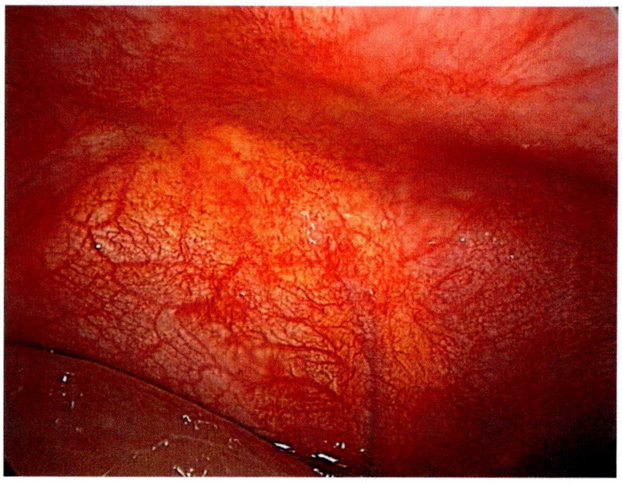

Figure 13 Irregular vessels with multiple anastomoses.

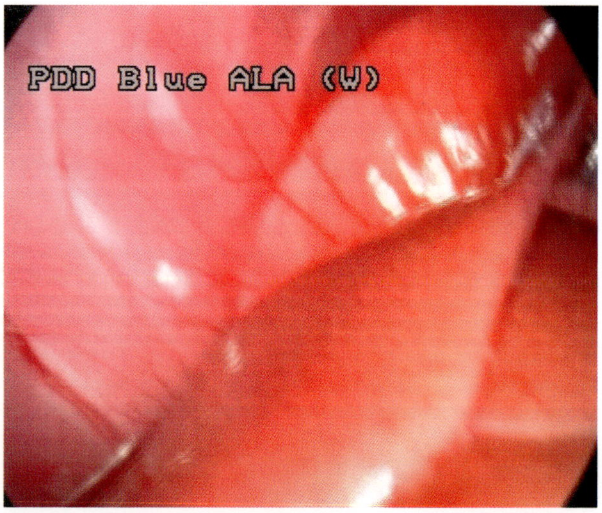

Figure 14 No visible lesion before use of fluorescence in an animal injected with aminolevulinic acid.

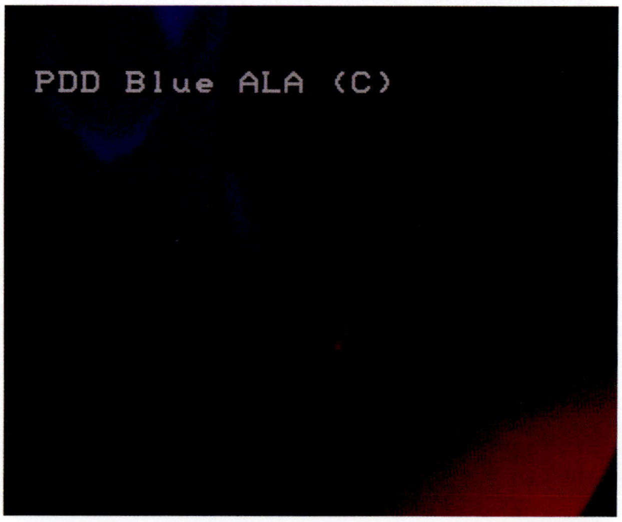

Figure 15 Tumor cells revealed with the use of fluorescent light.

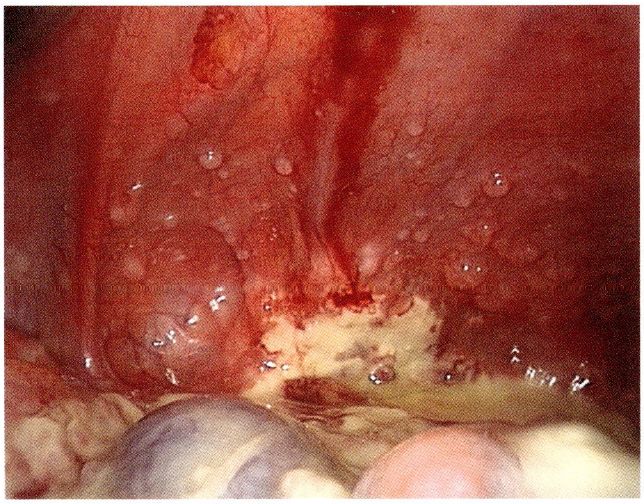

Figure 16 The pouch of Douglas, the vesicouterine fold.

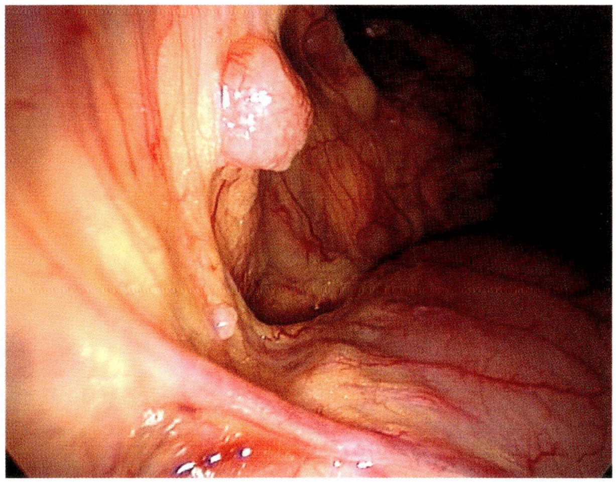

Figure 18 Minute deposits in the omentum.

Omentum

The omentum is a preferential site of peritoneal cancer. Minute (Fig. 18) or massive (Fig. 19) deposits can be observed.

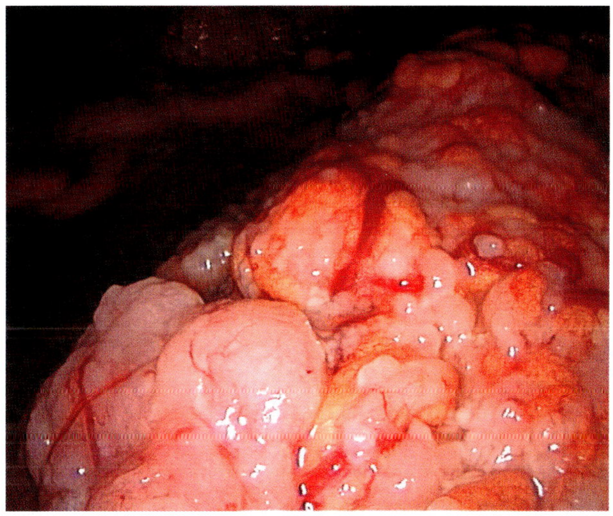

Figure 19 Massive deposits in the omentum.

Central Abdomen

The paracolic gutters, mesentery, small bowel, and large bowel must be observed. The mesentery only (Fig. 20), visceral peritoneum only (Fig. 21), or both may be involved.

Upper Abdomen

Diaphragm

The left hemidiaphragm (Fig. 11) and the right hemidiaphragm (Fig. 22) are completely explored. Actually, the laparoscope is probably the best tool to accomplish this, thanks to magnification and light. Special attention must be brought to the lesser omentum, which is observed after moving down

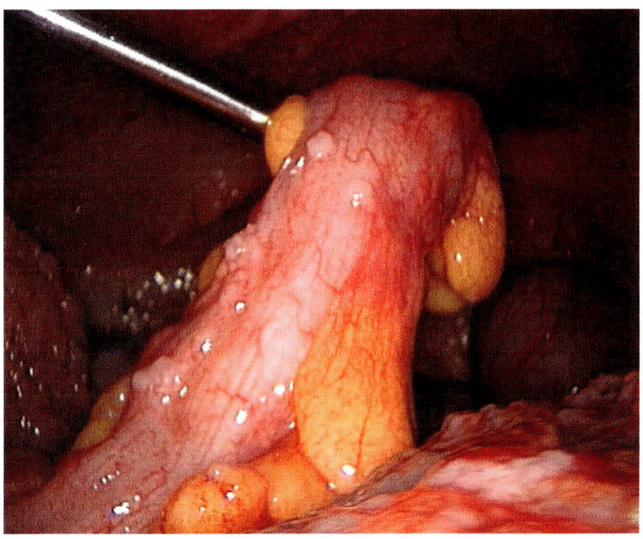

Figure 17 Sigmoid colon.

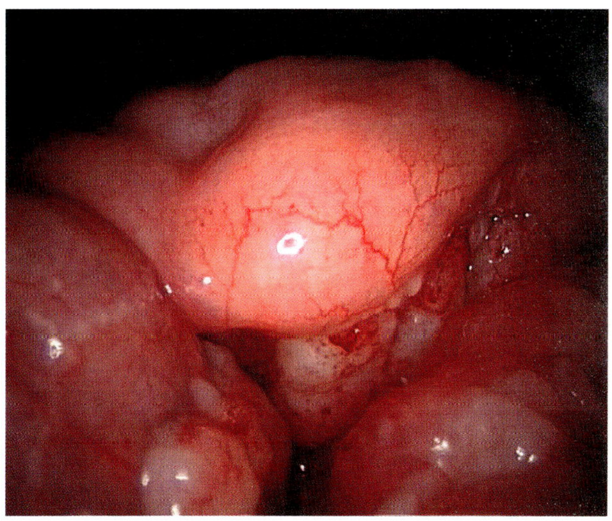

Figure 20 Involvement of the mesentery.

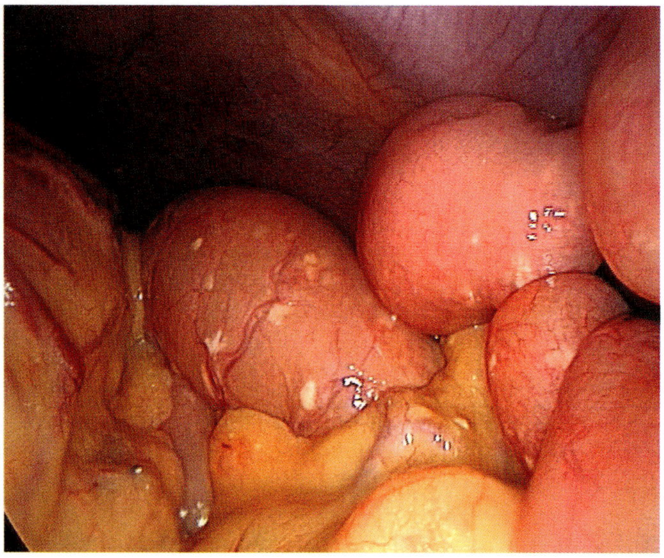

Figure 21 Involvement of the visceral peritoneum.

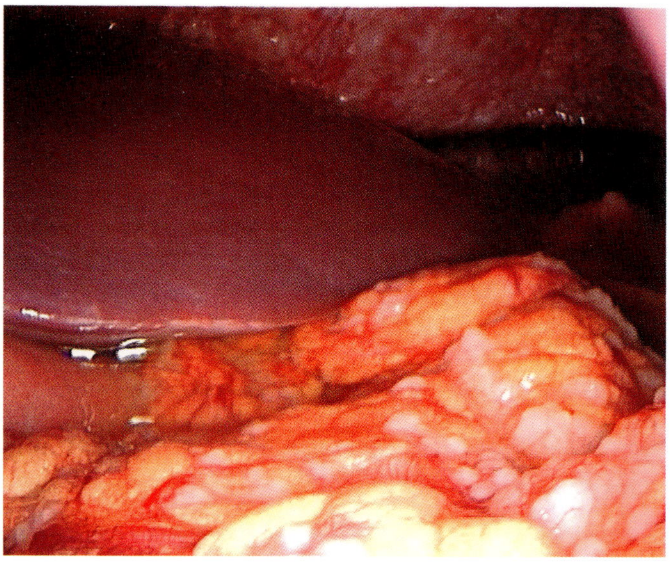

Figure 23 The lesser omentum.

the transverse colon and then the stomach (Fig. 23). The area of the hepatic pedicle is crucial, as massive involvement of this site is a contraindication to surgery (Fig. 24). In the same area of the abdomen, the round ligament of the liver is examined (Fig. 25).

Spleen and liver

The spleen (Fig. 26, see also Fig. 11) may be involved as a result of growth on the serosal surface or the extension of omental disease to the hilus. In the same way, the surface of the liver may be involved as any serosal surface of abdominal viscera or via an extension of disease of the smaller omentum (Fig. 27) or may demonstrate parenchymatous metastases (Fig. 28).

LAPAROSCOPIC LYMPH NODE DISSECTION

A new classification of lymph node dissection for cervical cancers, which is applicable to ovarian malignancies, has recently been proposed (1). Anatomically, the most stable landmarks are arteries. As a consequence, four areas or levels are defined according to the corresponding arterial anatomy: level 1, external/internal iliac; level 2, common iliac (including presacral); level 3, aortic inframesenteric; and level 4, aortic infrarenal. The techniques for these procedures have been described elsewhere (2).

Aortic Dissection

Aortic node dissection is a mainstay of surgical staging and management of ovarian or tubal carcinoma. Transperitoneal

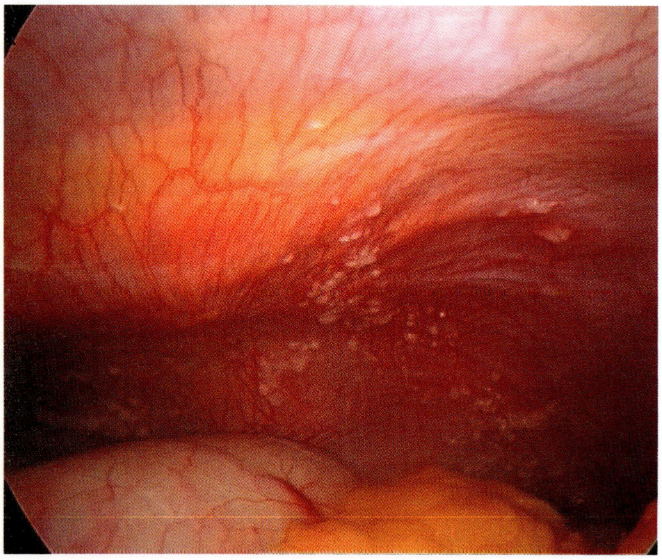

Figure 22 The right hemidiaphragm.

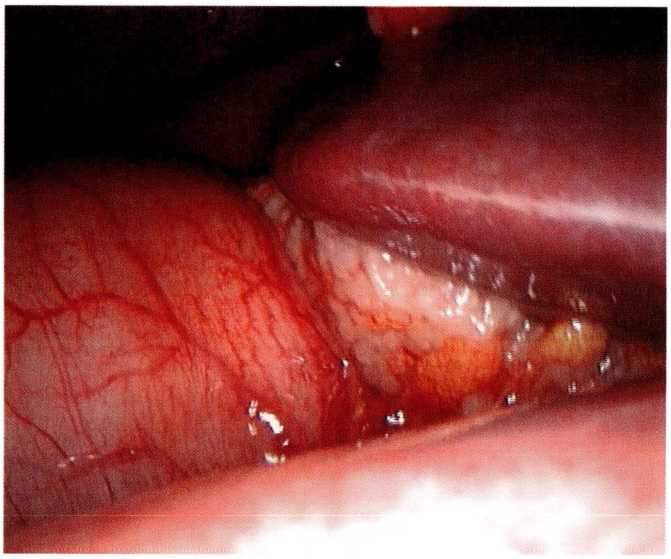

Figure 24 The hepatic pedicle.

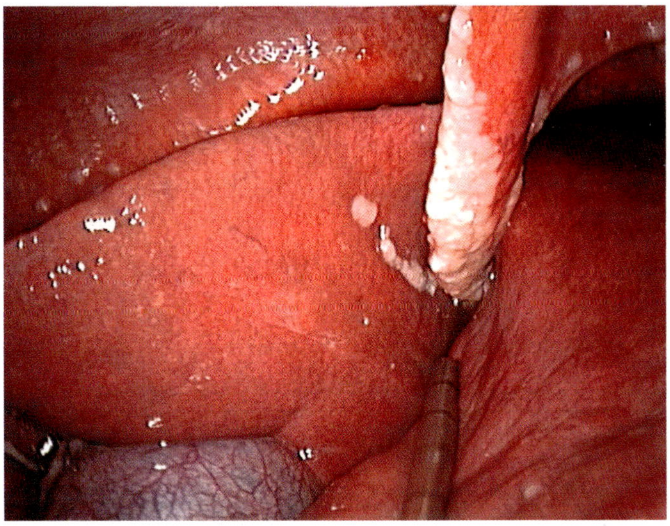

Figure 25 The round ligament of the liver.

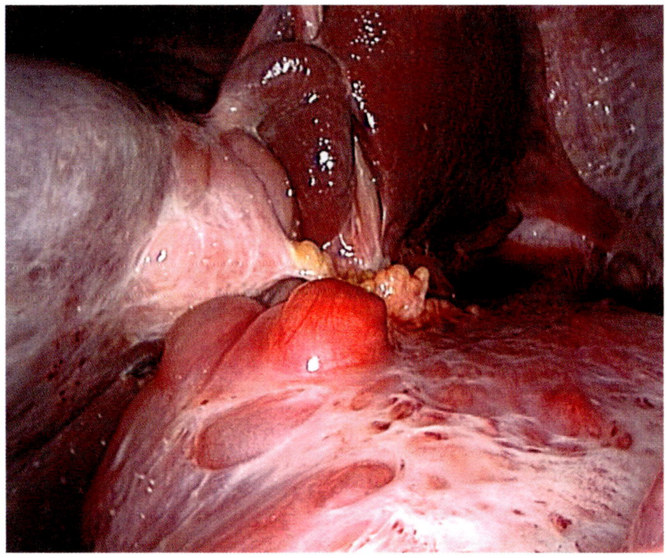

Figure 27 The surface of the liver.

dissection is the standard approach for aortic node dissection in case of ovarian tumor, although an extraperitoneal approach may be used when technically necessary. Levels 3 (Fig. 29) and 4 (Fig. 30) can be dissected laparoscopically.

Pelvic Dissection

Historically, pelvic dissection in gynecologic cancer was the first oncological operation performed laparoscopically (3). Level 1 (Fig. 31) is standard in the management of adnexal cancers.

INDICATIONS IN CLINICAL PRACTICE

This information is of use in clinical practice. The use of laparoscopic surgery at any stage of malignant adnexal disease has been documented in many reports since the pioneering era. Only outstanding papers presenting large series of patients or original research have been selected to document the various applications of the laparoscopic technique to ovarian disease.

Diagnostic Laparoscopy

The Clermont–Ferrand team published a large experience of laparoscopic diagnosis of adnexal masses, with long-term follow-up (4). The authors stated that the technique is safe and reliable, provided that cautious management and strict guidelines are respected. Sensitivity for malignant disease was 100% in a series of 757 patients. No patient had faulty laparoscopic surgery for undiagnosed ovarian cancer. Specificity was 97%, resulting in a 41% positive predictive value. As a result, only 27 patients in this series had unnecessary laparotomies. The most important issue in this setting is to avoid cyst rupture and consequent spillage of tumor cells in the peritoneal cavity, transforming a stage IA into a stage IC, resulting in the need

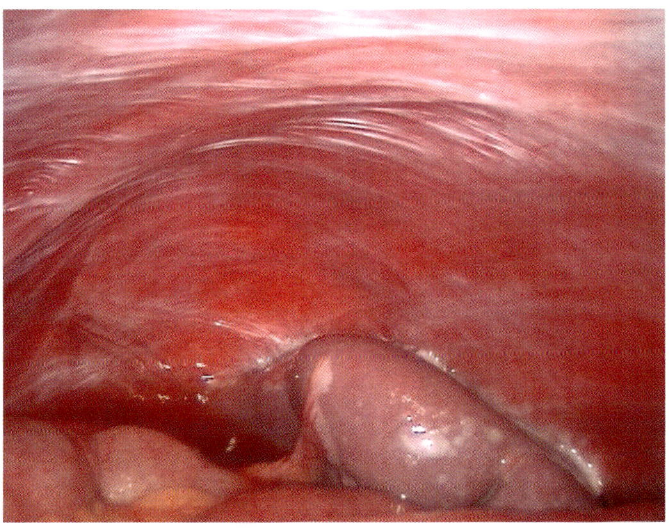

Figure 26 The spleen.

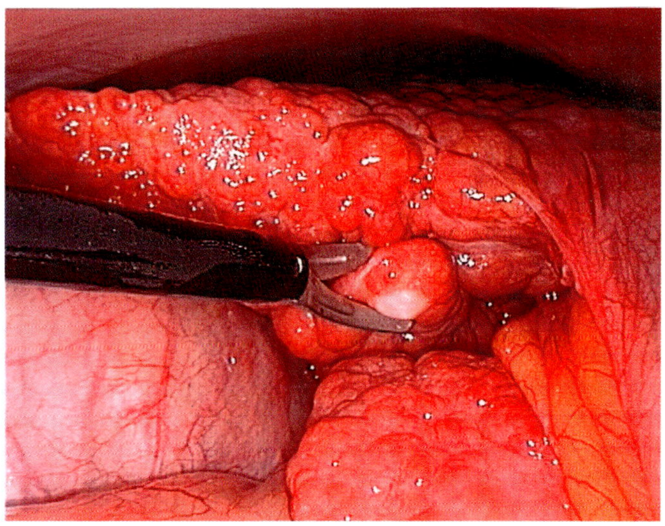

Figure 28 Parenchymatous liver metastasis.

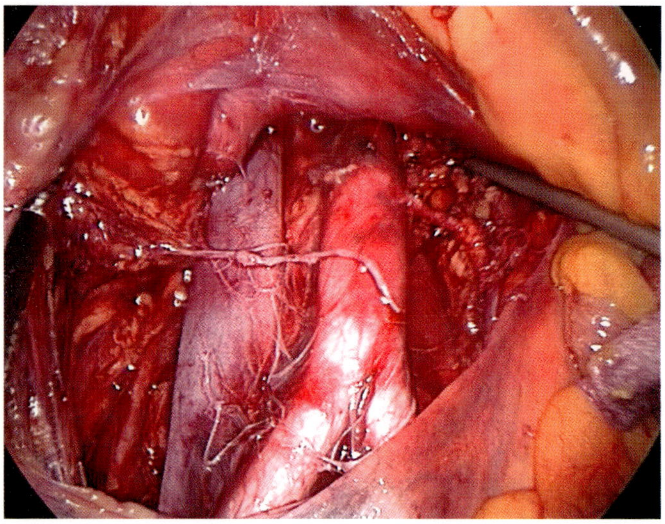

Figure 29 Level 3 aortic node dissection.

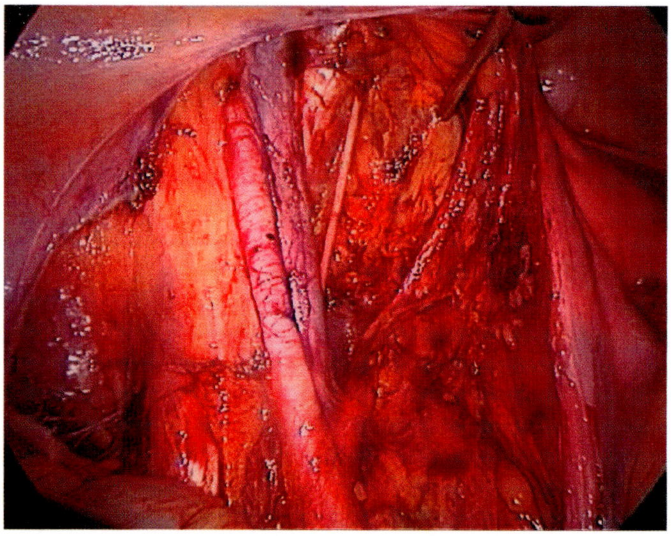

Figure 31 Level 1 pelvic dissection.

for adjuvant chemotherapy. Frozen section, with some limitations, adds to the diagnostic value of laparoscopy. In a series of 141 patients, the Clermont–Ferrand team observed only one false-negative result of frozen section (5).

Laparoscopic Reassessment of Early Ovarian Carcinomas

Leblanc et al. (6) published the largest series of comprehensive laparoscopic reassessment of apparently early ovarian or fallopian tube malignancies. All patients had full staging, including pelvic and infrarenal aortic lymph node dissection and omentectomy (Fig. 32). The long-term results are consistent with the data available after open staging.

Surgical Management of Early Ovarian Cancer

Tozzi et al. mentioned in their series a favorable outcome in a few cases of full laparoscopic management (one-step surgery including staging and surgical management) (7). However, patients had only partial omentectomy in this series. In a nationwide retrospective study in France, Lecuru et al. (8) indicated that laparoscopic approach is not detrimental to patients in early ovarian cancer, although staging was suboptimal in a significant proportion of cases.

Issue of Borderline Tumors

Laparoscopic surgery has become the mainstay of management of borderline ovarian tumors (9). This indication combines the advantages of laparoscopic surgery in diagnosis, peritoneal staging, and conservative surgery.

Decisional Laparoscopy in Advanced Ovarian Cancer

Laparoscopy has been proposed as a tool to select patients likely to benefit from upfront surgery, as opposed to neoadjuvant chemotherapy for advanced ovarian cancer. The best evidence supporting this concept has been published by Fagotti et al. (10). Ninety-five patients presenting with advanced ovarian malignancy had both laparoscopy and laparotomy.

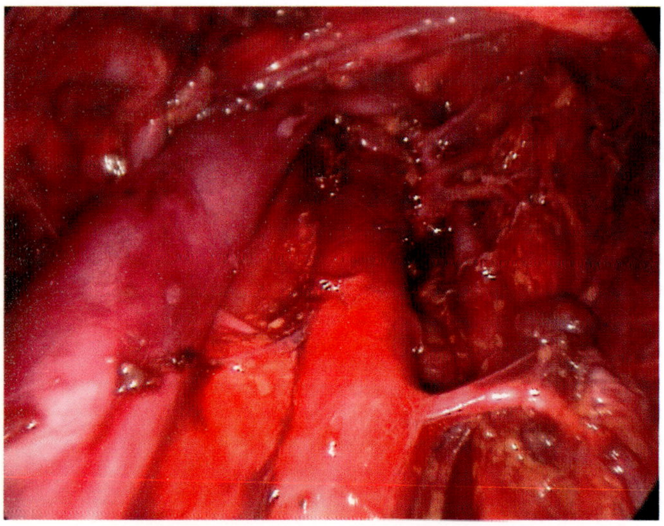

Figure 30 Level 4 aortic node dissection.

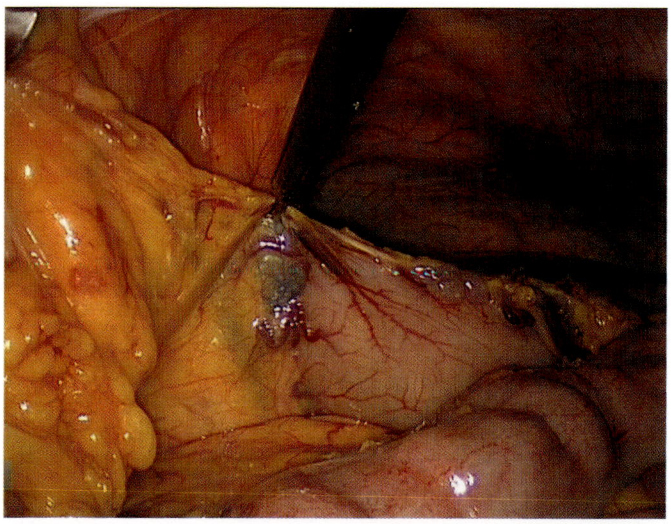

Figure 32 Omentectomy.

The negative predictive value of laparoscopic assessment of resectability was 100%; the judgment of unresectable disease obtained by laparoscopy was invariably confirmed at laparotomy. On the other hand, 5 of 39 cases judged as resectable at laparoscopy were not optimally resected.

Placement of Intraperitoneal Catheters

Laparoscopy may also be used to place intraperitoneal catheters in order to give intraperitoneal chemotherapy (11), which illustrates the fact that laparoscopy may be used at different stages of the disease and different steps of the management.

The Issue of Port-Site Metastasis

A major concern related to the introduction of new techniques is the de novo appearance of previously unknown complications. Mismanagement of ovarian cancer by laparoscopic surgery, or the use of laparoscopy in the presence of disseminated peritoneal malignancy, may lead to port-site metastases. Vergote et al. published the largest series documenting the incidence of port-site metastases after laparoscopy in the case of advanced ovarian cancer (12). They found an incidence of 17% port-site metastases in a series of 173 patients submitted to laparoscopy in the presence of advanced ovarian carcinoma. However, only 5% of patients had clinically identified port-site tumors. All port-site metastases disappeared during chemotherapy. As a result, the prognosis was not impaired in the group of patients with port-site metastases.

RECOMMENDATIONS FOR THE GENERAL GYNECOLOGIST

When the general gynecologist, not skilled in oncological surgery, has to deal with an unsuspected diagnosis of malignant or suspicious adnexal mass at the time of laparoscopy, several important recommendations may help to avoid faulty management:

- Take a sampling of peritoneal fluid or of washings.
- Fully observe and then describe in the operative report the peritoneal cavity, including the undersurface of hemidiaphragms, the mesentery, and the omentum.
- Avoid rupturing the mass in the peritoneal cavity.
- Biopsy only extracapsular disease.
- Biopsy at least one extraovarian implant if there are any.
- Use bags to remove any suspicious material from the peritoneal cavity.
- Avoid morcellation of the mass and contamination of the abdominal wall; if the laparoscopic approach is not 100% safe in this regard, prefer an adapted short midline laparotomy—never a transverse laparotomy.
- In parous patients, favor unilateral adnexectomy; in young patients, avoid definitive surgery.
- Take a blood sample as soon as possible to assess the Ca-125 plasma level.

The key issues are to avoid mismanagement and obtain a definitive pathology before counseling the patient or referring her to a gynecologic oncologist. There is no reason for rushing and performing an inadequate surgery and/or staging. Knowing that fertility-preserving surgery isacceptable with stage III borderline ovarian tumors, the decision to perform a total hysterectomy with bilateral salpingo-oophorectomy must await definitive pathology in young patients.

CONCLUSIONS

At the end, a few practical conclusions can be drawn. Laparoscopy is a performing diagnostic tool in the exploration of the peritoneal cavity and retroperitoneal space. It may be used at any time in the management of adnexal cancers. It allows careful examination of the peritoneal surface and precise description of peritoneal lesions. However, it should always be integrated in the oncological management and used by experienced gynecologic oncologists. The general gynecologist may liberally use laparoscopic diagnosis and surgery of adnexal masses, but should always be aware that any adnexal mass may be malignant. Contamination of the peritoneal cavity and seeding of the abdominal wall must be avoided. Although complete laparoscopic management of ovarian cancer is not documented enough to gain acceptance, reassessment of adnexal malignancies found on pathology specimens is a universally accepted indication for laparoscopic surgery.

REFERENCES

1. Querleu D, Morrow CP. Classification of radical hysterectomy. Lancet Oncol 2008; 9:297–300.
2. Querleu D, Leblanc E. Laparoscopic surgery in gynecologic cancer. In: Gomel V, Parker J, eds. Manual of Laparoscopic Surgery. Mosby: New York 1995:277–298.
3. Querleu D, Leblanc E, Castelain B. Laparoscopic pelvic lymphadenectomy in the staging of early carcinoma of the cervix. Am J Obstet Gynecol 1991; 164:579–581.
4. Canis M, Mage G, Pouly JL, et al. Laparoscopic diagnosis of adnexal cystic masses: A 12-year experience with long-term follow-up. Obstet Gynecol 1994; 85:707–712.
5. Canis M, Maschiach R, Wattiez A, et al. Frozen section in laparoscopic management of macroscopically suspicious ovarian masses. J Am Assoc Gynecol Laparosc 2004; 11:365–369.
6. Leblanc E, Sonoda Y, Narducci F, et al. Laparoscopic staging of early ovarian carcinoma. Curr Opin Obstet Gynecol 2006; 18: 408–412.
7. Tozzi R, Kohler C, Ferrara A, et al. Laparoscopic treatment of early ovarian cancer: Surgical and survival outcomes. Gynecol Oncol 2004; 93:199–203.
8. Lecuru F, Desfeux P, Camatte S, et al. Impact of initial surgical access on staging and survival of patients with stage I ovarian cancer. Int J Gynecol Cancer 2006; 16:87–94.
9. Camatte S, Morice P, Atallah D, et al. Clinical outcome after laparoscopic pure management of borderline ovarian tumors: Results of a series of 34 patients. Ann Oncol 2004; 15:605–609.
10. Fagotti A, Fanfani F, Ludovisi M, et al. Role of laparoscopy to assess the chance of optimal cytoreductive surgery in advanced ovarian cancer: A pilot study. Gynecol Oncol 2005; 96:729–735.
11. Anaf V, Gangji D, Simon P, et al. Laparoscopical insertion of intraperitoneal catheters for intraperitoneal chemotherapy. Acta Obstet Gynecol Scand 2003; 82:1140–1145.
12. Vergote I, Marquette S, Amant F, et al. Port-site metastasis after open laparoscopy: A study in 173 patients with advanced ovarian carcinoma. Int J Gynecol Cancer 2005; 15:776–779.

9

Treatment of endometriosis associated with infertility

Mauro Busacca and David L. Olive

INTRODUCTION

Endometriosis and infertility have had a long and controversial relationship. The two have been circumstantially linked for over a century, yet many of the aspects of the relationship have been clouded by bias, faulty assumption, and poor science. Today, many issues remain unresolved in the ongoing controversy of the relative importance of endometriosis as a causative factor for infertility.

There is no question that severe endometriosis, with substantial pelvic anatomic distortion, can decrease fertility substantially. Existing studies in animals support this notion (1,2). Additionally, the efficacy of surgical therapy to treat endometriosis-associated infertility with severe disease lends credence to this concept.

More intriguing are the roles of early-stage disease and endometriomas as causative agents of infertility. Animal studies have been equivocal, but most have failed to demonstrate a reduced fecundity secondary to lesions alone (in the absence of significant adhesions) (1,3). Clinical investigation has similarly provided conflicting evidence. Jansen, analyzing the results of women undergoing donor insemination, found early-stage endometriosis to significantly reduce fecundity (4). However, Rodriguez-Escudero et al. (5), Chauhan et al. (6), and Dunphy et al. (7) all failed to show an effect in their published research.

Endometriomas, too, have often been implicated as fertility-reducing entities; yet, existing studies have failed to provide a consistent picture. It has been claimed that large endometriomas affect anatomic relationships to an extent that normal reproductive processes can be disrupted (thus far unproven), whereas small endometriomas may produce a variety of chemokines that alter oocyte quality, embryo quality, or implantation (also yet to be demonstrated definitively).

Given the tenuous relationship between endometriosis and infertility, it has been left to treatment trials to define the likelihood of a cause–effect relationship and, if one exists, to elucidate the magnitude of the effect. This chapter will review the different types of treatment for endometriosis-associated infertility, their degree of efficacy, and their roles in clinical practice.

ISSUES OF TREATMENT TRIAL STUDY DESIGN AND ANALYSIS

Problem of Diagnosis

When studying endometriosis, it is imperative to have a clearly defined demarcation between those who have the disease and those who do not. Unfortunately, this line is blurred in most, if not all, investigations involving endometriosis. It would be ideal if a simple blood test or imaging study provided highly accurate classification of patients with and without the disease; unfortunately, while these modalities are of some value, their sensitivity, specificity, and accuracy are far too low to be reliable as a gold standard in classifying patients for a treatment trial (8). Similarly, relying upon symptoms and signs to accurately assign patients has proven less than ideal, due to their lack of specificity. Recently, attempts have been made to combine these factors into an algorithm for diagnosis, but this approach is both complex and thus far inadequate (9). Finally, recent work investigating results from invasive tests such as endometrial biopsy has shown promise but needs further study, confirmation, and actual clinical application (10).

Given these shortcomings of diagnostic tests, the traditional gold standard has been laparoscopy with visual identification of endometriosis. However, even this invasive and expensive approach is problematic. Although endometriosis was believed for many years to have a fairly characteristic appearance, reports by Jansen and Russell (11) and Stripling et al. (12) in the 1980s demonstrated that endometriosis can take on a variety of visual forms, varying in color, size, and structure. These atypical-appearing lesions in fact make up a majority of lesions present in the diseased patient, yet they are missed by many otherwise experienced surgeons. Furthermore, endometriosis may exist in a subperitoneal location, inaccessible to the surgeon's view via laparoscopy.

The converse situation also exists: what appears to be endometriosis may well not be. Two published studies have shown the positive predictive value of visualizing implants, even by well-experienced endometriosis surgeons, to be less than 50% when compared to histology (13,14). Thus, if you do not see endometriosis it may still be present, and if you do see it the disease may not actually be present! A proposed solution to this issue is excision of all lesions with histologic evaluation; unfortunately, this is difficult for many surgeons, poses significant surgical danger in some women, and still does not remedy the problem of "hidden" or subperitoneal disease. This limitation should be kept in mind when evaluating the veracity of treatment trials for endometriosis-associated infertility.

Issues with Study Design

Although many studies have been published regarding the treatment of endometriosis, it is important to realize that not all are of equal importance. A hierarchy of clinical trial design exists enabling the discerning reader to determine which studies should be relied on most heavily for validity and applicability (15). These study designs, and their place in the hierarchy, are listed in Table 1.

Table 1 Hierarchy of Evidence from Clinical Studies

I.	Meta-analysis or large randomized clinical trial
II.	Small randomized clinical trial
III.	Nonrandomized, concurrently controlled trial
IV.	Historically controlled trial
V.	Case–control study or cohort study
VI.	Time-series study or anecdotal case reports
VII.	Expert opinion

Uncontrolled trials have limited value other than to suggest hypotheses to be tested by more rigorous designs. The same is true for historically controlled studies and concurrently controlled nonrandomized trials, each of which introduces significant biases into the results. The gold standard today is the randomized clinical trial (RCT), where subjects are randomly allocated to one of several treatment groups, often in a blinded manner such that the assignment is unknown to the patient or the physician until the conclusion of the trial. This design is the least biased of all approaches and results in the most reliable conclusions.

Unfortunately, many RCTs are too small to reach a negative conclusion with any degree of confidence. The results of RCTs may also differ from one another, due to slight differences in study design, different patient populations, or even as a result of chance events. For these reasons, when multiple randomized trials exist, they can often be combined into a single evaluation called a meta-analysis (16). The meta-analysis allows us to gain a single best answer to a question with a higher level of confidence than is usually possible with individual studies. However, it is important to keep in mind that a meta-analysis is only as good as the studies included in it; if poor-quality trials are placed into a meta-analysis, the resulting conclusions are as tenuous as those of the component studies.

Issues with Outcome Measures

The value of a particular treatment upon endometriosis will vary depending on the therapeutic goal of the intervention. With regard to endometriosis, there are three outcomes that can be assessed to determine drug efficacy: (*i*) the anatomic manifestations of the disease, (*ii*) pain symptomatology, and (*iii*) infertility status. Only fertility as an outcome measure is relevant to the issues discussed in this chapter.

The basic issues regarding fertility enhancement include the degree of infertility, the many causative and contributing factors to infertility, and the time-dependent nature of fertility. Degree of infertility is a critically important factor that can substantially affect outcomes. For instance, subfertility that is due to an absolute factor (azospermia and obstructed fallopian tubes) would be expected to be easily reversed if the inciting factor is repaired. Thus, infertile women undergoing donor insemination due to a partner with azospermia have a higher monthly pregnancy rate than women undergoing the same procedure for unexplained infertility. Similarly, women who have problems that are sporadic but correctable (oligo-ovulation) will have a higher posttreatment success rate than women with unknown reasons for subfecundity (unexplained infertility). This confounder must be considered when examining two groups in a treatment trial.

Another basic issue in such studies is whether or not to attribute a treatment success to the treatment. This is easily done with absolute infertility, but less reasonable with relative subfertility. It is rare that the woman with endometriosis-associated infertility has absolute infertility due to the disease, as is the case with bilateral tubal blockage or azospermia. Instead, most women suffering from endometriosis-associated infertility have a relative reduction in fecundity. Thus, they are able to conceive, albeit at a slower rate. To demonstrate improved fertility status after intervention, a comparison group of similar, untreated women is clearly needed.

The final methodological issue in analyzing results of fertility treatments is the problem of time dependence of the outcome: pregnancy. Clearly, women followed for three months postintervention will likely have a far lower pregnancy rate than if they were followed for three years. This variability in length of follow-up must be considered and dealt with either by uniformity of the follow-up period or by appropriate correction for this confounding factor.

From the above discussion, it is clear that optimal trials are properly controlled and randomized. In addition, it is important to have studies with lengthy follow-ups so that we can determine the long-term course posttreatment. Studies such as these will primarily be relied upon in the subsequent discussion.

SURGICAL MANAGEMENT

When performing surgery for endometriosis, the surgeon is confronted with a number of technical issues regarding the performance of the surgery. These include the desired method of access, the method of treating implants, and the type of surgery done for endometriomas. Additionally, aside from treating endometriosis, the surgical approach to this disease frequently involves lysing adhesions to restore pelvic anatomy.

Surgical Techniques

Method of Access

When conservative surgery is desired, the first technical issue confronted is the method of access. Traditionally, laparotomy has been used for endometriosis surgery. However, recently, most surgeons performing extensive surgery for endometriosis have favored a laparoscopic approach. The reasons for this are several. First, laparoscopy is less invasive, with a much more rapid recovery time. In addition, the cost for a laparoscopic procedure is less than that for a major surgery. Finally, magnification by the laparoscope offers the possibility of a more precise technique.

Method of Destruction of Implants

Surgical destruction of endometriosis lesions can be accomplished in a variety of ways: excision, vaporization, and *electrosurgical* fulguration/desiccation/*coagulation* have all been used. Excision is generally thought to be the most complete of these techniques and can be accomplished with a variety of instruments ranging from the laser, to monopolar needles, to ultrasonic energy, to scissors. The technique is straightforward: the lesion margins are identified by close inspection of the peritoneum, and the mechanical or energized cutting instrument is used to outline the area to be excised. A relaxing incision is made between any vital anatomy and the lesion to minimize inadvertent traumatic or thermal injury. The implant is then lifted with atraumatic forceps and separated from the underlying normal fibroareolar tissue by careful dissection. Depending on the location, thickness, and size of the implant, this procedure may be simple or extremely difficult. Many surgeons favor hydrodissection, a technique of irrigating under pressure the tissue near the lesion, in an attempt to separate normal from abnormal. However, two dangers exist: first, fluid below the peritoneum frequently distorts anatomy, making a difficult dissection even more difficult, and second, structures fibrotically adherent to endometriosis such as the ureter will not separate and can be damaged if care is not taken to ensure their safety during excision of the lesion.

Vaporization is achieved using high power density energy over a short interval of time. This induces a rapid increase in water temperature, resulting in vaporization and volumetric tissue destruction. Energy density sufficient to vaporize can be created using the edge or tip of an electrosurgical electrode while sparking to the target lesion, avoiding carbonization (see Chapter 3). This can also be achieved using a focused, very high power density super- or ultrapulse CO_2 laser.

Techniques for desiccation and coagulation use lower energy densities and result in comparatively lower temperatures at the tissue level. At 60°C to 80°C for even very short periods of time, there is a loss of intracellular water and denaturation of protein, resulting in irreversible cellular destruction. This technique is considerably less precise than vaporization, as peripheral destruction to adjacent tissue and the depth of penetration are not always predictable. While lasers with lower energy density provide a rapid means of performing this method, bi- and monopolar electrosurgical contact techniques can be used as well.

Method of Treating Endometriomas

Endometriomas are commonly present in the patient with endometriosis, and the method by which they are surgically treated may be quite important to the outcome. The goals of treating ovarian endometriomas are to (*i*) remove all ectopic endometrium in the ovary, (*ii*) minimize ovarian trauma and preserve follicles, and (*iii*) minimize postoperative adhesion formation (17).

Two types of endometriomas are recognized. The first and least common type is one entirely within the interior of the ovary. More common, however, is an inverted anterior ovarian cortex with adhesions and implants on the surface, frequently adherent to the broad ligament. This latter type represents more than 90% of ovarian endometriomas (Fig. 1) (18).

When operating on endometriomas, the ovaries should first be freed of all adhesions by successively lysing cephalocaudally and lateromedially. The endometrioma may open spontaneously during this process; if not, incision and drainage are indicated. At this point, the cyst wall may be stripped, excised, or drained as indicated. Stripping involves separating the cyst wall from the ovary and slowly peeling them apart. One method, termed the Putman–Redwine technique, consists of circumscribing the opening to the endometrioma with a laser, electrosurgery, or ultrasonic energy, then dissecting down to the cyst wall. The two are then separated sharply and bluntly until the cyst wall is removed, frequently intact. Excision can also be accomplished by wedge resection; while removal of the endometrioma is invariably complete, the potential for adhesion formation is higher (19). Vaporization or coagulation of cyst walls has also been described.

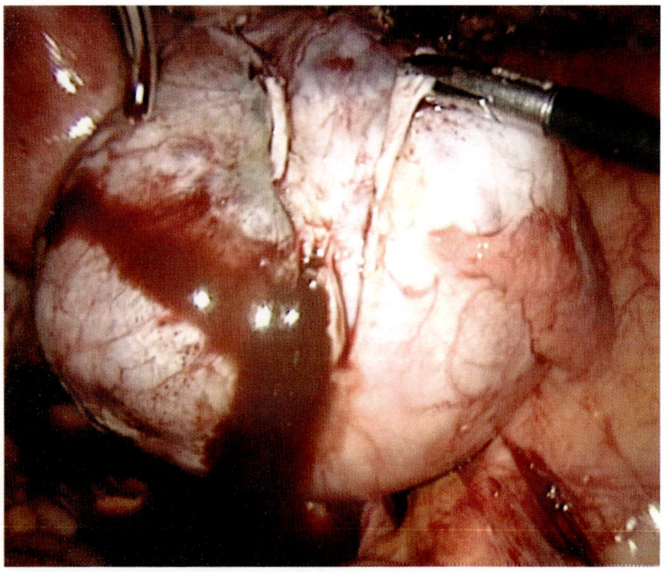

Figure 1 Right ovarian endometrioma.

The safety of the surgical removal of endometriomata in terms of damage to ovarian reserve has recently been questioned. In fact, the presence of healthy ovarian tissue adjacent to the cyst wall has been discovered in the majority of excised endometriomata, while this is an occasional finding in non-endometriotic benign ovarian cysts. The role of excisional surgery in damaging ovarian reserve, at least immediately after the procedure, has been reported in a recent trial, which studied 31 patients who underwent excision of unilateral ($n = 25$) or bilateral ($n = 6$) benign ovarian cysts. The authors showed a percentage of reduction of the ovarian volume of 33% (20).

The risk of ovarian reserve reduction should be considered especially when approaching bilateral endometriomata. In fact, a prevalence of postsurgical ovarian failure of 2.4% (95% CI: 0.5–6.8) has recently been reported in 126 patients operated for bilateral endometriotic ovarian cysts, two times higher than that in general population (21).

Lysis of Adhesions

Adhesiolysis is an important step in the restoration of normal pelvic and abdominal anatomy. While simple lysis of adhesions is adequate if they were formed following infection, most experts believe a more complete approach is required for the endometriosis-induced adhesion; the reason for this is the relatively high incidence of endometriosis present within the adhesion tissue itself. Thus, removal of the adhesion by lysing both boundaries of the scar tissue and connecting structures is preferable. The instrumentation is of little consequence, so long as precision and hemostasis are maintained.

To minimize adhesion reformation, adhesion prevention adjuvants can be used. All such currently available adjuvants have been demonstrated by RCTs to decrease the amount of adhesion reformation (22). These can be applied to the dissected tissue surfaces either laparoscopically or laparotomically.

Results of Surgical Treatment of Endometriosis-Associated Infertility

The surgical approach to endometriosis varies considerably based on the degree of disease present. While older, poorly constructed studies frequently lumped all patients together for surgical treatment trials, modern investigators have generally divided or limited their study population by stage of endometriosis.

Stages I and II (Early-Stage Endometriosis)

Several RCTs have investigated the value of surgically treating early-stage endometriosis (Fig. 2) in infertile women. The first involved 341 Canadian women undergoing laparoscopic surgery with or without the destruction of visible endometriotic lesions (23). A significantly higher pregnancy rate (30.7% vs. 17.7%; $p = 0.006$) was noted in those patients who had resection or ablation of all endometriotic lesions. A second trial, by the Gruppo Italiano per lo Studio dell'Endometriosi, involved 101 women with characteristics similar to the Canadian group trial, followed for 52 weeks after laparoscopy (24).

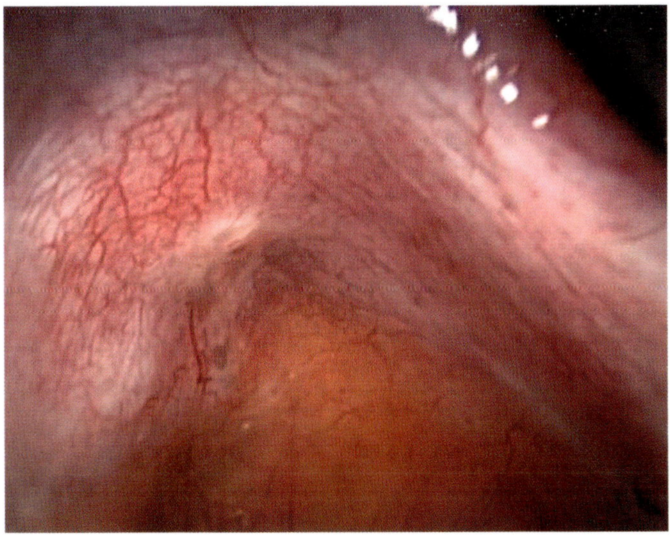

Figure 2 Superficial peritoneal endometriosis of cul-de-sac.

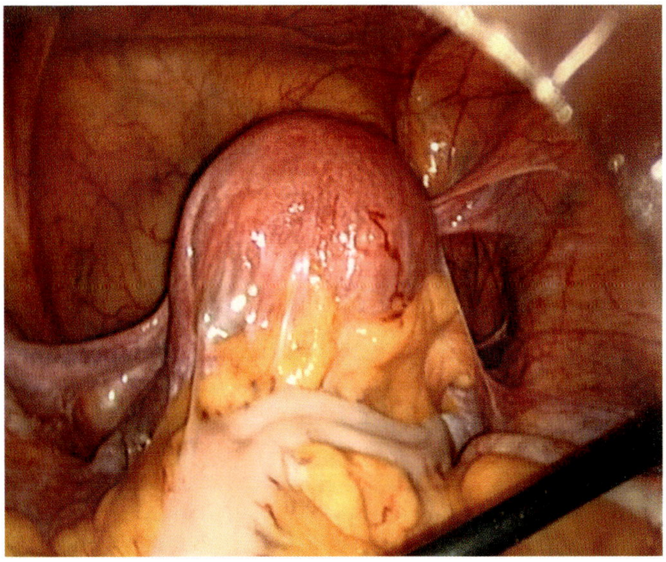

Figure 4 Uterine sigmoid adhesions.

The pregnancy rate observed in the two groups was no different statistically (24% vs. 29%), and fecundity was 0.016 and 0.019 in the ablated and untreated groups, respectively. Despite the disparate results from these two trials, when the studies are combined into a meta-analysis, there is a significant benefit to surgical treatment (OR for pregnancy, 1.7); for every 12 patients having minimal or mild disease at laparoscopy, there will be one additional successful pregnancy if ablation or resection of visible endometriosis is performed, with respect to no treatment (25). A third recent RCT by Elsheikh and associates recently confirmed this conclusion (26). Whereas adenomyosis is commonly present in women who also have endometriosis (Fig. 3), its significance as a "disease" and possible effect(s) on fertility are presently unknown.

Stages III and IV (Advanced Endometriosis)

In infertile patients affected by moderate and severe endometriosis, the intent of surgery is to restore normal anatomy through extirpation of the disease and careful adhesiolysis as further elucidated in Chapter 10, in order to facilitate fecundity. No RCTs exist to address this issue, but retrospective controlled studies support the concept that surgical treatment is beneficial (Figs. 4 and 5) (27).

Ovarian Endometriosis

The ovarian endometrioma, when found in the absence of significant adhesion formation, provides another therapeutic quandary. There are several studies suggesting that the presence of an ovarian endometriotic cyst might impair oocyte

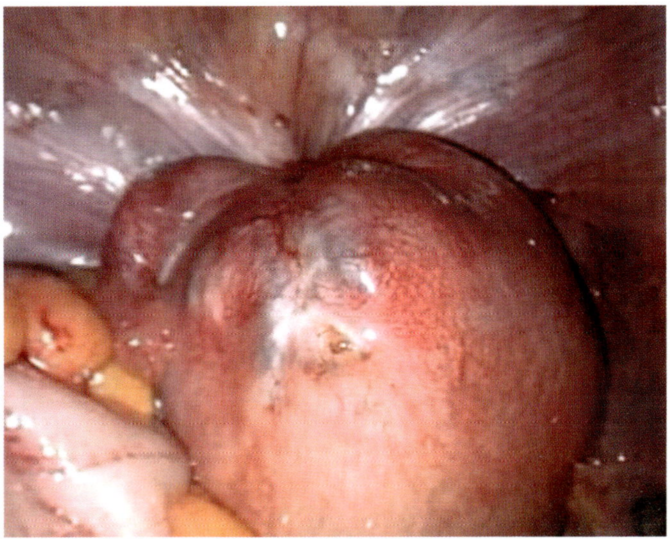

Figure 3 Adenomyosis.

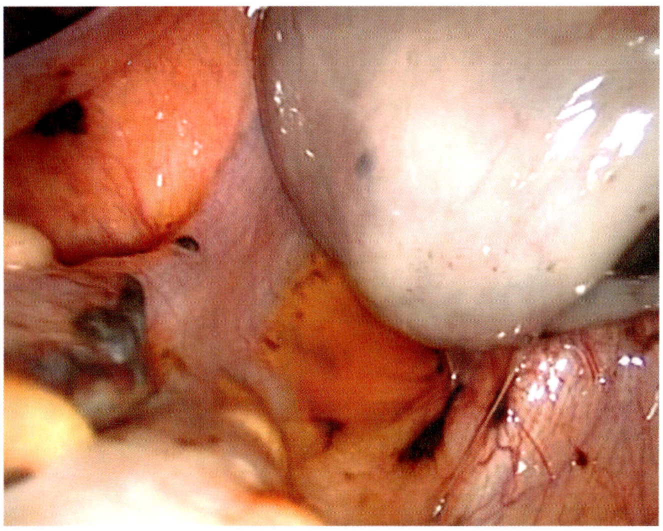

Figure 5 Endometriotic nodules on sigmoid serosa.

quality in the affected ovary and that the response to controlled ovarian hyperstimulation (COH), as well as fertilization and implantation rates, might be reduced. Fortunately, it has been reported by Redwine that the finding of endometriosis as only confined to the ovary is rare, about 1% (27).

Prospective study (28) and two randomized trials of removal of the cyst wall versus fenestration and aspiration of cyst contents clearly demonstrate improved results with removal, whether the outcome of interest is pain relief, fertility, or rate of reoperation (29,30). These data, recently supported by a Cochrane review (31), suggest that an excisional approach should be favored in the surgical management of endometriomata. When bleeding is encountered at the site of the excised cyst, data suggest that it is preferable to obtain hemostasis with sutures than with electrosurgery (32).

Deep Infiltrating Endometriosis

Deep infiltrating endometriosis, which penetrates below the surface of the peritoneum more than 5 mm (Figs. 6 and 7) (33), differs from other peritoneal and ovarian lesions in its particular histopathologic features and its strong correlation with pelvic pain and severe dyspareunia (34). Excision of such lesions has long been advocated; fortunately, it appears that such aggressive surgery rarely causes infertility due to postoperative adhesion formation, even after bowel and bladder resection (Figs. 8 and 9) (27,35–38).

A very recent paper of Fedele et al. (39) had focused on the odd phenomenon of infertility associated with deep endometriosis. The authors retrospectively studied 105 infertile women with rectovaginal endometriosis who underwent conservative surgery (44/105) or expectant management (61/105) according to a shared decision-making approach. The 12-month cumulative probability of conception was 20.5% and 34.7%, respectively. No statistically significant differences were noted even when considering the cumulative 24-month probabilities (44.9% and 46.8%, respectively; p = 0.38). These results suggest that radical conservative surgery for rectovaginal endometriosis should not be considered for infertility only, but for patients suffering from pain in addition to infertility.

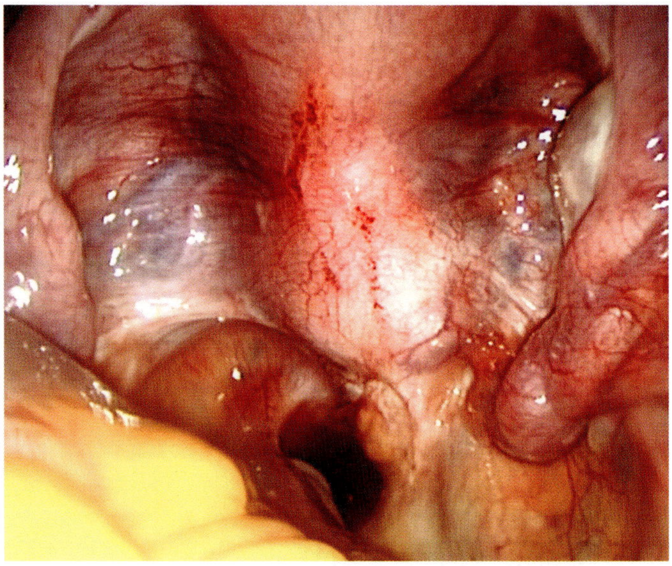

Figure 7 Endometriotic nodule of right posterior cul-de-sac.

Surgical Therapy: Conclusions

The surgical treatment of endometriosis-associated infertility appears to be of value in all stages of the disease, although the quality of data is severely limited in the advanced stages. However, the improvement may be only marginal in early-stage disease, thus making diagnostic laparoscopy to determine the presence or absence a questionable endeavor. For example, if one in three infertile women has endometriosis, then laparoscopy of all infertile women will require more than 30 procedures to produce a single additional pregnancy. Thus, it is most sensible to surgically investigate only those patients at high risk of disease (increasing pelvic pain and dyspareunia) or those who have another indication for surgical exploration (prior pelvic surgery, history of sexually transmitted disease, and abnormal hysterosalpingogram). We should all move toward a more judicious use of laparoscopy in the

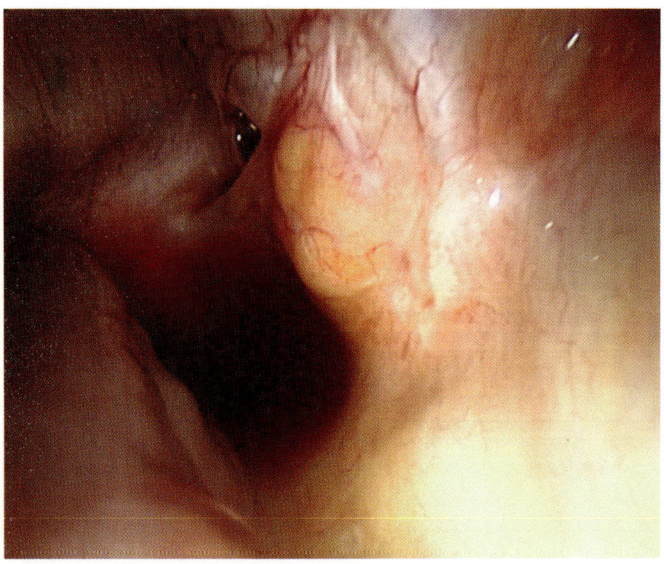

Figure 6 Rectovaginal endometriotic nodule.

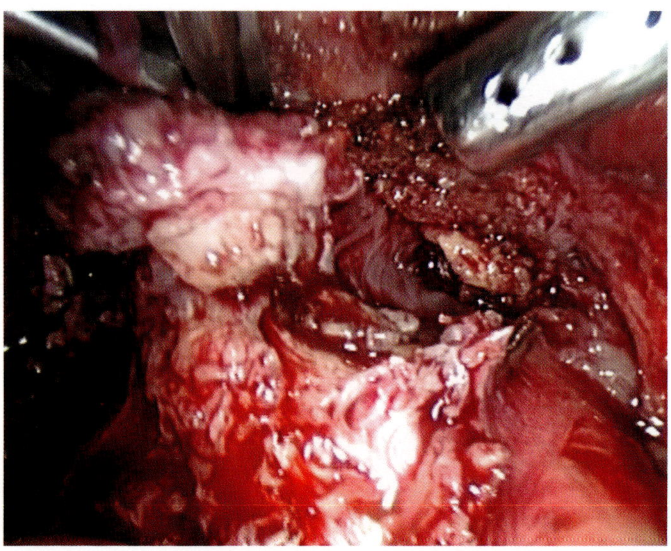

Figure 8 Anterior rectal wall nodule.

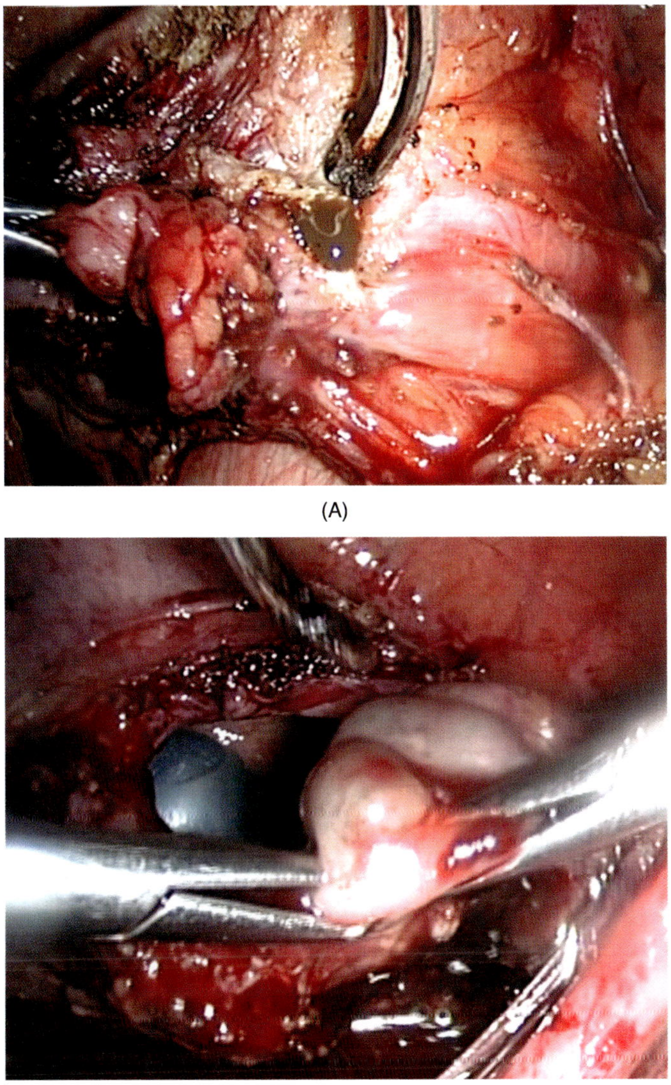

(A)

(B)

Figure 9 (A) Deep infiltrating endometriotic nodule of the bladder. (B) View of internal face of nodule in (A).

infertile woman when the sole rationale is the investigation of possible endometriosis.

MEDICAL THERAPY

The medical treatment of endometriosis has long played a major role in the therapeutic approach to this disorder. However, the approach to the design of medical therapeutics for endometriosis is evolving scientifically, as new strategies are aiding in the attack upon this disease. What once was an armamentarium of a handful of ovulation suppression agents is fast becoming a diverse array of finely directed treatment options.

The original development of medication to treat endometriosis was built upon several observations. First, endometriosis is infrequently encountered in the parous women, but much more often in the nulliparous female, suggesting a protective effect of the hormonal milieu of pregnancy. Second, endometrium is known to be estrogen dependent, with ectopic endometrium presumably behaving in much the same manner. Finally, endometriosis tends to occur nearly exclusively in menstruating, reproductive-age women, again suggesting hormonal dependence. These findings suggested the potential benefits of hormonal therapy to alter the normal menstrual cyclicity of the reproductive years, the mainstay of medical treatment for endometriosis.

Recently, however, the approach has changed. We now have a much greater depth of understanding of the pathogenesis, growth, and maintenance of ectopic endometrium, particularly at the molecular level. This has provided drug developers with new, precise molecular targets for treatment of the disease. Currently under development, these newer agents hold the potential of greater efficacy and flexibility with fewer systemic effects.

Established Treatments of Endometriosis

Danazol

The first drug to be approved for the treatment of endometriosis was danazol, an isoxazol derivative of 17-alpha-ethinyl testosterone. It was originally thought to produce a pseudomenopause, but subsequent studies have revealed the drug to act primarily by diminishing the midcycle luteinizing hormone (LH) surge, creating a chronic anovulatory state (40,41). Additional actions include inhibitor of multiple enzymes in the steroidogenic pathology (42) and increase in free serum testosterone (43). The recommended dosage of danazol for the treatment of endometriosis is 600 to 800 mg/day; however, these doses have substantial androgenic side effects such as increased hair growth, mood changes, adverse serum lipid profiles, deepening of the voice (possibly irreversible), and, rarely, liver damage (possibly irreversible and life threatening) and arterial thrombosis (44,45). Studies of lower doses as primary treatment for endometriosis-associated pain have been uncontrolled or in small numbers and thus contain information of limited value (46). However, due to many side effects of the drug, alternative routes of administration have been sought. Recently, the use of danazol vaginal suppositories and danazol-impregnated vaginal ring has been described in small, uncontrolled trials (47,48). Preliminary results suggest that side effects may be less severe with the transvaginal approach.

Progestogens

Progestogens are a class of compounds that produce progesterone-like effects upon endometrial tissue. A large number of progestogens exist, ranging from those chemically derived from progesterone (progestins) such as medroxyprogesterone acetate to 19-nortestosterone derivatives such as norethindrone and norgestrel. The proposed mechanism of action of these compounds is initial decidualization of endometrial tissue followed by eventual atrophy. This is believed to be due to a direct suppressive effect of progestogens upon the estrogen receptors of the endometrium. Recent evidence suggests that another mechanism of action at the molecular level is the suppression of matrix metalloproteinases, enzymes important in the implantation and growth of ectopic endometrium (49).

The most extensively studied progestational agent for the treatment of endometriosis is medroxyprogesterone. The drug was originally used orally for the treatment of endometriosis, with doses ranging from 20 to 100 mg daily; published randomized studies are limited to 100 mg daily. However, the depot formulation has also been used, in a dose of 150 mg every three months. Side effects of medroxyprogesterone are multiple and varied, yet, even in high doses, seems to be better tolerated metabolically than danazol. A common side effect is transient breakthrough bleeding, which occurs in 38% to 47% of patients. This is generally well tolerated and, when necessary, can be adequately treated with supplemental estrogen or an increase in the progestogen dose. Other side effects include nausea (0–80%), breast tenderness (5%), fluid retention (50%), and depression (6%) (50). In published trials, few patients have discontinued the medications secondary to side effects. In contradistinction to danazol, all of the abovementioned adverse effects resolve upon discontinuation of the drugs.

Other progestational agents have also been used in the occasional study, including lynestrenol, a gestagen used primarily in Europe. Levonorgestrel, the active ingredient of Norplant, has also been used recently, via an intrauterine device delivery system (51). The drug has been shown to effectively decrease vascular endothelial growth factor and blood vessel proliferation, providing rationale for its use in endometriosis (52). It has been touted recently as a desirable treatment for rectovaginal endometriosis, although evidence thus far is uncontrolled (51).

Progestogens may adversely affect serum lipoprotein levels (53–55). The 19-nortestosterone derivatives significantly decrease high-density lipoprotein, a change linked to an increased risk of coronary artery disease (54). Data on medroxyprogesterone acetate are less clear, with studies demonstrating either no effect or a slight decrease (54,55). It is likely that there is a decrease in high-density lipoprotein with all these agents, but the magnitude is related to the specific progestogen and the dose administered. Whether alterations in serum lipoprotein levels for four to six months have any clinical significance is unclear.

Oral Contraceptives (Combination Estrogen–Progestogen)

The combination of estrogen and progestogen for therapy of endometriosis, the so-called "pseudopregnancy" regimen, has been used for 40 years. Like progestational therapy alone, pseudopregnancy is believed to produce initial decidualization and growth of endometrial tissue, followed in several months by atrophy. This has been observed in women (56) but is in direct conflict with data obtained for the rhesus monkey (57), demonstrating larger implants with considerable local growth following such a therapeutic approach.

Pseudopregnancy regimens have been administered both orally and parenterally. Combination oral contraceptive pills such as norethynodrel and mestranol, norethindrone acetate and ethinyl estradiol, lynestrenol and mestranol, and norgestrel plus ethinyl estradiol have all been tried. Parenteral combinations have included 17-hydroxyprogesterone or depot medroxyprogesterone acetate paired with stilbestrol or conjugated estrogens.

Side effects of pseudopregnancy are often quite impressive and include those encountered with progestogens alone, as well as estrogenic- and androgenic-related effects. Estrogens may cause nausea, hypertension, thrombophlebitis, and uterine enlargement. The 19-nortestosterone-derived progestogens may cause androgenic effects such as acne, alopecia, increased muscle mass, decreased breast size, and deepening of the voice. Noble and Letchworth, in a comparative trial of norethynodrel and mestranol versus danazol, found that 41% of the pseudopregnancy group failed to complete their course of therapy due to side effects of the medication (58). However, the medications in this study used far higher doses than are found in modern contraceptive preparations. The oral contraceptives commonly prescribed today for combination therapy are most likely to produce a progestogen-dominant picture similar to that of progestogen alone.

Today, oral contraceptives are the most commonly prescribed treatment for endometriosis symptoms. Despite this, there are little data regarding the mechanism of action. One recent investigation suggests that oral contraceptives suppress proliferation and enhance programmed cell death (apoptosis) in endometrial tissue, perhaps providing a mechanistic clue for the action of these drugs (59).

GnRH Agonists

Gonadotropin-releasing hormone agonists (GnRH agonists) are analogs of the hormone GnRH. This hypothalamic hormone is responsible for stimulating the pituitary gland to secrete follicle-stimulating hormone (FSH) and LH, two hormones necessary for normal ovarian function. GnRH is secreted in a pulsatile manner; the correct pulse results in stimulation of FSH and LH release, while too high or too low a pulse rate results in a decrease in pituitary hormone secretion. GnRH agonists are modified forms of GnRH that bind to the pituitary receptors and remain for a longer period. Thus, they are identified by the pituitary as rapidly pulsatile GnRH and, after initial stimulation of FSH and LH secretion, result in a shutdown (down regulation) of the pituitary, and there is no resulting stimulation of the ovary. The result is a hypoestrogenic state similar to that of menopause, producing endometrial atrophy and amenorrhea. It is also possible that the drug affects ectopic endometrium via additional mechanisms: animal studies have suggested alterations in plasminogen activators and matrix metalloproteinases, factors important in endometriosis development (60).

The agonist can be given intranasally, subcutaneously, or intramuscularly depending on the specific product, with frequency of administration ranging from twice daily to every three months. The side effects are those of hypoestrogenism such as transient vaginal bleeding, hot flashes, vaginal dryness, decreased libido, breast tenderness, insomnia, depression, irritability and fatigue, headache, osteoporosis, and decreased skin elasticity; these are dose dependent (61).

A recent modification of GnRH agonist treatment is to "add back" small amounts of steroid hormone in a manner similar to that used in the treatment of postmenopausal women. The theory is that the requirement for estrogen is greater for endometriosis than is needed by the brain (to prevent hot flashes), the bone (to prevent osteoporosis), and other tissues deprived of this hormone (62). Interestingly, this "threshold hypothesis" appears to be true, with estrogen–progestogen or progestogen-only add-back therapy resulting in an equivalent rate of pain relief with far fewer side effects than GnRH agonist alone. Estrogen as a solitary add-back, however, is less effective and thus unindicated (63).

Gestrinone

Gestrinone (ethyl norgestrienone, R2323) is an antiprogestational steroid whose effects include androgenic, antiprogestogenic, and antiestrogenic actions, although the latter is not mediated by estrogen-receptor binding.

This steroid is believed to act by inducting a progesterone withdrawal effect at the endometrial cellular level, thus enhancing lysosomal degradation of the cellular structure. There is a rapid decrease in estrogen and progesterone receptors in normal endometrium following administration of gestrinone, as well as a sharp increase in 17 β-hydroxysteroid dehydrogenase. Interestingly, these cellular effects did not occur in samples of endometriotic tissue (64).

Table 2 Meta-analysis of Medical Therapy for Endometriosis-Associated Infertility

Study	Medical treatment	Placebo or no treatment	Relative risk	95% Confidence limits
Bayer et al. (66)	11/37	17/36	0.63	0.32–1.22
Fedele et al. (67)	17/35	17/36	1.03	0.60–1.76
Telimaa (68)	13/35	6/14	0.87	0.41–2.25
Thomas and Cooke (69)	5/20	4/17	1.06	0.28–4.29
Harrison and Barry-Kinsella (70)	0/50	3/50	0.00	0.00–2.18
Total	46/177	47/153	0.85	0.59–1.22

Gestrinone may also inhibit ovarian steroidogenesis. A 50% decrease in serum estradiol level is noted after administration, perhaps related to the associated significant decline in sex-hormone-binding globulin concentration (an androgenic or antiprogestogenic effect) (65). No effect on adrenal function or prolactin secretion has been noted.

Gestrinone is administered orally in doses of 2.5 to 10 mg weekly, on a daily, twice-weekly, or thrice-weekly schedule. Side effects include androgenic and antiestrogenic sequelae. Although most side effects are mild and transient, several, such as voice changes, hirsutism, and clitoral hypertrophy, are potentially irreversible.

Infertility Treatment Results

Most of the established medical therapies used to treat endometriosis have been applied to the problem of subfertility in women with endometriosis. These medications inhibit ovulation and thus are used to treat the disease for a period of time prior to allowing an attempt at conception. Five randomized trials with six treatment arms have compared one of these medical treatments directed at endometriosis to placebo or no treatment with fertility as the outcome measure (Table 2) (66–70). Another eight RCTs compared danazol to a second medication. These latter trials have been summarized recently by a meta-analysis by Hughes et al. (71). Clearly, no increase in fertility can be demonstrated with these medications when compared to expectant management, nor has any medication proven superior to danazol in this regard.

It is important to note, however, that some studies were placebo controlled, while others simply compared medication to no treatment. For this latter study design, follow-up of the patient was begun at the conclusion of therapy; thus, those receiving no treatment began attempting to conceive immediately after the diagnostic laparoscopy, while those placed on drug therapy were not allowed attempted conception until after the medication course was completed (generally six months). These studies were analyzed considering that the time began at the conclusion of the "treatment," but for the patient, the clock begins ticking at the time of diagnostic laparoscopy. The real question is not who gets pregnant faster after therapy is completed, but rather who gets pregnant faster from the time of diagnosis.

If we reanalyze the above data, with follow-up proceeding from the time of diagnosis instead of conclusion of treatment, a different image emerges (Table 3). Now, suppressive medical therapy proves significantly detrimental to fertility. In essence, the interval spent on medical therapy has been wasted time, merely serving to prolong the infertility in a number of couples. Thus, traditional medical therapy for endometriosis has not proven to be of value and in fact may be counterproductive to the subfertile patient.

Experimental Medical Therapy

Using the basic research that has recently uncovered many molecular aspects of the pathogenesis and pathophysiology of endometriosis, a number of new medical approaches have been studied or are under development. These drugs include selective estrogen receptor modulators, selective progesterone receptor modulators, GnRH antagonists, aromatase inhibitors, tumor necrosis factor α inhibitors, angiogenesis inhibitors, matrix metalloproteinase inhibitors, immunomodulators, and estrogen receptor β agonists.

Of the experimental treatment for endometriosis, only pentoxifylline (an immunomodulator) has been investigated as a treatment for endometriosis-associated infertility. This drug has the advantage of not inhibiting ovulation and thus can be used without delay of attempted conception. A single placebo-controlled RCT with 60 patients resulted in a 12-month pregnancy rate of 31% with pentoxifylline and 18.5% with placebo, a difference not statistically significant but intriguing nonetheless (72). Hopefully, additional, larger trials will further investigate this approach to help clarify the value of this and similar drugs.

Medical Therapy: Conclusions

Today, there is no good evidence that medical therapy to treat endometriosis is of any value in enhancing fertility; indeed, the data suggest that the delay produced by most treatment intervals actually deters fertility, an undesirable effect in the infertile couple.

Table 3 Meta-analysis of Medical Therapy for Endometriosis-Associated Infertility: Adjustment for Follow-Up from Time of Diagnosis

Study	Medical treatment	Placebo or no treatment	Relative risk	95% Confidence limits
Bayer et al. (66)	11/37	17/36	0.63	0.32–1.22
Fedele et al. (67)	10/35	13/36	0.79	0.36–1.68
Telimaa (68)	4/35	5/14	0.32	0.08–1.24
Thomas and Cooke (69)	4/20	4/17	0.85	0.20–3.69
Harrison and Barry-Kinsella (70)	0/50	3/50	0.00	0.00–2.18
Total	29/177	42/153	0.60	0.38–0.93

This is not to suggest, however, that medical therapy is incapable of playing a role in the treatment of the infertile couple with endometriosis. It is quite possible that a subgroup of infertile women exist who could be helped with drug therapy. This concept has been explored in two areas. The first is pre-ART medical therapy, which will be discussed in a later section of this chapter.

A second potential area of interest lies in selecting patients for treatment by morphologic appearance of the disease. Elsheikh and colleagues recently performed a randomized fertility treatment trial in women with stage I endometriosis comparing surgery, medical therapy (six months of GnRH agonist), and expectant management. The group being treated medically was further subclassified by type of lesion observed at laparoscopy: blue-black, red, or other. In patients with red lesions, fertility at two years was equivalent to surgery and exceeded that of expectant management (26). Such selective administration of medical therapy should be further investigated.

ASSISTED REPRODUCTION

A third treatment option for the infertile woman with endometriosis is assisted reproduction. This therapeutic class includes the use of COH, intrauterine insemination (IUI), and in vitro fertilization (IVF). Issues surrounding these treatment approaches include the following: (*i*) What is the efficacy of assisted reproduction in the patient with endometriosis-associated infertility? (*ii*) Is pretreatment of the patient undergoing ART with medical therapy for endometriosis of value?

COH with or Without IUI

COH can be performed with medications such as clomiphene, letrozole, and gonadotropins. These drugs can be used in both ovulatory and anovulatory patients, with the goal being to produce multiple ovulatory follicles. This is frequently followed by the use of IUI, an attempt to produce more functional sperm in the vicinity of the oocyte.

The use of these treatments in the couple with endometriosis and no other demonstrable pathology has been investigated. Three RCTs have examined the use of COH in women with endometriosis, and all have shown a three- to fivefold increase in pregnancy rates using this intervention (Table 4) (73–75). To our knowledge, no randomized study has specifically investigated the effectiveness of COH-IUI in endometriosis stages III and IV with patent tubes. However, retrospective analyses of large case series suggest that COH-IUI may increase the fecundity rate when compared to spontaneous conception.

Despite the apparent enhancement in fertility with COH and IUI, the resulting pregnancy rate is lower than that seen in women with chronic anovulation or couples with unexplained infertility (76). Thus, while this treatment may prove advantageous, it is also worthwhile to consider even more aggressive approaches.

Table 4 Randomized Trials Comparing COH and IUI to No Treatment in Women with Endometriosis

Author	Year	Stimulant	COH and IUI	EM
Deaton et al.	1990	CC	9.5%	3.3%
Tummon et al.	1997	FSH	11%	2%
Fedele et al.	1992	FSH/LH	14.8%	4.5%

EM: Expected management.

In Vitro Fertilization

IVF is widely recognized, despite the absence of randomized, controlled data, to be an effective treatment for endometriosis-associated subfertility (77). However, whether or not endometriosis has an adverse effect upon IVF success rates has been hotly debated in the medical literature. Numerous studies have retrospectively investigated the issue. Recently, Barnhart et al., in a meta-analysis of existing studies, documented an odds ratio (OR) for pregnancy rate of 0.56 (95% CI: 0.44–0.70) in patients with endometriosis when compared to those with tubal disease (78). An updated meta-analysis addressing the same issue by Collins gave similar results, but the analysis lost its statistical significance (OR: 0.72; 95% CI: 0.40–1.31) (Collins JA, personal communication).

The effect of disease stage on the success of IVF has also been examined. The aforementioned meat analysis by Barnhart suggested that the pregnancy rate was significantly lower for women with severe forms of the disease than for those with mild disease (OR = 0.60; 95% CI: 0.42–0.87) (78). This is supported by examining those trials that include only patients of a single stage: three examining only stage I patients revealed no difference in pregnancy, while the one study restricted to stage IV patients found a marked lowering of success in the presence of severe endometriosis.

If severe endometriosis can reduce the effectiveness of IVF, might we be able to increase that success rate with pretreatment using medical therapy directed at the endometriosis? Numerous studies of variable quality, ranging from randomized trials to retrospective chart reviews, have examined the issue. A recent meta-analysis based on three randomized controlled trials (with 165 women) supports this approach, showing that clinical pregnancy rate per woman was significantly higher in those receiving GnRH agonist for three to six months prior to IVF compared to the control group (OR: 4.3; 95% CI: 2.0–9.2) (Collins JA, personal communication).

One final issue regarding the management of endometriosis with IVF is that of the endometrioma. When faced with an otherwise asymptomatic endometrioma prior to IVF, options include surgical excision versus expectant management. While endometriomas may reduce success, it is also quite possible that surgery will similarly adversely affect IVF results.

Available evidence supports the notion that ovarian responsiveness in operated gonads is markedly reduced. Studies comparing operated and unoperated ovaries in women who previously underwent excision of unilateral endometriomas showed a mean reduction in the number of follicles and oocytes by about 50% (79,80). Moreover, a recent study emphasized that ovarian responsiveness is considerably altered in women operated on for bilateral endometriomas (81). Possible mechanisms leading to this damage include the accidental removal of ovarian tissue during cystectomy and the injury that may be inflicted on the ovarian stroma and vascularization by both surgery-related local inflammation and electrosurgical coagulation (80). It is noteworthy, however, that some evidence supports the possibility that the ovarian damage may, at least in part, precede surgery. Using pathological sections of the ovarian cortex surrounding ovarian endometriomas, Maneschi et al. found a reduced number of follicles antecedent to surgery (82). Moreover, the presence of an unoperated endometrioma is also associated with a reduced responsiveness to gonadotropins in IVF cycles (83).

Clinical studies aimed at determining whether surgical excision of endometriomas prior to initiation of an IVF cycle may be of benefit are scant. In general, available retrospective studies on this point do not support a benefit of surgery (84,85). To our knowledge, there is only one randomized study that has specifically investigated this point (86). The patients were randomized into two groups: 49 patients underwent conservative ovarian surgery before IVF and 50 patients underwent the IVF directly. In the ovarian surgery group, stimulation was significantly longer, total recombinant FSH dose was significantly higher, and mean number of mature oocytes was significantly lower. Operated and unoperated women did not differ in terms of implantation (16% and 18%, respectively) and pregnancy rate (34% and 38%, respectively). Overall, current available evidence does not support a strategy of systematic surgical treatment in women selected for IVF who have asymptomatic endometriomas.

SUMMARY

Endometriosis and infertility are irrevocably linked in the mind of most gynecologists. Indeed, many forms of endometriosis may well cause or contribute to a decrease in conception rates. However, care must be taken in consideration of how to manage such patients, for endometriosis is not a homogeneous disease with a simple treatment algorithm in the presence of infertility. Surgical therapy is clearly of value for most patients with endometriosis-associated infertility, but in some situations (early-stage disease that is otherwise asymptomatic) the benefit may be marginal and the value of exploratory laparoscopy is highly questionable. Assisted reproduction also appears beneficial, very likely for all stages of disease. The relative success of surgery versus ART has never been directly compared and likely depends on many confounding factors such as age, insurance coverage, desired family size, and degree of endometriosis. At the present time, there is no indication for medical therapy in endometriosis-associated infertility, aside from the woman with stage IV disease planning to undergo IVF. However, there may be a role for medical therapy in a defined subset of women wishing to conceive; this concept will require further study before it can be advised. Finally, new medical therapies may provide new options for enhancing fertility in these women. Ongoing and future trials should be closely followed and examined, to determine if this exciting prospect will ultimately benefit the couples afflicted with both endometriosis and infertility.

REFERENCES

1. Schenken RS, Asch RH, Williams RF, et al. Etiology of infertility in monkeys with endometriosis. Fertil Steril 1984; 41:122–130.
2. Werlin LB, DiZerega GS, Hodgen GD. Endometriosis: Effect of ovulation, ovum pickup, and transport in monkeys: An interim report [abstract]. Fertil Steril 1981; 35:263S.
3. Kaplan CR, Eddy CA, Olive DL, et al. Effect of ovarian endometriosis on ovulation in rabbits. Am J Obstet Gynecol 1989; 160:40–44.
4. Jansen RPS. Minimal endometriosis and reduced fecundability: Prospective evidence from an artificial insemination by donor program. Fertil Steril 1986; 46:141–143.
5. Rodriguez-Escudero FJ, Neyro JL, Corcosteugui B, et al. Does minimal endometriosis reduce fecundity? Fertil Steril 1988; 50:522–524.
6. Chauhan M, Barratt CLR, Cooke SMS, et al. Differences in the fertility of donor insemination recipients – A study to provide prognostic guidelines as to its success and outcome. Fertil Steril 1989; 51:815–819.
7. Dunphy BC, Kay R, Barratt CLR, et al. Female age: The length of involuntary infertility prior to investigation and fertility outcome. Hum Reprod 1989; 4:527–530.
8. Duleba AJ. Diagnosis of endometriosis. Obstet Gynecol Clin North Am 1997; 24:331–346.
9. Eskenazi B, Warner M, Bonsignore L, et al. Validation study of non-surgical diagnosis of endometriosis. Fertil Steril 2001; 76(5):929–935.
10. Hemmings R, Rivard M, Olive DL, et al. Evaluation of risk factors associated with endometriosis. Fertil Steril 2004; 81:1513–1521.
11. Jansen RPS, Russell P. Nonpigmented endometriosis: Clinical, laparoscopic, and pathologic definition. Am J Obstet Gynecol 1986; 155:1154–1159.
12. Stripling MC, Martin DC, Chatman DL, et al. Subtle appearance of pelvic endometriosis. Fertil Steril 1988; 49:427–431.
13. Walter AJ, Hentz JG, Magtibay PM, et al. Endometriosis: Correlation between histologic and visual findings at laparoscopy. Am J Obstet Gynecol 2001; 184:1407–1413.
14. Stratton P, Winkel CA, Premkumar A, et al. Diagnostic accuracy of laparoscopy, magnetic resonance imaging, and histopathologic examination for the detection of endometriosis. Fertil Steril 2003; 79:1078–1085.
15. Olive DL, Pritts EA, Morales AJ. Evidence-based medicine: Study design for evaluation and treatment. J Am Assoc Gynecol Laparosc 1998; 5:75–82.
16. Hughes EG. Systematic literature review and meta-analysis. Semin Reprod Endocrinol 1996; 14:161–169.
17. Guarnaccia MM, Silverberg K, Olive DL. Endometriosis and adenomyosis. In: Copeland LJ, ed. Textbook of Gynecology. Philadelphia, PA: W.B. Sanders, 2000:687–722.
18. Hughesdon PE. The structure of endometrial cysts of the ovary. J Obstet Gynaecol Br Emp 1957; 44:481–487.
19. Fayez JA, Vogel MF. Comparison of different treatment methods of endometriomas by laparoscopy. Obstet Gynecol 1991; 78: 660–665.
20. Candiani M, Barbieri M, Bottani B, et al. Ovarian recovery after laparoscopic enucleation of ovarian cysts: Insights from echographic short term post-surgical follow-up. J Minim Invasive Gynecol 2005; 12:409–414.
21. Busacca M, Riparini J, Somigliana E, et al. Postsurgical ovarian failure after laparoscopic excision of bilateral endometriomas. Am J Obstet Gynecol 2006; 195:421–425.
22. Farquhar C, Vandekerckhove P, Watson A, et al. Barrier agents for preventing adhesions after surgery for subfertility (Cochrane review). In: The Cochrane Library, Issue 1. Oxford: Update Software, 2000.
23. Marcoux S, Maheux R, Bèrubè S. Laparoscopic surgery in infertile women with minimal or mild endometriosis. N Engl J Med 1997; 337:217–222.
24. Parazzini F. Ablation of lesions or no treatment in minimal-mild endometriosis in infertile women: A randomized trial. Hum Reprod 1999; 14:1332–1334.
25. Olive DL, Pritts EA. Treatment of endometriosis. N Engl J Med 2001; 345(4):266–275.
26. Elsheikh A, Milingos S, Loutradis D, et al. Endometriosis and reproductive disorders. Ann N Y Acad Sci 2003; 997:247–254.
27. Redwine DB, Wright JT. Laparoscopic treatment of complete obliteration of the cul-de-sac associated with endometriosis: Long-term follow-up of en bloc resection. Fertil Steril 2001; 76:358–365.
28. Busacca M, Marana R, Caruana P, et al. Recurrence of ovarian endometrioma after laparoscopic excision. Am J Obstet Gynecol 1999; 180:519–523.

29. Pritts EA, Taylor RN. An evidence-based evaluation of endometriosis-associated infertility. Endocrinol Metab Clin North Am 2003; 32(3):653–667.
30. Beretta P, Franchi M, Ghezzi F, et al. Randomized clinical trial of two laparoscopic treatments of endometriomas: Cystectomy versus drainage and coagulation. Fertil Steril 1998; 70:1176–1180.
31. Alborzi S, Momtahan M, Parsanezhad ME, et al. A prospective, randomized study comparing laparoscopic ovarian cystectomy versus fenestration and coagulation in patients with endometriomas. Fertil Steril 2004; 82:1633–1637.
32. Fedele L, Bianchi S, Zanconato G, et al. Bipolar electrocoagulation versus suture of solitary ovary after laparoscopic excision of ovarian endometriomas. J Am Assoc Gynecol Laparosc 2004; 11:344–347.
33. Jones KD, Sutton CJ. Pregnancy rates following ablative laparoscopic surgery for endometriomas. Hum Reprod 2002; 17: 782–785.
34. Koninckx PR, Martin D. Treatment of deeply infiltrating endometriosis. Curr Opin Obstet Gynecol 1994; 6:231–241.
35. Koninckx PR, Meuleman C, Demeyere S, et al. Suggestive evidence that pelvic endometriosis is a progressive disease, whereas deeply infiltrating endometriosis is associated with pelvic pain. Fertil Steril 1991; 55:759–765.
36. Chapron C, Fritel X, Dubuisson DB, et al. Fertility after laparoscopic management of deep endometriosis infiltrating uterosacral ligaments. Hum Reprod 1999; 14:329–332.
37. Reich H, McGlynn F, Salvat J. Laparoscopic treatment of cul-de-sac obliteration secondary to retrocervical deep fibrotic endometriosis. J Reprod Med 1991; 36:516–522.
38. Possover M, Diebolder H, Plaul K, et al. Laparoscopically assisted vaginal resection of rectovaginal endometriosis. Obstet Gynecol 2000; 96:304–307.
39. Fedele L, Bianchi S, Zanconato G, et al. Is rectovaginal endometriosis a progressive disease? Am J Obstet Gynecol 2004; 191:1539–1542.
40. Goebel R, Rjosk HK. Laboratory and clinical studies with the new antigonadotropin, danazol [abstract]. Acta Endocrinol (Copenh) 1977; 85(Suppl 212):134.
41. Floyd WS. Danazol: Endocrine and endometrial effects. Int J Fertil 1980; 25:75–80.
42. Barbieri RL, Canick JA, Makris A, et al. Danazol inhibits steroidogenesis. Fertil Steril 1977; 28:809–813.
43. McGinley R, Casey JH. Analysis of progesterone in unextracted serum: A method using danazol [17 α-pregn-4-en 20 yno(2,3-d) osoxazol-17-ol] a blocker of steroid binding to proteins. Steroids 1979; 33:127–138.
44. Buttram VC Jr, Belue JB, Reiter R. Interim report of a study of danazol for the treatment of endometriosis. Fertil Steril 1982; 37:478–483.
45. Alvarado RG, Liu JY, Zwolak RM. Danazol and limb-threatening arterial thrombosis: Two case reports. J Vasc Surg 2001; 34: 1123–1126.
46. Vercellini P, Tresid L, Panazza S, et al. Very low dose danazol for relief of endometriosis-associated pelvic pain: A pilot study. Fertil Steril 1994; 62:1136–1142.
47. Janicki TI. Treatment of the pelvic pain associated with endometriosis using danazol vaginal suppositories. Two year followup. Fertil Steril 2002; 77:S52.
48. Igarashi M, Iizuka M, Abe Y, et al. Novel vaginal danazol ring therapy for pelvic endometriosis, in particular deeply infiltrating endometriosis. Hum Reprod 1998; 13:1952–1956.
49. Bruner KL, Eisenberg E, Gorstein F, et al. Progesterone and transforming growth factor-beta coordinately regulate suppression of endometrial matrix metalloproteinases in a model of experimental endometriosis. Steroids 1999; 64:648–653.
50. Olive DL. Medical treatment: Alternatives to danazol. In: Schenken RS, ed. Endometriosis: Contemporary Concepts in Clinical Management. Philadelphia, PA: J.B. Lippincott, 1989:189–211.
51. Fedele L, Bianchi S, Zanconato G, et al. Use of a levonorgestrel-releasing intrauterine device in the treatment of rectovaginal endometriosis. Fertil Steril 2001; 75:485–488.
52. Lau TM, Affandi B, Rogers PAW. The effects of levonorgestrel implants on vascular endothelial growth factor expression in the endometrium. Mol Hum Reprod 1998; 5:57–63.
53. Hamblen EC. Androgen treatment of women. South Med J 1957; 50:743.
54. Hirvonen E, Malkonen M, Manninen V. Effects of different progestogens on lipoproteins during postmenopausal replacement therapy. N Engl J Med 1981; 304:560.
55. Fahraeus L, Sydsjo A, Wallentin L. Lipoprotein changes during treatment of pelvic endometriosis with medroxyprogesterone acetate. Fertil Steril 1986; 45:503.
56. Andrews MC, Andrews WC, Strauss AF. Effects of progestin-induced pseudopregnancy on endometriosis; clinical and microscopic studies. Am J Obstet Gynecol 1959; 78:776.
57. Scott RB, Wharton LR Jr. The effect of estrone and progesterone on the growth of experimental endometriosis in rhesus monkeys. Am J Obstet Gynecol 1957; 74:852.
58. Noble AD, Letchworth AT. Medical treatment of endometriosis: A comparative trial. Postgrad Med J 1979; 55(Suppl 5):37.
59. Meresman GF, Auge L, Barano RI, et al. Oral contraceptives treatment suppresses proliferation and enhances apoptosis of eutopic endometrial tissue from patients with endometriosis. Fertil Steril 2001; 76:S47–S48.
60. Sharpe-Timms KL, Zimmer RL, Jolliff WJ, et al. Gonadotropin-releasing hormone agonist (GnRH-a) therapy alters activity of plasminogen activators, matrix metalloproteinases and their inhibitors in rat models for adhesion formation and endometriosis: Potential GnRH-a-regulated mechanisms reducing adhesion formation. Fertil Steril 1998; 69:916–923.
61. Dmowski WP. The role of medical management in the treatment of endometriosis. In: Nezhat CR, Berger GS, Nezhat FR, Buttram VC Jr, Nezhat CH, eds. Endometriosis: Advanced Management and Surgical Techniques. New York, NY: Springer-Verlag, 1995:229–240.
62. Barbieri RL. Endometriosis and the estrogen threshold theory, relation to surgical and medical treatment. J Reprod Med 1998; 43:287–292.
63. Hurst BS, Gardner SC, Tucker KE, et al. Delayed oral estradiol combined with leuprolide increases endometriosis-related pain. JSLS 2000; 4:97–101.
64. Cornillie FJ, Brosens IA, Vasquez G, et al. Histologic and ultrastructural changes in human endometriotic implants treated with the antiprogesterone steroid ethylnorgestienone (gestrinone) during 2 months. Int J Gynecol Pathol 1986; 5:95.
65. Robyn C, Delogne-Desnoeck J, Bourdoux P, et al. Endocrine effects of gestrinone. In: Raynaud J-P, Ojasoo T, Martini L, eds. Medical Management of Endometriosis. New York, NY: Raven Press, 1984:207.
66. Bayer SR, Seibel MM, Saffan DS, et al. Efficacy of danazol treatment for minimal endometriosis in infertile women: A prospective, randomized study. J Reprod Med 1988; 33:179–183.
67. Fedele L, Parazzini F, Radici E, et al. Buserelin acetate versus expectant management in the treatment of infertility associated with minimal or mild endometriosis: A randomized clinical trial. Am J Obstet Gynecol 1992; 166:1345–1350.
68. Telimaa S. Danazol and medroxyprogesterone acetate inefficacious in the treatment of infertility in endometriosis. Fertil Steril 1988; 50:872–875.
69. Thomas E, Cooke I. Successful treatment of asymptomatic endometriosis: Does it benefit infertile women? BMJ 1987; 294:1117–1119.
70. Harrison RF, Barry-Kinsella C. Efficacy of medroxyprogesterone treatment in infertile women with endometriosis: A prospective, randomized, placebo-controlled study. Fertil Steril 2000; 74: 24–30.
71. Hughes E, Ferorkow D, Collins J, et al. Ovulation suppression for endometriosis (Cochrane review). In: The Cochrane Library, Issue 1. Oxford, U.K.: Update Software, 2000.

72. Balasch J, Creus M, Fabregues F, et al. Pentoxifylline versus placebo in the treatment of infertility associated with minimal or mild endometriosis: A pilot randomized clinical trial. Hum Reprod 1997; 12:2046–2050.
73. Deaton JL, Gibson M, Blackmer KM, et al. A randomized, controlled trial of clomiphene citrate and intrauterine insemination in couples with unexplained infertility or surgically corrected endometriosis. Fertil Steril 1990; 54:1083–1088.
74. Fedele L, Bianchi S, Marchini M, et al. Superovulation with human menopausal gonadotropins in the treatment of infertility associated with minimal or mild endometriosis: A controlled randomized study. Fertil Steril 1992; 58:28–31.
75. Tummon IS, Asher LJ, Martin JSB, et al. Randomized controlled trial of superovulation and insemination for infertility associated with minimal or mild endometriosis. Fertil Steril 1997; 68: 8–12.
76. Peterson CM, Hatasaka HH, Jones KP, et al. Ovulation induction with gonadotropins and intrauterine insemination compared with in vitro fertilization and no therapy: A prospective, nonrandomized, cohort study and meta-analysis. Fertil Steril 1994; 62:535–540.
77. De Hondt A, Meuleman C, Tomassetti C, et al. Endometriosis and assisted reproduction: The role for reproductive surgery? Curr Opin Obstet Gynecol 2006; 18:374–379.
78. Barnhart K, Dunsmoor-Su R, Coutifaris C. Effect of endometriosis on in vitro fertilization. Fertil Steril 2002; 77:1148–1155.
79. Ragni G, Somigliana E, Benedetti F, et al. Damage to ovarian reserve associated with laparoscopic excision of endometriomas: A quantitative rather than a qualitative injury. Am J Obstet Gynecol 2005; 193:1908–1914.
80. Somigliana E, Vercellini P, Vigano P, et al. Should endometriomas be treated before IVF-ICSI cycles? Hum Reprod Update 2006; 12:57–64.
81. Esinler I, Bazdag G, Aybar F, et al. Outcome of in vitro fertilization/intracytoplasmic sperm injection after laparoscopic cystectomy for endometriomas. Fertil Steril 2006; 85:1730–1735.
82. Maneschi F, Marasa L, Incandela S, et al. Ovarian cortex surrounding benign neoplasms: A histologic study. Am J Obstet Gynecol 1993; 169:388–393.
83. Somigliana E, Infantino M, Benedetti F, et al. The presence of ovarian endometriomas is associated with a reduced responsiveness to gonadotropins. Fertil Steril 2006; 86:192–196.
84. Garcia-Velasco JA, Mahutte NG, Corona J, et al. Removal of endometriomas before in vitro fertilization does not improve fertility outcomes: A matched, case-control study. Fertil Steril 2004; 81:1194–1197.
85. Wong BC, Gillman NC, Oehninger S, et al. Results of in vitro fertilization in patients with endometriomas: Is surgical removal beneficial? Am J Obstet Gynecol 2004; 191:597–606.
86. Demirol A, Guven S, Baykal C, et al. Effect of endometrioma cystectomy on IVF outcome: A prospective randomized study. Reprod Biomed Online 2006; 12:639–643.

10

Treatment of endometriosis associated with pain

Paolo Vercellini, Giorgio Aimi, Fabio Amicarelli, Annalisa Abbiati, Raffaella Daguati, and Giussy Barbara

INTRODUCTION

For almost a century, the treatment of endometriosis has been based mainly on a straightforward oncologic principle, i.e., radical removal of lesions. This is still a mainstay of therapy in cases of bowel and ureteral stenosis or adnexal masses with ultrasonographic doubtful characteristics. However, endometriosis is not a cancer and, in the vast majority of patients, it does not cause intestinal or ureteral strictures. Moreover, in the past two decades, it became progressively evident that the overall "amount" of disease is correlated neither with frequency and severity of symptoms nor with long-term prognosis in terms of conceptions and recurrences (1,2). Furthermore, effective pharmacological alternatives have been developed to deal with a chronic inflammatory disease, such as endometriosis, that needs drug modulation for years, and not only for the arbitrary standard period of six months (3,4). Accordingly, a more pragmatic approach to the treatment of endometriosis was gradually developed, focusing more on the woman's needs than on the extension of lesions (3). In other words, the problems of patients with endometriosis are disease-related symptoms and not implants per se, and treatments should be centered on resolution of complaints, independently of a priori excision of lesions.

However, the two positions still coexist and the debate continues. On one hand, it has been stated that "the definitive treatment of endometriosis is simple: surgical eradication" and that "the success of surgical treatment is best assessed by determining how much disease, if any, remains after operative interventions" (5). On the other hand, it has been considered that "increasingly, the focus has been on using research outcomes that matter to patients" and that "patient oriented outcomes of relief of pain and pregnancy rate [. . .] are the outcomes considered to make a difference to the daily lives of women with endometriosis" (6).

Surgical and medical therapies for symptomatic endometriosis play their roles in this undefined clinical scenario. The purposes of the present chapter are to describe the most frequently encountered clinical conditions in terms of disease severity, discuss the principles on which to base a surgical approach with regard to techniques and results, and identify the most useful hormonal therapies to be used as an alternative or as a complement to surgery in women with endometriosis-associated pain.

LESION TYPES AND SURGICAL MODALITIES

Peritoneal and Ovarian Endometriosis

It is now well established that the results of surgery at laparoscopy or laparotomy are similar in the vast majority of cases (7–10). Consequently, laparoscopy is now considered the standard surgical approach for peritoneal and ovarian endometriosis. Conservative surgery at laparoscopy is generally performed with a three- or four-puncture technique, using mechanical instruments and electrosurgery. Adhesions are sectioned with microscissors, the ovaries are completely mobilized, and endometriomas are evacuated, rinsed with normal saline and excised by means of countertraction applied on the pseudocapsule and normal gonadal cortex with atraumatic microforceps. Peritoneal implants are excised or coagulated with low-power monopolar current. Hemostasis is finally achieved with limited application of bipolar current. Lasers are preferred by some surgeons, but, apart from theoretical advantages, it has not been definitively demonstrated that these costly tools are associated with better postoperative outcomes compared with mechanical or electrosurgical instruments. Accordingly, the use of lasers is more a matter of surgeon's preference and attitude than a matter of proven efficacy.

Deeply Infiltrating Lesions

The so-called infiltrating lesions consist mostly of dense, reactive fibrotic tissue, and usually little ectopic endometrium; it is found even in the most devastating forms of deep endometriosis. The pathogenetic pathway leading to anatomic distortion begins with superficial implantation of endometrial cells. This constitutes a strong inflammatory stimulus that triggers a common "protective" response: pelvic structures adhere to the site of ectopic implants with the "aim" of circumscribing the irritating lesion and excluding it from the peritoneal environment (11). Fibroblasts participate in the "burial" of endometrial foci, but any ensuing scar retraction may cause duplication and invagination of adjacent surfaces. In other words, the process involves folding of various structures around endometriotic implants with their final encirclement. If this occurs, the result differs according to the affected site. When the ovary is involved, an endometriotic cyst may develop (12), whereas duplication of the anterior cul-de-sac peritoneum initiates bladder detrusor endometriosis (13). When the process involves the sigmoid or, more rarely, the cecum, the surgeon may have the impression of a distinct, large, hard nodule, but often most of the palpated lesion consists of duplicated and invaginated intestinal wall with only very limited endometriotic tissue (11).

The specific technical problems associated with deeply infiltrating endometriosis of the antero- and posterouterine pouches may tip the balance in favor of laparoscopy or laparotomy depending on several factors, including the need for low anterior rectal resection, ureteral stenosis with indication for ureteroneocystotomy, and the availability of a colorectal endoscopist expert in severe endometriosis. In general, it is preferable to perform difficult and highly demanding surgery under conditions comfortable enough to minimize the risk of serious intra- and postoperative complications.

Posterior Cul-de-sac Disease

It has been suggested that deep endometriotic lesions of the posterior cul-de-sac originate from metaplasia of müllerian remnants located in the rectovaginal septum, thus constituting an entity different from peritoneal endometriosis (14). However, the vast majority of these fibrotic plaques are found in the retrocervical area. The rectovaginal septum is located caudally with respect to the posterior vaginal fornix and, based on normal anatomy, may not be the real site of deep nodular endometriosis. In fact, it has been demonstrated in a living anatomy study that the base of the posterior cul-de-sac extends to at least the level of the middle third of the posterior vaginal wall (15,16).

If the müllerian remnants metaplasia theory is true, the anatomy of the pouch of Douglas should be similar in women with and without the so-called "adenomyotic nodules" because these lesions, if they really originate in the rectovaginal septum, should be located extraperitoneally. Only if deep foci are a manifestation of intraperitoneal disease, the pouch of Douglas should be partly or completely obliterated.

The mean depth of the rectovaginal pouch in normal women, as measured from the upper border of the uterosacral ligaments to its base, has been demonstrated to be slightly over 5 cm regardless of parity or prolapse (15,16). In a laparoscopic study (17), findings in endometriosis patients without rectovaginal lesions and in subjects with conditions other than endometriosis or with a normal pelvis were substantially consistent with these observations. However, patients with the so-called deep endometriotic lesions had about a one-third reduction in depth of the pouch of Douglas. Partial obliteration by the anterior rectal wall is the cause of this apparent depth reduction and may give the false impression that nodules are subperitoneal. This is also supported by the reduced volume of the pouch of Douglas observed specifically in women with rectovaginal lesions (17).

The inflammation triggered by bleeding intraperitoneal endometriotic papules in the most dependent portion of the pouch of Douglas may result in adhesion between the adjacent peritoneal surfaces of the anterior rectal wall and posterior vaginal fornix, with subsequent infiltration of the muscular layers of both organs. In other words, what is called rectovaginal septum endometriosis is instead a massive disease of the deepest portion of the pouch of Douglas, which has been buried and excluded from the remaining pelvis by adhesions. The semilunar hard crest protruding through the posterior fornix, which is frequently palpated and observed in these situations, is the fibrotic "cast" of what was the bottom of the posterior cul-de-sac. Endometriotic plaques and nodules are found in the posterior vaginal fornix, cranially with respect to the rectovaginal septum (Fig. 1). Moreover, various forms of peritoneal and ovarian disease are usually present in patients with vaginal endometriosis, suggesting that the pathogenesis may not be different (19).

Excision of posterior deep lesions implies removal of a fibrotic cast of the cul-de-sac, which may or may not involve the entire vaginal wall thickness and the rectal muscular layer according to the severity of the lesion (20–23). MRI and transrectal ultrasonography have been proposed to define the extension and degree of infiltration of these lesions (24–27). However, endometriotic cul-de-sac plaques are easily reached by the gynecologist's examining fingers, and a careful recto-

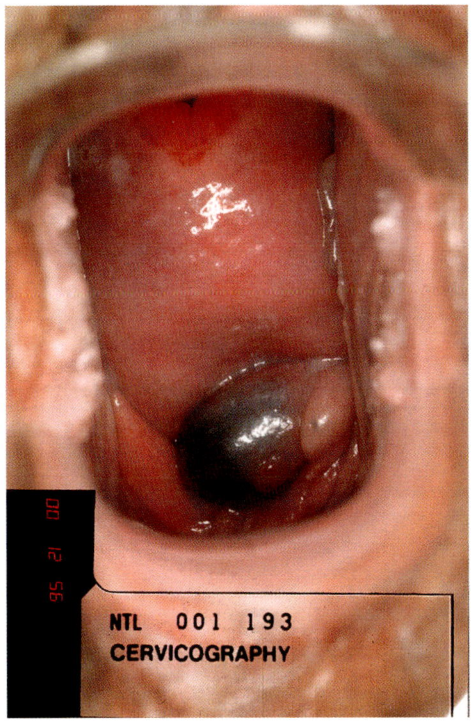

Figure 1 Colposcopic appearance of vaginal endometriosis of the posterior fornix with reddish vegetations and a bluish nodule. *Source*: From Ref. 18.

vaginal evaluation is usually informative enough (28–30). It is important to determine whether the lesion is situated in the midline or extends laterally, involving the parametria. From a surgical point of view, the former situation is generally easier to handle, whereas the latter may be rendered problematic by the proximity of the ureter as well as uterine and vaginal vessels (11). When lateral infiltration has occurred, the left side is more often affected than the right (31).

The left pelvic side wall seems to be the preferential site of really severe, deep infiltrating endometriosis, where dense, diffuse adhesions cause tenacious coalescence of several organs. The sigmoid may adhere to the tube, ovary, and left broad ligament, burying the adnexa partially or completely (11). In such cases, the rectum may also be involved, obliterating the pouch of Douglas and rendering recognition of the left uterosacral ligament difficult (32). The sigmoid must be gently, progressively, and amply mobilized to expose the adnexal area. Sometimes, the salpinx is stretched over and around an endometrioma, with the ampulla hidden under the ovary and fixed by dense adhesions. Adnexal mobilization must be done carefully, as in these conditions anatomical landmarks may be altered. In particular, it may be difficult to recognize the ureter, which can be dislocated superiorly and attached to the ovary, or medially and adjacent to the uterosacral ligament. When in doubt, it may be appropriate to adopt a retroperitoneal approach to identify, dissect, and mobilize the ureter (33). This increases peritoneal trauma but may avoid inadvertent lesions, which may become symptomatic during the postoperative period. Insertion of ureteric stents under cystoscopic control is suggested in severely altered anatomic conditions. Performance of laparoscopic uterosacral ligament resection by surgeons with limited endoscopic experience is not recommended when the pelvic anatomy is greatly altered (34,35).

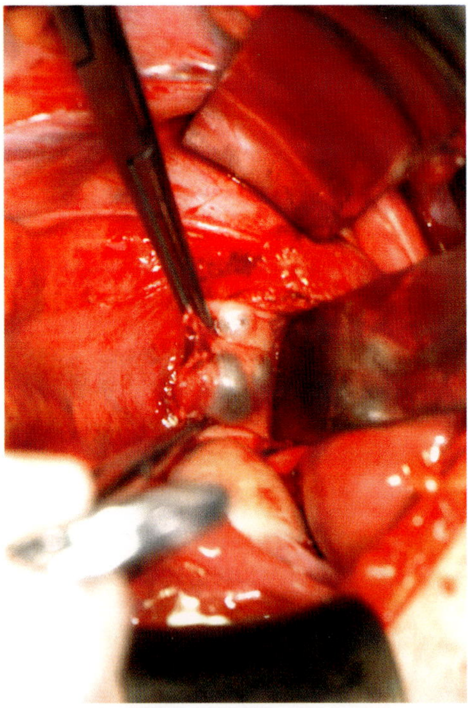

Figure 2 Treatment of rectovaginal endometriosis at laparotomy. The posterior vaginal fornix has been opened and extended with delicate grasping forceps, and a narrow blade retractor is inserted between cervix and vagina, pushing the uterus toward the pubis symphysis.

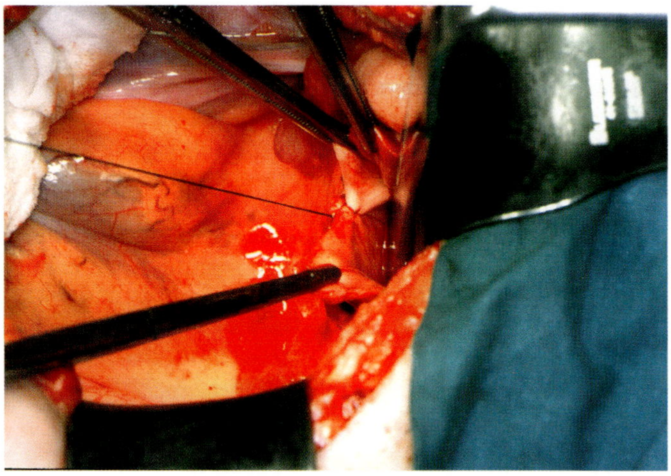

Figure 3 After excision of the endometriotic rectovaginal plaque, the vagina is reattached to the cervix by means of a "T2-shaped" suture.

Different techniques have been suggested to excise deep cul-de-sac endometriotic plaques at laparotomy or laparoscopy, or by the vaginal route (20–23,32,34,36,37). To be safe and effective, the surgical approach should take into account the pathogenesis of these lesions. When the ureters are not involved, the major operative risk is rectal perforation. In this regard, endometriosis of the pouch of Douglas should usually be considered a contraindication to an exclusively vaginal approach. Moreover, because most of the patients are nulliparous, vaginal accessibility may be suboptimal, especially in operations at the apex at an unfavorable site. Finally, pelvic fibrosis may considerably reduce uterine mobility, which is important in excision of tissue located just behind the cervix (11).

Laparoscopy is being increasingly chosen to excise deep rectovaginal endometriotic lesions. However, an abdominal approach at laparotomy can still be adopted in difficult conditions, as it renders a procedure relatively easy, rapid, and effective, which might otherwise be rather cumbersome (11,32). In this case, the patient's legs are then placed in Allen universal stirrups, with the thighs flexed approximately 15° in relation to the abdomen and the knees separated by 30°. After incision of the abdominal wall, the upper, accessible portion of the pouch of Douglas is first freed from any ovarian endometriomas. After exploration of what is the false bottom of the cul-de-sac, bilateral identification or dissection of the ureters, and development of the pararectal spaces, the surgeon inserts the index and middle fingers of the left hand into the vagina behind the cervix, pushing the posterior fornix upward. This results in optimal exposure of the operating field and enables the surgeon to detach the rectum from the posterior fornix with the scissors used by the right hand, directing the cuts towards the left fingertips in the vagina. The juxtaposition of the left fingers and the tip of the scissors' blades handled by the right hand gives a precise and continuous feeling of the plane of dissection being progressively developed, minimizing the risk of bowel perforation. The fornix is then opened by cutting along the attachment of the vaginal cuff to the posterior part of the cervix (Fig. 2). The incised posterior vaginal fornix is extended with delicate grasping forceps, and a narrow-blade retractor is inserted between cervix and vagina, pushing the uterus toward the pubic symphysis (Fig. 3). This allows direct inspection of the posterior vaginal wall and a precise estimate of the need for further rectal detachment. Once free margins are reached both laterally and caudally, the plaque is excised, usually with a "V"-shaped incision, which follows the original shape of the lower pouch of Douglas. The specimen removed is a sort of cast of the bottom of the cul-de-sac and usually involves part of the muscularis layer of the rectum (Figs. 4 and 5). The vagina is reattached to the cervix by means of a

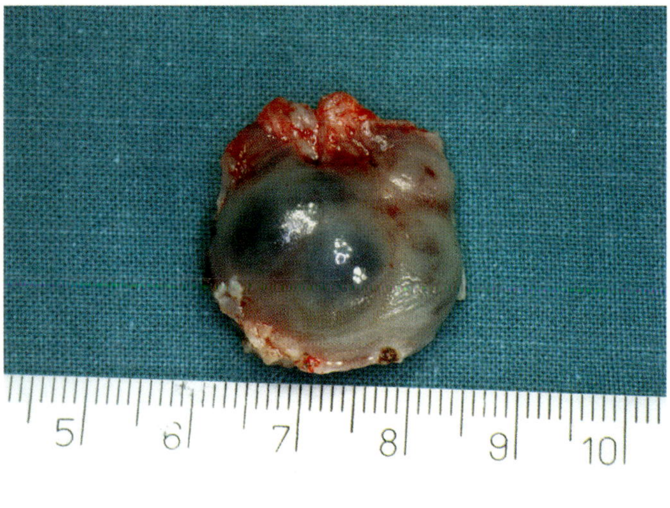

Figure 4 Vaginal side of the excised rectovaginal endometriotic nodule infiltrating the posterior fornix.

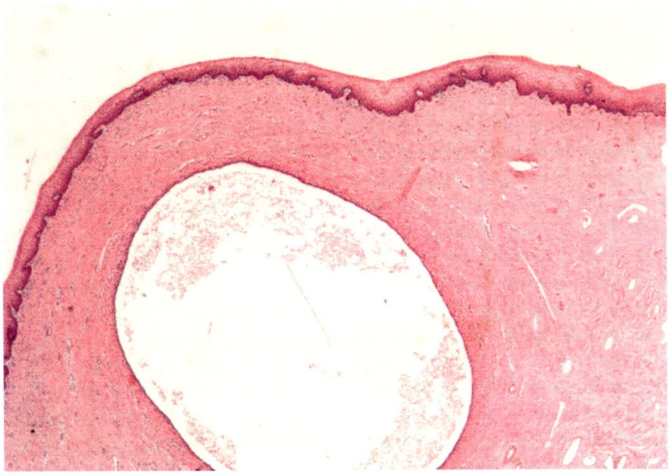

Figure 5 Histologic preparation of vaginal endometriosis. A cyst lined by endometrial-type mucosa and containing menstrual debris is evident under the stratified squamous epithelium. (Hematoxylin and eosin, magnification ×10.) *Source*: From Ref. 18.

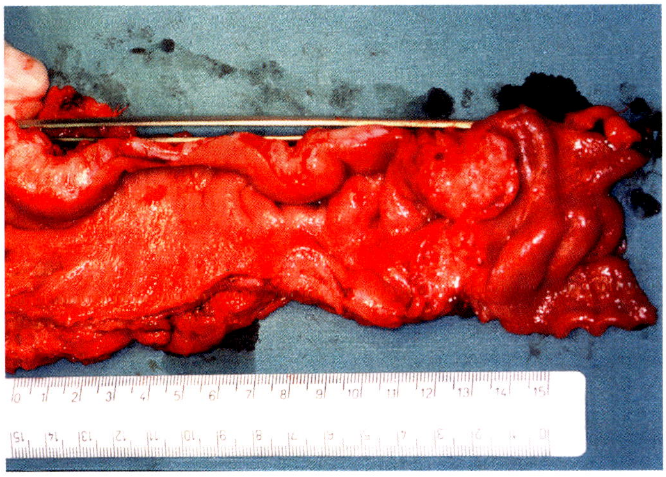

Figure 7 Same case as in Fig. 6. Bowel specimen opened after rectosigmoid resection for multiple endometriotic lesions, with a large nodule causing subocclusion.

"T"-shaped suture, and the anterior rectal wall is reinforced (11,32).

As an alternative, a combined laparoscopic and vaginal approach can be adopted according to Possover et al.'s technique (37). According to this modality, the posterior fornix is first exposed with two Breisky retractors and the cervix is pulled ventrally with two tenacula. An incision is made around the endometriotic plaque and the posterior cervix is dissected, leaving the excised portion of the vagina on the anterior rectal wall. To avoid bowel injury, the pouch of Douglas is not opened transvaginally. After suturing of the vagina to the posterior cervix, the procedure can then be completed laparoscopically.

Although opening of the rectal lumen should be avoided if at all possible, a rectal resection may be necessary (Figs. 6–8). Rectal endometriosis can be dealt with using three different modalities: superficial thickness excision, full-thickness discoid resection/anterior rectal wall excision, and segmental colorectal resection. Lesions less than 2 cm in size or less than one-third of the rectal circumference can be excised in a full-thickness manner, either transabdominally or laparoscopically. For lesions requiring segmental resection of the rectum, the proximal healthy colon should be mobilized and the ureters identified. The anterior rectal resection is defined high when the distance between the anastomosis and the anal verge is more than 10 cm, low when it is between 6 and 10 cm, and ultralow when it is less than 6 cm (38). The lower the

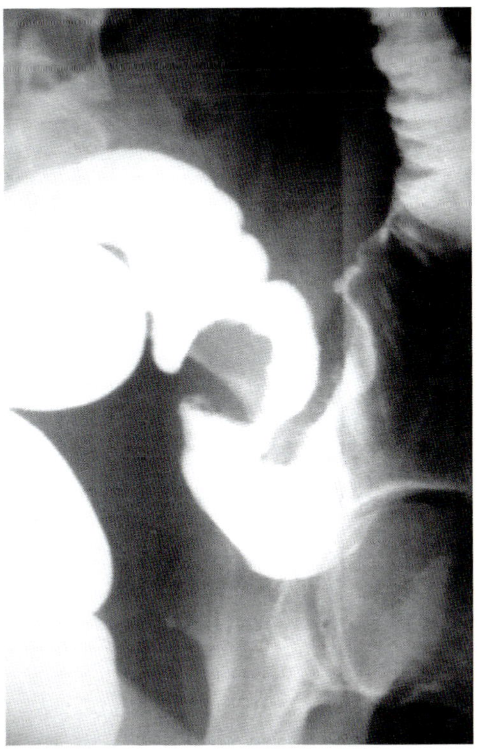

Figure 6 Barium enema showing stenosis of the rectosigmoid junction caused by a large endometriotic nodule.

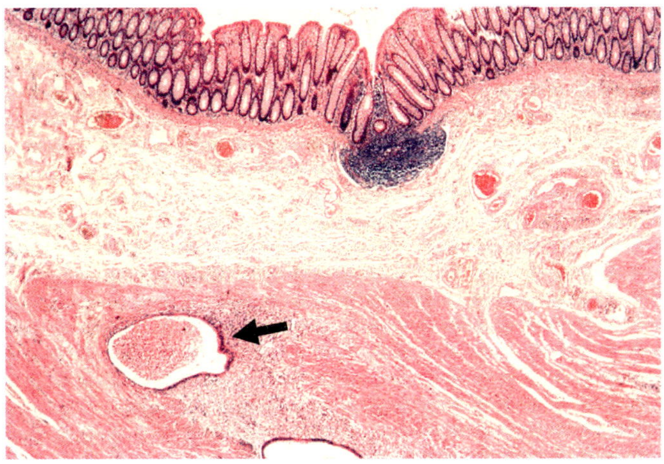

Figure 8 Histologic preparation of large bowel endometriosis showing nodules lined by endometrial-type mucosa and containing menstrual debris infiltrating the smooth muscle layer (*arrow*). (Hematoxylin and eosin, magnification ×8.)

anastomosis, the higher the probability of postoperative leakage and rectovaginal fistula formation (39).

Segmental rectal resection can be carried out transanally, transvaginally by a laparovaginal approach, and transabdominally, either at laparotomy or at laparoscopy. Description of these advanced techniques in detail is beyond the scope of the present chapter, and reference should be made to recent exhaustive reviews (38–40).

When endometriotic nodules are located above the rectosigmoid junction, the sigmoid colon usually is not mobilized to the splenic flexure, and division of the inferior mesenteric vessels at the level of the pelvic brim is generally sufficient to allow length for tension-free anastomosis. Because leakage and late functional problems are much less frequent after a sigmoid than after a rectum resection, an aggressive approach seems reasonable whenever subocclusive symptoms are present, double-contrast barium enema identifies a stricture of more than 50% of the bowel lumen, or intraoperative digital evaluation demonstrates stenosis with obstruction.

The support of an experienced colorectal surgeon and, when opportune, of an urological surgeon, increases the possibility of radical excision of all endometriotic lesions, reducing at the same time the risk of major intra- and postoperative complications.

Anterior Cul-de-sac Disease

Bladder detrusor endometriosis, once considered rare, is now increasingly recognized (13). Three different and mutually exclusive etiologic hypotheses have been proposed, namely, transtubal menstrual reflux of endometrial cells with implantation on the peritoneum covering the bladder dome (41), extension of adenomyosis from the anterior uterine wall to the bladder (42), and metaplasia of subperitoneal müllerian remnants located in the vesicovaginal septum (43). Imaging and surgical findings demonstrate that, in the vast majority of cases, bladder detrusor endometriosis originates intraperitoneally in the vesicouterine pouch and that the association with uterine adenomyosis is occasional (13,41). The pathogenesis of deep infiltrating vesical endometriosis is no different from that of rectovaginal endometriosis. That is, both forms are caused by intraperitoneal seeding of regurgitated endometrial cells, which collect and implant in the most dependent portions of the peritoneal cavity, namely the anterior and posterior cul-de-sac, and trigger an inflammatory process leading to adhesion of contiguous organs with creation of false peritoneal bottoms (12,13,17,41). Based on anatomical, surgical, and pathological findings, we suggest that infiltrating endometriotic lesions do not originate extraperitoneally, but intraperitoneally. Accordingly, the definition "deep" may be questioned.

Ultrasonography performed with a full bladder identifies a heterogeneous, hyperechoic, intraluminal, usually conical vegetation, sometimes with small transonic formations, protruding from the posterior vesical wall. A cleavage plane between the detrusor nodule and the anterior uterine wall is generally clearly detected, excluding a leiomyoma. At median longitudinal scans, the lesions are above the isthmus. The maximum lesion diameter varies between 1 and 5 cm. The uterine body is invariably anteflexed (13,41–44).

Cystoscopy demonstrates an intraluminal mass of the posterior bladder wall or dome, and, in patients not operated previously, the distance between the caudal border of the endometriotic lesion and the interureteric ridge is rarely less than 2 cm (41). Systematic endoscopic biopsy is critical to exclude epithelial neoplasia as well as detrusor mesenchymal tumors. However, with the exception of transurethral resection procedures, biopsy at cystoscopy is not always diagnostic for endometriosis. The typical bluish nodules are present in about half of the cases, and the urothelium is not ulcerated (13,41).

Intravenous pyelography classically reveals a filling defect of the bladder dome, suggesting the presence of a "high" extravesical lesion, and is decisive in ruling out ureteral involvement. MRI and CT scans confirm the ultrasonographic findings but usually do not add different or more precise information to ultrasonography, cystoscopy, and pyelography, as they identify a supracervical lesion, with a cleavage plane with the anterior uterine wall.

At surgery, the uterus is anteflexed and the anterior cul-de-sac is obliterated partially or totally due to extensive adhesions between the peritoneum of the bladder fold and the uterine wall and fundus (Fig. 9). Very often one or both round ligaments are distorted and involved in the adhesive process. The detrusor nodule is almost always palpated medially in the posterior wall or dome of the bladder, adherent to the anterior uterine wall, well above the isthmus, trigone, and vesicovaginal septum (Figs. 10 and 11). Additional pelvic endometriotic lesions are usually present (13,41). Vesical endometriosis is usually not observed in women with a retroverted uterus. This is in agreement with the postulate of Jenkins et al. (45), as in this condition no dependent anterior cul-de-sac is present. The imaging and surgical findings are not compatible with the development of endometriosis in the vesicovaginal septum, which is anatomically much more caudal. By definition, the vesicovaginal (and vesicocervical) septum does not extend beyond the cervix (46), whereas detrusor nodules are usually found adherent to the uterine body.

A wrong pathogenetic view may have major unfavorable consequences, as patients may undergo transurethral resection of endometriosis with short-term recurrence of both symptoms and detrusor disease. This is to be expected if the lesion originates outside the vesical wall, developing later into a full-thickness nodule. In this condition, radical cystoscopic surgery would involve bladder perforation. On the other hand, avoiding this complication renders urologic resection obviously nonradical.

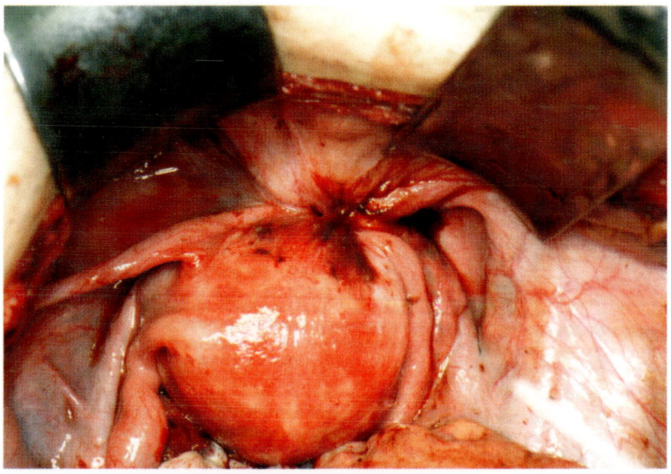

Figure 9 Detrusor endometriosis. At laparotomy, the vesicouterine pouch is partially obliterated by dense adhesions between the peritoneum that covers the bladder dome and the anterior uterine wall. Both round ligaments are retracted and distorted by the endometriotic process. *Source*: From Ref. 41.

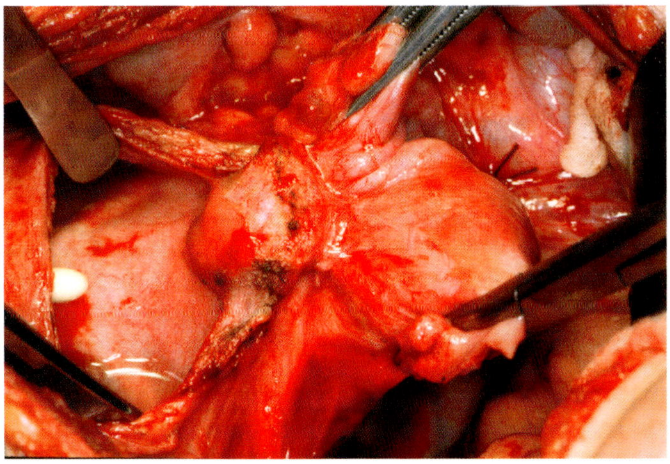

Figure 10 Abdominal hysterectomy with concomitant partial cystectomy. Margins of incision on the bladder dome are opened to demonstrate the presence of a full-thickness endometriotic nodule that adheres to the anterior uterine wall and well above the uterine cervix. The tip of the Folley catheter is visible on the left side of the photograph. *Source*: From Ref. 41.

There are two distinct forms of bladder detrusor endometriosis, spontaneous and iatrogenic (47) (after a cesarean section), with clearly different pathogenesis and clinical implications. In the former case, the vesical nodule represents only one site of a more generalized disease (13,41), whereas in the latter the lesion is usually isolated and may be caused by intraoperative dissemination of endometrial cells or a suboptimal surgical technique for closure of the low transverse uterine incision (47). About 1% of women with spontaneous pelvic endometriosis have urinary tract lesions, involving the bladder in 84% of the cases (48,49). Vesical endometriosis may present with variable symptoms and insidious onset, often mimicking recurrent cystitis (13,49). The classic clinical features are catamenial frequency, urgency, and pain at micturition with vesical tenesmus of varying severity (13,49). Urine cultures are usually negative. As endometriosis rarely infiltrates and ulcerates the mucosal layer of hollow viscera, hematuria is rare. Prompt recognition of the condition is important to avoid prolonged morbidity and erroneous treatments.

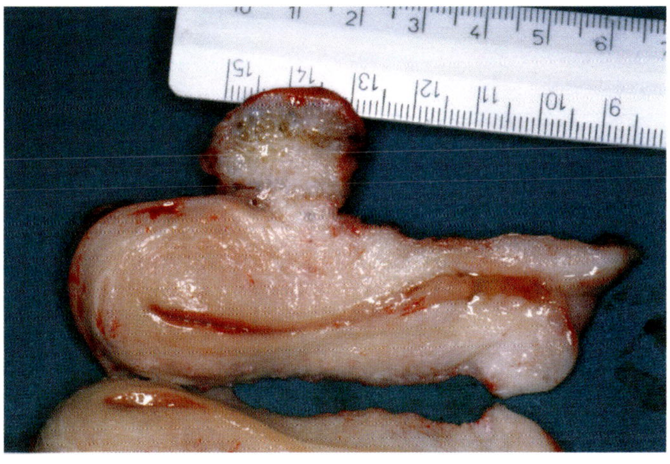

Figure 11 Surgical specimen from the same case as in Fig. 10. A sagittal incision of uterine body and bladder detrusor nodule together clearly demonstrates the supra-isthmic location of the endometriotic lesion. The cervix is intact. *Source*: From Ref. 41.

A strong association between vesical and ureteral endometriosis has not been demonstrated (50). Bladder and ureteral endometriosis may have different pathogeneses, as the latter usually develops from ovarian implants or fibrotic rectovaginal plaques (51). Thus, concomitant pelvic endometriotic disease, but not the detrusor nodule per se, may constitute a risk factor for additional urologic lesions.

The definitive solution for bladder endometriosis is transperitoneal abdominal surgery at laparoscopy (52–54) or laparotomy (13,41). The procedure begins with careful identification of the limits of the nodule, which is generally anterior to the uterine isthmus along the midline. First, any adhesions between the anterior uterine wall and the vesicouterine fold peritoneum must be lysed. As it is usually not possible to remove the detrusor nodule without opening the bladder lumen, an intentional perinodular incision through the vesical dome is suggested (11). The lesion is excised with mechanical scissors or unipolar electricity, and the bladder is finally oversewn with two transverse watertight fine synthetic absorbable sutures (13,41).

At first-line surgery, the endometriotic vegetation is usually located on the posterior bladder wall well above the trigonal area. Consequently, ureteral cannulation is generally not indispensable. A different situation may exist in patients with recurrent lesions, which may infiltrate down the bladder approaching the ureteral orifi (11).

Generally, segmental bladder resection for detrusor endometriosis is a relatively simple and safe procedure. In fact, differently from the bowel, vesical content is sterile, bladder sutures heal easily due to abundant vascularization, and fistula formation is almost always prevented by sufficiently prolonged urine drainage. Several reports demonstrated the excellent surgical outcomes of resection of bladder endometriosis in terms of symptom relief and recurrence rate, whether the procedure is carried out at laparotomy or laparoscopy (55–58).

Due to its position far from the adnexa, isolated bladder detrusor endometriosis may not always interfere with fertilization processes (53). Consequently, it is not unusual to observe conceptions also in women not undergoing surgery. However, in the event that a cesarean section is indicated, one should not be tempted to schedule partial cystectomy on the same occasion, as the considerable increase in blood flow renders the procedure hemorrhagic. Furthermore, unexpectedly, pregnancy status does not facilitate development of cleavage planes between the uterus and the bladder due to the firm fibrotic nature of the adhesions. Unfortunately, symptoms usually reappear when ovulation resumes, and surgery is only deferred.

Ureteral Disease

The prevalence of ureteral endometriosis ranges from 0.01% to 1% of all women with the disease (48). Although ureteral lesions are relatively rare, they may cause major morbidity, as silent loss of renal function is not infrequent in these patients. Obstructive uropathy is associated with both ovarian endometriosis and extensive rectovaginal lesions (51). In these circumstances, even silent loss of renal function may occur. When preoperative rectovaginal examination reveals severe endometriotic infiltration of the lateral parametria, an ultrasound scan of the urinary apparatus or an intravenous urography is opportune to detect a ureteral stricture preoperatively, to allow adequate counseling about the type of surgery required and its potential sequelae, to schedule intraoperative urologic consultation timely (11,51), and to avoid possible medicolegal disputes on whether the stenosis was caused by endometriosis or by surgical procedures.

According to a systematic review (51), ureteral endometriosis is significantly more frequent on the left pelvic side (left lesions, 72%; 95% CI: 61–83%). This is in line with the hypothesized origin of the "left hemipelvis endometriotic complex," which is caused by the presence of the sigmoid and may involve the left ovary, pelvic peritoneum, uterosacral ligament, the ureter, and the large bowel itself (59).

The affected ureter must be identified through the pelvic peritoneum high on the pelvic sidewall. The ureteral dissection commences by incising the peritoneum at the level of the pelvic brim to enter the retroperitoneal space. The ureter can then be swept off the peritoneum in a healthy and nonadherent tract (Fig. 12). The peritoneum is retracted medially, whereas the ureter is bluntly dissected of surrounding tissue using delicate scissors and bipolar pinpoint coagulation. After completion of ureterolysis, endometriotic implants and fibrotic areas are excised (Fig. 13). When as much as possible of the disease is resected, based on the final ureteral conditions a decision must be made on a conservative approach or on resection of the stenotic tract with end-to-end anastomosis or, more properly, a ureteroneocystostomy by Politano–Leadbetter technique with bladder–psoas hitch (Figs. 13 and 14). The last technique is indicated whenever the stenosis is not clearly relieved by ureterolysis. In fact, the possibility of endometriosis infiltrating the ureteral wall (intrinsic ureteral endometriosis) renders persistence of hydronephrosis highly probable.

A few reports on laparoscopic management of ureteral endometriosis have been published. In the series by Nezhat et al. (54), only 4 of 21 patients required segmental ureteral resection and anastomosis. All women conservative surgery for a partial obstruction had a patent ureter at postoperative intravenous pyelography, and no recurrence occurred after a mean follow-up of 22 months.

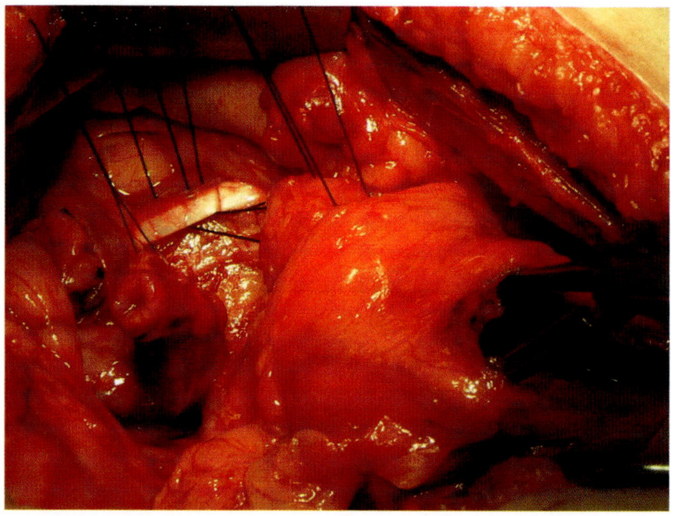

Figure 13 Same case as in Fig. 12. The left ureter has been restricted and the bladder, after mobilization and opening of the dome, is being fixed to the psoas muscle using three interrupted Vicryl 2-0 sutures.

Donnez et al. (60) evaluated retrospectively the outcome of 18 patients with ureteral endometriosis, 16 of which were managed conservatively. Postoperative resolution of urinary obstruction was observed in all cases, and no reintervention for disease recurrence was performed during a follow-up period of 3 to 38 months.

More recently, laparoscopic ureterolysis was evaluated by Ghezzi et al. (62) in a group of 33 patients with moderate to severe hydronephrosis on preoperative intravenous pyelography. A partial ureteral resection was necessary in one case and a segmental resection with bladder–psoas hitch in another one. Thirty-two patients (97%) had a patent ureter at three-month postoperative intravenous pyelography. After a median follow-up of 16 months, the reoperation rate for

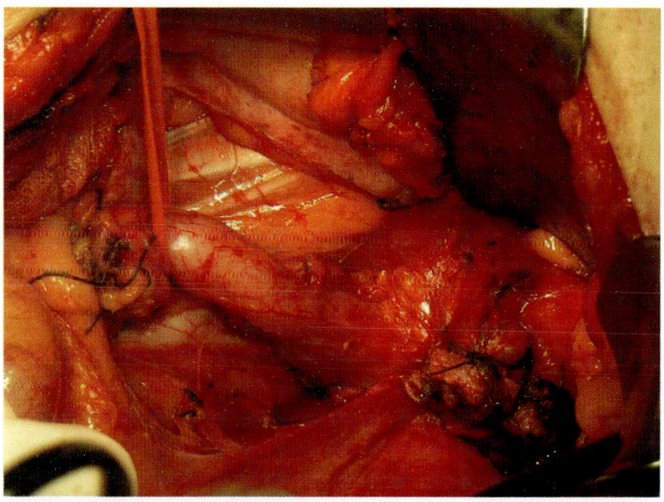

Figure 12 Treatment of ureteral endometriosis at laparotomy. After removal of the left adnexa, the dilated portion of the left ureter is isolated up to its entrance in the parametrial tunnel.

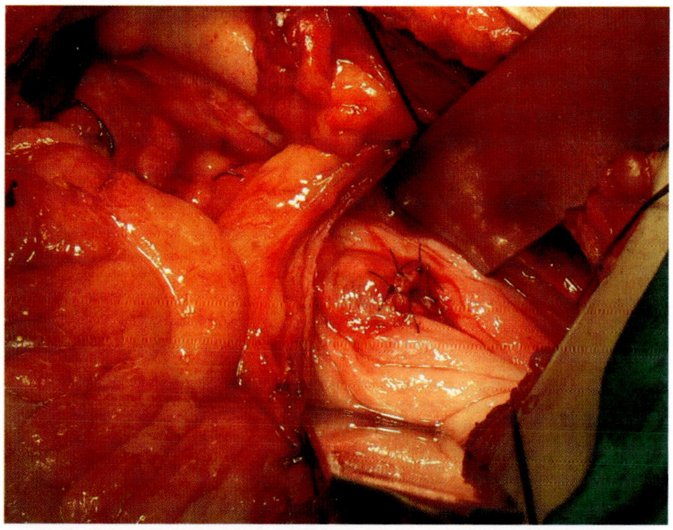

Figure 14 Same case as in Fig. 12. The ureter passes through the bladder wall while maintaining a linear course. A submucous path three to five times wider than the ureter has been created to avoid postureteroneocystostomy reflux. *Source*: From Ref. 61.

disease recurrence was 15% (5/33). Also Frenna et al. (33) reported successful laparoscopic ureterolysis in three patients with ureteral stenosis.

However, Antonelli et al. (63) consider that ureterolysis should be limited to women with localized extrinsic lesions, confined to a small ureteral portion. These investigators suggest that performance of segmentary ureterectomy should be the treatment of choice for pelvic endometriosis involving the ureter, as a definite distinction between intrinsic and extrinsic forms is possible only on histologic basis. Given the very limited available evidence supporting the safety and efficacy of laparoscopic ureterolysis, the major clinical importance of ureteral strictures with potential loss of kidney function, and the not negligible recurrence and reoperation rates observed by some authors after a laparoscopic conservative procedure (62), we recommend a radical approach with resection of the stenotic ureteral tract and performance of reimplantation with accurate antireflux vesicoureteral plasty.

EFFECT OF SURGERY FOR STAGE I–IV DISEASE: NONCOMPARATIVE STUDIES

Several case series have been published, defining the purported efficacy of conservative surgery for endometriosis in terms of pain relief (1,64–75).

Redwine (65) evaluated the long-term results of laparoscopic excision of endometriosis in a series of 359 women operated in a 10-year period. The cumulative rate of recurrent or persistent disease was 19% at 5-year follow up. Of notice, no adjuvant medical treatment was used. A similar rate of pain recurrence (22%), two years after laparoscopic surgery for stage III–IV disease, was reported by Busacca et al. (66) in a group of 141 patients.

Garry et al. (67) introduced the evaluation of health-related quality of life after radical laparoscopic excision of endometriosis. In 57 patients with severe preoperative pain symptoms, a significant improvement in quality of life based on the EuroQOL and SF 12 questionnaires was observed four months after conservative surgery, with the exception of mental health scores. Substantial reductions in dysmenorrhea, deep dyspareunia, and pelvic as well as rectal pain were recorded using a visual analog scale. Unfortunately, due to the very limited length of follow-up, it is not possible to exclude that the overall results are partly determined by a placebo effect.

Jones and Sutton (68) studied pain variation and patient satisfaction for 3 to 12 months following ablative laparoscopic surgery using CO_2 and potassium-titanic-phosphate (KTP) lasers and bipolar coagulation in a series of 73 women with stage III–IV endometriosis. Significant reductions in dysmenorrhea, dyspareunia, and nonmenstrual pain scores, as measured by means of a 10-cm visual analog scale, were observed at three-month evaluation. Pain relief did not vary significantly during the following nine months. According to the authors, 64/73 (89%) subjects were satisfied or very satisfied at final assessment. However, the cutoff points chosen on a 10-point scale to define different satisfaction categories have not been validated.

Abbott et al. (69) investigated the outcomes of laparoscopic excision of endometriosis up to five years after surgery in 176 women with severe pain symptoms. The median visual analog scores decreased from nine to three for dysmenorrhea, from eight to three for nonmenstrual pelvic pain, from seven to zero for dyspareunia, and from seven to two for dyschezia. Quality of life, as measured by three different and validated instruments, significantly improved. Significant ameliorations in sexual functioning as well as decrease in discomfort were also observed. Importantly, the five-year cumulative probability of requiring further surgery was 36%.

Vignali et al. (70) evaluated the risk of pain and disease recurrence after conservative surgery for endometriosis in a series of 115 women with deep infiltrating lesions. After a minimum follow-up of 12 months, recurrence of pain was observed in 28 (24%) and recurrence of lesions in 15 (13%) patients. Twelve subjects (10%) underwent repetitive surgery. Multivariate analysis demonstrated that only age was a significant predictor of pain recurrence, enhancing the risk in younger patients. Recurrence of lesions was predicted by obliteration of the Douglas pouch, and reoperation was predicted by nonradical first-line surgery.

Ferrero et al. (71) examined the effect of laparoscopic excision of endometriosis on deep dyspareunia and quality of sex life in a group of 73 women with intensity of pain ≥ 6 on a 10-cm visual analog scale. Only 52 subjects completed the 12-month follow-up. At intention-to-treat analysis, an improvement in the intensity of deep dyspareunia of ≥ 4 points at 12-month evaluation was achieved in 56% of the study population (41/74), in 59% (27/46) of the patients with endometriosis infiltrating the uterosacral ligaments, and in 56% (14/25) of those without such involvement. Significant improvements in several aspects of sex life were observed at the end of follow-up in the former subjects.

Wykes et al. (72) evaluated by means of postal questionnaires 62 women with chronic pelvic pain (CPP) who underwent laparoscopic excision of peritoneal endometriosis. After an average follow-up of 13 months, 67% of assessed subjects reported improvement in pain symptoms and 71% were satisfied with the results of treatment. However, 40% of women still reported regular use of analgesics, and one-third noted deterioration in initial symptom relief within 12 months. One in six women required repeat surgical intervention for persistent symptoms. The impact of surgery on health-related quality of life was less clear, and deterioration in subjective response over time was observed. Finally, the 70% response rate to postal questionnaires, the lack of a control group, and the relatively short-term and varied length of follow-up probably result in overestimation of the treatment effect.

The largest surgical series published included 729 consecutive women with endometriosis undergoing first-line conservative surgery at laparoscopy (1). To evaluate variations in pelvic pain, only subjects with moderate or severe symptoms of more than six months' duration before surgery were considered. Pain symptoms were graded according to a zero- to three-point multidimensional categorical rating scale and a 100-mm visual analog: a score of 1 to 50 was considered mild pain, 51 to 80 moderate pain, and 81 to 100 severe pain.

A total of 425 subjects had moderate or severe dysmenorrhea before surgery. The crude pain recurrence rate in these women was 91/425, 21% (33/117, 28%, at stage I; 15/66, 23%, at stage II; 22/113, 20%, at stage III; and 21/129, 16%, at stage IV). The overall cumulative probability of moderate or severe dysmenorrhea recurrence at three years from surgery was 24% (32% at stage I, 24% at stage II, 21% at stage III, and 19% at stage IV; log rank test, $\chi^2_3 = 6.39$, $P = 0.094$). Cumulative dysmenorrhea recurrence curves by stages are shown in Fig. 15. At multivariate proportional hazards regression analysis, the only covariate significantly associated with recurrence of dysmenorrhea was age at surgery. In particular, endometriosis stage was not associated with the risk of recurrence of

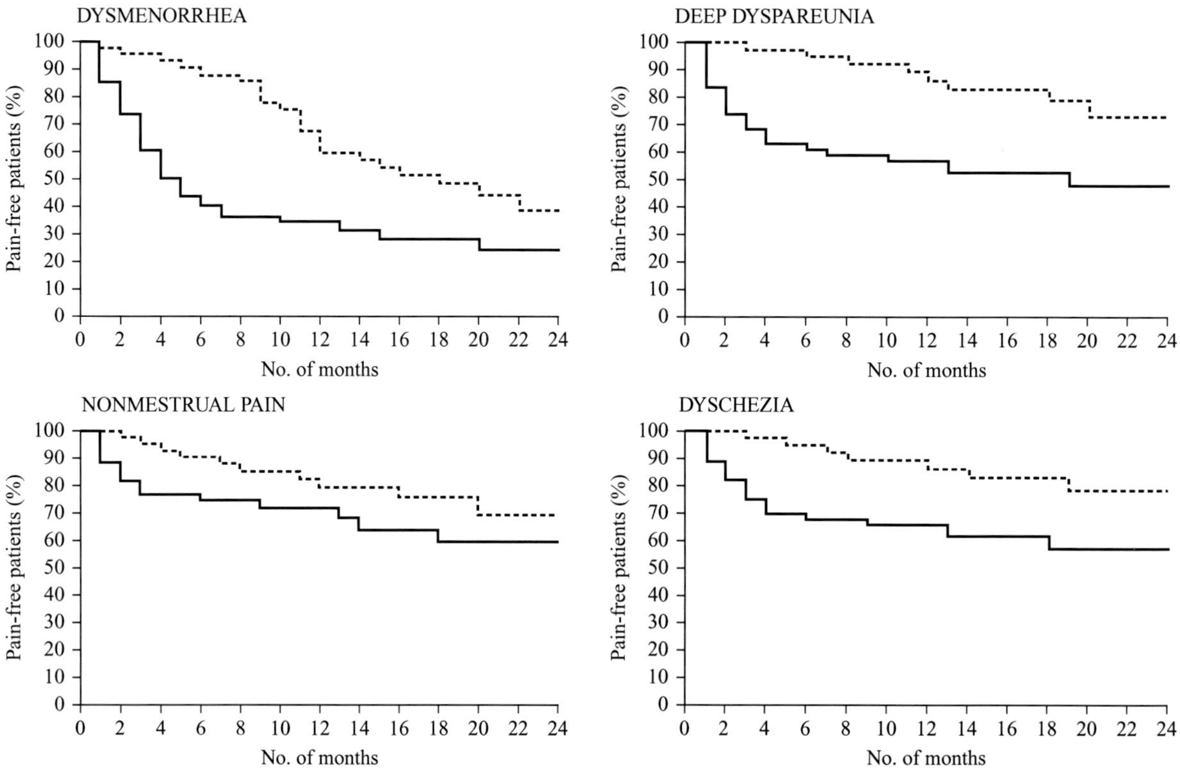

Figure 15 Twenty-four-month symptom-free survival analysis in 105 women with rectovaginal endometriosis undergoing conservative surgery at laparotomy (- - -) or expectant management (——). *Source*: From Ref. 76.

moderate or severe menstrual pain. Deep dyspareunia and nonmenstrual pain were reported before surgery by, respectively, 110/729 (15%) and 167/729 (23%) patients. Recurrence of moderate or severe pain at intercourse was reported by 8 women (7%) and of nonmenstrual pain by 24 (14%). After surgery, de novo dysmenorrhea occurred in only eight subjects, de novo deep dyspareunia in seven, and de novo nonmenstrual pain in eight (1).

In general, major methodological drawbacks limit the validity of the data presented in observational, noncomparative studies. Indeed, several factors could influence the available evidence, such as the criteria adopted for the diagnosis of symptoms or disease recurrence, the duration of follow-up of a chronic disease with a high relapse rate, and the exclusion of dropouts, a subgroup with a potentially worse prognosis. Publication bias seems probable, as the estimate of recurrence rate derives mainly from retrospective trials that tend to over-represent optimistic results. Surgeons with suboptimal long-term outcomes may be less willing to submit their data or have those published. The real incidence of pain symptoms recurrence may thus be undefined due to misdiagnosis and under-reporting.

The modality to treat peritoneal endometriosis appears inconsequential with regard to pain relief. Wright et al. (73) conducted a randomized, double-blind trial comparing laparoscopic excision and ablation of peritoneal lesions in 24 patients with symptomatic endometriosis. After six-month follow-up, about two-thirds of subjects in each study group reported substantial reduction of pain. No significant difference was observed in postoperative pelvic signs also.

In contrast, the modality adopted to treat ovarian endometriomas has a major impact on surgical outcomes (74,75). Hart et al. (77) conducted a systematic literature review in order to determine the most effective technique of treating endometriotic cysts: either excision of the cyst pseudocapsule or drainage and electrocoagulation of the pseudocyst wall, with regard to relief of pain, recurrence of the endometrioma, recurrence of symptoms, and the subsequent spontaneous pregnancy rate. Laparoscopic excision of the pseudocyst wall was associated with a reduced rate of recurrence of the endometrioma (OR: 0.41; 95% CI: 0.18–0.93), reduced requirement for further surgery (OR: 0.21; 95% CI: 0.05–0.79), reduced recurrence rate of dysmenorrhea (OR: 0.15; 95% CI: 0.06–0.38), dyspareunia (OR: 0.08; 95% CI: 0.01–0.51), and nonmenstrual pelvic pain (OR: 0.10; 95% CI: 0.02–0.56). Excision was also associated with a subsequent increased rate of spontaneous pregnancy in women who had documented prior subfertility (OR: 5.21; 95% CI: 2.04–13.29). Consequently, excision of the endometrioma pseudocapsule should be the favored surgical approach (74,75). Moreover, only excisional treatment allows histological examination of surgical samples.

EFFECT OF SURGERY FOR STAGE I–IV DISEASE: CONTROLLED STUDIES

The results of three randomized controlled trials (RCTs) are available in order to evaluate properly the effect of surgery on endometriosis-associated pain.

Sutton et al. (78) performed a double-blind study on 63 women with minimal to moderate endometriosis undergoing laparoscopy for pelvic pain symptoms. The subjects were allocated intraoperatively to laser destruction of endometriotic lesions plus uterosacral nerve ablation ($n = 32$) or expectant management ($n = 31$). At six-month follow-up, 20 patients in the laser group were better (63%) compared with 7 (23%) in the expectant management group.

Three years later, Sutton et al. (79) reported the results observed at one-year follow-up. The authors maintain that symptom relief continued in 90% of those who initially responded. However, based on an intention-to-treat analysis, this translates in a success rate of 56% (18/32) in the active management group versus 23% (7/31) in the control group, with a pain recurrence rate of 44% after laser surgery. In other words, one year after laparoscopy, the absolute benefit increase of surgery is 33%.

A further, long-term report on the same population has been published in 2001 (80). However, no additional information on the two separate study groups is obtainable, as 24 patients in the expectant management arm eventually underwent laser laparoscopy, and their data were mixed with those originally allocated to the surgical arm. Unfortunately, 25 subjects of the resulting cohort of 56 patients have been lost to follow-up. After a mean period of 73 months since the procedure, 21 of the remaining 38 women (55%) experienced satisfactory symptom relief, whereas 17 (45%) described continued painful symptoms. Again, inclusion of dropouts in the final analysis, according to a conservative and probably more realistic approach, would modify the optimistic view of the authors, because only 21 of the 56 (37%) women treated with laser laparoscopy have actually been demonstrated to experience a substantial symptomatic benefit.

A second, small, blinded RCT was conducted by Abbott et al. (81) on 39 symptomatic women undergoing laparoscopy for minimal to severe endometriosis. Twenty of them were allocated to immediate excision of lesions, whereas in 19 no surgical procedure was performed. A second laparoscopy was scheduled after six months, with the aim of excising all the visible lesions in both study groups. At six-month follow-up, 16 subjects (80%) in the surgery group reported symptomatic improvement compared with 6 (32%) in the expectant management group. The increase in benefit of 48% is similar to the 40% observed by Sutton et al. (78) after the same, short, follow-up period. A total of 33 women underwent a second laparoscopy, 15 in the surgery group and 18 in the expectant management group. After a further six-month follow-up, 8 subjects in the former (53%) and 15 in the latter (83%) groups reported improvement in pain. This demonstrates that the second-line surgery is less effective than the first-line one, as the proportions of nonresponders were 47% and 20%, respectively. In both groups, amelioration in health-related quality of life was demonstrated after excisional surgery.

The third blind study on the effectiveness of surgery for endometriosis was conducted by Jarrell et al. (82) who allocated 29 women with severely symptomatic minimal to moderate endometriosis to laparoscopic excision ($n = 15$) or sham surgery ($n = 14$). The subjects completed pain diaries at baseline and then at three-month intervals for one year. Only seven women in the excisional surgery group and eight in the control group completed the entire follow-up period. No significant difference was observed in visual analog scale pain score reduction (45% vs. 33%, respectively). Similar proportional reductions were observed also in dropouts at their last evaluation (42% vs. 35%, respectively).

Recently, Jarrell reported long-term follow-up data of the above study population in order to determine the predictors of subsequent surgery (83). The overall repeat surgical operation rate 12 to 14 years after the original trial was 52% in the excision group and 48% in the sham surgery group. Only the reported measurement of pain prior to the initial trial was a significant covariate in the prediction of repeat surgery among all subjects. Age, stage of disease, and excision of endometriosis were not associated with an improvement in pain, as measured by the time to repeat surgery.

Several conclusions can be drawn based on the results of these few formal, comparative studies on the effectiveness of laparoscopic surgery for symptomatic endometriosis: the absolute benefit increase compared with sham surgery in terms of proportion of women reporting pain relief is probably between 30% and 40%; this difference, observed a few months after surgery, tends to decrease over time; and the reoperation rate because of pain recurrence can be as high as 50%.

The authors of the above trials are to be commended for the enormous efforts necessary for the conduction of randomized, blinded, comparative studies including a sham surgery arm. However, even these methodologically valuable trials are afflicted by some methodological drawbacks, such as limited sample size (78,81,82), short follow-up period (81), and a substantial number of dropouts (82). This partly limits the precise measurement of the treatment effect. Any therapy for a chronic inflammatory disease such as endometriosis should be evaluated in the context of long-term strategies. Accordingly, in all future RCTs on the outcome of surgery for endometriosis-associated pain, long-term data should be provided to allow for dropouts and smaller likely effect sizes as a result of declining treatment effect (72,84).

EFFECT OF SURGERY FOR DEEP INFILTRATING DISEASE

Endometriosis infiltrating the posterior vaginal and anterior rectal walls usually causes severe organic-type symptoms, such as deep dyspareunia and dyschezia, in addition to dysmenorrhea (85–87). Incomplete lesion resection in this technically demanding condition generally does not achieve benefits, whereas radical interventions carry an occasional risk of major complications, and ureteral and rectal injuries with associated sequelae are not exceptional (Table 1) (84,88,114).

The diagnosis of rectovaginal endometriosis is based on vaginal and rectal examinations, transvaginal and transrectal ultrasonography, pelvic MRI, and histological demonstration of endometriosis in biopsy of the posterior fornix. The preoperative workup must also include kidney and urinary tract ultrasonography as well as rectosigmoidoscopy.

Table 1 Major Intra- and Postoperative Complications of Radical Surgery for Rectovaginal Endometriosis. Literature Data, 2000–2008 (37,38,55,70,76,84,88–113)

Complication	Observed incidence (%)
Neurogenic bladder dysfunction	4–10
Rectovaginal fistula formation	2–10
Blood transfusion	2–6
Inadvertent rectal perforation	1–3
Anastomotic leakage	1–2
Pelvic abscess	1–2
Temporary diverting loop ileostomy/colostomy	0.5 1.5
Intraoperative ureteral lesion	0.5–1
Postoperative ureteral fistula formation	0.5–1
Postanastomotic rectal stenosis	0.5–1
Postanastomotic ureteral stenosis	0.5–1

Since 2000, the results of more than 30 case series have been published in English language, peer-reviewed journals, with the aim of evaluating the effect of radical conservative surgery for rectovaginal endometriosis on pelvic pain symptoms (37,38,55,70,76,84,88–113). With one exception (76), all the available studies are observational and noncomparative, most of them including a limited number of patients; the criteria used to define presence and extension of deeply infiltrating endometriosis are not always clearly described; the surgical access is inconsistent (i.e., laparotomy alone, laparoscopy alone, a combination of laparotomy or laparoscopy, and a vaginal approach); the proportion of women undergoing colorectal surgery is highly variable, as some groups advocate an aggressive strategy whereas others discourage bowel resection whenever possible; colorectal surgery has been performed differently, as some authors support simple nodulectomy (disk resection) and other low anterior resection; in many reports, it is not stated if resection of the posterior vaginal fornix has been performed systematically; rates of major intra- and postoperative complications vary widely, ranging from 0% to 13%; the follow-up is very different but, in the vast majority of the considered studies, unusually short (even a few months); in general, dropouts are not included in the efficacy analysis; and the proportion of patients who used postoperative medical treatment is usually not reported. Such an extreme clinical heterogeneity virtually impedes data pooling as well as generalization of the observed results.

Controlled data have been reported in a single trial (76). Women with infertility and pain symptoms were offered surgery at laparotomy or expectant management. The study was conducted according to an informed and shared medical decision-making approach. Therefore, the selected therapeutic option was not by random allocation but in accordance with the patient's preference.

Of the 105 patients evaluated, 44 preferred surgical treatment and 61 chose expectant management. Seven patients underwent a low anterior rectal resection; ureterolysis was necessary in six subjects and a segmental bladder resection for a full-thickness detrusor nodule in one. No severe intraoperative complication occurred. Postoperatively, a left ureteroperitoneal fistula with urinary extravasation developed in a woman who underwent extensive ureterolysis because of dense fibrosis.

After a mean follow-up of >2 years, a statistically significant difference in time to moderate or severe pain experience in favor of the surgery group was observed. The benefit of surgery was particularly evident with regard to deep dyspareunia and dyschezia. Dysmenorrhea was the most frequent type of pain reported. The 12-month cumulative proportion of subjects free from moderate or severe dysmenorrhea was 59.8% in the surgery group compared with 34.6% in the expectant management group. Corresponding figures at 24 months were, respectively, 38.9% and 24.5% ($P = 0.001$). At the same time points, the cumulative proportions of women free from moderate or severe deep dyspareunia were, respectively, 86.2% and 72.9% in the surgery group compared with 57.1% and 48.2% in the expectant management group ($P = 0.001$). The cumulative proportions of patients free from dyschezia at 12 and 24 moths were, respectively, 86.3% and 78.1% in the surgery group versus 65.3% and 57.4% in the expectant management group ($P = 0.008$) (Fig. 16). No significant between-group difference was observed in nonmenstrual pain-free survival time.

The mean ± SD number of naproxen sodium tablets used each month throughout the study period was 2.3 ± 1.5 in the conservative surgery group and 5.4 ± 3.3 in the expectant management group (mean difference, 3.1; 95% CI: 2.0–4.2), and the mean ± SD monthly number of days on analgesics was, respectively, 1.6 ± 1.1 and 3.5 ± 2.6 (mean difference, 1.9; 95% CI: 1.1–2.7).

Overall, based on the bulk of the available evidence (37,38,55,70,76,84,88–113) and taking into consideration all the methodological drawbacks, several assumptions may be drawn. Following surgery for rectovaginal endometriosis, major variations are observed in several health-related quality-of-life indicators; substantial pain relief is experienced by about 70% to 80% of patients; such a proportion usually declines with time, and at one-year follow-up about half of the women need analgesics or hormonal treatments; major complications are observed in 3% to 10% of patients (including hemoperitoneum, rectovaginal fistula, anastomotic

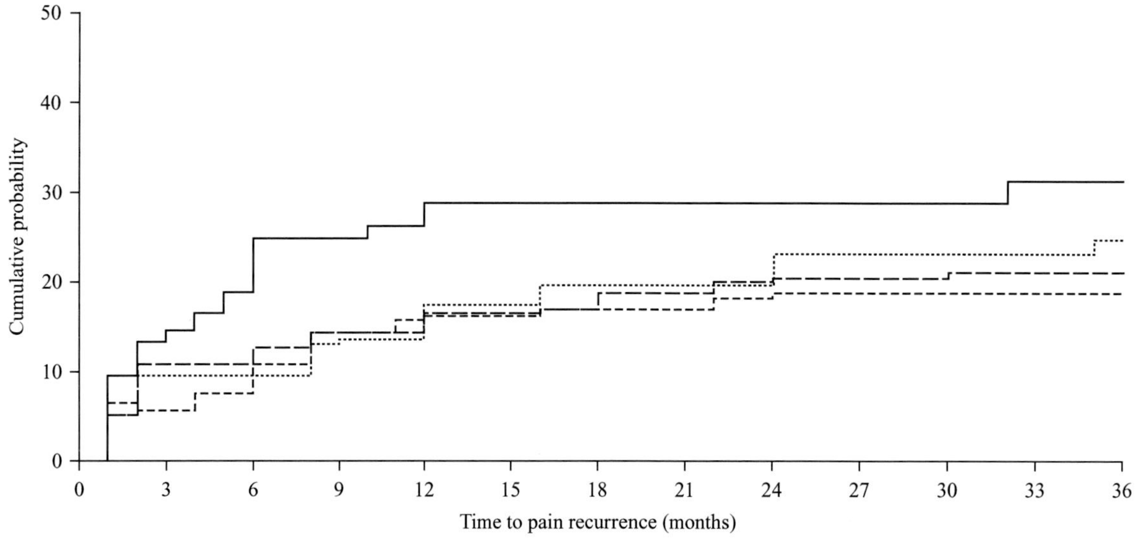

Figure 16 Cumulative 36-month probability of recurrence of moderate or severe dysmenorrhea by disease in 425 symptomatic women who underwent conservative surgery for endometriosis (———, stage I; . . . ., stage II; - - - - -, stage III; and -.-.-.-., stage IV). *Source*: From Ref. 1.

Table 2 Reported Incidence of Rectovaginal Fistula Formation After Radical Surgery for Deeply Infiltrating Endometriosis with Colorectal Resection

Source	Year	% with fistula
Koninckx et al. (113)	1996	3.1
Camagna et al. (114)	2004	6.9
Ford et al. (83)	2004	1.6
Marpeau et al. (115)	2004	6.3
Darai et al. (96)	2005	7.5
Dubernard et al. (103)	2006	10.3
Landi et al. (104)	2006	6.6
Mareu et al. (116)	2007	2.6

Source: From Ref. 118.

leakage/fistula, ureteral fistula/uroperitoneum, bowel perforation, pelvic abscess, need for temporary loop ileostomy, postoperative bowel or ureteral anastomotic stenosis, neurogenic bladder dysfunction, constipation, and peripheral sensory disturbance) (Table 1); concomitant resection of the anterior rectal wall and posterior vaginal fornix increases the risk of rectovaginal fistula formation, due to juxtaposition of sutures of bacteria-containing organs (Table 2) (118); excision of the posterior vaginal fornix is suggested in order to increase the probability of pain relief; performance of low or ultralow anterior rectal resection, although sometimes unavoidable, should be carefully weighed against the major increase in the risk of severe complications; medium-term recurrence of lesions is observed in about one-fifth of the cases; one-fourth of the operated subjects will undergo repetitive conservative or definitive surgery; and all the above outcomes are strictly dependent on surgical experience and radicality, and such results are observed only in tertiary-care referral centers for the treatment of endometriosis.

The most frequent postoperative complication is urinary retention probably due to damage to the parasympathetic plexus, resulting in temporary bladder denervation. This complication is associated with, but not exclusive to, colorectal resection (119). Recently, nerve-sparing techniques have been suggested with substantial reductions in time to resumption of spontaneous voiding, residual urine volume, and need for self-catheterization at discharge (94,101,105).

Rectovaginal endometriosis is a benign condition with limited tendency to progress. In a series of 88 women who underwent watchful waiting for a mean period of six years, Fedele et al. (120) demonstrated that rectovaginal endometriosis is a nonprogressive disease, as an increase in the volume of endometriotic plaques was not observed at transrectal ultrasonography in more than 90% of the subjects. This seems logical based on the intraperitoneal origin of the lesion. In fact, the inflammatory cascade triggered by retrouterine endometriotic implants induces the formation of a fibrotic cast of the deepest portion of the Douglas pouch. In this condition, ectopic endometrial glands may undergo cystic changes with typical bluish nodule formation, but, once buried in dense connective tissue, they cannot easily infiltrate further the surrounding structures (17,86,87).

Hence, the decision to undergo conservative surgery should be undertaken in selected conditions, tailored to the patient's needs, and based on convincing evidence (121). This is particularly important when radical conservative surgery may be challenging and the risk of intra- and postoperative morbidity not negligible (84,87,88,114). Unbearable pain in women wanting pregnancy and refusing IVF constitutes a reasonable indication for excisional treatment, as medical therapies invariably suppress ovulation. Surgery is also a valid alternative in patients not responding to or not tolerating progestogens and estrogen–progestogen combinations. In particular, subjects suffering from severe deep dyspareunia and dyschezia should be considered good candidates for surgery, as excision of deep lesions is usually more effective than medical therapy in relieving organic-type pain.

PELVIC DENERVATING PROCEDURES

Sensory innervation of the pelvic organs is from the superior hypogastric plexus or presacral nerve, the nervi erigentes or pelvic nerves, and the ovarian plexuses (122). The segmental derivation of the presacral nerve is T11-L2. Sympathetic effector fibers and most sensory fibers from the pelvic organs enter the superior hypogastric plexus. This latter usually consists of interlaced nerve bundles lying on the L4 and L5 bodies and the sacral promontory extending over most of the interiliac triangle (122). The nervi erigentes originate from S2-S4 and consist of parasympathetic effector and sensory fibers.

Both sympathetic and parasympathetic fibers run in and around the uterosacral folds and reach the parametrium, posterolateral to the uterine cervix, where they unite to form the plexuses of Frankenhauser. The latter may be considered a "clearing station" for these fibers, which enter the plexuses, intermingle, and then proceed together to innervate the upper part of the vagina, uterus, proximal portion of the tubes, bladder, urethra, and rectum (122). Innervation of the tubal ampullae and ovaries is instead from the ovarian plexus, which is formed mainly of sympathetic fibers of T9-T10 derivation that run along the vessels of the infundibulopelvic ligament. Although the uterine body is innervated mainly by fibers of the hypogastric plexus, the fundus also receives fibers from the ovarian plexuses (122).

Severe, disabling dysmenorrhea is, by far, the most frequent problem in women with endometriosis (85). Accordingly, the addition of uterine denervation to lesion destruction has been suggested to improve long-term antalgic results (123). Two types of pelvic denervating procedures have been proposed in women with CPP, namely presacral neurectomy (PSN) and uterosacral ligament resection (i.e., laparoscopic uterosacral nerve ablation—LUNA). The efficacy of both interventions has been assessed in a few RCTs (124).

Efficacy of PSN

The results of the three published RCTs on PSN in women with endometriosis are inconsistent (Fig. 17). Tjaden et al. (125) recruited eight subjects who were randomly allocated to PSN in addition to conservative surgery ($n = 4$) or to conservative surgery only ($n = 4$) for moderate or severe midline dysmenorrhea associated with stage III–IV endometriosis. Eighteen other women wanting ($n = 13$) or refusing ($n = 5$) PSN were included in the evaluation. At six-month follow-up, 15/17 subjects who underwent PSN experienced dysmenorrhea relief (four randomized and 11/13 nonrandomized), whereas all the subjects who underwent conservative surgery only remained symptomatic. This led the monitoring committee to stop the study because it was considered unethical to continue to deprive patients of the evident benefit of PSN.

In the second RCT by Candiani et al. (126), 71 women with moderate or severe midline dysmenorrhea were allocated to conservative surgery at laparotomy and PSN ($n = 35$) or conservative surgery only ($n = 36$). Recurrence of moderate or severe dysmenorrhea at one-year follow-up was observed in

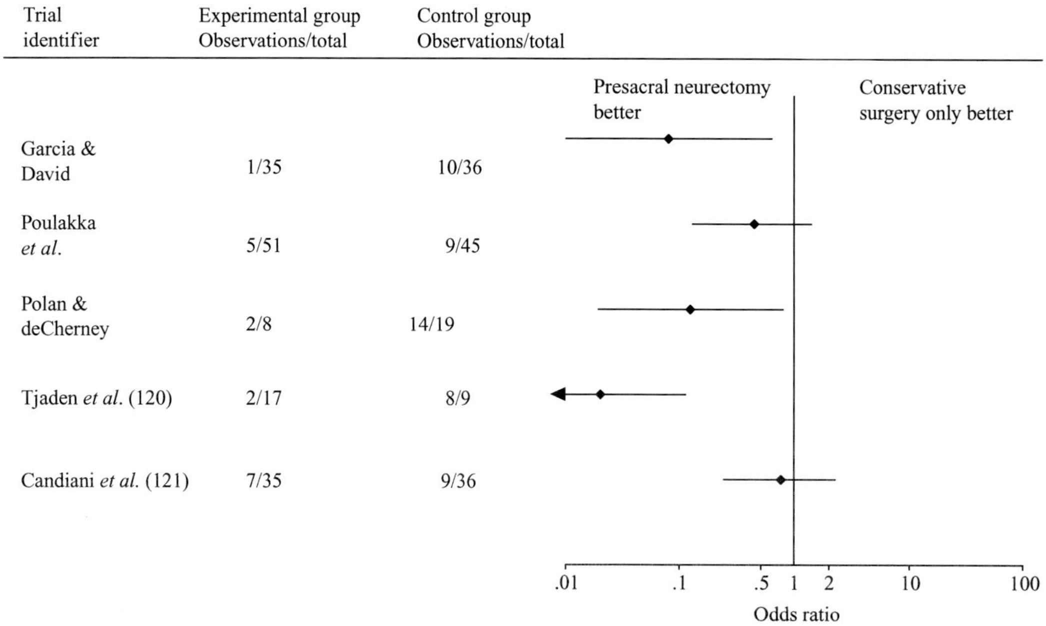

Figure 17 Results of studies comparing conservative surgery plus presacral neurectomy with conservative surgery only for dysmenorrhea associated with endometriosis. Diamonds represent odds ratio of nonresponse and horizontal lines represent 95% confidence intervals. Breslow–Day test for heterogeneity: $\chi^2_4 = 12.36$, $P = 0.014$. *Source*: From Ref. 122. Figure elaborated with GraphPad Prism 4 Project.

6/35 (17%) in the experimental group and 9/36 (25%) in the control group according to a linear analog scale and, respectively, 5/35 (14%) and 7/36 (19%) according to a multidimensional verbal rating scale, the differences not being statistically significant. In the PSN group, constipation developed or worsened in 13 patients and urinary urgency occurred in three.

In the third, more recent, RCT (127), 141 subjects with severe dysmenorrhea were allocated to laparoscopic surgery for endometriosis plus PSN or laparoscopic surgery only. Sixty-three women in each study group were included in the efficacy analysis. At 6- and 12-month follow-ups, the cure rate in terms of dysmenorrhea relief was significantly higher in the PSN group than in the surgery-only group (respectively, 87% vs. 60% and 86% vs. 57%). At the end of the study period, also the frequency and severity of deep dyspareunia and nonmenstrual pain were significantly lower in women in the former group than in those in the latter group.

One year later, Zullo et al. (128) published the 24-month follow-up data observed in 120 women (60 in each study group) enrolled in the original trial (127). The severity of dysmenorrhea, dyspareunia, and nonmenstrual pelvic pain was significantly lower and health-related quality of life significantly better in subjects who underwent PSN in addition to laparoscopic treatment of endometriotic lesions. The cure rate was 83% (50/60) in the PSN group compared with 53% (32/60) in the surgery-only group. However, 11 women who underwent PSN experienced long-term complications such as de novo constipation ($n = 9$, 15%) and urinary urgency ($n = 3$, 5%).

Efficacy of Uterosacral Ligament Resection/Ablation

The efficacy of LUNA has been evaluated in RCTs conducted in women with pain associated with endometriosis as well as in those without obvious pathology.

In the study by Sutton et al. (129), 27 subjects were randomly allocated to laparoscopic surgery for endometriosis plus LUNA and 24 to laparoscopic surgery only. Significant differences in favor of the surgery-only group were observed in dysmenorrhea as well as in nonmenstrual pain scores at three- and six-month follow-up. Results were similar with regard to deep dyspareunia.

The largest RCT on the efficacy of LUNA for endometriosis-associated moderate to severe dysmenorrhea was conducted in Milan on 180 women undergoing first-line surgery for stage I–IV disease (35). Among the patients who could be evaluated one year after operative laparoscopy, 23 of 78 (29%) women who had LUNA and 21 of 78 (27%) women who had conservative surgery only reported recurrent dysmenorrhea. The corresponding number of patients at three years were 21 of 59 (36%) and 18 of 57 (32%) women, respectively (Fig. 18). Pain was substantially reduced, and subjects in both groups experienced similar and significant improvements in health-related quality of life, psychiatric conditions, and sexual satisfaction. Overall, 68 of 90 (75%) patients in the LUNA group and 67 of 90 (75%) patients in the conservative surgery-only group were satisfied at one year.

Johnson et al. (130) designed a double-blind RCT recruiting 67 women with and 56 without endometriosis. The addition of LUNA to laparoscopic surgical treatment of endometriosis was not associated with a significant difference in any pain outcomes. However, a significantly greater relief from dysmenorrhea was observed at 12-month follow-up in women without endometriosis who underwent LUNA, 42% versus 14% experiencing a successful treatment defined as a 50% or greater reduction in VAS score. No significant between-group difference was observed in relief from nonmenstrual pelvic pain, deep dyspareunia, or dyschezia.

The results of Johnson et al. (130) confirm the findings of Lichten and Bombard (131), who were the first to conduct a randomized trial, albeit small, on the effect of LUNA in 21 subjects, with no demonstrable pelvic pathology at

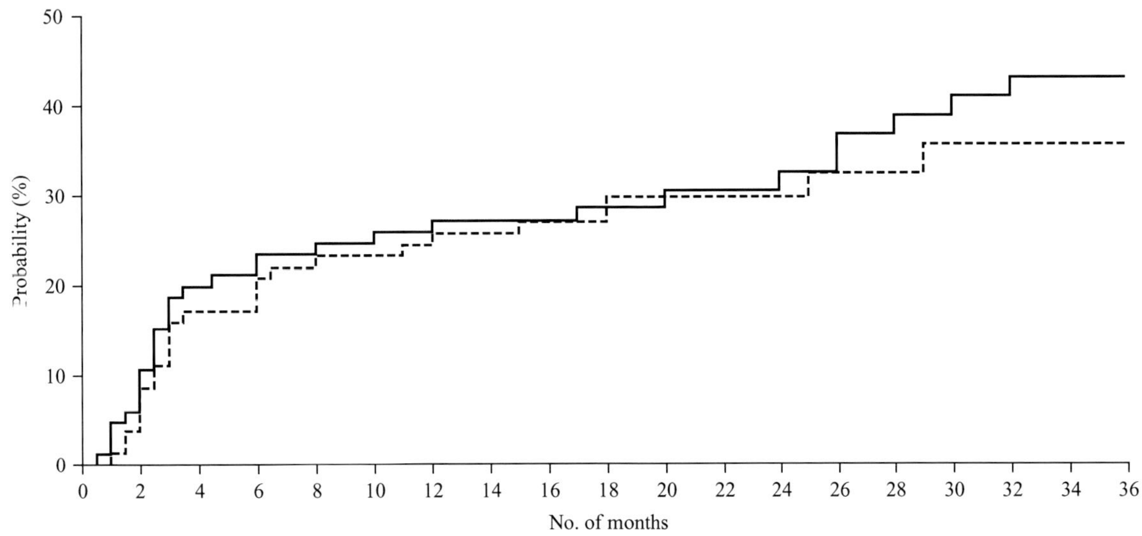

Figure 18 Cumulative 36-month probability recurrence of moderate or severe dysmenorrhea, as assessed by a linear analog scale in 180 symptomatic women with endometriosis who had laparoscopic surgery with (*solid line*) or without (*dashed line*) uterosacral ligament resection (log-rank test, $\chi^2_1 = 0.28$, $P = 0.59$). *Source*: From Ref. 35.

laparoscopy performed because of severe dysmenorrhea. Nine of the 11 patients (81%) allocated to LUNA reported postoperative relief of menstrual pain, compared with none in the control arm.

Meta-analysis of Data on Pelvic Denervating Procedures

Latthe et al. (132) recently published the results of a meta-analysis conducted by the Cochrane Menstrual Disorders and Subfertility Group. After pooling of the results of the above-considered RCTs, the authors concluded that, for the treatment of primary dysmenorrhea, LUNA was better than a control or no treatment at 12 months after surgery (OR: 6.12; 95% CI: 1.78–21.03). However, in secondary dysmenorrhea, along with laparoscopic surgical treatment of endometriosis, the addition of LUNA did not improve the pain relief (OR: 0.77; 95% CI: 0.43–1.39), whereas PSN did (OR: 3.14; 95% CI: 1.59–6.21). The authors conclude that the evidence for nerve interruption in the management of dysmenorrhea is limited and that further, methodologically adequate RCTs are needed. A further meta-analysis on the effectiveness of LUNA is currently being performed by collecting individual patient data from the existing trials (133).

Complications and Side Effects of Pelvic Denervations

Some women who underwent PSN experienced complications and side effects, postoperative constipation being the most frequent disturbance (122,132). It cannot be excluded that in some trials side effects were considered only if sufficiently severe to cause withdrawal of the patient or that only spontaneously reported and not regularly assessed side effects were included. The inconveniences caused by uterosacral ligament resection are generally rare and of limited severity; this may be the result of a more selective uterine denervation or, alternatively, an indirect proof that such a localized neurotomy does not affect the overall innervation and function of pelvic organs.

PSN is carried out in a complex anatomic area, and great care must be taken to avoid damaging major as well as midsacral vessels and also the right ureter. Fatal venous sacral hemorrhages have been reported, and postoperative bowel and bladder dysfunctions are not infrequent. In the absence of robust evidence of a treatment effect, PSN should be performed only by expert surgeons in highly selected women who specifically report midline, hypogastric pain without lateral components.

Performance of laparoscopic uterosacral ligament resection appears simple and quick and gives the impression that everything that is surgically feasible has been done, including an intervention on the peripheral nervous system. This may be gratifying for both gynecologists and patients, but it is not possible to exclude that this type of neurotomy is of little or no benefit. Contrary to the case of PSN, almost all laparoscopic surgeons feel that they are able to carry out uterosacral ligament resection safely. However, complications have also been reported after this apparently easy operation, including hemorrhages, ureteral damage, and pelvic support disorders (126,134–138).

Although the main anatomic pathways through which pelvic pain impulses are transmitted are known, precise relations between site of pain sensation, area of corresponding innervation, and afferent fibers are difficult to define (85,86,139). The old clinical tenet that lateral, adnexal pain cannot be influenced by pelvic denervations and that only central, hypogastric pain may be reduced or abolished must clearly be borne in mind. However, uterine sensory innervation may also be neither simple nor schematic. Nerve fibers may be distributed more widely or may have more complex interconnections than previously thought. Finally, a chronic inflammatory status, such as that associated with endometriosis, may cause stimulation of pain sensory fibers innervating a vast area of the pelvic peritoneum (85,86,140). This incomplete knowledge makes surgical treatment of pelvic pain by denervations empirical.

Although the results of conservative surgery only for endometriosis are suboptimal in terms of long-term pain relief, routine complementary performance of denervating procedures cannot be recommended based on the quality of the available information.

ADJUVANT THERAPY

As a result of the increasing surgical approach to endometriosis, the combination of medical treatment with laparoscopic procedures, either pre- or postoperatively, represents a growing field of application of drugs. Unfortunately, little information is available on the potential benefits of hormonal treatments in combination with conservative surgery for endometriosis (141).

Preoperative Medical Treatment

The theoretical advantages of medical treatment before surgery are reduced inflammation and vascularization and shrinkage of implants. According to some authors, these effects may contribute to easier, quicker, and less traumatic surgery, with more chance of complete eradication of the disease and a reduced risk of postoperative adnexal adhesions (142–148). Practical advantages include avoidance of operating in the secretory phase with the disturbing presence of the corpus luteum and the possibility of hospital admission at any time (149). This may be important in large, busy, public hospitals. The carryover effect of most drugs used preoperatively prevents short-term ovulation in a recently traumatized gonad (149). Finally, with preoperative treatment lasting a few weeks, the differential diagnosis between endometriotic and corpus luteum cysts can be made easily, avoiding an untimely intervention when a functional formation is present. On the other hand, under medical suppression, small endometriotic foci may temporarily regress and thus escape laparoscopic recognition and ablation. Delaying surgery may be inopportune in some circumstances, especially when the nature of the cyst is not completely defined and serum CA-125 levels are particularly elevated. Indisputable disadvantages are the increase in the overall cost of the treatment and drug-related side effects.

Apart from general considerations, only limited data are available to evaluate the effect of preoperative medical treatments on surgical aspects and long-term outcome. According to the extensive evaluations of preoperative medical therapies by Donnez et al. (148,150,151), a gonadotropin-releasing hormone (GnRH) agonist in depot formulation proved superior to progestins, danazol, gestrinone, and the same GnRH agonist as nasal spray in terms of reduction of inflammation, vascularization, AFS score, mean endometrioma diameter, and mitotic index. In a randomized trial, Donnez et al. (147) demonstrated that goserelin administration for three months after drainage of endometriomas partially prevented the regrowth to the original dimensions observed in the subjects who were not medically treated between first- and second-look laparoscopy. Whether all these factors lead to easier, quicker, and more effective surgery remains debatable, however. When Muzii et al. (152) compared the intraoperative results of 20 patients who underwent laparoscopy after three months of GnRH agonist treatment with the results of 21 women who were allocated to immediate surgery for unilateral ovarian endometriomas, no significant difference could be demonstrated in total operating time, cyst wall stripping time, and time needed to obtain complete hemostasis. Audebert et al. (153) did not observe significant differences in surgical feasibility when using a GnRH agonist before laparoscopy. In pretreated women, 6/25 (24%) of the procedures were classified as difficult or very difficult compared with 8/28 (28%) in the subjects who underwent immediate surgery.

With regard to the effect on pelvic pain after surgery, Donnez et al. (154) reported that the combination of preoperative progestin therapy and surgery at laparotomy for moderate and severe endometriosis in a series of 50 patients resulted in complete relief of pain in 45% and improvement in 42% of previously symptomatic women. Corresponding figures for dyspareunia were 16% and 58%, respectively. These data are of doubtful value, given the noncomparative study design. When Napolitano et al. (155) retrospectively reviewed their series of 117 women operated for moderate or severe endometriosis, they observed that 64% of previously symptomatic women who underwent combined medical and surgical treatment experienced complete pain relief, and 16% experienced partial improvement. Corresponding figures in the surgery-only group were 55% and 18%, without significant differences.

In the absence of convincing evidence of a treatment effect in terms of surgical advantages and symptomatic relief, preoperative medical treatment seems unjustified, especially if this modality includes the performance of two surgical procedures some months apart. In these circumstances, the increase in morbidity and costs seems to far outweigh the hypothetical benefits. Based on the results of a systematic literature review, Yap et al. (156) maintain that there is insufficient available evidence to conclude that hormonal suppression combined with surgery for endometriosis is associated with a significant clinical advantage. Presurgical medical therapy decreases the AFS classification scores, but whether this results in better outcomes for the patients is questionable.

Postoperative Medical Treatment

The hypothetical advantages of postoperative medical treatment include resorption of residual visible lesions whose surgical removal was considered inopportune or not possible, "sterilization" of microscopic implants, and reduction in the risk of disease dissemination when endometriomas rupture during mobilization. These advantages should reduce postoperative lesions and symptoms recurrence rate (142–146). The effect of systemic short-term medical treatment after surgery has been reviewed by Vercellini et al. (141).

In the study by Telimaa et al. (157), medroxyprogesterone acetate (MPA) and danazol given postoperatively reduced pelvic pain scores more effectively than placebo, the difference being significant at six months of therapy. It is unclear if the difference in symptomatic relief persisted even after the withdrawal of medical therapy. Absolute numbers of responders/nonresponders were not indicated—a limit that applies also to the trial by Parazzini et al. (158). The latter study assessed the analgesic effect of nasal nafarelin for three months after surgery using a seven-point multidimensional verbal rating scale and a ten-point linear analog scale. At 12-month follow-up, the mean reduction of the multidimensional score was 3.6 and 4.0, respectively, in women allocated to nafarelin or placebo, and the mean reduction of the 10-point linear scale score was 7.0 and 6.9, respectively. These differences were not statistically significant.

The assessment of effect in terms of pelvic pain relief at the end of follow-up for other five available trails (159–163) is shown in Fig. 19. The pooled odds ratio was 0.54 (95% CI: 0.34–0.82), which suggests an effect of postoperative medical treatment in reducing the rate of pain symptoms recurrence (141). More information is needed to confirm these findings, however, particularly in view of the discordant results obtained by Parazzini et al. (158), Vercellini et al. (161), and Busacca et al. (163).

Slightly different conclusions were drawn by Yap et al. (156) after conducting a systematic literature review with the

Trial Identifier	Pain Recurrences / Patients	
	Experimental	Control
Hornstein *et al.* (154)	15/49	25/44
Bianchi *et al.* (155)	7/31	9/29
Vercellini *et al.* (156)	19/81	27/74
Muzii *et al.* (157)	3/33	6/35
Busacca *et al.* (158)	10/44	11/45
Common odds ratio		

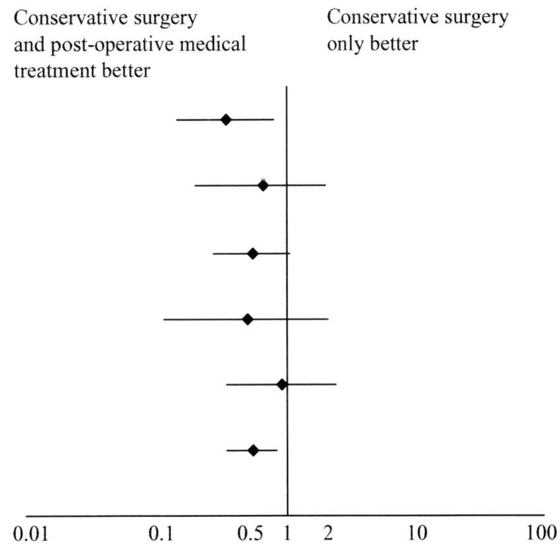

Breslow-Day = 2.12 (P = 0.71)

Figure 19 Overview of randomized, controlled trials that compare conservative surgery for endometriosis with or without postoperative medical treatment. Diamonds represent odds ratio of symptoms recurrence, and horizontal lines are 95% CI. *Source*: From Ref. 141. Figure elaborated with GraphPad Prism 4 Project.

objective of assessing if adjunctive medical treatment postoperatively prolong the symptom-free interval. According to the author (155), postsurgical hormonal suppression of endometriosis compared to surgery alone (either no medical therapy or placebo) in the eight considered trials showed no benefit for the outcome of pain recurrence rate, but a significant improvement in disease relapse.

The observed differences among various drugs used after surgery are limited in clinical terms and, in the absence of formal randomized comparisons, are difficult to interpret. If and when postoperative medical treatment is deemed opportune, progestins with or without estrogens should be considered first because of their tolerable side effects, limited costs, and antalgic efficacy similar to GnRH agonists and danazol. This allows prolonged use in women not wanting pregnancy immediately after surgery, offering a real benefit compared with short-term treatments. In fact, it seems rather naïve to hypothesize an enduring effect of hormonal treatments, which have been repeatedly demonstrated to act only symptomatically. In endometriosis, drugs work until they are used, not after withdrawal.

Moreover, an important additional advantage of prolonged postoperative contraceptive use is the recently demonstrated major reduction in the risk of endometrioma recurrence after surgery (164). The authors observed a crude cyst recurrence rate of 9% (9/103) in the oral contraceptive (OC) users and 56% (26/46) in the never users. The adjusted OR for OC use was 0.04 (95% CI: 0.02–0.13). The 36-month cumulative proportion of subjects free from endometrioma recurrence was 94% in the always users, compared with 51% in the never users (log-rank test, $\chi^2_1 = 36.2$; $P < 0.001$). The adjusted incidence rate ratio was 0.10 (95% CI: 0.04–0.24). The absolute risk reduction of endometrioma recurrence in always users compared with never users was 47% (95% CI: 37–57%). This means that regular postoperative use of an estrogen–progestin combination prevented endometrioma recurrence in one out of two patients (95% CI: 0.2–7) three years after surgery, with a relative risk reduction of 80%. However, the protective effect of estrogen–progestin combination tends to vanish rapidly after discontinuation.

An alternative modality to offer prolonged postoperative progestin treatment consists in the insertion of a levonorgestrel-releasing intrauterine device (Lng-IUD) at the end of laparoscopy for symptomatic endometriosis. Vercellini et al. (165) designed a pilot study to verify if the frequency and severity of dysmenorrhea recurrence are reduced at one-year follow-up in women in whom an Lng-IUD is inserted immediately after laparoscopic surgery for endometriosis compared with women treated with laparoscopic surgery only.

After complete excision or coagulation of all endometriotic lesions, 20 subjects were randomized to Lng-IUD insertion and 20 to postoperative expectant management. Median (interquartile range) dysmenorrhea visual analog scale scores fell by 50 mm (35–65 mm) in the postoperative Lng-IUD group and by 30 mm (25–40 mm) in the surgery-only group (P = 0.012 and 0.021). According to an intention-to-treat analysis, postoperative moderate or severe dysmenorrhea recurrence was less frequent in the former group (2/20 subjects, 10%) than in the latter (9/20, 45%; P = 0.03; relative risk = 0.22; 95% CI: 0.05–0.90). An Lng-IUD should be inserted postoperatively in three patients to avoid moderate or severe dysmenorrhea recurrence in one of them one year after surgery. Also dyspareunia and nonmenstrual pain scores were reduced to a greater extent with the postoperative use of Lng-IUD. Insertion of the medicated device after conservative surgery for endometriosis may constitute an innovative, effective, safe, and convenient adjuvant treatment for the reduction of risk of dysmenorrhea recurrence. However, this local measure does not inhibit ovulation and may not protect from endometrioma reappearance.

RECURRENT DISEASE

Very limited information is available on the effect of repetitive surgery for recurrent symptomatic endometriosis in terms of postoperative pain relief.

Candiani et al. (166) evaluated the relief of pain symptoms in 42 women undergoing repetitive conservative surgery at laparotomy for recurrent endometriosis. At second-line operation, the disease was at stage IV in 14, stage III in 25, and stage I in 3 women. After a mean follow-up of 42 months, dysmenorrhea and deep dyspareunia reappeared in eight women and noncyclical pelvic pain in seven. A third operation was necessary in six subjects.

Busacca et al. (167) compared surgical outcomes in 81 women reoperated at laparotomy ($n = 41$) and laparoscopy ($n = 40$). The 24-month cumulative probability of recurrence of dysmenorrhea (34% and 43%, respectively) and of noncyclical pelvic pain was not significantly different in the two groups. However, the rate of recurrence of deep dyspareunia was higher in the patients operated at laparotomy as was the number requiring a third intervention. The authors conclude that laparoscopy should be considered the surgical approach of choice in cases of recurrent disease also.

More recently, Fedele et al. (168) compared the postoperative results observed after laparoscopic excision of primary ($n = 305$) versus recurrent ($n = 54$) ovarian endometrioma in the same ovary of the primary cyst. The five-year cumulative pain recurrence rate was 20% after the first surgical procedure and 17% after the second one, and re-treatment requirement was, respectively, 19% versus 17%. According to the authors, the effect on pain of repetitive laparoscopic surgery is similar to that observed after first-line surgery.

More data are urgently needed in this specific area of endometriosis management because the widespread performance of laparoscopy, combined with the relapsing tendency of the disease, has profoundly changed the clinical scenario, especially in referral centers, where patients with recurrent lesions and symptoms now constitute the burden of everyday clinical activity. It is a common tenet that reoperations for endometriosis are technically more demanding and potentially more risky, and these drawbacks should be balanced by acceptable postoperative results.

DEFINITIVE SURGERY

Approximately 10% to 18% of hysterectomies are performed because of CPP (169). In a recent survey by Learman et al. (170), presence of multiple pelvic symptoms, previous use of a GnRH agonist, and absence of symptom resolution predicted the likelihood of subsequent hysterectomy, which reached 95% if all three predictors were simultaneously present. Definitive surgery in women with chronic pain of various origins is a controversial procedure, especially in young women. Patient self-reported outcomes of hysterectomy generally have revealed high levels of satisfaction with treatment in various clinical conditions. However, careful preoperative assessment and discussion of alternative therapeutic choices with examination of risk-to-benefit ratio are mandatory, and the patient's preference regarding treatment alternatives must be considered carefully (171,172).

Although anecdotal clinical experience support the efficacy of hysterectomy for severe pelvic pain associated with endometriosis, formal literature evidence is difficult to interpret. In fact, most reports include patients with several causes of pain and not only endometriosis. Moreover, extrapolating data relative to hysterectomy with or without bilateral oophorectomy is unfeasible. However, this factor should be carefully evaluated in order to offer a reliable prognosis to women affected by an estrogen-responsive disease.

Stovall et al. (173) reviewed the long-term outcome in 99 women who underwent hysterectomy for CPP of presumed uterine origin. After a mean follow-up of 22 months, 77 women reported the absence of notable symptoms. The remaining 22 had persistent pelvic pain, which was however improved in 5 of them.

Carlson et al. (169) reported the results of the Maine Women's Health Study, a prospective cohort study of 418 patients aged 25–50 years undergoing hysterectomy for nonmalignant conditions. A total of 199 of 355 evaluated subjects experienced very frequent pelvic pain at baseline; of those, only 11 (6%) claimed that symptoms persisted 12 months after surgery. The women operated for pelvic pain referred a marked improvement in physical as well as psychological symptoms and sexual dysfunction. Significant improvements in mental and general health index scores and activity were also observed. However, only one-half of these women had specific diagnosis, such as endometriosis, fibroids, or adhesions.

Hillis et al. (174) assessed variations in symptoms one year after hysterectomy for CPP of at least six months' duration. Of the 279 evaluated subjects, 206 (74%) reported no pain, 58 (21%) decreased pain, and 15 (5%) unchanged or increased pain. An increased probability of persistent pain was observed among women who had no identified pelvic disease. In this group, complete symptom relief was achieved in 62% of the cases.

Tay and Bromwich (175) studied retrospectively 228 women who underwent hysterectomy for pelvic pain associated with mixed conditions. Almost half of the patients had multiple diseases. Of 98 subjects with pain as the only or main indication for hysterectomy, 71 responded to an outcome survey 12 or more months after surgery, which showed that 62 of them (87%) were satisfied with the intervention, 8 (11%) were unsure, and 1 (1%) was dissatisfied; 68 (96%) women reported relief from their symptoms.

The results of the Maryland Women's Health Study, a prospective cohort study conducted on 1299 women who underwent hysterectomy in 28 hospitals (176), demonstrated that symptom severity, depression, and anxiety levels decreased significantly after surgery and quality of life improved. A total of 657 patients out of the 745 who referred CPP before hysterectomy (88%) were relieved from symptoms at one-year follow-up. The proportion did not vary at two-year assessment (644/720, 89.4%). The percentage of subjects who developed new clinical problems after surgery was, respectively, 3.6% and 2.8%. Therapy for emotional or psychological problems, depression, and low income were associated with lack of symptom relief.

Hartmann et al. (177) examined differences in quality of life and sexual function after hysterectomy among the women enrolled in the Maryland Women's Health Study who had preoperative pain and depression. At 24 months, women with pain and depression had reduced prevalence of pelvic pain (from 97% to 19%), limited physical function (from 66% to 34%), impaired mental health (from 93% to 38%), and limited social function (from 41% to 15%). Women with pelvic pain only improved in pelvic pain (from 95% to 9%) and limited activity level (from 74% to 24%). The group with depression only had improvement in impaired mental health (from 85%

to 33%). Dyspareunia decreased in all groups. In the authors' experience, women with pelvic pain and depression fare less well 24 months after hysterectomy than women who have either disorder alone or neither. Nevertheless, these women improve substantially over their preoperative baseline in all the quality-of-life and sexual function areas assessed.

Two studies addressed the advantages of definitive surgery, specifically in patients with severely symptomatic endometriosis. MacDonald et al. (178) compared surgical outcomes in women who underwent hysterectomy for pelvic pain in endometriosis at less than 30 ($n = 16$) or more than 40 years of age ($n = 27$). Although similar proportion reported alleviation of pain (80% and 87%, respectively), younger subjects were significantly more likely to report residual symptoms, such as dyspareunia and dysuria. They also more often reported a sense of loss after hysterectomy and more overall disruption in different aspects of life. However, the low response rate to mailed questionnaires (less than 30%), the small sample size, and some atypical clinical characteristics (sexual abuse in 31% and current psychiatric counseling in 25% of women younger than 30 years) limit the usefulness of the data presented.

Fedele et al. (179) compared the outcome of standard extrafascial hysterectomy ($n = 26$) and radical hysterectomy, with the removal of deeply infiltrating endometriosis ($n = 12$) as a definitive treatment for recurrent deep endometriosis in 38 women. During the postoperative unbalanced estradiol treatment, pain recurred in eight (31%) women in the standard hysterectomy group and in none in the modified radical hysterectomy group. These results stress the importance of complete deep lesion removal in order to achieve optimal postoperative symptomatic outcome (180), especially if hormonal replacement therapy is planned (181,182).

The information available suggests that the outcome of hysterectomy for pelvic pain at one- to two-year follow-up is consistently satisfactory. However, in several studies the definition of CPP is somewhat vague and a number of clinical conditions have been included. Preoperative patient assessment must obviously be complete, including testing for bowel dysmotility, urologic disorders, musculoskeletal lesions, and psychosocioenvironmental factors. When no other possible cause of pain is identified in addition to endometriosis and the woman has completed her family, hysterectomy can be considered as an alternative with the hypothesis that this will improve health-related quality of life. This is particularly true when the uterus is exquisitely tender, its palpation or mobilization causes excruciating pain, and several courses of medical therapies have failed. However, women should be adequately informed on the expected probability of success, and they should specifically be aware that almost 20% of subjects will have persistent pain after hysterectomy. As women with chronic pain symptoms are often hyperalgesic, the possibility of unrecognized comorbid disorders should not be disregarded even in the presence of documented endometriosis. A minority of patients (3–5%) will experience even worsening of pain or will develop new symptoms after surgery. This should be specifically included in the preoperative informed consent form.

MEDICAL ALTERNATIVES TO SURGERY

A major misunderstanding that undermines the entire concept of medical therapy of endometriosis lies in the conviction that ectopic implants may regress, degenerate, and ultimately disappear because of an unfavorable hormonal milieu.

Unfortunately, it is well established that hormonal drugs do not cure endometriosis but only induce temporary quiescence of active lesions (183) and that in most cases of advanced disease surgery is the final solution (87). However, there are several situations in which medical treatments are still useful. Some women who have already undergone several operations might prefer to avoid further surgery but need pain relief, and others may only want to postpone surgery because of study, work, or family problems. Furthermore, drugs may be chosen as an alternative to surgery in the rare and very difficult cases in which the risks of morbidity and complications outweigh the benefits of a radical operation. Nonetheless, surgery for ovarian cysts or pelvic lesions of doubtful nature should never be deferred on the assumption that they are endometriotic in origin. The results of testing transvaginal ultrasonography for the diagnosis of endometriotic cysts are impressive but obtained by expert observers working in tertiary-care referral centers. Moreover, although elevated CA-125 serum levels are not unusual in the presence of endometriosis, they may be associated with ovarian cancer even in a young woman.

Endometriosis is a chronic inflammatory disease that responds to steroidal manipulation. Creation of a steady hormonal environment with inhibition of ovulation temporarily suppresses the ectopic implants and reduces the inflammatory status as well as the associated pain symptoms. The pharmacologic management of endometriosis must be set within the framework of long-term therapeutic strategies. Because the available drugs are not curative, treatments should be prolonged even for years or until women desire a pregnancy. The various therapies studied have shown similar efficacy. Consequently, based on a more favorable profile in terms of safety, tolerability, and cost, combined OCs and progestins should be considered the first-line option, both as an alternative to surgery and as a postoperative adjuvant measure. GnRH analogs, danazol, and gestrinone should be used when progestins and OCs fail, are not tolerated, or are contraindicated. Future therapies for endometriosis must compare favorably with the existing drugs before hypothesizing their implementation in current practice. Medical treatment is not indicated in women seeking conception because reproductive prognosis is not ameliorated.

Stage I–IV Disease

The Birth Control Pill

For many years, OCs have been extensively used in clinical practice for the reduction of pelvic pain and dysmenorrhea associated with endometriosis. Although their effectiveness has been recognized by all gynecologists, only a limited number of formal studies have quantified their effects or compared these with those obtained during administration of other drugs (184,185).

In the 1990s, GnRH analogs were considered the therapeutic standard reference for medical treatment of endometriosis. To test this notion, Vercellini et al. compared the efficacy of a six-month treatment with a monophasic OC (desogestrel 0.15 mg and ethinyl estradiol 0.02 mg, 28 patients) administered cyclically versus goserelin depot (3.6 mg subcutaneously every 28 days, 29 patients) (184). At the end of the treatment, a significant reduction in deep dyspareunia was observed in both groups, with goserelin assessed as superior to the OC. Nonmenstrual pain was diminished without differences between treatments. Women taking the OC experienced a significant reduction in dysmenorrhea. With respect to the latter symptom, a comparison with GnRH is impracticable due to amenorrhea secondary to hypoestrogenism. Symptoms recurred unaltered six months after drug withdrawal.

Parazzini et al. (185) investigated whether a GnRH analog (triptorelin 3.75 mg IM every 28 days, 47 patients) administered for four months before starting the treatment with a cyclic OC would improve results compared with the immediate use of an estrogen–progestin combination (gestodene 0.75 mg and ethinyl estradiol 0.03 mg, 55 patients) for 12 months. One year after randomization, the two treatment modalities showed similar relief of pelvic pain in women with endometriosis. No data are available to support the belief that estrogen–progestin combinations are to be considered as second-line drugs. When a long-term use is indicated, an OC may be prescribed without the need of "preparation" with a GnRH analog.

OCs used cyclically are the only treatment for endometriosis that permits monthly uterine bleeding. Dysmenorrhea is known as the most frequent and most severe complaint in women with this disease. The symptom may therefore not subside completely during administration of an OC. Recent studies have demonstrated that women with menstrual-related problems during cyclic use of an OC may benefit from a shift to continuous administration (186–188). Although elimination of the seven-day interval is recommended by various experts (189), there are no specific data regarding women with endometriosis. Consequently, Vercellini et al. prescribed a monophasic OC (desogestrel 0.15 mg and ethinyl estradiol 0.02 mg) continuously to 50 patients with dysmenorrhea recurring after conservative surgery for endometriosis and not responding to the cyclic use of the same OC (190). During the two-year study period, 38% of women reported amenorrhea, 36% spotting, and 26% breakthrough bleeding. The mean score of menstrual pain, evaluated according to a 100-mm visual analog scale, showed a reduction from 75 ± 13 to 31 ± 17 (Fig. 20). Moderate or severe side effects were reported by 14% of the women. At final evaluation, 26% of subjects were very satisfied, 54% satisfied, 2% uncertain, 16% unsatisfied, and 2% very unsatisfied.

When cyclic use of OCs does not resolve pain associated with monthly bleeding, continuous administration might constitute a simple, effective, safe, and well-tolerated option for the long-term treatment in women not wanting children.

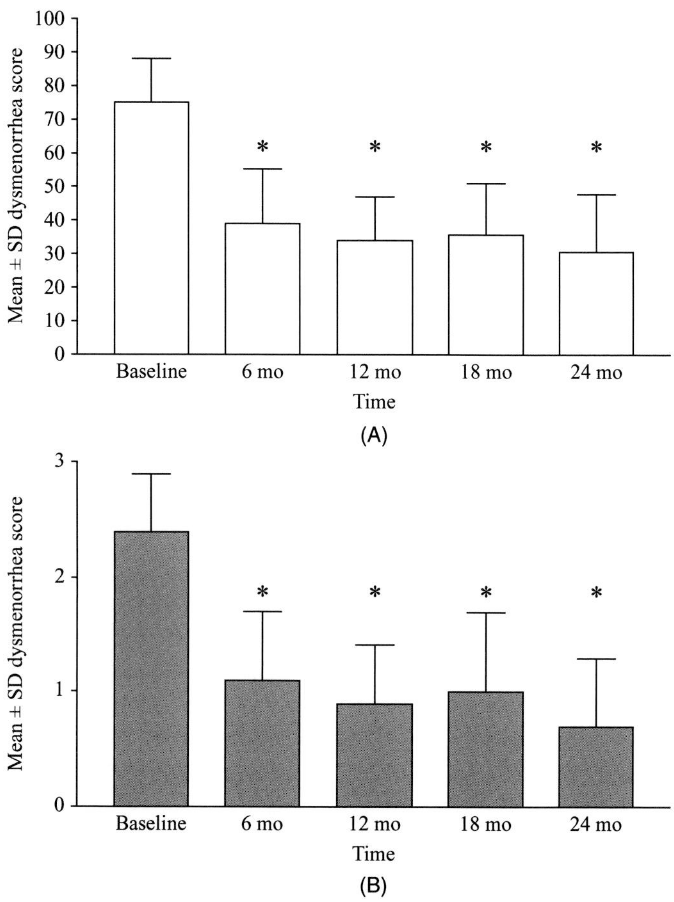

Figure 20 Variation of intensity of dysmenorrhea after switch from cyclic to continuous oral contraceptive use. **(A)** Visual analog scale scores. **(B)** Verbal rating scores. Values are mean ± SD; $P < 0.001$ compared with corresponding baseline value, paired *t* test. *Source*: From Ref. 190.

Cyproterone Acetate

Cyproterone acetate (CPA), a derivative of 17-hydroxyprogesterone with antiandrogenic and antigonadotropic properties, has been first used in the treatment of endometriosis by Fedele et al. (191) at the dosage of 27 mg/day.

A reduced dosage (12.5 mg/day) administered continuously was tested in a randomized study that compared its effects to those of an OC (desogestrel 0.15 mg and ethinyl estradiol 0.02 mg), given continuously for six months (192). Ninety women were recruited with moderate to severe pelvic pain that recurred after conservative surgery for symptomatic endometriosis. The main outcome of the study was patients' degree of satisfaction, which was deemed important in order to be able to consider their point of view in the evaluation of drug efficacy, as well as the impact of side effects. At six months, dysmenorrhea, deep dyspareunia, and nonmenstrual pelvic pain were considerably reduced (Fig. 21). In addition, the health-related quality of life, psychological profile, and sexual satisfaction improved significantly, with no major differences between groups. Metabolic and subjective side effects were limited. According to an intention-to-treat analysis, 33/45 (73%) women in the CPA group and 30/45 (67%) in the OC group were satisfied with the treatment received. CPA may be used when subjective and metabolic effects of estrogens need to be avoided, or in women unwilling to use contraception because of cultural or religious objections. On the other hand, the continuous use of a low-dose monophasic OC is most probably the preferred option to prevent the effects of estrogen deprivation in women for whom a long period of therapy is expected.

Depot Medroxyprogesterone Acetate

The depot formulation of MPA (DMPA) has been widely evaluated for contraceptive purposes and is currently being used by approximately 12 million women worldwide (193). The administration modality is extremely convenient and consists of a single 150-mg intramuscular injection every three months. The increase in risk of breast cancer in users of DMPA is not superior to that of OCs (194). Literature data suggest that bone demineralization secondary to hypoestrogenism may develop in chronic users (195–198).

Results from the first formal study on the use of DMPA in patients with endometriosis have been published in 1996 (199). The progestin was compared to an association of a monophasic OC pill with low-dose danazol (50 mg/day). After a one-year treatment, 29/40 women (72%) allocated to DMPA were satisfied versus 23/40 (57%) of those randomized to receive the OC plus danazol. A significant reduction in pain symptoms

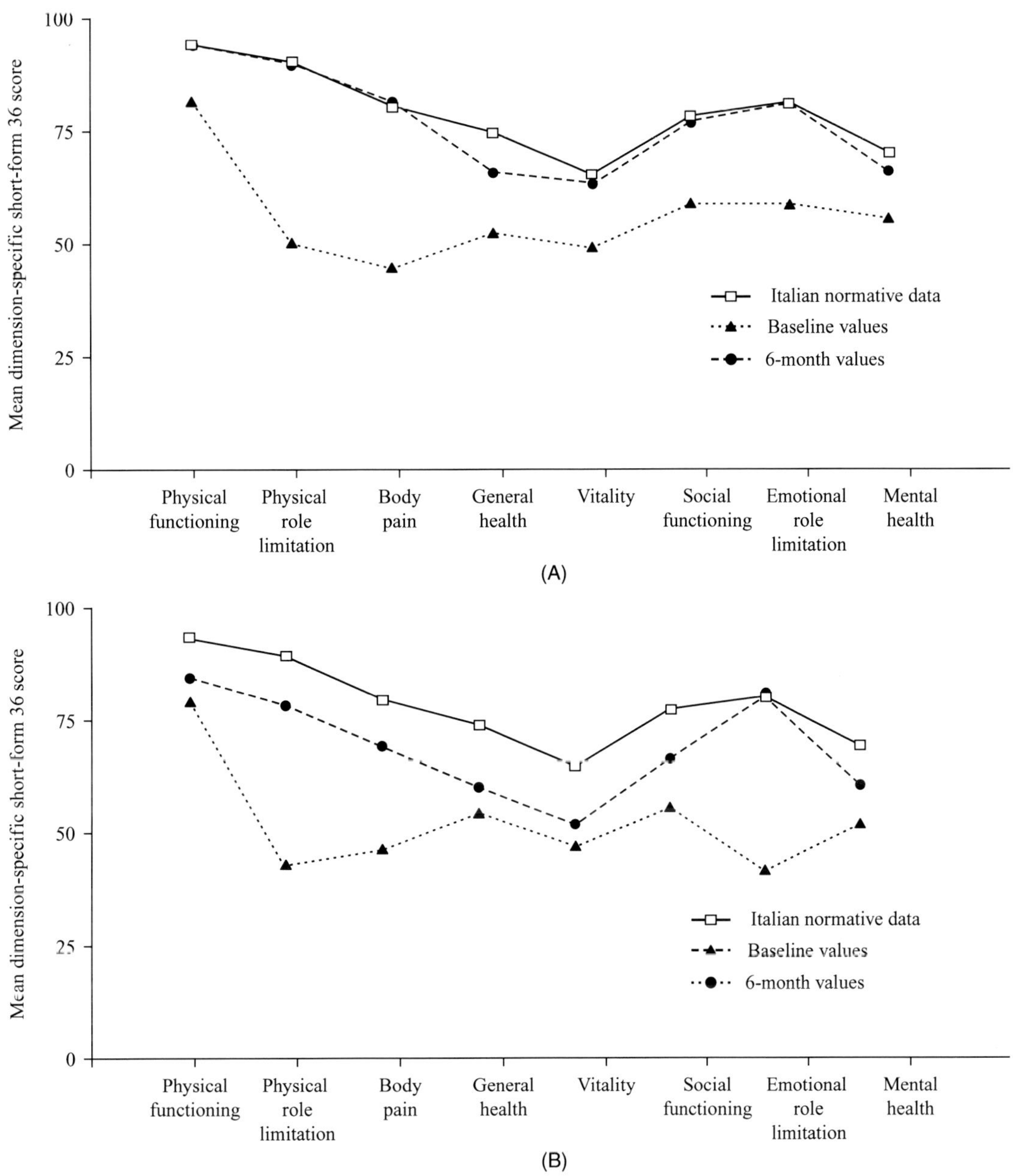

Figure 21 Short Form-36 general health survey profile of dimension-specific scores in patients with endometriosis-associated pain before and at six-month treatment, compared with 1032 healthy Italian women 25 to 34 years of age. (**A**) Cyproterone acetate group ($n = 39$). (**B**) Oral contraceptive group ($n = 36$). *Source*: From Ref. 192.

evaluated with a visual analog and multidimensional scale had been observed in both groups. However, patients in the combined OC/danazol group complained of a greater frequency and severity of dysmenorrhea, which is a logical consequence of cyclic administration. Both treatments induced a similar, significant reduction in serum HDL cholesterol levels, whereas an increase in LDL cholesterol levels was only observed in subjects allocated to the OC plus danazol treatment. The incidence of side effects was greater in DMPA users. In these, the mean delay in appearance of a regular menstrual cycle after suspension was seven months to a maximum of one year.

The efficacy of DMPA as a therapy for endometriosis was recently confirmed in two RCTs (200,201) conducted in order to investigate a new, subcutaneous formulation of DMPA 104 mg and to assess its equivalence (noninferiority) to leuprolide acetate 11.25 mg chosen as the standard comparator. Both drugs were injected during a menstrual cycle and then after three months, for an overall study period of six months. In one trial, 300 women with surgically diagnosed endometriosis were recruited in Europe, Asia, Latin America, and New Zealand (200), and in the other trial 274 subjects with similar characteristics were recruited in Canada and United States (201). The DMPA subcutaneous preparation proved statistically equivalent to leuprolide in reducing pain symptoms both at the end of the treatment and at 12-month follow-up. Patients in the DMPA-SC 104 group showed significantly less bone mineral density loss than did leuprolide patients. Bone mineral density returned to pretreatment levels 12 months posttreatment in the progestin but not in the GnRH analog group. Compared with leuprolide, DMPA-SC 104 was associated with fewer hypoestrogenic symptoms but more irregular bleeding. In the former study (200), continuation rate was 90% in the DMPA-SC 104 group and 93% in the leuprolide group, whereas in the second study (201), the percentages were 65% and 74%, respectively. Total productivity and health-related quality of life improved in both groups.

DMPA is an effective, safe, and extremely economic alternative for the treatment of symptomatic endometriosis. However, because of some of its characteristics, candidates for treatment need to be selected carefully. In fact, prolonged delay in resumption of ovulation is a contraindication to the use of DMPA in women wanting children in the near future. Additionally, uterine breakthrough bleeding may be prolonged, repeated, and troublesome to correct. More in general, treatment cannot be interrupted in the event of side effects, rendering clinical management complicated when these are severe or scarcely tolerable. Its indication of choice is residual symptomatic endometriosis following definitive surgery. In such circumstances, there are no problems regarding future conception or irregular uterine bleeding, and use of DMPA allows a simple and well-tolerated suppression of persistent foci after nonradical operations, with no need to opt for daily administration of drugs or further surgery.

Rectovaginal Disease

In current practice, it is erroneously taken for granted that medical treatments are not efficacious for rectovaginal endometriosis (84,87,88). This uncritical belief, based on a reportedly different receptor pattern from eutopic endometrium (84), leads to the obvious conclusion that surgery is the only reasonable therapeutic choice and thus exposes women to potentially severe morbidity, especially if procedures are performed by gynecologists not specifically trained in this difficult and technically demanding field. This clinical approach should be challenged, as in these patients good results are obtainable with safe, tolerable, and inexpensive drugs that can be used for prolonged periods of time. Deep infiltrating endometriosis has been treated successfully with danazol, GnRH analogs, progestins, and estrogen–progestin combinations.

Igarashi et al. (202) treated 42 women with deep infiltrating endometriosis of the posterior cul-de-sac with danazol for 2 to 16 months. They used a vaginal delivery system consisting of a silicon rubber doughnut-shaped ring containing 1500 mg of the drug, which was replaced every 4 to 8 weeks until pregnancy was established or endometriotic lesions regressed. During treatment, serum danazol concentrations were undetectable, ovulation was not inhibited, and menstrual cycles remained regular. Dysmenorrhea was relieved in 32/42 subjects, cul-de-sac lesions disappeared in 36/42 of them, and conception was achieved by 17/31 women seeking pregnancy.

Recently Razzi et al. (203) reported the results of vaginal treatment of deeply infiltrating endometriosis with danazol capsules (200 mg/day) self-administered for 12 months in 21 symptomatic women. Dysmenorrhea, dyspareunia, and noncyclic pelvic pain significantly decreased within three months of therapy and disappeared after six months, with a persistent effect during the entire study period. A relief of dyschezia was also observed. Ultrasound examination demonstrated a reduction of rectovaginal nodules, and few local vaginal adverse effects were reported. According to the authors, long-term vaginal danazol therapy may be proposed as an alternative to surgery in women with deeply infiltrating endometriosis.

Depot leuprolide acetate (3.75 mg IM every 28 days for 6 months) was used by Fedele et al. (204) to treat 15 patients with symptomatic rectovaginal endometriosis. Two subjects dropped out because of persistent pain, whereas the other 13 showed a marked improvement but had early symptom recurrence after drug suspension. Transrectal ultrasonography revealed that the endometriotic lesions underwent a significant size reduction during therapy, but they returned to the original volume within six months of follow-up.

With the aim of overcoming the problem of the limited period allowed for GnRH analog treatment, several studies have been performed on the combination of GnRH agonist with different types of steroidal add-back therapy (205). The combination schemes are better tolerated and consistently induce less side effects as well as limited or no bone resorption. However, the use of GnRH agonists plus add-back regimens in routine practice would greatly increase the cost of therapy and may limit patients' compliance.

An Lng-IUD was used in the treatment of persistent rectovaginal endometriosis in 11 patients who underwent nonradical conservative surgery (206). Dysmenorrhea, which had been moderate or severe in all cases, and nonmenstrual pelvic pain were absent one year after IUD insertion. Of notable interest was the reduction of deep dyspareunia, which had been moderate or severe in eight cases prior to IUD insertion, to absent or mild in all subjects throughout treatment. Rectal tenesmus was also substantially alleviated. Furthermore, transrectal ultrasound scans demonstrated a progressive reduction in size of rectovaginal lesions. The results of this study are of particular clinical importance because they prove the efficacy of a progestinic treatment in a type of lesion generally considered as nonresponsive to medical therapy. Relief of organic symptoms such as deep dyspareunia and rectal tenesmus is due not only to size reduction of the fibronodular rectovaginal plaques but also to decrease in the intra- and perilesional inflammatory condition. Intrauterine administration of levonorgestrel with a possible direct distribution to pelvic tissues would imply a local concentration greater than its plasma levels. This could translate into a superior effectiveness with limited side effects, also due to absence of the hepatic first-pass effect following oral administration of the drug.

Recently, an RCT was conducted (18) in 90 women with recurrent moderate or severe pelvic pain after unsuccessful conservative surgery for symptomatic rectovaginal endometriosis, who were allocated to 12-month continuous treatment with oral ethinyl estradiol 0.01 mg plus CPA 3 mg/day, or norethindrone acetate (NETA) 2.5 mg/day. Seven subjects in the ethinyl estradiol plus CPA arm and five in the NETA arm withdrew because of side effects ($n = 5$), treatment inefficacy ($n = 6$), or loss to follow-up ($n = 1$). At 12 months, dysmenorrhea, deep dyspareunia, nonmenstrual pelvic pain, and dyschezia scores were substantially reduced, without major between-group differences. In particular, moderate to severe deep dyspareunia was reported at baseline by 12 women in the ethinyl estradiol and CPA group, and by 13 in the NETA group (Fig. 22). The symptom was not relieved in two subjects in each group. Moderate to severe dyschezia was present before treatment in, respectively, 10 and 15 patients and regressed under therapy in all cases.

Among the women who completed the study, 17/38 (45%) who took the ethinyl estradiol plus CPA combination achieved amenorrhea compared with 29/40 (72%) given NETA. Twenty-one women in the former group and 11 in the latter experienced erratic bleeding episodes (spotting in 14 and 9 subjects, respectively; breakthrough bleeding in seven and

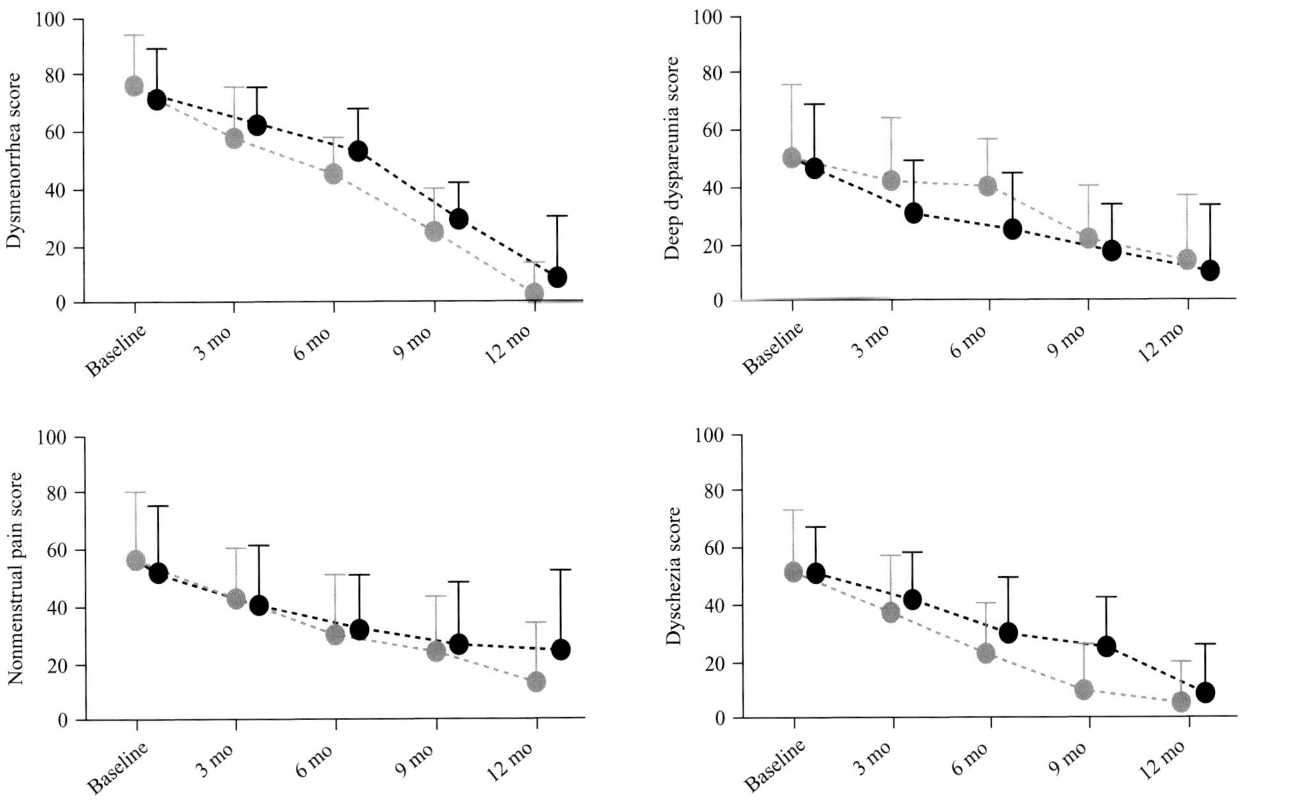

Figure 22 Variation of intensity of pain symptoms as assessed on a visual analog scale during the study period. Values are mean ± SD shown by vertical bars. *Violet*, ethinyl estradiol E_2 plus cyproterone acetate group; *red*, norethindrone acetate group. *Source*: From Ref. 18.

two). These patients were advised to interrupt treatment for one week.

Side effects were reported by 16/41 (39%) subjects allocated to ethinyl estradiol plus CPA, and by 21/42 (50%) of those taking NETA. The mean gain in the patients reporting a weight increase was 2.3 ± 1.0 kg (+4.1%) in seven subjects in the former group, and 3.6 ± 2.3 kg (+6.7%) in 12 subjects in the latter group. Both regimens induced minor unfavorable variations in serum lipid profile.

At transrectal ultrasonography, the mean ± SD volume of rectovaginal plaques dropped from a baseline value of 3.1 ± 1.4 mL in the ethinyl estradiol plus CPA group and of 3.0 ± 1.3 mL in the NETA group to, respectively, 2.2 ± 1.0 and 1.9 ± 1.1 mL at the end of the treatment.

According to an intention-to-treat analysis, 28/45 (62%) patients in the ethinyl estradiol plus CPA group and 33/45 (73%) in the NETA group were satisfied with the treatment received. In Italy, the monthly cost of treatment with NETA 2.5 mg daily is about €1.5. Consequently, low-dose NETA has been indicated by the authors as the treatment of choice for patients with recurrent or persistent deeply infiltrating lesions after failure of conservative surgery who do not want to conceive. The ethinyl estradiol plus CPA combination was slightly less effective but well tolerated, and could be suggested for women with acne or hypertrichosis and those who experience androgenic side effects with NETA.

Norethisterone acetate (or NETA) is a strong progestin derivative of 19-nortestosterone. NETA offers various advantages for the long-term treatment of endometriosis. This progestin allows good control of uterine bleeding as compared with other compounds, has a positive effect on calcium metabolism by producing greater increases in bone mineral density than alendronate, and at low dosages has no negative effects on the lipoprotein profile (207). NETA administered continuously to treat endometriosis is approved by the U.S. Food and Drug Administration and the Italian Ministry of Health.

There is no conclusive evidence that danazol or GnRH agonists produce significantly better pain relief in women with deep infiltrating endometriosis than progestins or estrogen–progestogen combinations, although the considerable differences in safety and tolerability should obviously be taken into account. Besides opinions on the most beneficial drug, the available evidence clearly supports the efficacy of medical treatment in women with symptomatic rectovaginal endometriosis and patients' consent to surgery should no longer be sought based solely on the purported uselessness of medical therapies.

Vesical Disease

Westney et al. (208) treated 13 subjects with symptomatic full-thickness bladder detrusor endometriosis. Women of child-bearing age were placed on a low-dose OC. In postmenopausal patients already on hormonal replacement therapy, the dose of estrogen was decreased or stopped, while a progestational agent was given to those not taking hormones. The patients were followed at least every three months after an initial evaluation for a mean period of 18.6 months (8–24). Twelve women reported partial or complete resolution of symptoms, and pain relief was sufficient for them not to require more aggressive therapy. The remaining subject discontinued the progestational agent because of excessive breast tenderness.

All antiendometriosis medical therapies are temporarily successful in the treatment of bladder detrusor disease, but recurrence of symptoms is the rule at drug withdrawal. However, a preoperative course of medical therapy may be helpful to support the diagnosis in doubtful cases.

Hormone Replacement Therapy in Women with Past History of Endometriosis

The issue of initiating hormone replacement therapy (HRT) may arise in young patients after pelvic clearance or in women with a previous diagnosis of endometriosis who reach the physiologic menopause. The risk of recurrence of endometriosis during HRT remains unknown. Of more concern is the risk of malignant transformation of residual foci. Soliman and Hillard (209) have recently reviewed literature data on the topic, concluding that the available evidence does not suggest denying HRT in subjects with hypoestrogenic symptoms. The authors are in favor of a continuous instead of cyclic therapy, as symptoms of endometriosis are known to be stimulated by hormone fluctuations. In their opinion, the lowest effective dose should always be used, commencing HRT shortly after definitive surgery or as soon as menopausal symptoms arise, without delays of unproven benefit. Avoidance of estrogen-only treatments and the use of combined preparations or tibolone are strongly suggested.

Tibolone is a synthetic steroid with weak estrogenic, progestinic, and androgenic activity. The effect of tibolone on the endometrium is inhibitory, as the progestinic–androgenic activity is prevalent. In vitro, tibolone is metabolized by endometrial Δ-4 isomerase/dehydrogenase to its Δ-4 metabolite, which is characterized by strong progestinic activity. This explains its endometrial tissue-specific progestinic effect as well as a positive effect on calcium metabolism.

Fedele et al. (210) compared the effects of treatment with transdermal estradiol (50 mg twice weekly $\pm$ cyclic MPA 10 mg/day) to those of tibolone (2.5 mg/day p.o.), given for a minimum of 12 months to 21 women with residual pelvic endometriosis after bilateral oophorectomy with or without hysterectomy. Residual endometriosis was found in the bowel wall in four, in the rectovaginal septum in six, and deep in the retroperitoneal pelvic space in six subjects. All women were symptomatic before definitive surgery. Moderate to severe pain recurred in four subjects in the transdermal estradiol arm versus one in the tibolone arm. These results suggest that tibolone may be considered the drug of choice as postmenopausal replacement treatment for women with pelvic endometriosis. In addition, tibolone may constitute an optimal choice as an add-back therapy in candidates selected for prolonged treatment with GnRH analog (211).

CONCLUSIONS

Symptomatic endometriosis is a nonmalignant condition that usually affects young women with high expectations in terms of well-being and health-related quality of life. In women not seeking pregnancy, results of treatment are functional, and therapeutic indications should be based mainly on complaints and anticipated pain relief. Thus, the approach should be "problem oriented" and not "lesion oriented," and before suggesting systematic resection one should be reasonably confident that the chances of overcoming the main clinical issue are substantial and the benefits long lasting.

When discussing any type of therapy, a woman should know the specific objectives of treatments, the evidence on which to base the alleged advantages, and the frequency and severity of side effects or morbidity and, more importantly, she should be able to measure, to "weigh," the purported benefits. A shared medical decision-making approach should be implemented in each center caring for endometriosis patients. Detailed and thorough information is always of utmost importance when choosing among therapeutic alternatives. This is especially true when dealing with benign chronic diseases not interfering with general health, in case of major differences in terms of risks and morbidity between treatment options, and when the outcomes of an invasive procedure are undetermined. Uncertainties deriving from lack of reliable evidence should be discussed openly. Many medical decisions, typically including elective surgical procedures for benign chronic diseases, fall into a grey area where the optimal choice for an individual patient may be unclear and where reasonable people might choose differently.

The diagnosis of endometriosis per se is somewhat vague because, apart from implying the presence of ectopic endometrium, it does not define a specific clinical pattern. Extremely different conditions are grouped under the vast umbrella of the endometriosis label, including women with major anatomic complications such as bowel or ureteral stenosis, large and complex adnexal masses, as well as girls with dysmenorrhea associated with limited peritoneal implants. Consequently, different treatment alternatives should be taken into account, based on the different characteristics of the patients and the specific therapeutic objective identified. The choice of treatment should never be swayed by fear of not prescribing the latest fashion drug, technical limits, conflicts of interest, and even established but unproven "gold standards."

The first operation is usually crucial for the prognosis. Unduly traumatic or nonradical procedures greatly reduce the chance of spontaneous pregnancy and increase the risk of disease and symptoms recurrence (or persistence). Second-line interventions cannot always or completely reverse previous iatrogenic damage, particularly in cases of deep infiltrating endometriosis. Radical excision of rectovaginal disease is almost invariably a traumatic procedure that entails extensive adhesiolysis, systematic vaginal opening, occasional rectal perforation or incidental resection, and wide pelvic deperitonealization. When adequate endoscopic experience is not available locally to deal with all forms of deep endometriosis, the woman should be referred to tertiary-care specialized centers. If this is not feasible, it may be preferable for the "traditional" surgeon to perform a safe and effective intervention at laparotomy rather than operate incompletely at laparoscopy.

A thorough preoperative diagnostic investigation and careful, detailed counseling are of major importance. Involvement of the intestinal and urologic apparatuses should be known in advance, to schedule intraoperative consultation if necessary and to inform the woman about the type of surgery required and its potential sequelae. This will also help to make patients and their families understand the clinical severity of the condition and balance the risks and benefits of the proposed treatments.

Poor communication and lack of information can lead to unrealistic expectations, and patients will be unprepared to face problems and treatment failures if they arise. In young and otherwise healthy women, intra- and postoperative complications are perceived and tolerated with difficulty, and invalidating pain recurrence and persistent infertility are particularly frustrating. Awareness of the real possibilities of different treatments will enhance the patient's collaboration, facilitating acceptance of what may be revealed as a reasonable compromise but might otherwise appear as a partial therapeutic debacle.

If the woman has already completed her family and disabling pain is the major problem, definitive surgery could be the best solution. However, prolonged progestin administration may be preferred when hysterectomy or castration are psychologically intolerable (206,212).

Management of endometriosis with OCs or progestins is safe, effective, and well tolerated and should constitute the first-line medical treatment modality in symptomatic women not wanting children. This pharmacologic option is relatively unexpensive and suitable for prolonged periods of therapy, with the additional advantage of being available all over the world with reproducible results. After attending updating courses, even general practitioners could prescribe and monitor treatments, thus limiting the medical costs of the disease.

Several other drugs for endometriosis have been studied, usually for the almost standard six-month period. However, the objectives of these short-term treatments are far from clear, as women with endometriosis may benefit marginally from such a limited time span without pain. Furthermore, the major side effects caused by GnRH analogs, danazol, and gestrinone may impact substantially on the health-related quality of life of patients, tipping the balance toward unfavorable final outcomes. Major international gynecologic organizations have clearly stated in their official guidelines that the analgesic efficacy of the various drugs used for endometriosis, including OCs and progestins, is equivalent and that only side-effect profiles and costs differ (213–216).

In the majority of women not seeking pregnancy, symptomatic endometriosis could be controlled, although not cured, in a noninvasive manner. About one patient out of four using OCs or progestins will still need an intervention because of lack of response or intolerance to side effects, but the overall impact of surgery would be limited greatly, with reduction in morbidity and, possibly, long-term complications. In fact, the outcomes of surgery are strictly operator dependent, and optimal results can be assured only in tertiary-care and referral centers.

The unverified clinical tenet according to which "it is better for the patients to undergo a single surgical procedure than decades of hormonal treatments" should be viewed with skepticism. Pain recurrence afflicts a substantial proportion of the women undergoing conservative surgery for severely symptomatic endometriosis, and reoperations seem to be the rule rather than the exception. Consequently, as far as pain is considered, in most circumstances the concrete alternative is among surgery plus long-term adjuvant medical therapy versus drugs alone. Obviously, choices may well be different in women seeking conception. In fact, medical treatments for symptomatic endometriosis generally inhibit ovulation.

The common belief that a preliminary laparoscopy must always be performed in order to definitely diagnose as well as stage the disease should be challenged, as the nonsurgical diagnosis of endometriosis has been demonstrated to be highly reliable (217). Moreover, the current staging system has a limited clinical impact due to the lack of predictive value in terms of reproductive performance, risk of posttreatment symptoms' reappearance, and lesions recurrences (1). Furthermore, it has not been demonstrated that an early visual identification results in a substantial limitation of lesion progression or, more importantly, a more favorable prognosis.

Finally, a diagnosis of endometriosis commonly imposes a great psychological burden on a young woman, as she may envisage a future of chronic pain, infertility, difficulties in coping with daily activities, marital distress, serial laparoscopic procedures, and repeated courses of scarcely tolerated pharmacological therapies until menopause or definitive surgery will put an end to her illness. This pessimistic scenario is quite often unfounded, and helping patients view their condition in the right perspective avoiding counterproductive dramatizations must be a fundamental aim of the caring gynecologist who should encourage resumption of a lifestyle as "normal" as possible.

REFERENCES

1. Vercellini P, Fedele L, Aimi G, et al. Reproductive performance, pain recurrence and disease relapse after conservative surgical treatment for endometriosis: The predictive value of the current classification system. Hum Reprod 2006; 21:2679–2685.
2. Vercellini P, Fedele L, Aimi G, et al. Association between endometriosis stage, lesion type, patient characteristics and severity of pelvic pain symptoms: A multivariate analysis over 1000 patients. Hum Reprod 2007; 22:266–271.
3. Vercellini P, Fedele L, Pietropaolo G, et al. Progestogens for endometriosis: Forward to the past. Hum Reprod Update 2003; 9:387–396.
4. Vercellini P, Somigliana E, Viganò P, et al. Endometriosis: Current and future medical therapies. Best Pract Res Clin Obstet Gynecol 2008; 22:275–306.
5. Redwine D, Mann CH, Wright JT. Evidence on endometriosis. Elitism about randomised controlled trials is inappropriate. BMJ 2000; 321:1077–1078.
6. Farquhar CM. Extracts from the "clinical evidence". Endometriosis. BMJ 2000; 320:1449–1452.
7. Fayez JA, Collazo LM. Comparison between laparotomy and operative laparoscopy in the treatment of moderate and severe stages of endometriosis. Int J Fertil 1990; 35:272–279.
8. Bateman BG, Kolp LA, Mills S. Endoscopic versus laparotomy management of endometriomas. Fertil Steril 1994; 62:690–695.
9. Catalano GF, Marana R, Caruana P, et al. Laparoscopy versus microsurgery by laparotomy for excision of ovarian cysts in patients with moderate or severe endometriosis. J Am Assoc Gynecol Laparosc 1996; 3:267–270.
10. Crosignani PG, Vercellini P, Biffignardi F, et al. Laparoscopy versus laparotomy in conservative surgical treatment for severe endometriosis. Fertil Steril 1996; 66:706–711.
11. Vercellini P, Pisacreta A, De Giorgi O, et al. Management of advanced endometriosis. In: Kempers RD, Cohen J, Haney AF, Younger JB, eds. Fertility and Reproductive Medicine. Amsterdam: Elsevier Science B.V., 1998:369–386.
12. Brosens IA, Puttemans P, Deprest J, et al. The endometriosis cycle and its derailments. Hum Reprod 1994; 9:770–772.
13. Vercellini P, Meschia M, De Giorgi O, et al. Bladder detrusor endometriosis: Clinical and pathogenetic implications. J Urol 1996; 155:84–86.
14. Nisolle M, Donnez J. Peritoneal endometriosis, ovarian endometriosis, and adenomyotic nodules of the rectovaginal septum are three different entities. Fertil Steril 1997; 68:585–596.
15. Kuhn RJP, Hollyock VE. Observations on the anatomy of the rectovaginal pouch and septum. Obstet Gynecol 1982; 59:445–447.
16. Baessler K, Schuessler B. The depth of the pouch of Douglas in nulliparous and parous women without genital prolapse and in patients with genital prolapse. Am J Obstet Gynecol 2000; 182:540–544.
17. Vercellini P, Aimi G, Panazza S, et al. Deep endometriosis conundrum: Evidence in favor of a peritoneal origin. Fertil Steril 2000; 73:1043–1046.

18. Vercellini P, Pietropaolo G, De Giorgi O, et al. Treatment of symptomatic rectovaginal endometriosis with an estrogen-progestogen combination versus low-dose norethindrone acetate. Fertil Steril 2005; 84:1375–1387.
19. Somigliana E, Infantino M, Candiani M, et al. Associated ratio between deep peritoneal endometriosis and other forms of the disease: Pathogenetic implications. Hum Reprod 2004; 19:168–171.
20. Martin DC. Laparoscopic and vaginal colpotomy for the excision of infiltrating cul-de-sac endometriosis. J Reprod Med 1988; 33:806–808.
21. Reich H, Mc Glynn F, Salvat J. Laparoscopic treatment of cul-de-sac obliteration secondary to retrocervical deep fibrotic endometriosis. J Reprod Med 1991; 36:516–522.
22. Redwine DB. Laparoscopic en bloc resection for treatment of the obliterated cul-de-sac in endometriosis. J Reprod Med 1992; 37:695–698.
23. Nezhat C, Nezhat F, Pennington E. Laparoscopic treatment of infiltrative rectosigmoid colon and rectovaginal septum endometriosis by the technique of videolaparoscopy and the CO_2 laser. Br J Obstet Gynaecol 1992; 99:664–667.
24. Chapron C, Dumontier I, Dousset B, et al. Results and role of rectal endoscopic ultrasonography for patients with deep pelvic endometriosis. Hum Reprod 1998; 13:2266–2270.
25. Fedele L, Bianchi S, Portuese A, et al. Transrectal ultrasonography in the assessment of rectovaginal endometriosis. Obstet Gynecol 1998; 91:444–448.
26. Kinkel K, Chapron C, Balleyguier C, et al. Magnetic resonance imaging characteristics of deep endometriosis. Hum Reprod 1999; 14:1080–1086.
27. Chapron C, Liaras E, Fayet P, et al. Magnetic resonance imaging and endometriosis: Deeply infiltrating endometriosis does not originate from the rectovaginal septum. Gynecol Obstet Invest 2002; 53:204–208.
28. Martin DC, Hubert G, Levy B. Depth of infiltration endometriosis. J Gynecol Surg 1989; 5:55–59.
29. Ripps BA, Martin DC. Correlation of pelvic tenderness with implant dimension and stage of endometriosis. J Reprod Med 1990; 37:620–624.
30. Ripps BA, Martin DC. Focal pelvic tenderness, pelvic pain and dysmenorrhea in endometriosis. J Reprod Med 1991; 36:470–476.
31. Chapron C, Fauconnier A, Dubuisson JB, et al. Does deep endometriosis infiltrating the uterosacral ligaments present an asymmetric lateral distribution? BJOG 2001; 108:1021–1024.
32. Candiani GB, Vercellini P, Fedele L, et al. Conservative surgical treatment of rectovaginal septum endometriosis. J Gynecol Surg 1992; 8:177–182.
33. Frenna V, Santos L, Ohana E, et al. Laparoscopic management of ureteral endometriosis: Our experience. J Minim Invasive Gynecol 2007; 14:169–171.
34. Chapron C, Dubuisson JB. Laparoscopic treatment of deep endometriosis located on the uterosacral ligaments. Hum Reprod 1996; 11:868–873.
35. Vercellini P, Aimi G, Busacca M, et al. Laparoscopic uterosacral ligament resection for dysmenorrhea associated with endometriosis: Results of a randomized, controlled trial. Fertil Steril 2003;80:310–319.
36. Donnez J, Nisolle M, Gillerot S, et al. Rectovaginal septum adenomyotic nodules: A series of 500 cases. Br J Obstet Gynecol 1997; 104:1014–1018.
37. Possover M, Diebolder H, Plaul K, et al. Laparoscopic assisted vaginal resection of rectovaginal endometriosis. Obstet Gynecol 2000; 96:304–307.
38. Brouwer R, Woods RJ. Rectal endometriosis: Results of radical excision and review of published work. ANZ J Surg 2007; 77:562–571.
39. Ret Davalos ML, De Cicco Carlo, D'Hoore A, et al. Outcome after rectum resection: A review for gynecologists. J Minim Invasive Gynecol 2007; 14:33–38.
40. Darai E, Bazot M, Rouzier R, et al. Outcome of laparoscopic colorectal resection for endometriosis. Curr Opin Obstet Gynecol 2007; 19:308–313.
41. Vercellini P, Frontino G, Pisacreta A. The pathogenesis of bladder detrusor endometriosis. Am J Obstet Gynecol 2002; 187:538–542.
42. Fedele L, Piazzola E, Raffaelli R, et al. Bladder endometriosis: Deep infiltrating endometriosis or adenomyosis? Fertil Steril 1998; 69:972–975.
43. Donnez J, Spada F, Squifflet J, et al. Bladder endometriosis must be considered as bladder adenomyosis. Fertil Steril 2000; 74:1175–1181.
44. Fedele L, Bianchi S, Raffaelli R, et al. Pre-operative assessment of bladder endometriosis. Hum Reprod 1997; 12:2519–2522.
45. Jenkins S, Olive DL, Haney AF. Endometriosis: Pathogenetic implications of the anatomic distribution. Obstet Gynecol 1986; 67:335–338.
46. De Lancey JOL. Surgical anatomy of the female pelvis. In: Rock JA, Thompson JD, eds. Te Linde's Operative Gynecology, 8th ed. Philadelphia, PA: Lippincott – Raven, 1997:63–93.
47. Buka NJ. Vesical endometriosis after cesarean section. Am J Obstet Gynecol 1988; 158:1117–1118.
48. Jubanyik KJ, Comite F. Extrapelvic endometriosis. Obstet Gynecol Clin North Am 1997; 24:411–440.
49. Stanley KE Jr, Utz DC, Dockerty MB. Clinically significant endometriosis of the urinary tract. Surg Gynecol Obstet 1965; 120:491–502.
50. Abrao MS, Dias JA, Bellelis P, et al. Endometriosis of the ureter and bladder are not associated diseases. Fertil Steril 2008; epub ahead of print.
51. Vercellini P, Pisacreta A, Pesole A. Is ureteral endometriosis an asymmetric disease? BJOG 2000; 107:559–561.
52. Nezhat CR, Nezhat FR. Laparoscopic segmental bladder resection for endometriosis: A report of two cases. Obstet Gynecol 1993; 81:882–884.
53. Dubuisson JB, Chapron C, Aubriot FX, et al. Pregnancy after laparoscopic partial cystectomy for bladder endometriosis. Hum Reprod 1994; 9:730–732.
54. Nezhat C, Nezhat F, Nezhat C, et al. Urinary tract endometriosis treated by laparoscopy. Fertil Steril 1996; 66:920–924.
55. Chapron C, Jacob S, Dubuisson J, et al. Laparoscopic assisted vaginal management of deep endometriosis infiltrating the rectovaginal septum. Acta Obstet Gynecol Scand 2001; 80:349–354.
56. Nezhat CH, Malik S, Osias J, et al. Laparoscopic management of 15 patients with infiltrating endometriosis of the bladder and a case of primary intravesical endometrioid adenosarcoma. Fertil Steril 2002; 78:872–875.
57. Seracchioli R, Mannini D, Colombo FM, et al. Cystoscopy-assisted laparoscopic resection of extramucosal bladder endometriosis. J Endourol 2002; 16:663–666.
58. Fedele L, Bianchi S, Zanconato G, et al. Long term follow-up after conservative surgery for bladder endometriosis. Fertil Steril 2005; 83:1729–1733.
59. Vercellini P, Abbiati A, Viganò P, et al. Asymmetry in distribution of diaphragmatic endometriotic lesions: Evidence in favour of the menstrual reflux theory. Hum Reprod 2007; 22:2359–2367.
60. Donnez J, Nisolle M, Squifflet J. Ureteral endometriosis: A complication of rectovaginal endometriotic (adenomyotic) nodules. Fertil Steril 2002; 77:32–37.
61. Carmignani L, Vercellini P, Spinelli M, et al. Pelvic endometriosis and hydroureteronephrosis. Fertil Steril 2010; 93:1741–1744.
62. Ghezzi F, Cromi A, Bergamini V, et al. Outcome of laparoscopic ureterolysis for ureteral endometriosis. Fertil Steril 2006; 86:418–422.
63. Antonelli A, Simeone C, Frego E, et al. Surgical treatment of ureteral obstruction from endometriosis: Our experience with thirteen cases. Int Urogynecol J Pelvic Floor Dysfunct 2004; 15:407–412.
64. Porpora MG, Gomel V. The role of laparoscopy in the management of pelvic pain in women in reproductive age. Fertil Steril 1997; 68:765–779.

65. Redwine DB. Conservative laparoscopic excision of endometriosis by sharp dissection: Life table analysis of reoperation and persistent or recurrent disease. Fertil Steril 1991; 56: 628–634.
66. Busacca M, Bianchi S, Agnoli B, et al. Follow-up of laparoscopic treatment of stage III–IV endometriosis. J Am Assoc Gynecol Laparosc 1999; 6:55–58.
67. Garry R, Clayton R, Hawe J. The effect of endometriosis and its radical laparoscopic excision on quality of life indicators. BJOG 2000; 107:44–54.
68. Jones KD, Sutton C. Patient satisfaction and changes in pain scores after ablative laparoscopic surgery for stage III–IV endometriosis and endometriotic cysts. Fertil Steril 2003; 79:1086–1090.
69. Abbott JA, Hawe J, Clayton RD, et al. The effects and effectiveness of laparoscopic excision of endometriosis: A prospective study with 2–5 year follow-up. Hum Reprod 2003; 18:1922–1927.
70. Vignali M, Bianchi S, Candiani M, et al. Surgical treatment of deep endometriosis and risk of recurrence. J Minim Invasive Gynecol 2005; 12:508–513.
71. Ferrero S, Abbamonte LH, Giordano M, et al. Deep dyspareunia and sex life after laparoscopic excision of endometriosis. Hum Reprod 2007; 22:1142–1148.
72. Wykes CB, Clark TJ, Chakravati S, et al. Efficacy of laparoscopic excision of visually diagnosed peritoneal endometriosis in the treatment of chronic pelvic pain. Eur J Obstet Gynecol Reprod Biol 2006; 125:129–133.
73. Wright J, Lotfallah H, Jones K, et al. A randomized trial of excision versus ablation for mild endometriosis. Fertil Steril 2005; 83:1830–1836.
74. Chapron C, Vercellini P, Barakat H, et al. Management of ovarian endometriomas. Hum Reprod Update 2002; 8:591–597.
75. Vercellini P, Chapron c, De Giorgi O, et al. Coagulation or excision of ovarian endometriomas? Am J Obstet Gynecol 2003; 188:606–610.
76. Vercellini P, Pietropaolo G, De Giorgi O, et al. Reproductive performance in infertile women with rectovaginal endometriosis: Is surgery worthwhile? Am J Obstet Gynecol 2006; 195:1303–1310.
77. Hart RJ, Hickey M, Maouris P, et al. Excisional surgery versus ablative surgery for ovarian endometriomata. Cochrane Database Syst Rev 2005; 5:CD004992.
78. Sutton CJG, Ewen SP, Whitelaw N, et al. Prospective, randomized, double-blind, controlled trial of laser laparoscopy in the treatment of pelvic pain associated with minimal, mild, and moderate endometriosis. Fertil Steril 1994; 62:696–700.
79. Sutton CJG, Pooley AS, Ewen SP, et al. Follow-up report on a randomized controlled trial of laser laparoscopy in the treatment of pelvic pain associated with minimal to moderate endometriosis. Fertil Steril 1997; 68:1070–1074.
80. Kones KD, Haines P, Sutton CJG. Long-term follow-up of a controlled trial of laser laparoscopy for pelvic pain. JSLS 2001; 5:111–115.
81. Abbott J, Hawe J, Hunter D, et al. Laparoscopic excision of endometriosis: A randomized, placebo-controlled trial. Fertil Steril 2004; 82:878–884.
82. Jarrell J, Mohindra R, Ross S, et al. Laparoscopy and reported pain among patients with endometriosis. J Obstet Gyaecol Can 2005; 27:477–485.
83. Jarrell J, Brant R, Leung W, et al. Women's pain experience predicts future surgery for pain associated with endometriosis. J Obstet Gyaecol Can 2007; 29:988–991.
84. Ford J, English J, Miles WA, et al. Pain, quality of life and complications following the radical resection of rectovaginal endometriosis. BJOG 2004; 111:353–356.
85. Vercellini P, Trespidi L, De Giorgi O, et al. Endometriosis and pelvic pain: Relation to disease stage and localization. Fertil Steril 1996; 65:299–304.
86. Vercellini P. Endometriosis: What a pain it is. Semin Reprod Endocrinol 1997; 15:251–261.
87. Vercellini P, Frontino G, Pietropaolo G, et al. Deep endometriosis: Definition, pathogenesis, and clinical management. J Am Assoc Gynecol Laparosc 2004; 11:153–161.
88. Fedele L, Bianchi S, Zanconato G, et al. Long term follow-up after conservative surgery for rectovaginal endometriosis. Am J Obstet Gynecol 2004; 190:1020–1024.
89. Anaf V, Simon P, El Nakadi I, et al. Impact of surgical resection of rectovaginal pouch of Douglas endometriotic nodules on pelvic pain and some elements of patients' sex life. J Am Assoc Gynecol Laparosc 2001; 8:55–60.
90. Redwine DB, Wright JT. Laparoscopic treatment of complete obliteration of the cul-de-sac associated with endometriosis: Long-term follow-up of en bloc resection. Fertil Steril 2001; 76:358–365.
91. Wright JT, Shafic A. Quality of life following radical excision of rectovaginal endometriosis associated with complete obliteration of the posterior cul-de-sac. J Gynaecol Endosc 2001; 10:107–110.
92. Duepreee HJ, Senagore AJ, Delaney CP, et al. Laparoscopic resection of deep pelvic endometriosis with rectosigmoid involvement. J Am Coll Surg 2002; 195:754–758.
93. Thomassin I, Bazot M, Detchev R, et al. Symptoms before and after surgical removal of colorectal endometriosis that are assessed by magnetic resonance imaging and rectal endoscopic sonography. Am J Obstet Gynecol 2004; 190:1264–1271.
94. Volpi E, Ferrero A, Sismondi P. Laparoscopic identification of pelvic nerves in patients with deep infiltrating endometriosis. Surg Endosc 2004; 18:1109–1112.
95. Campagnacci R, Perretta S, Guerrieri M, et al. Laparoscopic colorectal resection for endometriosis. Surg Endosc 2005; 19:662–664.
96. Chopin N, Vieira M, Borghese B, et al. Operative management of deeply infiltrating endometriosis: Results on pelvic pain symptoms according to a surgical classification. J Minim Invasive Gynecol 2005; 12:106–112.
97. Darai E, Thomassin I, Barranger E, et al. Feasibility and clinical outcome of laparoscopic colorectal resection for endometriosis. Am J Obstet Gynecol 2005; 192:394–400.
98. Fleisch MC, Xafis D, De Bruyne F, et al. Radical resection of invasive endometriosis with bowel or bladder involvement. Long-term results. Eur J Obstet Gynecol Reprod Biol 2005; 123:224–229.
99. Keckstein J, Weisinger H. Deep endometriosis, including intestinal involvement – the interdisciplinary approach. Minim Invasive Ther Allied Technol 2005; 14:160–166.
100. Mohr C, Nezhat FR, Nezhat CH, et al. Fertility considerations in laparoscopic treatment of infiltrative bowel endometriosis. JSLS 2005; 9:16–24.
101. Possover M, Quakernack J, Chiantera V. The LANN technique to reduce postoperative functional morbidity in laparoscopic radical pelvic surgery. J Am Coll Surg 2005; 21:913–917.
102. Angioni S, Peiretti M, Zirone M, et al. Laparoscopic excision of posterior vaginal fornix in the treatment of patients with deep endometriosis without rectum involvement: Surgical treatment and long-term follow-up. Hum Reprod 2006:21:1629–1634.
103. Ayroza Ribeiro PA, Rodrigues FC, Kehdi IPA, et al. Laparoscopic resection of intestinal endometriosis: A 5-year experience. J Minim Invasive Gynecol 2006; 13:442–446.
104. Dubernard G, Piketty M, Rouzier R, et al. Quality of life after laparoscopic colorectal resection for endometriosis. Hum Reprod 2006; 21:1243–1247.
105. Landi S, Ceccaroni M, Perutelli A, et al. Laparoscopic nerve-sparing complete excision of deep endometriosis: Is it feasible? Hum Reprod 2006; 21:774–781.
106. Langebrekke A, Istre O, Busund B, et al. Endoscopic treatment of deep infiltrating endometriosis (DIE) involving the bladder and rectosigmoid colon. Acta Obstet Gynecol 2006; 85:712–715.
107. Lyons SD, Chew SSB, Thomson AJM, et al. Clinical and quality-of-life outcomes after fertility-sparing laparoscopic surgery

with bowel resection for severe endometriosis. J Minim Invasive Gynecol 2006; 13:436–441.
108. Kristensen J, Kjer KJ. Laparoscopic laser resection of rectovaginal pouch and rectovaginal septum endometriosis: The impact on pelvic pain and quality of life. Acta Obstet Gynecol 2007; 86:1467–1471.
109. Mereu L, Ruffo G, Landi S, et al. Laparoscopic treatment of deep endometriosis with segmental colorectal resection: Short-term morbidity. J Minim Invasive Gynecol 2007; 14:463–469.
110. Secchiaroli R, Poggioli G, Pierangeli F, et al. Surgical outcome and long-term follow-up after laparoscopic rectosigmoid resection in women with deep infiltrating endometriosis. BJOG 2007; 114:889–895.
111. Dubernard G, Rouzier R, David-Montefiore E, et al. Use of SF-36 questionnaire to predict quality-of-life improvement after laparoscopic colorectal resection for endometriosis. Hum Reprod 2008; 23:846–851.
112. Matsuzaki S, Houlle C, Botchorishvili R, et al. Excision of the posterior vaginal fornix is necessary to ensure complete resection of rectovaginal endometriotic nodules of more than 2 cm in size. Fertil Steril 2008; epub ahead of print.
113. Zanetti-Dallenbach R, Bartley J, Muller C, et al. Combined vaginal-laparoscopic-abdominal approach for the surgical treatment of rectovaginal endometriosis with bowel resection: A comparison of this new technique with various established approaches by laparoscopy and laparotomy. Surg Endosc 2008; 22:995–1001.
114. Koninckx PR, Timmermans B, Meuleman C, et al. Complications of CO_2 laser endoscopic excision of deep endometriosis. Hum Reprod 1996; 10:2263–2268.
115. Camagna O, Dhainaut C, Dupuis O, et al. Surgical management of rectovaginal septum endometriosis from a continuous series of 50 cases. Gynecol Obstet Fertil 2004; 32:199–209.
116. Marpeau O, Thomassin I, Barranger E, et al. Laparoscopic colorectal resection for endometriosis: preliminary results. J Gynecol Obstet Biol Reprod 2004; 33:600–606.
117. Mereu L, Ruffo G, Landi S, et al. Laparoscopic treatment of deep endometriosis with segmental colorectal resection: Short-term morbidity. J Minim Invasive Gynecol 2007; 14:463–469.
118. Slack A, Child T, Lindsey I, et al. Urological and colorectal complications following surgery for rectovaginal endometriosis. BJOG 2007; 114:1278–1282.
119. Dubernard G, Rouzier R, David-Montefiore E, et al. Urinary complications after surgery for posterior deep infiltrating endometriosis are related to the extent of dissection and to uterosacral ligaments resection. J Minim Invasive Gynecol 2008; 15:235–240.
120. Fedele L, Bianchi S, Zanconato G, et al. Is rectovaginal endometriosis a progressive disease? Am J Obstet Gynecol 2004; 191:1539–1542.
121. Emmanuel KR, Davis C. Outcomes and treatment options in rectovaginal endometriosis. Curr Opin Obstet Gynecol 2005; 17:399–402.
122. Vercellini P, De Giorgi O, Pisacreta A, et al. Surgical management of endometriosis. Baillieres Best Pract Res Clin Obstet Gynaecol 2000; 14:501–523.
123. Vercellini P, Fedele L, Bianchi S, et al. Pelvic denervation for chronic pelvic pain associated with endometriosis: Fact or fancy? Am J Obstet Gynecol 1991; 165:745–749.
124. Proctor ML, Latthe PM, Farquhar CM, et al. Surgical interruption of pelvic nerve pathways for primary and secondary dysmenorrhoea. Cochrane Database Syst Rev 2005; 4:CD001896.
125. Tjaden B, Schla WD, Kimball A, et al. The efficacy of presacral neurectomy for the relief of midline dysmenorrhea. Obstet Gynecol 1990; 76:89–91.
126. Candiani GB, Fedele L, Vercellini P, et al. Presacral neuroectomy for the treatment of pelvic pain associated with endometriosis: A controlled study. Am J Obstet Gynecol 1992; 167:100–103.
127. Zullo F, Palomba S, Zupi E, et al. Effectiveness of presacral neurectomy in women with severe dysmenorrhea caused by endometriosis who were treated with laparoscopic conservative surgery: A 1-year prospective randomized double-blind controlled trial. Am J Obstet Gynecol 2003; 189:5–10.
128. Zullo F, Palomba S, Zupi E, et al. Long-term effectiveness of presacral neurectomy for the treatment of severe dysmenorrhea due to endometriosis. J Am Assoc Gynecol Laparosc 2004; 11:23–28.
129. Sutton C, Pooley AS, Jones KD, et al. A prospective, randomized, double-blind controlled trial of laparoscopic uterine nerve ablation in the treatment of pelvic pain associated with endometriosis. Gynecol Endosc 2001; 10:217–222.
130. Johnson NP, Farquhar CM, Crossley S, et al. A double-blind randomized controlled trial of laparoscopic uterine nerve ablation for women with chronic pelvic pain. BJOG 2004; 111:950–959.
131. Lichten EM, Bombard J. Surgical treatment of primary dysmenorrhea with laparoscopic uterine nerve ablation. J Reprod Med 1987; 32:37–41.
132. Latthe PM, Proctor ML, Farquhar CM, et al. Surgical interruption of pelvic nerve pathways in dysmenorrhoea: A systematic review of effectiveness. Acta Obstet Gynecol 2007; 86:4–15.
133. Xiong T, Daniels J, Middleton L, et al. Meta-analysis using individual patient data from randomised trials to assess the effectiveness of the laparoscopic uterosacral nerve ablation in the treatment of chronic pelvic pain: A proposed protocol. BJOG 2007; 114:1580–1587.
134. Grainger DA, Soderstrom RM, Schiff SF, et al. Ureteral injuries at laparoscopy: Insights into diagnosis, management, and prevention. Obstet Gynecol 1990;75:839–843.
135. Good MC, Copas PR, Doody MC. Uterine prolapse after laparoscopic uterosacral transection. J Reprod Med 1992; 37:995–996.
136. Davis GD. Uterine prolapse after laparoscopic uterosacral transection in nulliparous airborne trainees. A report of three cases. J Reprod Med 1996; 41:279–282.
137. Chen FP, Lo TS, Soong YK. Management of chylous ascites following laparoscopic presacral neurectomy. Hum Reprod 1998; 13:880–883.
138. Lo TS, Chen FP, Chu KK, et al. Successful management of chylous ascites after laparoscopic presacral neurectomy. J Am Assoc Gynecol Laparosc 1998; 5:431–433.
139. Vercellini P, Daguati R, Abbiati A. Chronic pelvic pain. In: Arici A, Seli E, eds. Non-invasive Management of Gynecologic Disorders. London: Taylor and Francis Publishing Group, 2008:33–51.
140. Vercellini P, Bocciolone L, Vendola N, et al. Peritoneal endometriosis: Morphologic appearance in women with chronic pelvic pain. J Reprod Med 1991; 36:533–556.
141. Vercellini P, Frontino G, De Giorgi O, et al. Endometriosis preoperative and postoperative medical treatment. Obstet Gynecol Clin North Am 2003; 30:163–180.
142. Thomas EJ. Combining medical and surgical treatment foe endometriosis: The best of both worlds? Br J Obstet Gynaecol 1992; 99:5–8.
143. Hemmings R. Combined treatment for endometriosis: GnRH agonists and laparoscopic surgery. J Reprod Med 1998; 43:316–320.
144. Winkel CA. Combined medial and surgical treatment for women with endometriosis. Clin Obstet Gynecol 1999; 42:645–663.
145. Kettel LM, Mrphy AA. Combination medical and surgical therapy for infertile patients with endometriosis. Obstet Gynecol Clin North Am 1989; 16:167–177.
146. Malinak LR, Wheeler JM. Combination medical-surgical therapy for endometriosis. In: Shaw RW, ed. Endometriosis. London: Carnfoth Pertheneon Publishing Group, 1990:85–91.
147. Donnez J, Nisolle M, Gillerot S, et al. Ovarian endometrial cysts: The role of gonadotropin-releasing hormone against and/or drainage. Fertil Steril 1994; 62:63–66.
148. Donnez J, Nisolle M, Clerckx F, et al. Advanced endoscopic techniques used in dysfunctional bleeding, fibroids and endometriosis, and the role of gonadotropin-releasing hormone against treatment. Br J Obstet Gynaecol 1994; 101:2–12.
149. Malinak LR. Surgical treatment and adjunct therapy of endometriosis. Int J Gynecol Obstet 1993; 40(Suppl):316–320.

150. Donnez J, Nisolle-Pochet M, Clerckx-Braun F, et al. Administration of nasal buserelin as compared with subcutaneous buserelin implant for endometriosis. Fertil Steril 1989; 52:27–30.
151. Donnez, Nisolle M, Casanas-Roux F. Endometriosis-associated infertility: Evaluation of preoperative use of danazol, gestrinone and buserelin. Int J Fertil 1990; 35:297–301.
152. Muzii L, Marana R, Caruana P, et al. The impact of preoperative gonadotropin-releasing hormone against treatment on laparoscopic excision of ovarian endometriotic cysts. Fertil Steril 1996; 65:1253–1257.
153. Audebert A, Deschamps P, Marret H, et al. Pre or post-operative medical treatment with nafarelin in stage III–IV endometriosis: A French multicenter study. Eur J Obstet Gynecol Reprod Biol 1998; 79:145–148.
154. Donnez J, Lemaire-Rubbers M, Karaman Y, et al. Combined (hormonal and microsurgical) therapy in infertile women with endometriosis. Fertil Steril 1987; 48:239–242.
155. Napolitano C, Marziani R, Mossa M, et al. Management of stage III and IV endometriosis: A 10-year experience. Eur J Obstet Gynecol Reprod Biol 1994; 53:199–204.
156. Yap C, Furness S, Farquhar C. Pre and post operative medical therapy for endometriosis. Cochrane Database Syst Rev 2004; 3:CD003678.
157. Telimaa S, Ronnberg L, Kauppila A, et al. Placebo-controlled comparison of danazol and high-dose medroxyprogesterone acetate in the treatment of endometriosis after conservative surgery. Gynecol Endocrinol 1987; 1:363–371.
158. Parazzini F, Fedele L, Busacca M, et al. Postsurgical medical treatment of advanced endometriosis: Results of a randomized clinical trial. Am J Obstet Gynecol 1994; 171:1205–1207.
159. Hornstein MD, Hemmings R, Yuzpe AA, et al. Use of nafarelin versus placebo after reductive laparoscopic surgery for endometriosis. Fertil Steril 1997;68:860–864.
160. Bianchi S, Busacca M, Agnoli B, et al. Effects of 3 month therapy with danazol after laparoscopic surgery for stage III–IV endometriosis: A randomized study. Hum Reprod 1999; 14:1335–1337.
161. Vercellini P, Crosignani PG, Fadini R, et al. A gonadotrophin releasing hormone agonist versus expectant management after conservative surgery for symptomatic endometriosis. Br J Obstet Gynaecol 1999; 106:672–677.
162. Muzii L, Marana R, Caruana P, et al. Postoperative administration of monophasic combined oral contraceptives after laparoscopic treatment of ovarian endometriomas: A prospective, randomized trail. Am J Obstet Gynecol 2000; 183:588–592.
163. Busacca M, Somigliana E, Bianchi S, et al. Post-operative GnRH analogue treatment after conservative surgery for symptomatic endometriosis stage III-IV: A randomized controlled study. Hum Reprod 2001; 16:2399–2402.
164. Vercellini P, Somigliana E, Daguati R, et al. Postoperative oral contraceptive exposure and risk of endometrioma recurrence. Am J Obstet Gynecol 2008; epub ahead of print.
165. Vercellini P, Frontino G, De Giorgi O, et al. Comparison of a levonorgestrel-releasing intrauterine device versus expectant management after conservative surgery for symptomatic endometriosis: A pilot study. Fertil Steril 2003; 80:305–309.
166. Candiani M, Fedele L, Vercellini P, et al. Repetitive conservative surgery for recurrence of endometriosis. Obstet Gynecol 1991; 77:421–424.
167. Busacca M, Fedele L, Bianchi S, et al. Surgical treatment of recurrent endometriosis: Laparotomy versus laparoscopy. Hum Reprod 1998; 13:2271–2274.
168. Fedele L, Bianchi S, Zanconato G, et al. Laparoscopic excision of recurrent endometriomas: Long-term outcome and comparison with primary surgery. Fertil Steril 2006; 85:694–699.
169. Carlson KJ, Miller BA, Fowler FJ Jr. The Maine Women's Health Study: I. Outcome of hysterectomy. Obstet Gynecol 1994; 83:556–565.
170. Learman LA, Kuppermann M, Gates E, et al. Predictors of hysterectomy in women with common pelvic problems: A uterine survival analysis J Am Coll Surg 2007; 204:633–641.
171. Jarrell JF, Vilos GA, Allaire C, et al. Chronic Pelvic Pain Working Group; SOGC. Consensus guidelines for the management of chronic pelvic pain. J Obstet Gynaecol Can 2005; 27:869–887.
172. Gomel V. Chronic pelvic pain: A challenge. J Minim Invasive Gynecol 2007; 14:521–526.
173. Stovall TG, Ling FW, Crawford DA. Hysterectomy for chronic pelvic pain of presumed uterine etiology. Obstet Gynecol 1990; 75:676–679.
174. Hillis SD, Marchbanks PA, Peterson HB. The effectiveness of hysterectomy for chronic pelvic pain. Obstet Gynecol 1995; 86:941–945.
175. Tay SK, Bromwich N. Outcome of hysterectomy for pelvic pain in premenopausal women. Aust N Z J Obstet Gynaecol 1998;38:72–76.
176. Kjerulff KH, Lagenberg PW, Rhodes JC, et al. Effectiveness of hysterectomy. Obstet Gynecol 2000; 3:319–326.
177. Hartmann KE, Cindy MA, Lamvu GM, et al. Quality of life and sexual function after hysterectomy in women with preoperative pain and depression. Obstet Gynecol 2004; 104:701–709.
178. MacDonald SR, Klock SCK, Milad MP. Long-term outcome of nonconservative surgery (hysterectomy) for endometriosis-associated pain in women <30 years old. Am J Obstet Gynecol 1999; 180:1360–1363.
179. Fedele L, Bianchi S, Zanconato G, et al. Tailoring radicality in demolitive surgery for deeply infiltrating endometriosis. Am J Obstet Gynecol 2005; 193:114–117.
180. Magos A. Endometriosis: Radical surgery. Baillieres Clin Obstet Gynecol 1993; 7:849–864.
181. Clayton RD, Hawe JA, Love JC, et al. Recurrent pain after hysterectomy and bilateral salpingo-oophorectomy for endometriosis: Evaluation of laparoscopic excision of residual endometriosis. Br J Obstet Gynaecol 1999; 106:740–744.
182. Goumenou AG, Chow C, Taylor A, et al. Endometriosis arising during estrogen and testosterone treatment 17 years after hysterectomy: A case report. Maturitas 2003; 46:239–241.
183. Prentice A. Endometriosis. BMJ 2001; 323:93–95.
184. Vercellini P, Trespidi L, Colombo A, et al. A gonadotropin-releasing hormone agonist versus a low-dose oral contraceptive for pelvic pain associated with endometriosis. Fertil Steril 1993; 60:75–79.
185. Parazzini F, Di Cintio E, Chatenoud L, et al. Estroprogestin vs. gonadotropin agonists plus estroprogestin in the treatment of endometriosis-related pelvic pain: A randomized trial. Eur J Obstet Gynecol Reprod Biol 2000; 88:11–14.
186. Sulak PJ, Cressman BE, Waldrop E, et al. Extending the duration of active oral contraceptive pills to manage hormone withdrawal symptoms. Obstet Gynecol 1997; 89:179–183.
187. Sulak P, Thomas J, Ortiz M, et al. Acceptance of altering the standard 21-day/7-day oral contraceptive regimen to delay menses and reduce hormone withdrawal symptoms. Am J Obstet Gynecol 2002; 186:1142–1149.
188. Coffee AL, Sulak PJ, Kuehl TJ. Long-term assessment of symptomatology and satisfaction of an extended oral contraceptive regimen. Contraception 2007; 75:444–449.
189. Duleba AJ, Keltz MD, Olive DL. Evaluation and management of chronic pelvic pain. J Am Assoc Gynecol Laparosc 1996; 3:205–227.
190. Vercellini P, Frontino G, De Giorgi O, et al. Continuous use of an oral contraceptive for endometriosis-associated recurrent dysmenorrhoea that does not respond to a cyclic pill regimen. Fertil Steril 2003; 80:560–563.
191. Fedele L, Arcaini L, Bianchi S, et al. Comparison of cyproterone acetate and danazol in the treatment of pelvic pain associated with endometriosis. Obstet Gynecol 1989; 73:1000–1004.
192. Vercellini P, De Giorgi O, Mosconi P, et al. Cyproterone acetate versus a continuous monophasic oral contraceptive in the treatment of recurrent pelvic pain after conservative surgery for symptomatic endometriosis. Fertil Steril 2002; 77:52–61.
193. Kaunitz AM. Long-acting injectable contraception with depot medroxyprogesterone acetate. Am J Obstet Gynecol 1994; 170:1543–1549.

194. Skegg DCG, Noonan EA, Paul C, et al. Depot medroxyprogesterone acetate and breast cancer: A pooled analysis of the World Health Organization and New Zealand Studies. JAMA 1995; 273:799–804.
195. Cundy T, Evans M, Roberts H, et al. Bone density in women receiving depot medroxyprogesterone acetate for contraception. BMJ 1991; 303:13–16.
196. Scholes D, LaCroix AZ, Ichikawa LE, et al. Injectable hormone contraception and bone density: Results from a prospective study. Epidemiology 2002; 13:581–587.
197. Clark MK, Sowers MR, Nichols S, et al. Bone mineral density changes over two years in first-time users of depot medroxyprogesterone acetate. Fertil Steril 2004; 82:1580–1586.
198. Shaarawy M, El-Mallah SY, Seoudi S, et al. Effect of long-term use of depot medroxyprogesterone acetate as hormonal contraceptive on bone mineral density and biochemical markers of bone remodeling. Contraception 2006; 74:297–302.
199. Vercellini P, De Giorgi O, Oldani S, et al. Depot medroxyprogesterone acetate versus an oral contraceptive combined with very-low-dose danazol for long-term treatment of pelvic pain associated with endometriosis. Am J Obstet Gynecol 1996; 175:396–401.
200. Crosignani PG, Luciano A, Ray A, et al. Subcutaneous depot medroxyprogesterone acetate versus leuprolide acetate in the treatment of endometriosis-associated pain. Hum Reprod 2006; 21:248–256.
201. Schlaff WD, Carson SA, Luciano A, et al. Subcutaneous injection of depot medroxyprogesterone acetate compared with leuprolide acetate in the treatment of endometriosis-associated pain. Fertil Steril 2006; 85:314–325.
202. Igarashi M, Iizuka M, Abe Y, et al. Novel vaginal danazol ring therapy for pelvic endometriosis, in particular deeply infiltrating endometriosis. Hum Reprod 1998; 13:1952–1956.
203. Razzi S, Luisi S, Calonaci F, et al. Efficacy of vaginal danazol treatment in women with recurrent deeply infiltrating endometriosis. Fertil Steril 2007; 88:789–794.
204. Fedele L, Bianchi S, Zanconato G, et al. Gonadotropin-releasing hormone agonist treatment for endometriosis of the rectovaginal septum. Am J Obstet Gynecol 2000; 183:1462–1467.
205. Pickersgill A. GnRH agonists and add-back therapy: Is there a perfect combination? Br J Obstet Gynaecol 1998; 105:475–485.
206. Fedele L, Bianchi S, Zanconato G, et al. Use of a levonorgestrel-releasing intrauterine device in the treatment of rectovaginal endometriosis. Fertil Steril 2001; 75:485–488.
207. Riis BJ, Lehmann HJ, Christiansen C. Norethisterone acetate in combination with estrogen: Effects on the skeleton and other organs: A review. Am J Obstet Gynecol 2002; 187:1101–1106.
208. Westney OL, Amundsen CL, McGuire EJ. Bladder endometriosis: Conservative management. J Urol 2000; 163:1814–1817.
209. Soliman NF, Hillard TC. Hormone replacement therapy in women with past history of endometriosis. Climateric 2006; 9:325–335.
210. Fedele L, Bianchi S, Raffaelli R, et al. Comparison of transdermal estradiol and tibolone for the treatment of oophorectomized women with deep residual endometriosis. Maturitas 1999; 32:189–193.
211. Lindsay PC, Shaw RW, Bennink HJ, et al. The effect of add-back treatment with tibolone (Livial) on patients treated with the gonadotropin-releasing hormone agonist triptorelin (decapeptyl). Fertil Steril 1996; 65:342–348.
212. Vercellini P, Cortesi I, Crosignani PG. Progestins for symptomatic endometriosis: A critical analysis of the evidence. Fertil Steril 1997; 68:393–401.
213. The American College of Obstetricians and Gynecologists. Medical management of endometriosis. Number 11, December 1999. Int J Gynaecol Obstet 2000; 71:183–196.
214. Practice Committee of the American Society for Reproductive Medicine. Endometriosis and infertility. Fertil Steril 2006; 86:S156–S160.
215. Kennedy S, Bergqvist A, Chapron C, et al. ESHRE Special Interest Group for Endometriosis and Endometrium Guideline Development Group. ESHRE guideline for the diagnosis and treatment of endometriosis. Hum Reprod 2005; 20:2698–2704.
216. Royal College of Obstetricians and Gynaecologists. The Investigation and Management of Endometriosis. Guideline No. 24. London: RCOG Press, 2006.
217. Eskenazi B, Warner M, Bonsignore L, et al. Validation study of nonsurgical diagnosis of endometriosis. Fertil Steril 2001; 76:929–935.

11

Invasive endometriosis: investigation and medical and surgical treatment

Mauricio S. Abrão, Grace Janik, and Victor Gomel

Endometriosis is a prevalent disease, and specific attention was paid to its diagnostic and therapeutic aspects following the classification of endometriosis according to its depth by Cornillie et al. in 1990. Nodules affecting the pouch of Douglas, retrocervical area, bladder, ureter, intestinal wall, and, less frequently, the rectovaginal septum constitute the most severe form of endometriosis, which is considered an invasive disease. This chapter discusses the classifications, diagnosis, and specific treatment of deep endometriosis.

DEFINITIONS OF DEEP ENDOMETRIOSIS

A number of different classification systems have been suggested to describe deep endometriosis. These systems are not necessarily comparable, since they assume different physiopathological mechanisms for the condition. Deep or infiltrative endometriosis is defined as the presence of implants at a depth of more than 5 mm below the peritoneal surface, affecting the uterine ligaments, the retrouterine region, pouch of Douglas, and intestinal and urinary tracts, in decreasing order of frequency (1). Koninckx and Martin (2) later proposed that this disease be classified in accordance with the type of infiltration, thereby establishing three types of infiltrative endometriosis (Fig. 1):

- Type I—Pelvic area of a typical or atypical, cone-shaped lesion surrounded by scar tissue; depth being diagnosed following surgical removal
- Type II—Lesion formed by retraction of the rectum surrounding a typical lesion
- Type III—Endometriotic nodule deeply infiltrating the posterior cul-de-sac. The pelvis appears to be lesion free when observed laparoscopically

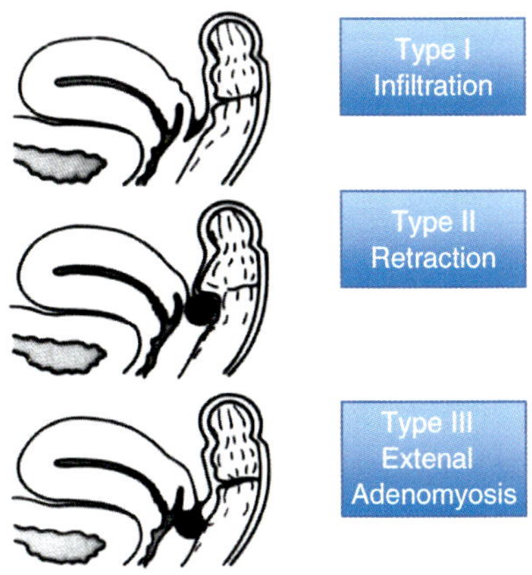

Figure 1 Classification of deep endometriosis according to the depth of the lesion (2).

Donnez et al. (3) described two different types of deep endometriosis. The first is deep infiltrative endometriosis, characterized by invasion of a deep, active peritoneal lesion into the retroperitoneal space. In cases of lateral peritoneal invasion, the uterosacral ligaments and the anterior wall of the rectum may be affected, resulting in a process of retraction, adhesion, and secondary obliteration of the pouch of Douglas. The second type is the result of pseudoinfiltration, also referred to as adenomyosis of the rectovaginal septum, in which the lesions originate in the tissue of the rectovaginal septum itself and consist of smooth muscle with active glandular epithelium or stroma and are therefore less invasive.

In 2001, Martin and Batt (4) pointed out that the term endometriosis of the rectovaginal septum referred to endometriosis affecting the connective tissue located between the vagina and the rectum, usually extending from the middle to the lower third of the vagina, differing, therefore, from the deep form of the disease, which is situated higher up, at the level of the posterior cervix, and is referred to as retrocervical endometriosis. Nodules reaching the rectovaginal septum (less frequent) and the intestinal wall constitute the most severe form of endometriosis, and this should be borne in mind in patients with clinical complaints of pelvic pain unrelated to the menstrual cycle, deep dyspareunia, and cyclic bowel alterations that include an increase in intestinal transport, pain on evacuation, and/or bloody feces during menstruation. In these cases, digital vaginal examination associated with diagnostic imaging methods, such as transvaginal tenderness-guided sonography and nuclear magnetic resonance, may be helpful in diagnosing this form of endometriosis (5).

Due to the severity of symptoms and the difficulty of treatment, deep invasive endometriosis presents an important challenge. In fact, Brosens and Brosens (6) proposed that deep infiltrating endometriosis had characteristics that differed from those present when peritoneum and ovary were affected. In this case, lesions are less frequent; they affect central regions of the pelvis and develop as a result of coelomic tissue metaplasia into endometrial tissue and not from the implantation of menstrual reflux to the peritoneal cavity. In general, they are more symptomatic, progressive, and less responsive to hormonal treatment.

This chapter deals with the treatment of infiltrative endometriosis, in particular with cases in which the ovaries and urinary and intestinal tracts are affected, and highlights diagnostic aspects of this condition.

PREDICTING SEVERE ENDOMETRIOSIS

The definitive diagnosis of deep endometriosis is most commonly reached during surgery. However, some clinical characteristics identified from the physical examination, laboratory tests, and diagnostic imaging may provide clues to the diagnosis of this form of endometriosis, after which surgery is recommended for diagnostic confirmation and treatment.

Although digital vaginal examination may provide evidence of thickening and/or painful nodules at the posterior cul-de-sac or along the uterosacral ligaments, as reported by some investigators (5), in a certain proportion of patients the physical examination may appear normal or nonspecific, but clinical examination during menses significantly increases the detection rate. Although none of the tests for predicting rectovaginal endometriosis are perfect (7), the following markers, especially in combination, may help to identify candidates at a need of specialist referral: dyspareunia is strongly related to posterior cul-de-sac lesions [$p = 0.0001$; odds ratio (OR) = 2.64, 95% confidence interval (CI) = 1.68–4.24], and intensity of dysmenorrhea (8). Moreover, nonmenstrual pain increases with endometriosis stage (7). Dyspareunia (positive predictive prevalence of 87%) and, interestingly, nausea and bloating are also good predictors of rectovaginal endometriosis (9).

Clinical examination should include inspection of the retrocervical and posterior vagina and palpation of the uterosacral ligaments for nodules and pain (10). If physical examination is performed during menstruation, the detection rate of these lesions is increased by a factor of 5 (11), when dyschezia is also most severe (12). Rectovaginal examination may provide additional information about the status of the cul-de-sac and also allows better evaluation of the rectovaginal septum.

Transvaginal ultrasound (TVUS) scan (Fig. 2) is more sensitive and specific in diagnosing deep retrovaginal endometriosis than digital vaginal examination, magnetic resonance imaging (MRI, Fig. 3) (13), and rectal ultrasound (Fig. 4) (14), when carried out by a trained professional and preferably following a simple rectal enema one hour prior to TVUS, and may provide useful information for therapeutic management (15). A modified scanning technique, taking into account subjective areas of tenderness during scanning, can improve the detection of rectovaginal, retrocervical, and cul-de-sac endometriosis (specificity of 95%; sensitivity of 90%) (5). MRI is becoming a useful adjunct to ultrasound scanning, especially in predicting severe endometriosis (16), and there seems to be a role for using additional endocavitary coils placed in the vagina together with the conventional pelvic-phased array coil (17).

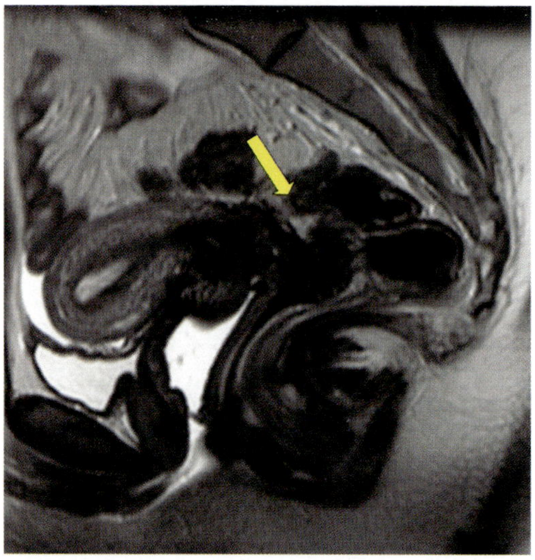

Figure 3 Nuclear magnetic resonance image suggestive of deep endometriosis affecting the rectum.

The preoperative diagnosis of bladder endometriosis, which is present in about 1% of endometriosis patients, remains a challenge. In a small series of patients with severe endometriosis, only 62% had urinary symptoms and ultrasound scanning predicted bladder involvement in only 38% of cases (18). Interestingly, dysuria is dependent on the location of the lesion(s) within the bladder and is increased when the bladder base is affected. In a group of women at high risk of endometriosis, a questionnaire based on the American Urologic Association Symptom Index showed good sensitivity (93%) and specificity (88%) in predicting bladder involvement.

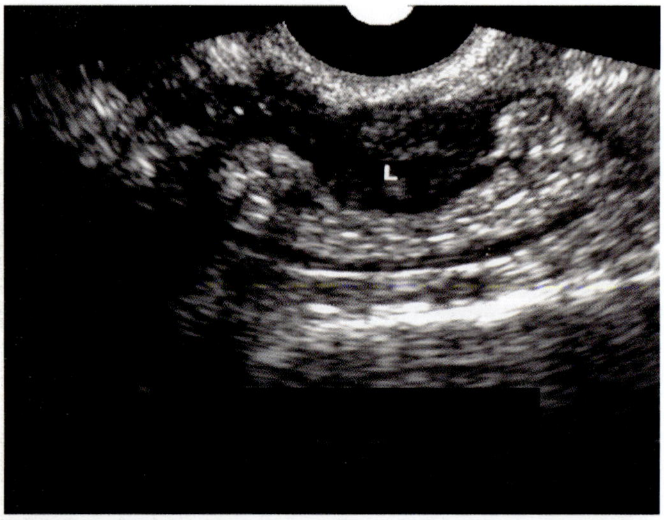

Figure 2 Image suggestive of endometriosis affecting the bowel: transvaginal ultrasonography with prior bowel preparation.

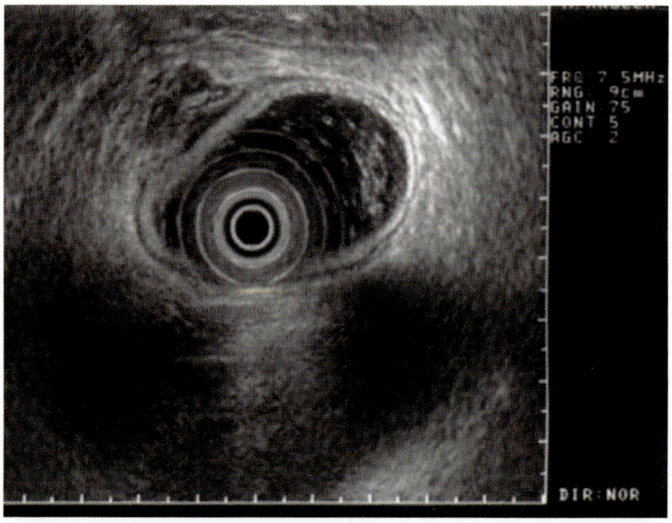

Figure 4 Image in a honeycomb-like pattern, suggestive of deep endometriosis affecting the bowel, diagnosed by rectal echoendoscopy.

Currently, CA-125 is not routinely used in the diagnosis of endometriosis because it is not specific enough. Therefore, serum levels of CA-125 >100 IU/mL and amyloid A protein >50 g/mL may predict diagnosis when associated with clinical complaints and a physical examination suggestive of the presence of the disease in the rectovaginal septum (19). However, in severe endometriosis, these markers, in combination with additional ones such as macrophage chemotactic protein-1, leptin, and macrophage migration inhibitory factor, may play a greater role in the future (20).

THERAPEUTIC ASPECTS OF OVARIAN ENDOMETRIOSIS

Patients with ovarian endometriomas may be asymptomatic or may have symptoms such as pain and/or infertility. The decision regarding therapy depends on the patient's age, her symptoms, the preoperative diagnosis, and her wishes regarding future fertility.

Reasons for recommending surgical treatment of endometriomas are

- pain relief (dysmenorrhea, acyclic pain, and dyspareunia) (21);
- treatment of infertility (3);
- lower probability of recurrence with surgical treatment compared to medical treatment (3);
- possibility of malignant transformation (22).

The guidelines of the European Society of Human Reproduction and Embryology state that histology specimens should be obtained from cysts >3 cm in diameter and with characteristics of endometriomas (23).

Laparoscopy is the method of choice for the treatment of endometriomas. Compared to laparotomy, this method results in shorter duration of hospitalization, lower costs, reduced postoperative pain intensity, and a lower incidence of postoperative adhesions. Cumulative pregnancy rates following surgery and recurrence rates of cysts are comparable irrespective of whether laparoscopy or laparotomy is used for surgical access (21).

Endometriomas may be managed as follows.

Puncture and Aspiration

This procedure can be carried out either by laparoscopy or transvaginally under ultrasonographic vision. Due to the high recurrence rate and low incidence of clinical improvement, this procedure is not normally recommended.

For the procedures described below, laparoscopic access is achieved as follows: A 10-mm incision is made within the umbilical fossa to permit the introduction of a 10-mm laparoscope and an incision at each iliac fossa for the introduction of auxiliary instruments of 5 mm.

Oophorectomy

Since endometriosis usually affects women of reproductive age and infertility is one of its principal symptoms, oophorectomy would not be the desirable treatment option, since most of these women would like to preserve their fertility. Oophorectomy may be indicated in climacteric and postmenopausal women.

From a technical point of view, lysis of any adhesions is first performed; rupture of the endometrioma usually occurs at this time. The utero-ovarian and infundibulopelvic ligaments are then identified, thoroughly desiccated using bipolar current, and divided. Next, oophorectomy is carried out using monopolar current. Extreme care should be taken with the ipsilateral ureter (which must be identified first) during the desiccation of the infundibulopelvic ligament.

Puncture, Aspiration, and Cauterization of the Endometrioma Lining

Once laparoscopic access has been achieved, a thorough evaluation of abdomen and pelvis is made to stage the endometriosis (24). Existing adhesions are then removed, and associated peritoneal lesions are treated by resection and/or cauterization of the lesions. When mobilizing the ovary containing the endometrioma, rupture usually occurs at the site of adherence with the pelvic wall or uterus. The chocolate-colored fluid that escapes is suctioned, and the cyst is drained by introducing the cannula through the ruptured site. Next, the cyst lining is carefully inspected; a fragment of the capsule is removed for histological examination, following which the capsule is cauterized using bipolar current or laser energy (25). The rationale of removing only a fragment of the cyst lining is to prevent loss of ovarian reserve. This, however, is not our preferred mode of treatment.

Resection of the Endometrioma Capsule

For this procedure, depending on the size of the endometrioma, we may elect to insert a 10-mm portal in one of the iliac fossa to enable removal of the specimen. The technique for puncturing and resecting the capsule of the endometrioma and cauterization of the ovarian bed has been described in 1991 by Reich et al. (26). We use the same approach. The ovary is retracted to release adhesions between this organ and the pelvic wall or uterus. Then an incision is made to open the endometrioma if not previously ruptured. This allows visualization of the capsule and the healthy ovarian tissue. To remove the capsule, the ovarian cortex is grasped with appropriate graspers and the endometrioma lining is similarly grasped with another forceps. This permits application of bilateral traction to resect the capsule from the adjacent ovarian tissue (Fig. 5). Following excision of the capsule, hemostasis of the surgical bed is obtained by coagulating individual bleeders. Bleeding from the ovarian bed is variable from case to

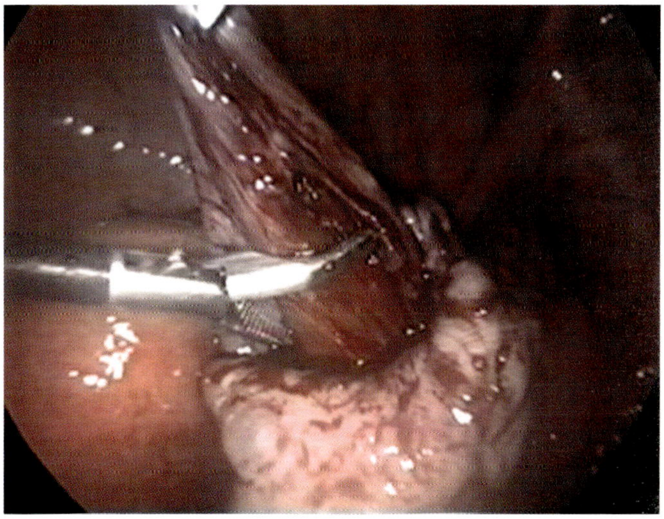

Figure 5 Traction to resect the capsule from the ovarian endometrioma.

case; cauterization should be minimized to protect the ovarian reserve. Initial application of pressure to the ovary with the help of graspers reduces the bleeding sites and the need of subsequent cauterization. We must emphasize that cauterization, if required, should be carried out carefully in bipolar mode, under close-range vision, while irrigating the cyst bed with saline solution; this permits more accurate cauterization of the bleeding sites and lessens adjacent tissue damage.

THERAPEUTIC ASPECTS OF ENDOMETRIOSIS OF THE URINARY TRACT

Endometriosis of the urinary tract is a rare condition and is present in approximately 1% of patients with endometriosis (27). The site most frequently affected is the bladder, in approximately 84% of cases, followed by the ureter in 15%, kidney in 4%, and urethra in 2% (28). The lesions are known to be extrinsic; in other words, they affect structures such as the ureter or bladder, always originating in the outermost layers.

Classification of urinary tract endometriosis as "deep endometriosis" requires the lesion(s) to be more than 5 mm deep and/or involves the muscular layer of the affected organ. This is imperative in order to properly classify the extent of the disease. For example, superficial endometriotic lesions, located in the uterovesical peritoneal reflection, must be classified as peritoneal endometriosis and not as bladder endometriosis.

Endometriosis of the urinary tract may be treated medically or surgically. The various medications currently available induce temporary quiescence of active foci and improve the patients' symptoms. However, with true deep urinary tract endometriosis, medical treatment rarely provides sufficient improvement of symptoms, making surgical treatment the therapeutic choice in such cases (29). Description of surgical treatment of endometriosis affecting the bladder and ureter follows.

Bladder Endometriosis

Proper management of this condition requires understanding of its pathophysiology. It must be emphasized that endometriosis is a disease that is extrinsic to the bladder; it originates in the uterovesical peritoneal reflection either by implantation or by metaplasia. Therefore, cystoscopic treatment of this type of lesion, when it extends to the mucosa of the bladder, will be incomplete or will lead to bladder perforation. According to Vercellini et al. (30), treatment should be carried out by laparoscopy or laparotomy, depending on the surgeon's experience. Surgical treatment should be carried out in a specialized center with a multidisciplinary team and should preferably be performed by laparoscopy. This approach is technically feasible and permits better evaluation and treatment of other sites affected by the disease.

Bladder lesions are usually located in the roof or on the posterior wall of the bladder; they are frequently adherent to the uterine corpus or isthmus. A preliminary cystoscopy permits better planning of the surgical strategy and allows ureteral catheterization, if required. It also permits to monitor the bladder during resection and suturing.

The procedure should be carried out with an urologist, competent at performing laparoscopic procedures. Once laparoscopic access is established, lesions suggestive of endometriosis are identified and removed. Bladder lesions may be removed by securing the nodule with a grasper and resecting it mechanically with either scissors or a monopolar electrode using pure cut mode to minimize damage to the surrounding tissues. After excision, the defect in the bladder wall is repaired with 3-0 Vycril continuous sutures. If excision extends into the bladder, the defect is closed in two layers, using continuous 3-0 Vycril for the inner layer and interrupted one for the outer layer. At the end of the procedure, the bladder must be distended using blue dye solution to identify any leakage, following which a Foley catheter is placed in the bladder. The catheter is left in place for 7 to 14 days.

Endometriosis Affecting the Ureter

Endometriosis affecting the ureter is often a part of an extensive form of the disease that generally makes surgical treatment challenging. Prior to surgery, it is often difficult to determine whether the ureter is compromised by extrinsic compression, distortion of the anatomy, or intrinsic disease. Therefore, careful evaluation of the ureteral anatomy is essential even when the obstruction appears to result from extrinsic compression, such as an endometrioma adherent to the pelvic side wall. After proper identification of the ureter, which may be facilitated by prior insertion of illuminated catheters, commencing at the pelvic brim this organ is carefully examined for any lesions and/or factors causing constriction. Depending on the findings, the ureter is liberated from extrinsic adhesions or diseases and any intrinsic lesions excised.

Adhesiolysis should be performed mechanically, without the use of electrical energy, in order not to compromise the ureter. Superficial lesions are treated by simple excision of the nodule, which is accomplished mechanically using sharp scissors. Lesions involving the muscularis are better treated by segmental excision of the affected portion using scissors without any energy. This is followed by end-to-end anastomosis of the two segments of ureter, using interrupted sutures of 5-0 absorbable monofilament. Rarely, the length of the excised segment may not permit an end-to-end anastomosis of the remaining segments and may require the reimplantation of the ureter into the bladder using the Boari flap or psoas hitch technique.

THERAPEUTIC ASPECTS OF RETROCERVICAL AND BOWEL ENDOMETRIOSIS

Bowel involvement may be present in 3% to 37% of all cases of endometriosis (31), affecting the rectosigmoid in 90% (Fig. 6) and, less frequently, other bowel segments such as the cecum, appendix (Fig. 7), terminal ileum, and jejunum (32,33).

In cases of suspected bowel endometriosis, it is mandatory to carry out a thorough preoperative assessment of the clinical data and imaging to avoid facing a situation the surgical team cannot treat fully. Imaging should be carried out by professionals with specific knowledge of this disease. It primarily includes TVUS, which provides clear evidence about ovarian endometriosis, deep endometriosis involving the retrocervical region, the rectovaginal septum, and the rectum itself. A TVUS, performed by a trained specialist, can demonstrate the size and site of the lesion and, if the rectum is involved, the layers of the organ that are affected by the disease (Fig. 8); it can also predict the distance between the lesion and the anal border (13,15). MRI also has an important place, especially in determining the morphologic characteristics of the lesion, when a trained ultrasonographer is not available for the TVUS.

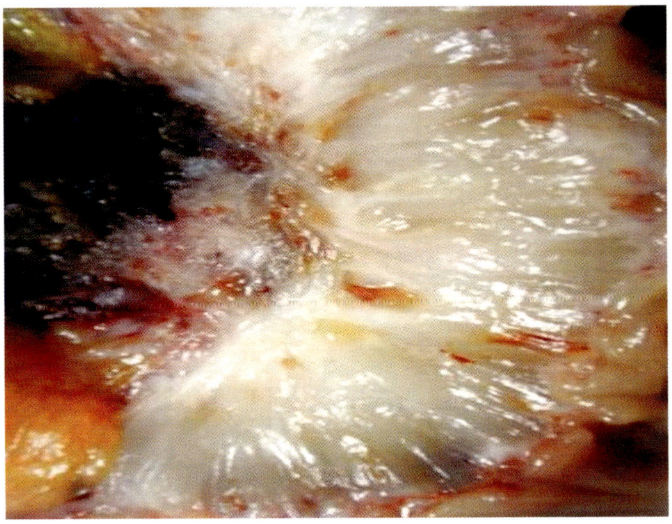

Figure 6 Endometriosis affecting the rectum.

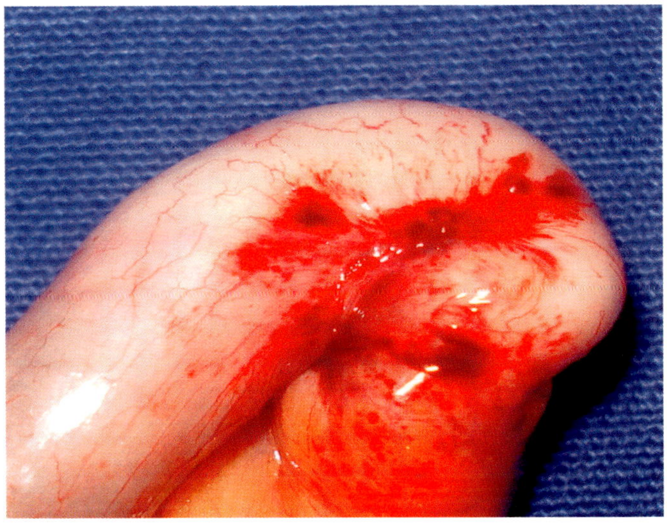

Figure 7 Appendix endometriosis.

We demonstrated that the sensitivity and specificity for bowel and retrocervical endometriosis are lower with MRI in comparison to that with TVUS (13). The aim of imaging is to determine the appropriate procedure for the patient and anticipate its level of complexity. The surgical procedure may require a multidisciplinary team including gynecologists, urologists, and bowel surgeons, since only excision of all visible and palpable lesions of the disease, avoiding complications, will result in a real benefit to the patient.

Evaluating the symptoms of 70 patients with bowel endometriosis undergoing laparoscopic treatment, Abrão et al. (34) reported complaints of dysmenorrhea in all cases, and in 38.8% the severity of the pain prevented them from carrying out their routine activities. Deep dyspareunia, likely caused by local lesions, was present in 72.2% of cases and acyclic pelvic pain in 66.7%. Cyclical bowel symptoms were present in 88.9% of cases and were significantly related to bowel endometriosis. Cyclical bowel symptoms were the principal complaint in 50% of patients ($n = 35$) and included pelvic pain at evacuation and/or diarrhea during menstruation and, more characteristically, blood in the feces during menstrual periods. Physical examination was suggestive of deep endometriosis in 73.3% of cases. In view of this observation, the value of the physical examination should not be underestimated; this examination should be carried out systematically, as it may result in identification of areas of thickness and nodules in the anterior and posterior cul-de-sac and in the uterosacral ligaments as well as in the rectovaginal septum.

The medical treatment of deep endometriosis and endometriosis of the rectovaginal septum remains controversial. Fedele et al. (35) reported an important improvement in pain during six months of treatment with gonadotropin-releasing hormone (GnRH) analogs; however, there was early recurrence after discontinuing the treatment. The discrete but significant reduction in the size of the endometriotic lesions

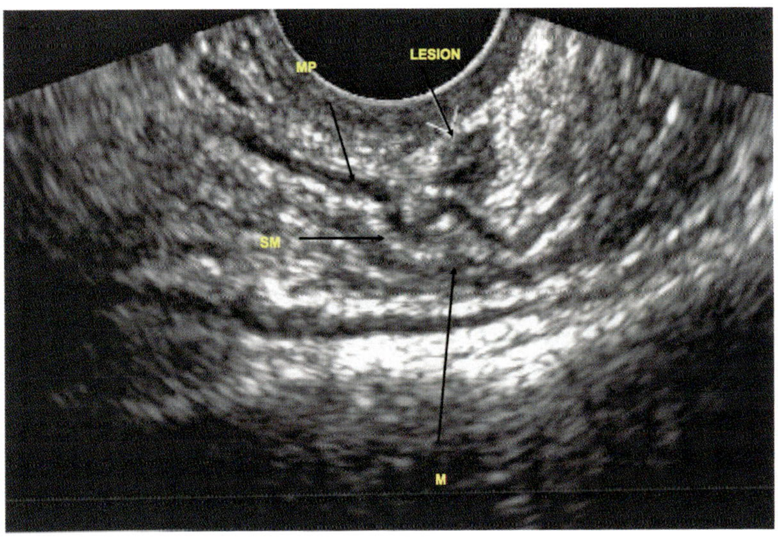

Figure 8 Transvaginal ultrasound with bowel preparation showing the layers of endometriosis infiltrated by the lesion. MP, muscularis; SM, submucosa; M, Mucosa.

during therapy disappeared six months after the treatment with GnRH. The guidelines published by the European Society of Reproductive Medicine offer recommendations with respect to this subject: In cases of deep endometriosis, there is no evidence that hormonal suppression of ovarian function is effective for the treatment of infertility. Furthermore, the patient is unable to achieve pregnancy during the treatment and thereafter until normal ovulatory function is reestablished. However, for the sole treatment of pelvic pain, this alternative, irrespective of the drug used (combined oral hormonal contraceptives, danazol, gestrinone, medroxyprogesterone acetate, or GnRH agonists), is effective when used for a period not greater than six months (23).

With regard to deep endometriosis associated primarily with pain, there appears to be a consensus in the literature that the treatment of choice is surgical (36–41). Surgical access may be achieved by laparotomy or laparoscopy, depending on the surgeon's experience and the extent of the disease.

In infertility patients with deep endometriosis, there are no randomized controlled studies or meta-analyses to support that the surgical treatment is preferable.

Abrão et al. (42) evaluated cases of bowel endometriosis and observed that endometriosis lesions that compromise the rectum deeper than the inner muscularis layer have more than 40% of the circumference of the rectum affected by the disease. On the other hand, when the superficial or serous layer of the bowel wall is affected, these same authors recommend resection of the nodule only.

Whenever deep endometriosis is clinically suspected, adequate preoperative bowel preparation is recommended. Antibiotic prophylaxis should be administered at the induction of anesthesia, using preferably a second-generation cephalosporin administered intravenously.

The surgical technique we employ for laparoscopic segmental resection of rectum affected by endometriosis comprises the following successive steps:

- Placement of an umbilical incision.
- Insufflation of CO_2 through the Veres needle to obtain proper pneumoperitoneum and subsequent insertion of a 10-mm trocar and optics.
- Insertion of three auxiliary trocars, two at the iliac fossa (10/12 mm on the right and 5 mm on the left) and a 5 mm trocar in the left flank.
- Examination of the abdominal and pelvic cavity and identification of all the sites affected by endometriosis.
- Lysis of the any adhesions affecting adnexal regions, uterine fundus, posterior cul-de-sac, uterosacral ligaments, and relevant bowel adhesions.
- Release of the sigmoid from the left lateral abdominal wall and from the retroperitoneum; identification of the left ureter up to the level of the pelvic brim.
- Opening of the mesosigmoid.
- Mobilization of the rectum by dissecting its anterior wall from the posterior surface of the cervix, following which a linear stapler is applied distal to the area affected by the disease (Fig. 9).
- Thereafter, the 10/12-mm incision on the right iliac fossa is enlarged sufficiently to exteriorize the divided bowel enclosing the diseased portion. The proximal stump is sutured to form a pouch; the ogive of the circular stapler is placed inside the stump (Fig. 10).
- The bowel containing the ogive is reintroduced into the abdominal cavity, and the abdominal incision is closed.

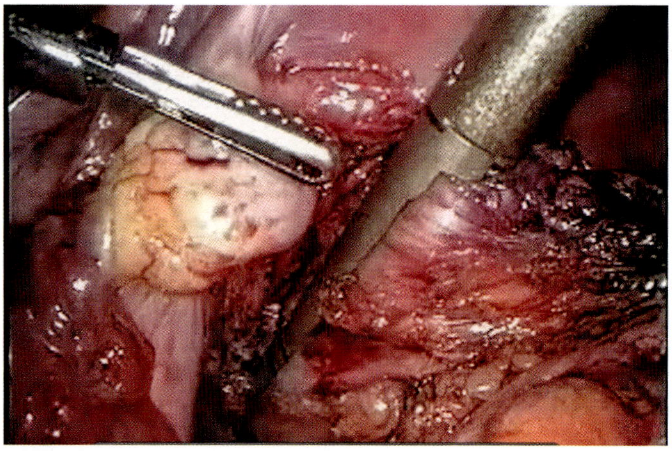

Figure 9 Linear stapler applied to the rectum, distal to the area affected by the disease.

- The circular stapler is then introduced through the anus and connected to the ogive, and the stapler is activated to form the end-to-end anastomosis.

The next step is to ascertain the integrity of the ureters and the anastomotic site. The latter is checked under laparoscopic control, by injecting 120 mL of air into the rectum, which is submerged in irrigation fluid to ensure that there is no leakage. In addition, a dilute solution of methylene blue or Betadine is introduced into the rectum to confirm absence of leakage. This procedure is performed in many other institutions, as evident from Table 1.

The principal issue with regard to surgical treatment of bowel endometriosis is why segmentary bowel resection should be carried out rather than simple resection of nodules when the lesions are deep. Published evidence in support of resection includes the following studies: Remorgida et al. (43) investigated 16 patients with bowel endometriosis and an indication for segmentary bowel resection based on an analysis of the depth of lesions. At surgery, they initially resected the individual endometriotic nodules from the bowel and thereafter performed a segmental resection of the affected portion

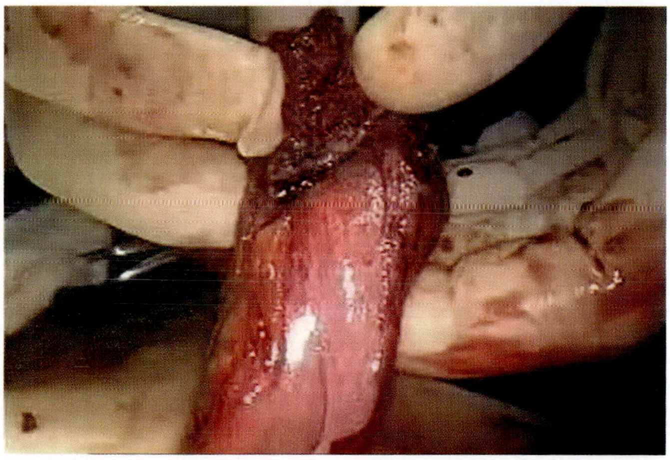

Figure 10 Rectum with endometriosis exteriorized on the right iliac fossa.

Table 1 Surgical Treatment of Bowel Endometriosis

	N	Surgery	Laparoscopy N (%)	Complications N (%)
Garry, 2000 (44)	57	Shaving	57 (100)	-
Duepree, 2002 (39)	51	26 shavings 5 disk excisions 18 segmentary resections	47 (92.1)	5(9.8)
Varol, 2003 (49)	169	132 shavings 12 disk excisions 25 segmentary resections	145 (85.8)	21 (12.4)
Ford, 2004 (50)	60	48 shavings 2 disk excisions 10 segmentary resections	48 (80)	
Dubernard, 2006 (56)	58	Segmentary resection	51 (87.9)	9 (15.5)

of bowel, as previously planned. In 7 of the 16 cases (43.8%), endometriotic tissue was found in the bowel wall adjacent to the site of nodule resection. This study confirms that nodule resection alone frequently leaves behind the diseased tissue.

Postoperative quality of life has been shown to be directly related to complete resection of deep lesions of the intestinal tract and other sites. Similar studies carried out by Garry et al. (44), Varol et al. (45), Ford et al. (46), and Dubernard et al. (47) used quality-of-life questionnaires to analyze the response of patients to "radical" surgical treatment for deep endometriosis. All concluded that there was a significant improvement in the parameters analyzed in the questionnaires, with rates of improvement in quality of life ranging from 85% to 90% and reported 36-month recurrence rates of around 10% to 15%.

Possover et al. (48) recommended that, irrespective of the access route, dissection of the uterine arteries and both ureters is essential to ensure that the subadjacent tissues are free of endometriosis (48). Laparoscopic palpation of tissues, prior to resection, should also be performed in order to select an adequate dissection plane for complete removal of the infiltrated area.

More recently, the possibility of lymph node involvement has been described in cases of endometriosis affecting the rectum and sigmoid. In a series of 40 consecutive segmentary resections, Abrão et al. (33) reported that, during pathologic examination of the specimens, in 19 of the 40 cases lymph nodes were detected in the surgical specimens, and in 26% of these 19 cases the lymph nodes were found to have endometriosis. It must be noted that positive lymph nodes were present in 100% of the cases, in which the disease was affecting more than 80% of the circumference of the rectum; the thicker the lesion, the greater the probability of lymph node involvement. These data illustrate the aggressive nature of this disease.

Since laparoscopic bowel resection is a complex surgical procedure, patients should be frequently monitored during the postoperative period for any complications. In an initial series of 100 cases, Reich et al. (26) reported four cases of rectal perforation, all successfully treated by laparoscopy. In a series of 225 women who underwent surgery for deep endometriosis, Koninckx et al. (49) reported injury of the uterine artery in two patients and inadvertently bisection of the ureter in one. In addition, there were six patients with bowel perforations, all of whom were diagnosed postoperatively (49). The two arterial lesions were repaired with a clip, the ureter was anastomosed, and in two of the six cases of bowel perforation the defects were sutured laparoscopically. As per the experience of the Endometriosis Division of Sao Paulo University (Brazil), out of 170 patients with severe endometriosis compromising the rectum submitted to a segmental resection of the bowel due to the extension of the disease, the laparoscopy was converted into laparotomy in 2 cases and there were 3 (1.8%) cases of leakage of the anastomosis, 1 case of postoperative abscess (0.6%), and 1 case (0.6%) of urinary retention that was reverted after three months.

CONCLUSIONS

Deep endometriosis requires a thorough preoperative investigation and an appropriate subsequent surgical planning. It is imperative to perform a careful, thorough, and critical preoperative analysis of the clinical data and the findings of the imaging techniques used to plan the appropriate treatment and surgical approach. Thereafter, the surgical approach for the various parts of the procedure will depend on the symptoms of the patient and the extent of invasion of each organ involved by the disease. The surgical team must be multidisciplinary and composed of gynecologists, urologists, and digestive tract surgeons, as necessary, since all visible and palpable lesions of the disease must be excised for the patient to reap any real benefits, bearing in mind that the concept of "one-shot surgery" is the best option to avoid persistence of lesions and minimize the rate of recurrence of the disease following surgery.

REFERENCES

1. Cornillie FJ, Oosterlynck D, Lauweryns JM, et al. Deeply infiltrating pelvic endometriosis: Histology and clinical significance. Fertil Steril 1990; 53(6):978–983.
2. Koninckx PR, Martin DC. Deep endometriosis: A consequence of infiltration or retraction or possibly adenomyosis externa? Fertil Steril 1992; 58(5):924–928.
3. Donnez J, Nisolle M, Casanas-Roux F, et al. Rectovaginal septum, endometriosis or adenomyosis: Laparoscopic management in a series of 231 patients. Hum Reprod 1995; 10(3):630–635.
4. Martin DC, Batt RE. Retrocervical, retrovaginal pouch, and rectovaginal septum endometriosis. J Am Assoc Gynecol Laparosc 2001; 8(1):12–17.
5. Guerriero S, Ajossa S, Gerada M, et al. Diagnostic value of transvaginal 'tenderness-guided' ultrasonography for the prediction of location of deep endometriosis. Hum Reprod 2008; 23(11):2452–2457.
6. Brosens IA, Brosens JJ. Redefining endometriosis: Is deep endometriosis a progressive disease? Hum Reprod 2000; 15(1): 1–3.

7. Vercellini P, Fedele L, Aimi G, et al. Association between endometriosis stage, lesion type, patient characteristics and severity of pelvic pain symptoms: A multivariate analysis of over 1000 patients. Hum Reprod 2007; 22(1):266–271.
8. Chêne G, Jaffeux P, Lasnier C, et al. Are there anatomical and clinical correlations between minimal and deep endometriosis? First results of Auvergne's Registry of Endometriosis. Gynecol Obstet Fertil 2008; 36(1):17–22.
9. Griffiths AN, Koutsouridou RN, Penketh RJ. Predicting the presence of rectovaginal endometriosis from the clinical history: A retrospective observational study. J Obstet Gynaecol 2007; 27(6):605–607.
10. Panel P, Renouvel F. Management of endometriosis: Clinical and biological assessment. J Gynecol Obstet Biol Reprod (Paris) 2007; 36(2):119–128.
11. Koninckx PR, Meuleman C, Oosterlynck D, et al. Diagnosis of deep endometriosis by clinical examination during menstruation and plasma CA-125 concentration. Fertil Steril 1996; 65(2):280–287.
12. Chapron C, Barakat H, Fritel X, et al. Presurgical diagnosis of posterior deep infiltrating endometriosis based on a standardized questionnaire. Hum Reprod 2005; 20(2):507–513.
13. Abrão MS, Goncalves MO, Dias JA Jr, et al. Comparison between clinical examination, transvaginal sonography and magnetic resonance imaging for the diagnosis of deep endometriosis. Hum Reprod 2007; 22(12):3092–3097.
14. Bazot M, Malzy P, Cortez A, et al. Accuracy of transvaginal sonography and rectal endoscopic sonography in the diagnosis of deep infiltrating endometriosis. Ultrasound Obstet Gynecol 2007; 30(7):994–1001.
15. Goncalves MO, Dias JA Jr, Podgaec S, et al. Transvaginal ultrasound for diagnosis of deeply infiltrating endometriosis. Int J Gynaecol Obstet 2009; 104(2):156–160.
16. Stratton P, Winkel C, Premkumar A, et al. Diagnostic accuracy of laparoscopy, magnetic resonance imaging, and histopathologic examination for the detection of endometriosis. Fertil Steril 2003; 79(5):1078–1085.
17. Roy C, Balzan C, Thoma V, et al. Efficiency of MR imaging to orientate surgical treatment of posterior deep pelvic endometriosis. Abdom Imaging 2009; 34(2):251–259.
18. Salvatores M, Landi S, Ceccaroni M, et al. The laparoscopic treatment of bladder endometriosis. A retrospective analysis of 21 cases. Minerva Ginecol 2007; 59(1):19–25.
19. Abrão MS, Podgaec S, Filho BM, et al. The use of biochemical markers in the diagnosis of pelvic endometriosis. Hum Reprod 1997; 12(11):2523–2527.
20. Seeber B, Sammel MD, Fan X, et al. Panel of markers can accurately predict endometriosis in a subset of patients. Fertil Steril 2008; 89(5):1073–1081.
21. Hart R, Hickey M, Maouris P, et al. Excisional surgery versus ablative surgery for ovarian endometriomata: A Cochrane review. Hum Reprod 2005; 20(11):3000–3007.
22. Nishida M, Watanabe K, Sato N, et al. Malignant transformation of ovarian endometriosis. Gynecol Obstet Invest 2000; 50(Suppl 1):18–25.
23. Kennedy S, Bergqvist A, Chapron C, et al. ESHRE guideline for the diagnosis and treatment of endometriosis. Hum Reprod 2005; 20(10):2698–2704.
24. Revised American Society for Reproductive Medicine. Classification of endometriosis: 1996. Fertil Steril 1997; 67(5):817–821.
25. Wyns C, Donnez J. Laser vaporization of ovarian endometriomas: The impact on the response to gonadotrophin stimulation. Gynecol Obstet Fertil 2003; 31(4):337–342.
26. Reich H, McGlynn F, Salvat J. Laparoscopic treatment of cul-de-sac obliteration secondary to retrocervical deep fibrotic endometriosis. J Reprod Med 1991; 36(7):516–522.
27. Generao SE, Keene KD, Das S. Endoscopic diagnosis and management of ureteral endometriosis. J Endourol 2005; 19(10):1177–1179.
28. Vercellini P, Meschia M, De Giorgi O, et al. Bladder detrusor endometriosis: Clinical and pathogenetic implications. J Urol 1996; 155(1):84–86.
29. Vercellini P, Frontino G, Pietropaolo G, et al. Deep endometriosis: Definition, pathogenesis, and clinical management. J Am Assoc Gynecol Laparosc 2004; 11(2):153–161.
30. Vercellini P, Frontino G, Pisacreta A, et al. The pathogenesis of bladder detrusor endometriosis. Am J Obstet Gynecol 2002; 187(3):538–542.
31. Zwas FR, Lyon DT. Endometriosis. An important condition in clinical gastroenterology. Dig Dis Sci 1991; 36(3):353–364.
32. Abrão MS, Podgaec S, Carvalho FM, et al. Bowel endometriosis and mucocele of the appendix. J Minim Invasive Gynecol 2005; 12(4):299–300.
33. Abrão MS, Podgaec S, Dias JA Jr, et al. Deeply infiltrating endometriosis affecting the rectum and lymph nodes. Fertil Steril 2006; 86(3):543–547.
34. Abrão MS, Neme RM, Averbach M. Rectovaginal septum endometriosis: A disease with specific diagnosis and treatment. Arq Gastroenterol 2003; 40(3):192–197.
35. Fedele L, Bianchi S, Zanconato G, et al. Gonadotropin-releasing hormone agonist treatment for endometriosis of the rectovaginal septum. Am J Obstet Gynecol 2000; 183(6):1462–1467.
36. Jerby BL, Kessler H, Falcone T, et al. Laparoscopic management of colorectal endometriosis. Surg Endosc 1999; 13(11):1125–1128.
37. Redwine DB, Wright JT. Laparoscopic treatment of complete obliteration of the cul-de-sac associated with endometriosis: Long-term follow-up of en bloc resection. Fertil Steril 2001; 76(2):358–365.
38. Varol N, Maher P, Woods R. Laparoscopic management of intestinal endometriosis. J Am Assoc Gynecol Laparosc 2000; 7(3):405–409.
39. Duepree HJ, Senagore AJ, Delaney CP, et al. Laparoscopic resection of deep pelvic endometriosis with rectosigmoid involvement. J Am Coll Surg 2002; 195(6):754–758.
40. Minelli L, Barbieri F, Fiaccavento A, et al. Complete laparoscopic removal of endometriosis for the management of pain symptomatology. J Am Assoc Gynecol Laparosc 2003; 10(S):11.
41. Senagore AJ, Duepree HJ, Delaney CP, et al. Results of a standardized technique and postoperative care plan for laparoscopic sigmoid colectomy: A 30-month experience. Dis Colon Rectum 2003, 46(4):503–509.
42. Abrão et al (2008). Endometriosis lesions that compromise the rectum deeper than the inner muscularis layer have more than 40% of the circumference of the rectum affected by the disease. J Am Gynecol Laparosc 2008; 1(3):280–285.
43. Remorgida V, Ragni N, Ferrero S, et al. How complete is full thickness disc resection of bowel endometriotic lesions? A prospective surgical and histological study. Hum Reprod 2005; 20(8):2317–2320.
44. Garry R, Clayton R, Hawe J. The effect of endometriosis and its radical laparoscopic excision on quality of life indicators. BJOG 2000; 107(1):44–54.
45. Varol N, Maher P, Healey M, et al. Rectal surgery for endometriosis – should we be aggressive? J Am Assoc Gynecol Laparosc 2003; 10(2):182–189.
46. Ford J, English J, Miles WA, et al. Pain, quality of life and complications following the radical resection of rectovaginal endometriosis. BJOG 2004; 111(4):353–356.
47. Dubernard G, Piketty M, Rouzier R, et al. Quality of life after laparoscopic colorectal resection for endometriosis. Hum Reprod 2006; 21(5):1243–1247.
48. Possover M, Diebolder H, Plaul K, et al. Laparoscopically-assisted vaginal resection of rectovaginal endometriosis. Obstet Gynecol 2000; 96(2):304–307.
49. Koninckx PR, Poppe W, Deprest J. Carbon dioxide laser for laparoscopic enterocele repair. J Am Assoc Gynecol Laparosc 1995; 2(2):181–185.

12

Surgical treatment of intraperitoneal adhesions

Dingeman J. Swank and Victor Gomel

Adhesions are found in 68% to 100% of patients who have had abdominal surgery (1–3). Fortunately, most patients with intra-abdominal adhesions have no complaints. However, 35% of approximately 30,000 patients who had open abdominal surgery were readmitted to hospital for adhesion-related disorders during the five years that followed the initial intervention (4). The rate was similar for patients who had open gynecological surgery, with an average of two readmissions per patient (4,5). After abdominal surgery, 3% to 5% of patients will suffer from the specific consequences of these abdominal adhesions (6), which include bowel obstructions (1,7), chronic abdominal pain (8), and infertility (9).

SURGICAL TREATMENT OF INTRAPERITONEAL ADHESIONS

General Considerations

Undertaking surgery for adhesions seems contradictory, since adhesions do develop after each laparotomy; the number and extent of abdominal adhesions are related to the number and type of previous laparotomies (10). In humans, there is limited, but not convincing, evidence that surgical access by laparoscopy is associated with less adhesion formation compared to laparotomy (11,12). In a retrospective study by Polymeneas and coworkers, a significantly lower adhesion rate was noted in a laparoscopic cholecystectomy patient group compared to open cholecystectomy. Their analysis was performed many years after the cholecystectomy during a repeat laparotomy for various indications (13). This study also demonstrated de novo adhesion formation (adhesions at sites where these were not present at the first operation and distant from the operative field) after laparoscopic surgery, although less than with open surgery. Repeat laparoscopy for recurrent chronic abdominal pain after previous laparoscopic adhesiolysis demonstrated decreased adhesion formation between organs and abdominal wall (8). A review by Gutt and coworkers concluded that laparoscopic surgery caused fewer adhesions compared to open surgery in most clinical and experimental studies (14).

There is sufficient evidence to suggest that laparoscopy is associated with lesser de novo adhesions, away from the principal surgical site, compared with laparotomy. This is not the case at the site of primary surgery. This was assessed in an experimental animal study by Filmar et al. (15). Using microsurgical technique, a standard trauma, in the form of three incisions at approximately 1-cm intervals, was placed through the serosa and superficial muscularis of one of the uterine horns, either by laparotomy or by laparoscopy. Postoperative adhesions were assessed two weeks later by second-look laparotomy during which the adhesions involving the uterine horn were lysed using microscissor under the magnification of an operating microscope. The resulting raw patches on the uterine surface were stained with methylene blue solution and measured with a millimeter-graded transparency and expressed in millimeter square (mm^2). All surgical procedures were carried out by the same investigator. The mean surface area of uterine adhesions in the laparotomy group was 4.29 mm^2 versus 8.88 mm^2 in the laparoscopy group. This outcome surprised us since we expected the opposite to occur. Although the difference did not reach statistical significance, this we believe was due to the limited total sample size of 31 animals (15). Subsequent clinical evidence corroborated these findings (16).

Indications for Surgical Treatment

Nearly all patients of both sexes develop intra-abdominal adhesions after abdominal surgery. Five percent of these patients will ever suffer from the consequences of these adhesions with conditions such as bowel obstruction, strangulation, chronic pain, and infertility. Little doubt exists about the indication of adhesiolysis for bowel obstruction, but adhesiolysis by open surgery for chronic pain or infertility is subject for criticism. Laparoscopic approach is both adequate and safe for adhesiolysis. A repeat laparotomy will likely aggravate the extent of pre-existing adhesions and therefore not recommended for adhesiolysis, except for acute bowel obstruction.

Bowel Obstruction

Bowel obstruction generally involves the small intestine and occurs in 1% to 12% of cases after a laparotomy (1), especially after colorectal surgery, appendectomy, and gynecological procedures (17). Surgical access is predominantly by laparotomy, because laparoscopic approach is usually difficult due to the existing abdominal distension that limits the extent of the pneumoperitoneum, which in turn limits free space and proper handling of the abdominal organs. Most of the adhesions causing the obstruction are situated between the bowel on the one side and the retroperitoneum on the other side. Recurrent small bowel obstruction occurs in 28% of patients after adhesiolysis. Mortality figures for acute bowel obstruction exceed 10% (3)

Infertility

Pelvic and periadnexal adhesions may cause infertility in reproductive-age women. Adhesions frequently are the sequel of pelvic inflammatory disease (PID). These adhesions may be broad or shallow; they are usually not too vascular and extend from one structure to another, from tube to ovary, uterus to adnexa, pelvic side wall to adnexa, etc. In doing so, they tend to leave a space or potential space between the involved structures, a characteristic that facilitates adhesiolysis. When PID progresses to abscess formation, the resulting adhesions are dense and organs may be intimately adherent to one another. This type of adhesions may also result from endometriosis and prior pelvic surgery. When adjacent structures are intimately conglutinated, the adherent area is devoid of the superficial, mesothelial layer of peritoneum. In other words, the underlying stromal layers of the two structures coalesce. The lysis of such an adhesive process is technically difficult and is associated with a very high percentage of recurrence, unless the two denuded surfaces can be separated or an effective antiadhesive barrier is placed between the two apposing surfaces.

Periadnexal adhesions may be the sole abnormality causing infertility; they encapsulate an otherwise patent tube and/or the ovary and prevent the oocyte to be captured by the fimbriae. Periovarian adhesions may also adversely affect follicular development, as has been demonstrated in both animal and human studies. The association of postoperative adhesions and infertility is well recognized. Gomel reported a series of laparoscopic salpingo-ovariolysis of 90 patients, whose primary cause of infertility was periadnexal adhesions. In 40 (44%) of these 90 women, the cause of periadnexal adhesions and resulting infertility was secondary to prior surgical procedures such as ovarian surgery, myomectomy, removal of ectopic pregnancy, etc. (18).

One of the major causes of failure of reconstructive surgery for tubal infertility has been postoperative adhesions: de novo adhesions and reformation of existing adhesions following lysis. This was one of the major reasons for the introduction of microsurgical techniques in reproductive surgery and their application by both open and laparoscopic access (19).

Salpingo-ovariolysis by laparoscopic access in women in whom periadnexal adhesions are the primary cause of infertility yields a live birth rate of around 50% to 60% (20–23). For detailed description of this technique, see chapter 23.

Chronic Pain

Laparoscopic adhesiolysis for chronic pain remains controversial. Some authors deny that adhesions can cause chronic abdominal pain (24–29), while many others believe the contrary and report good results after laparoscopic adhesiolysis (Table 1). The presence of sensory nerve fibers in adhesions was demonstrated in 2001, postulating pain conduction to be a product of their own stimulation, and not pain indirectly induced by peritoneal traction. However, in these series, 20% of the patients had nerve fibers in their adhesions but had no history of chronic abdominal pain (30). Laparoscopic adhesiolysis for chronic pain results in a significant reduction of the extent, type, and severity of the adhesions between the abdominal organs and the abdominal wall, as demonstrated at second-look laparoscopy. De novo adhesions occur in approximately 20% of patients subjected to laparoscopic adhesiolysis (31).

Table 1 Outcome of Laparoscopic Adhesiolysis in Patients with Chronic Abdominopelvic Pain and No Other Cause for Their Pain Than Adhesions (29)

Study	Number of patients	Cured or improved
Klingensmith et al. (25)	19	14 (75%)
Miller et al. (49)	19	16 (84%)
Nezhat et al. (50)	48	22 (46%)
Lavonius et al. (52)	24	17 (71%)
Nezhat et al. (51)	48	36 (67%)
Schietroma et al. (53)	45	34 (75%)
Schmidbauer et al. (54)	44	37 (84%)
Swank et al. (55)	167	134 (80%)
Swank et al. (8)	200	148 (74%)
Swank et al. (28)	52	30 (57%)
Onders and Mittendorf (27)	45	32 (71%)
Dunker and Bemelman (56)	23	10 (44%)

Surgical Technique

Critical in the procedure of laparoscopic adhesiolysis are the insertion of the insufflation needle, placement of the trocar, and the adhesiolysis itself.

Pneumoperitoneum

In patients who had previous abdominal surgery, the choice of the site and technique of initial access to the peritoneal cavity is very important. The traditional technique is transumbilical, blind insertion of the Veress needle. Such an approach causes bowel perforations in 0.04% and major bleeding in 0.04% of patients, whereas the open laparoscopy technique of surgically entering the peritoneal cavity through the umbilical site is rarely associated with vascular injuries but does not guard against bowel injuries (0.11%) (32). Elevation of the abdominal wall prior to needle introduction increases the distance to the major vessels but does not guard against injury of the bowel adherent to the abdominal wall (33).

With patients at risk, it is much safer to introduce the Veress needle through the Palmer point, in the left upper quadrant of the abdomen, 3 cm distal from the subcostal margin in the midclavicular line; create the pneumoperitoneum; and visualize the peritoneal cavity by inserting a mini endoscope through the same point. This approach permits the visualization of the peritoneal cavity and sites in which omentum and bowel are adherent to the anterior abdominal wall and select an appropriate safe site to introduce the principal trocar and laparoscope (34). This technique was used in a study reported by Audebert and Gomel (34); it included 814 consecutive patients undergoing laparoscopy. The purpose of the study was to determine the incidence of umbilical adhesions and the potential risk of bowel injury with blind insertion of the umbilical (principal) trocar. The subjects were divided into four groups: those in group I had no previous abdominal surgery, group II had prior laparoscopic surgery, group III had previous laparotomy with a horizontal suprapubic incision, and group IV had previous laparotomy with a midline incision. Patients who had adhesions were assessed as to whether or not they were at significant risk of injury from blind insertion of the principal trocar. The rates of umbilical adhesions were as follows: group I, 0.68%; group II, 1.6%; group III, 19.8%; and group IV, 51.7%. Severe adhesions with potential risk of bowel injury with blind insertion of the umbilical trocar in the four groups were 0.42%, 0.80%, 6.87%, and 31.46%, respectively. The study clearly demonstrated that subjects with previous laparotomy have a higher incidence of umbilical adhesions, especially in case of midline incision (34). The findings of this study have been subsequently confirmed by others (35). The point of initial entry in the left upper quadrant of the abdomen is a relatively safe site, since the parietal peritoneum here is fixed to the abdominal wall, the bowel is covered with omentum, and the spleen is situated 5 inches away, cranially (36).

Peritoneal hyperdistention with a pressure up to 25 mm Hg was performed to elevate the abdominal wall in order to create a larger space for trocar insertion (37). Phillips et al. found that using a downward force of 3 kg, the distance between the tip of the trocar and the abdominal organs increased from 0.6 to 5.6 cm when the insufflation pressure used was 25 versus 10 mm Hg (38). Once the trocar was inserted, the pressure was reduced to 16 mm Hg. No complications related to peritoneal entry were noted; no untoward physical changes happened (37).

Introduction of the Primary Trocar

A significant percentage of the major complications with laparoscopic surgery are associated with the insertion of the primary trocar through which the laparoscope will be introduced. More than half of these bowel lesions are not recognized during the procedure, when they are gastrointestinal or urinary, and diagnosed postoperatively when the patient returns with an acute abdomen as a result of peritonitis.

The so-called "safety shield trocars" do not reduce the rate of trocar injury (39). Radially dilating trocars have the advantage of less abdominal wall bleeding and less trocar site hernias, but do not reduce vascular or bowel risks. An optic trocar provides visual control of all abdominal layers during the introduction and has all the advantages of the radially dilating trocar. Visual control will permit the surgeon to notice presence of organs that are adherent at the entry site and to select another site. The optic trocar can be inserted directly into the abdominal cavity without prior pneumoperitoneum. This can be a solution for patients prone to Veress needle injuries such as obese patients and those with previous laparotomies (40).

Adhesiolysis

Adhesiolysis can be performed with various energy forms including sharp dissection. Some authors report good results with use of the CO_2 laser (41), although laser has been shown to be associated with more tissue damage compared to electrosurgery (42). Sharp dissection is the safest mode, especially close to bowel and major vessels; despite the disadvantage of the multiple small bleedings that may obscure visibility for further dissection. The use of a true microelectrode permits precise and effective dissection without touching the tissue and very limited adjacent damage; however, next to bowel or major vessels, the safest approach is indeed sharp dissection using an appropriate type of sharp scissors. This avoids necrosis due to thermal injury, which will cause delayed perforation of the vessel or bowel (43).

Since the year 2000, Swank has used ultrasonic dissection (Ultracision, Ethicon Endo-surgery, Cincinnati, Ohio) for laparoscopic adhesiolysis. The application of ultrasound to the tissues, with this equipment, produces three effects: cavitation, coagulation, and cutting, which act synergistically. This technique combines good hemostasis and dissection and, as a consequence, significantly reduces the need to change instruments (40). Ultrasonic adhesiolysis may be applicable to many types of abdominal adhesions. In 98% of 105 patients with chronic abdominal pain, simple as well as broad adhesions could be almost completely lysed with ultrasonic technique. Interloop or interorgan adhesions are more prone for perforations during lysis, but the risk is less with ultrasonic compared with electrical technique (40).

Results

Chronic abdominal pain remains a diagnostic challenge. Laparoscopy can visualize pathology that could not be diagnosed otherwise. If adhesions per se have to be considered as "pathological," the diagnostic value of laparoscopy can be as high as 96% in patients who had prior abdominal surgery. If adhesions are to be considered as physiological, other pathology will be found in 5% to 50% of patients with chronic abdominal pain (44). Twelve studies of laparoscopic adhesiolysis (1996–2006) were reviewed. In these retrospective analyses, pain relief after laparoscopic adhesiolysis varied from 46% to 84% (Table 1).

Table 2 The Influence of Several Factors on the Results of Laparoscopic Adhesiolysis for Chronic Pain in 200 Patients

	Pain-free number (%)	Not pain-free number (%)	*P*-value
Patients	79 (40%)	121 (60%)	
Factors:			
Gender (%)			0.02[a]
Male	28 (54%)	24 (46%)	
Female	51 (34%)	97 (65%)	
Age median (yr)	44 (9-79)	47 (6-81)	0.02
Duration of pain Median (mo)	12 (1-132)	12 (1-180)	0.24
Number of previous operations (median)	2 (0-23)	2 (0-18)	0.77
Type of previous operation (%)[b]			
Appendectomy	39 (49%)	56 (46%)	0.77
Gynecological procedures[c]	21 (41%)	54 (56%)	0.12-0.24
Others	41 (52%)	74 (61%)	
Instrument (%)[d]			0.12
Argon laser	19 (24%)	15 (13%)	
Scissors	25 (34%)	46 (40%)	
Electrocoagulation	15 (20%)	33 (28%)	
Ultracision	15 (20%)	22 (19%)	
Completeness (%)			0.19
Complete	69 (87%)	96 (79%)	
Almost complete	7 (9%)	12 (10%)	
Incomplete	3 (4%)	13 (11%)	
Major complications number (%)	3 (4%)	9 (7%)	0.37

Pain-free patients (disappearance of pain) versus not pain free patients (less pain, unchanged pain, or worse pain) (8).
[a]Subgroup analysis: gender difference was only significant comparing males with females with previous gynecological operations ($P = 0.005$)
[b]Total percentage more than 100% because of more previous operations in many patients.
[c]Percentages related to female patients only.
[d]Total number of patients is 190, treated with only one single technique.

The influence of several factors, on the results of laparoscopic adhesiolysis for chronic pain, was analyzed in a prospective study. Three months after the laparoscopic adhesiolysis, 40% of patients were pain free and 60% were not (they had less, unchanged, or worse pain). Multivariate analysis showed that age and being a female with prior gynecological operations were both independent factors related to the probability of becoming pain free (Table 2). It is noteworthy that the results for patients whose adhesions were completely lysed were not different from those who had incomplete lysis of their adhesions (Table 3).

Swank et al. designed a blinded, randomized study in 116 patients suffering from chronic abdominal pain. These patients underwent diagnostic laparoscopy, and those in whom the only abnormal finding was adhesions were randomly assigned to either diagnostic laparoscopy only (control group) or laparoscopic adhesiolysis. During the study, patients did not know their randomization outcome. After one

Table 3 Pain Relief in 174 Patients After Laparoscopic Adhesiolysis, and the Relation of the Relief with the Completeness of the Adhesiolysis (45)

	Good result[a]	Bad result[a]	Total
Incomplete adhesiolysis	31 (80%)	8 (20%)	39
Complete adhesiolysis	103 (80%)	25 (20%)	128
	134	33	167[b]

[a]Good result was defined as pain free and less pain, bad result as unchanged and more pain.
[b]Seven patients with conversion after laparoscopy without adhesiolysis were not evaluated.

year, the patients who had adhesiolysis, experienced significant improvement in their pain, as evident from significantly reduced VAS pain scores, MOS SF-36 scores, they required significantly less analgesics and experienced improvement of their quality of life. However, it is noteworthy that the results of treated patients were not statistically different from those in the control group (28). These outcomes suggest a substantial placebo effect. Other authors have stressed that the *therapeutic* value of *diagnostic* laparoscopy is underestimated and can be as high as 42% (25,27,28). The fact that incompleteness of the adhesiolysis did not significantly affect the pain relief supports a great role for placebo surgery. Relapse of chronic abdominal pain is as high as 26% (46) and seems more frequent the longer the follow-up (47). This relapse can be explained by regrowth of adhesions and de novo adhesion formation, but also by the wearing of a placebo effect (27).

Complications

Complications associated with laparoscopic adhesiolysis for chronic pain are comparable to those that occur during laparotomy or laparoscopy after previous abdominal surgery. In case of iterative laparotomy, bleeding, prolonged surgery, bowel perforations, an increased morbidity must be expected. The risk of bowel perforation or serosal bowel damage is 20% if a subsequent laparotomy is performed through the same incision (48).

Of 174 patients treated with laparoscopic adhesiolysis for chronic pain, major complications occurred in 16 (9%) (45); 3 patients suffered from intra-abdominal blood loss, 2 patients had postoperative strangulation and pseudoperitonitis, and 11 patients had visceral perforations. In 4 of these 11 patients, the perforation was not noticed during laparoscopy; all 4 developed generalized peritonitis and 2 of them died. This study demonstrated that older age and greater number of previous laparotomies were significantly correlated with more complications (Table 4) (45).

In 104 patients operated for chronic abdominal pain, adhesiolysis was performed with ultrasonic dissection. A complete lysis with the ultrasonic device was achieved in 98% of patients, and no additional electrocoagulation was necessary in all but two patients. In these series, four (4%) bowel perforations occurred; they were all recognized intraoperatively and repaired. There were no late perforations (40).

Table 4 Factors Associated with Complications of Laparoscopic Adhesiolysis (45)

Major complications	No	Yes	*P* value
Number of operations	158	16	
Factors			
• Gender m.%	30	19	NS
• Age mean (yr)	44 (SD 16)	55 (SD 18)	0.009
• Duration of pain			
(mo)	17	21	NS
(median)	9 (1-150)	8 (1-72)	
• Number of previous operations (median)	2 (0-21)	3 (1-23)	0.002
• Kind of previous operation (%)[a]			
○ Appendectomy	41	31	NS
○ Genecology procedure[b]	44	69	NS
○ Others	58	75	NS
• Instrument (%)[c]			
○ Argon laser	20	25	NS
○ Scissors	71	50	NS
○ Electrocoagulation	25	19	NS
• Surgical experience—First 15 patient%	26	25	NS

[a]Total percentage more than 100% because of more previous operations in many patients.
[b]Among women.
[c]In some patients, more than one technique was used.

CONCLUSIONS

Laparoscopic adhesiolysis may be indicated for adhesion-induced bowel obstruction with mild bowel distention.

Laparoscopic access is suitable to perform adhesiolysis for chronic pelvic pain. The reported rates of major complications and mortality, with this approach, are 9% and 1%, respectively. The incidence of complications can be decreased by using a primary entrance site that is away from the previous laparotomy incision. Initial visualization through the left upper quadrant of the abdomen, as described above, allows a relatively safe initial entry, which permits selection of a site for the insertion of the "primary trocar" that will house the laparoscope. The ultracision technique permits to perform an adequate adhesiolysis without thermal necrosis and diminishes postoperative bowel perforations secondary to thermal injury.

Laparoscopic adhesiolysis provides no additional pain relief in chronic pain, compared with diagnostic laparoscopy alone. Pain relief appears to be due to the diagnostic part of the procedure and not to the adhesiolysis. The observation of similar outcomes in patients with complete lysis of adhesions and those with incomplete lysis supports this conclusion. The only randomized study reported to date shows no differences in the results between the treated and the sham group, except for the complications that were more frequent in the treated group.

Laparoscopic adhesiolysis may be indicated in tubal infertility. Salpingo-ovariolysis by laparoscopic access in women in whom periadnexal adhesions are the primary cause of infertility yields a live birth rate of around 50% to 60%.

REFERENCES

1. Menzies D, Ellis H. Intestinal obstruction from adhesions – how big is the problem? Ann R Coll Surg Engl 1990; 72:60–63.
2. Luijendijk RW, de Lange DC, Wauters CC, et al. Foreign material in postoperative adhesions. Ann Surg 1996; 223:242–248.
3. Ellis H. The clinical significance of adhesions: Focus on intestinal obstruction. Eur J Surg Suppl 1997; 577:5–9.
4. Ellis H, Moran BJ, Thompson JN, et al. Adhesion-related hospital readmissions after abdominal and pelvic surgery: A retrospective cohort study. Lancet 1999; 353;1476–1478.
5. Lehmann-Willenbrock E, Mecke H, Riedel HH. Sequelae of appendectomy, with special reference to intra-abdominal adhesions, chronic abdominal pain, and infertility. Gynecol Obstet Invest 1990; 29:241–245.
6. Hershlag A, Diamond MP, DeCherney AH. Adhesiolysis. Clin Obstet Gynecol 1991; 34:395–402.
7. Al-Took S, Platt R, Tulandi T. Adhesion-related small-bowel obstruction after gynaecologic operations. Am J Obstet Gynecol 1999; 180:313–315.
8. Swank DJ, Van Erp WFM, Repelaer van Driel OJ, et al. A prospective analysis of predictive factors on the results of laparoscopic adhesiolysis in patients with chronic abdominal pain. Surg Laparosc Endosc Percutan Tech 2003; 13:88–94.
9. Vrijland WW, Jeekel J, Van Geldorp HJ, et al. Abdominal adhesions: Intestinal obstruction, pain and infertility. A review. Surg Endosc Ultrasound Interv Tech 2003; 17:1017–1022.

10. Van Den Tol MP, van Stijn I, Bonthuis F, et al. Reduction of intraperitoneal adhesion formation by use of non-abrasive gauze. Br J Surg 1997; 84:1410–1415.
11. Gerrand CL, Clements RH, Nannay L, et al. Adhesion formation is reduced after laparoscopic surgery. Surg Endosc 1999; 13: 10–13.
12. Jacobi CA, Sterzel A, Braumann C, et al. The impact of conventional and laparoscopic colon resection (CO_2 or helium) on intraperitoneal adhesion formation in a rat peritonitis model. Surg Endosc 2001; 15:380–386.
13. Polymeneas G, Theodosopoulos T, Stamatiadis E, et al. A comparative study of postoperative adhesion formation after laparoscopic vs. open cholecystectomy. Surg Endosc 2001, 15. 41–43.
14. Gutt CN, Oniu T, Schemmer P, et al. Fewer adhesions induced by laparoscopic surgery. Surg Endosc. 2004; 18(6): 898–906.
15. Filmar S, Gomel V, McComb PF. Operative laparoscopy versus open abdominal surgery: A comparative study on postoperative adhesion formation in the rat model. Fertil Steril 1987; 48: 486–489.
16. Wiseman DM, Trout JR, Diamond MP. The rates of adhesion development and the effects of crystalloid solutions on adhesion development in pelvic surgery. Fertil Steril 1998; 70:702–711.
17. Barkan H, Webster S, Ozeran S. Factors predicting the recurrence of adhesive small-bowel obstruction. Am J Surg 1995; 70:361–365.
18. Gomel V. Reconstructive tubal surgery. In: Rock HA, Jones HW III, eds. Te Linde's Operative Gynecology, 9th ed. Philadelphia., PA: Lippincott Williams & Wilkins, 2003:557–593.
19. Gomel V. Microsurgery in Female Infertility. Boston: Little, Brown and Co., 1983:3–5 and 147–149.
20. Gomel V. Laparoscopic tubal surgery in infertility. Obstet Gynecol 1975; 46:47–49.
21. Gomel V. Salpingo-ovariolysis by laparoscopy, in infertility. Fertil Steril 1983; 40:607–611.
22. Diamond E. Lysis of postoperative pelvic adhesions in infertility. Fertil Steril 1979; 31:287–295.
23. Franszen C, Schlosser HW. Microsurgery and postinfectious tubal infertility. Fertil Steril 1982; 38:397–340.
24. Ikard RW. There is no current indication for laparoscopic adhesiolysis to treat abdominal pain. South Med J 1992; 85:939–940.
25. Klingensmith ME, Soybel DI, Brooks DC. Laparoscopy for chronic abdominal pain. Surg Endosc 1996; 10:1085–1087.
26. Schietrauma M, Carlei F, Altilia F. The role of laparoscopic adhesiolysis in chronic abdominal pain. Minerva Chir 2001; 56:461–465.
27. Onders MP, Mittendorf EA. Utility of laparoscopy in chronic abdominal pain. Surgery 2003; 134:549–554.
28. Swank DJ, Swank-Bordewijk SCG, Hop WCJ, et al. Laparoscopic adhesiolysis in patients with chronic abdominal pain: A blinded randomized controlled multi-center trial. Lancet 2003; 361:1247–1251.
29. Swank DJ. Laparoscopic adhesiolysis for chronic abdominal pain is not indicated. Int Congr Ser 2005; 1279:85–89.
30. Sulaiman H, Gabella G, Davis C, et al. Presence and distribution of sensory nerve fibres in human peritoneal adhesions. Ann Surg 2001; 234:256–261.
31. Swank DJ, Hop WCJ, Jeekel J. Reduction, regrowth, and de novo formation of abdominal adhesions after laparoscopic adhesiolysis: A prospective analysis. Dig Surg 2004; 21:66–71.
32. Molloy D, Kaloo PD, Cooper M, et al. Laparoscopic entry: A literature review and analysis of techniques and complications of primary port entry. Aust N Z J Obstet Gynaecol 2002; 42(3):246–254.
33. Briel JW, Plaisier PW, Meijer WS, et al. Is it necessary to lift the abdominal wall when preparing a pneumoperitoneum? A randomised study. Surg Endosc 2000; 14(9):862.
34. Audebert AJ, Gomel V. Role of microlaparoscopy in the diagnosis of peritoneal and visceral adhesions and in the prevention of bowel injury associated with blind trocar insertion. Fertil Steril 2000; 73:631–635.
35. Agarwala N, Liu CY. Safe entry techniques during laparoscopy: Left upper quadrant entry using the ninth intercostal space—a review of 918 procedures. J Minim Invasive Gynecol 2005; 12(1):55–61.
36. Childers JM, Brzechffa PR, Surwit EA. Laparoscopy using the left upper quadrant as the primary trocar site. Gynecol Oncol 1993; 50(2):221–225.
37. Tsaltas J, Pearce S, Lawrence A, et al. Safer laparoscopic trocar entry: It's all about pressure. Aust N Z J Obstet Gynecol 2004; 44(4):349–350.
38. Phillips G, Garry R, Kumar C, et al. How much gas is required for initial insufflation at laparoscopy? Gynecol Endosc 1999; 8:327–334.
39. Vilos GA, Ternamian A, Dempster J, et al. Laparoscopic entry: A review of techniques, technologies and complications. J Obstet Gynecol Can 2007; 29(5):433–465.
40. Swank DJ, Bonjer HJ, Jeekel J. Safe laparoscopic adhesiolysis with optical access trocar and ultrasonic dissection; a prospective study. Surg Endosc 2002; 16:1796–1801.
41. Sutton C, MacDonald R. Laser laparoscopic adhesiolysis. J Gynecol Surg 1990; 6:155–159.
42. Luciano AA, Frishman GN, Maier DB. A comparative analysis of adhesion reduction, tissue effects, and incising characteristics of electrosurgery, CO_2 laser, and Nd:YAG laser at operative laparoscopy: An animal study. J Laparoendosc Surg 1992; 2:287–292.
43. Gomel V. Fertility promoting procedures and assisted reproductive technology. In: Gomel V, Taylor PJ, eds. Diagnostic and Operative Gynecologic Laparoscopy. St Louis: Mosby, 2000:169–176.
44. Salky BA, Edye MB. The role of laparoscopy in the diagnosis and treatment of abdominal pain syndromes. Surg Endosc 1998; 12:911–914.
45. Swank DJ, van Erp WFM, Repelaer van Driel OJ, et al. Complications and feasibility of laparoscopic adhesiolysis in patients with chronic abdominal pain. Surg Endosc 2002; 10:1468–1473.
46. Saravelos HG, Li TC, Cooke ID. An analysis of the outcome of microsurgical and laparoscopic adhesiolysis for chronic pelvic pain. Hum Reprod 1995; 10:2895–2901.
47. Kolmorgen K, Schulz AM. Results of laparoscopic lysis of adhesions in patients with chronic pelvic pain. Zentralbl Gynaekol 1991; 113:291–295.
48. Van Goor H. Iatrogenic bowel perforations due to adhesions in reoperated patients. Presentation ECCP Biennial Malmö: Sweden, 1998.
49. Miller K, Mayer E, Moritz E. The role of laparoscopy in chronic and recurrent abdominal pain. Am J Surg 1996; 172:353–357.
50. Nezhat CR, Nezhat FR, Swan AE. Long-term outcome after laparoscopic adhesiolysis in women with chronic pelvic pain after hysterectomy. J Am Assoc Gynecol Laparosc 1996; 3:S33–S34.
51. Nezhat FR, Chrystal RA, Nezhat CH, et al. Laparoscopic adhesiolysis and relief of chronic pelvic pain. JSLS 2000;4:281–285.
52. Lavonius M, Gullichsen R, Laine S, et al. Laparoscopy for chronic abdominal pain. Surg Laparosc Endos 1999; 9(1): 42–44.
53. Schietroma M, Risetti A, Altilia F, et al. The role of laparoscopic adhesiolysis in chronic abdominal pain. Minerva Chir 2001; 56:461–465.
54. Schmidbauer S, Hallfeldt KK. Laparoscopic adhesiolysis in the treatment of chronic abdominal pain. Surgery 2001; 129:513–514.
55. Swank DJ, van Erp WFM, Repelaer van Driel OJ, et al. Complications and feasibility of laparoscopic adhesiolysis in patients with chronic abdominal pain. A retrospective study. Ultrasound and Interventional Techniques. Surg Endosc 2002; 10:1468–1473.
56. Dunker M, Bemelman WA, Vijn A, et al. Long-term outcomes and quality of life after laparoscopic adhesiolysis for chronic abdominal pain. J Am Assoc Gynecol Laparosc 2004; 11(1):36–41.

13

Surgical options for pelvic pain

Fred M. Howard

INTRODUCTION

Pain is defined as an "unpleasant sensory and emotional experience associated with actual or potential tissue damage or described in terms of such damage" (1). This definition avoids tying pain to any stimulus, because pain is always subjective and may be present with or without the presence of tissue damage or any likely pathophysiological cause. Furthermore, the severity of pain may or may not correlate with the severity of any tissue damage. For example, viral gastroenteritis usually results in severe abdominal pain, whereas ovarian cancer rarely causes pain until very late in the course. The lack of correlation of severity of pain and that of disease is mechanistic, which means that one cannot conclude that severe pain in the presence of minimal disease signifies a psychological etiology. It is important that this principle be remembered during the clinical evaluation and treatment of patients with pain.

Pelvic pain is one of the most common reasons for which women seek gynecological care. Pelvic pain usually refers to abdominal pain below the umbilicus, but may also apply to pain at the lumbosacral back, buttocks, or vulva. Pelvic pain may be classified as acute, recurrent (or intermittent), or chronic. Recurrent pelvic pain refers to pain of sustained duration that occurs episodically or at regular intervals, with pain-free time between episodes of pain. Dysmenorrhea and dyspareunia are common examples of recurrent pelvic pain. Acute pelvic pain refers to pain of short duration that rarely lasts more than one month without crisis, resolution, or cure. Chronic pelvic pain (CPP) is usually defined by duration of more than three or more than six months. Although the disorders leading to acute, intermittent, and CPP tend to differ, there is some overlap. One major distinction between acute and CPP is that acute pelvic pain is a symptom of a visceral or somatic injury or disease, whereas CPP is often a diagnosis related to neurological and/or psychological disorders. Thus, treatment of acute pelvic pain is always directed to the pathological etiology, but treatment of CPP may be directed to an associated disorder or to pain itself.

In the initial evaluation, it is important to identify the locations of pain and of referred pain, especially with visceral and chronic pain. A useful technique is to have the patient to do a "pain map" on a human anatomy diagram (Fig. 1). The patient is asked to fill in the areas where she has pain. Sometimes, the pain map may also be useful in showing a distribution of pain suggesting a dermatomal distribution or a myotomal pattern, thus directing the subsequent evaluation toward the musculoskeletal or nervous systems. For example, pain located in the distribution of a cutaneous nerve may suggest an entrapped nerve or mononeuropathy. With the iliohypogastric or ilioinguinal nerve, this pain radiation is medially along the lower abdomen and the upper aspect of the thigh.

When pain is of visceral origin, the location of CPP is useful in differential diagnosis, but by itself is rarely diagnostic. A major reason for this is that true visceral pain is not as well localized as somatic pain, so patients with chronic pain related to visceral pathology may have trouble localizing their pain. Furthermore, as the cervix, uterus, and adnexae have the same metameric innervation as the bladder, distal ureter, lower ileum, colon, and rectosigmoid, it is often difficult to determine if abdominopelvic pain of visceral cause is of gynecological, urological, or intestinal origin (2). Lateral pelvic pain is commonly of adnexal or sigmoid colonic origin. However, due to the long mesentery of the sigmoid colon, pain associated with it may be variable in location and be right, left, or even midline lower abdominal pain. Midline or central infraumbilical pain may be secondary to the uterus, uterosacral ligaments, posterior cul-de-sac, or cervix but may also be due to distention of either the left or the right hemicolon. Pain associated with pathology of the small bowel is usually localized to the periumbilical area, but this may clearly be confused with pain from the reproductive or urinary tract. Pain from the bladder or vagina may localize over the mons pubis, pubic bone, or groin. Back pain in the lower sacral and midline areas may be from the uterosacral ligaments, posterior cul-de-sac, or cervix. Complaints of pain both ventrally and dorsally often suggest intrapelvic pathology, whereas only dorsal low back pain suggests an orthopedic or musculoskeletal origin.

There are a number of disorders that can cause pelvic pain, which are amenable to surgical treatment. Of these disorders, only those of the reproductive tract are discussed in this chapter (Tables 1–3).

ABORTION (SPONTANEOUS MISCARRIAGE)

Abortion is a common cause of acute pelvic pain. Outcomes of randomized clinical trials suggest that women with missed or incomplete abortion can effectively be managed surgically, medically, or expectantly. Surgical management more rapidly completes evacuation of the uterus but may have a slightly higher risk of infection than medical or expectant management (3,4). Surgical management is preferred in cases of septic abortion, in combination with antibiotic treatment. Only surgical management will be discussed in this chapter.

Surgical treatment is usually dilatation and curettage or dilatation and evacuation in the first and early second trimesters. Anesthesia is usually needed and may be local, regional, or general. Surgical risks are uterine perforation, intrauterine adhesions, cervical trauma, and infection, but these are not common. Postoperative risk of infection can be minimized by antibiotic prophylaxis, such as doxycycline 100 mg orally for two doses 12 hours apart on the day of the surgery (5). This recommendation is based on studies of induced abortion, whereas a randomized trial of doxycycline prophylaxis before curettage for incomplete abortion did not show a significant decrease in infection rates (6).

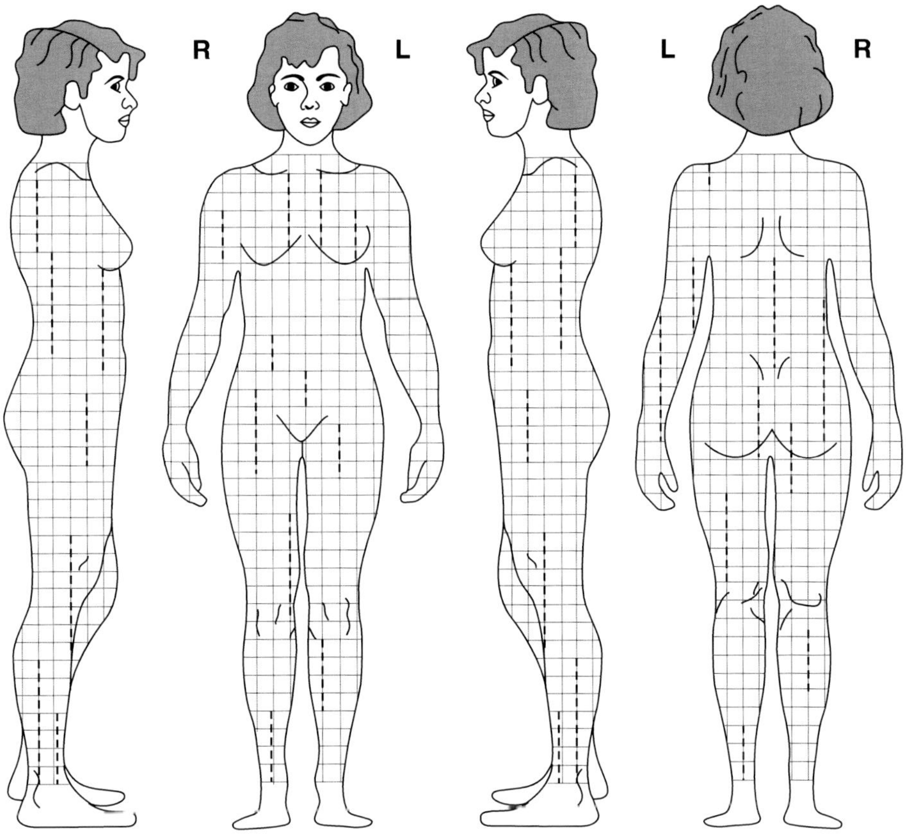

Figure 1 Example of a human figure on which the patient may "map" her areas of pain.

Suction curettage is the most commonly used method to surgically complete a first trimester miscarriage in the United States. This procedure can safely be used up to 13 menstrual weeks; after this gestation, extraction procedures are often needed to successfully complete a miscarriage surgically. Surgical dilatation is not always necessary in cases of spontaneous abortion, as the cervix is often already dilated. The diameter of the suction cannula can usually be correlated to the gestational weeks; for example, at eight weeks an 8-mm cannula can be used. In early miscarriages, a 50- or 60-mL syringe can be attached to the cannula for aspiration of the products of conception (Fig. 2). Electrical vacuum devices are preferable at 10 or more weeks of gestation. The cannula is introduced without suction, and the vacuum suction is applied to about

Table 1 Disorders Leading to Acute Pelvic Pain That Can Be Treated Surgically

Gynecological
Abortion
Adnexal torsion
Degenerating leiomyoma
Ectopic pregnancy
Endometriosis
Ovarian tumor
Pelvic inflammatory disease
Ruptured ovarian cyst

Table 2 Gynecological Disorders Leading to Recurrent Pelvic Pain That May Be Treated Surgically

Adnexal torsion
Endometriosis
Primary dysmenorrhea
Uterine retroversion

Table 3 Gynecological Disorders Associated with Chronic Pelvic Pain That May Be Treated Surgically

Adenomyosis[a]
Adhesions[b]
Adnexal cysts (nonendometriotic)[a]
Benign cystic mesothelioma[b]
Cervical stenosis[a]
Endometrial or cervical polyps[a]
Endometriosis[c]
Endosalpingiosis[a]
Gynecological malignancies (especially late stage)[c]
Leiomyomata[b]
Ovarian remnant syndrome[c]
Ovarian retention syndrome (residual ovary syndrome)[c]
Pelvic congestion syndrome[c]
Pelvic inflammatory disease[c]
Postoperative peritoneal cysts[b]
Residual accessory ovary[a]
Symptomatic pelvic relaxation (genital prolapse)[a]
Tuberculous salpingitis[c]

[a]Level C: causal relationship to chronic pelvic pain based on expert opinions.
[b]Level B: limited or inconsistent scientific evidence of causal relationship to chronic pelvic pain.
[c]Level A: good and consistent scientific evidence of causal relationship to chronic pelvic pain.

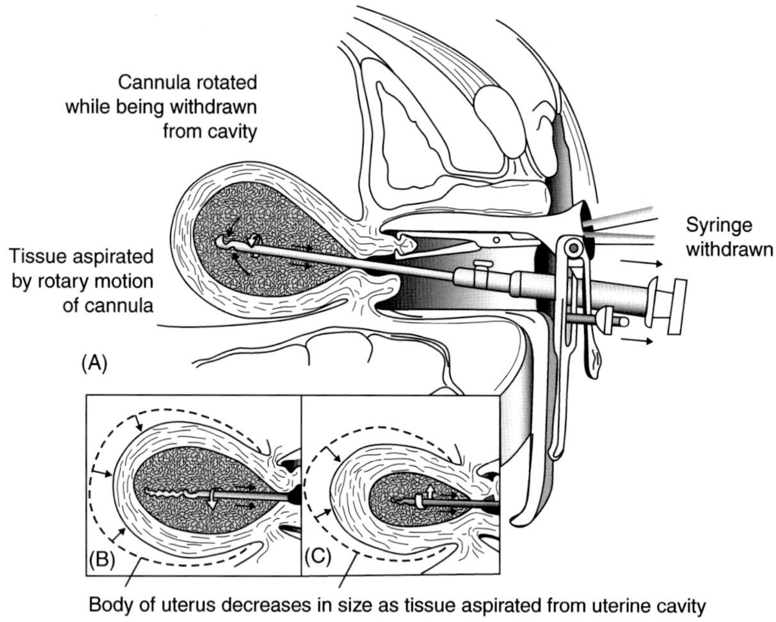

Figure 2 Procedure for suction curettage. (A to C) Rotation of the suction curette. Little rotation should occur when the instrument is near the uterine wall, to avoid perforation.

60 mm Hg. The cannula is rotated in a 360° arc until evacuation of the uterus appears to be complete. In-and-out movement of the cannula is discouraged, as this may increase the chance of perforation. The catheter is removed from the uterus under continuous negative pressure when no further tissue can be aspirated. A metal curette can be introduced to gently palpate the uterine sidewall for the gritty sensation that suggests complete evacuation, but this is not always necessary. It is important to avoid vigorous sharp curettage, as this may lead to uterine synechiae and Asherman's syndrome.

Tissue is best submitted for histological evaluation to exclude a complete or partial molar pregnancy. Genetic studies may be indicated in some cases.

ADENOMYOSIS

Adenomyosis is the presence of benign endometrial glands and stroma at least 2 to 3 mm deep in the myometrium. There is some controversy about the definition, however. An adenomyoma is a nodule of hypertrophic myometrium and ectopic endometrium. Adenomyomas may clinically be confused with intramural leiomyomas, although they are darker in color and not quite as firm.

The incidence of adenomyosis ranges from 5% to 70%, varying with the scrutiny of histological evaluation and patients' symptoms, ages, and parities (7–9). Adenomyosis is most often correlated with recurrent menstrual pain and less often is a cause of chronic pain. The etiology of pain with adenomyosis is not clear. In fact, there is a debate about the correlation of adenomyosis and pelvic pain symptoms. It is estimated that symptoms of adenomyosis are menorrhagia in 40% to 50% and dysmenorrhea in 15% to 30% of cases. One-third of patients are asymptomatic (10). Both menorrhagia and dysmenorrhea are found in about 20% of patients. There are some data suggesting that pelvic pain correlates with diffuse, widely spread disease, but not with the depth of invasion (11). The physical examination of a woman with adenomyosis usually shows a symmetrically enlarged uterus less than 14 weeks' size when an examination is performed just prior to or during menses (10). The uterus is enlarged in 60% to 80% of cases, but it rarely exceeds a size of 12 weeks' gestation. The uterus is diffusely boggy to palpation or it may have a nodular consistency, reminiscent of multiple small intramural fibroids. In patients with painful adenomyosis, the uterus is usually tender to palpation. Imaging studies, particularly transvaginal ultrasound and magnetic resonance imaging (MRI), may be useful in preoperative evaluation (12–16).

Transvaginal sonography may show an enlarged uterus, irregular vascular spaces within the myometrium, and an acoustically enlarged posterior wall with cystic eyelets in the myometrium. All these ultrasonic characteristics may be useful in making the preoperative diagnosis of this entity (12–14). Subendometrial myometrial cysts, subendometrial echogenic nodules, subendometrial echogenic linear striations, and poor definition of the endometrial–myometrial junction are other sonographic findings that suggest adenomyosis (17). Overall, the sensitivity of transvaginal ultrasound is about 80%, the specificity about 40%, the positive predictive value about 70%, and negative predictive value about 80% (18).

T2-weighted MRI scans of diffuse adenomyosis show distortion of normal zonal anatomy of the uterus with enlargement of the functional zone, seen as a wide band with low signal intensity, adjacent to the endometrium. Adenomyosis appears as a diffuse, ill-defined lesion extending adjacent to the endometrium. Adenomyomas may readily be identified with MIR imaging (Fig. 3).

Medical treatment with either progestational or combined estrogen and progestin medications may be effective for bleeding abnormalities, as may be the insertion of a levonorgestrel-releasing intrauterine device (19,20). Gonadotropin suppression with gonadotropin-releasing hormone (GnRH) agonists has been shown to provide at least temporary relief of symptoms of adenomyosis. Leuprolide (21,22), triptorelin (23), goserelin (23), and nafarelin (24) have shown effectiveness in case reports.

Surgical treatment is commonly used in suspected cases of adenomyosis. Initial excitement about the use of endometrial ablation to successfully control menorrhagia and pain associated with adenomyosis has dissipated with longer-term

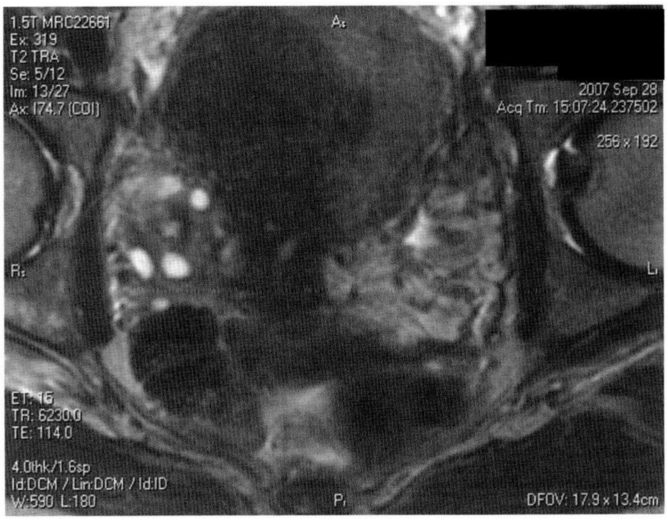

Figure 3 Magnetic resonance image of a large adenomyoma of the uterus in a patient with a history of endometriosis and chronic pelvic pain.

follow-up after such procedures (25–27). Deep adenomyosis of greater than 2.5 mm endometrial penetration is the major cause of failures. Uterine artery occlusion by uterine artery embolization (28–30), laparoscopic uterine artery ligation (31), or temporary occlusion of the uterine arteries by placement of Doppler-guided transvaginal clamp (32) has been discussed, but data are limited. In cases of adenomyomas, surgical adenomyomectomy, similarly to myomectomy, may be an effective approach (33). However, with adenomyomectomy there is no pseudocapsule and no clear plane of dissection between normal myometrium and adenomyosis, so the procedure may be far more difficult and bloody than myomectomy. Hysterectomy represents definitive therapy for adenomyosis. Whether supracervical hysterectomy is appropriate is not well established, as there may be nests of adenomyosis in the cervix and lower uterine segment (34).

ADHESIONS

An adhesion is a fibrous tissue by which anatomic structures abnormally adhere to one another. Adhesions are well accepted as causes of intestinal obstruction (35–37) and infertility (38), but their role as a cause of CPP is controversial. Intra-abdominal and pelvic adhesions are often found at laparoscopies in women with CPP (39). If adhesions cause CPP, then adhesiolysis might be expected to relieve pain. However, two published randomized trials of adhesiolysis failed to show any significant improvement in pain symptoms after lysis of adhesions, and a third study showed improvement. One study used laparoscopic adhesiolysis for chronic abdominal, not pelvic, pain and found that at one year pain relief was obtained in 57% of treated patients, compared to 42% in the control group. This difference was not statistically significant with their sample size (40). The other negative study used laparotomic adhesiolysis for pelvic pain and found that only a subgroup of 15 women with severe, stage IV adhesions showed improvement in pain that could be attributed to adhesiolysis (41). The third study, a randomized clinical trial of lysis of right paracolic adhesions in women with CPP, showed that right lower quadrant pain was decreased to a significantly greater degree than left lower quadrant or suprapubic pain (42). Right lower quadrant pain was also decreased significantly more in patients with right paracolic adhesiolysis than in those with right paracolic adhesions that were not lysed at the time of laparoscopic surgery. A number of observational studies have also shown significant improvement in pain in women with CPP after adhesiolysis (43–46). A major problem with adhesiolysis as a treatment for pelvic pain is that adhesiolysis does not eliminate adhesions. At least 70% of lysed adhesions reform postoperatively.

Adhesions are generally believed to cause pelvic pain that is exacerbated by sudden movements, intercourse, or certain physical activities. Often the pain is consistent in its location, although over time the area of involvement may expand. A history of one of the classic causes of adhesions—pelvic inflammatory disease (PID), endometriosis, perforated appendix, prior abdominopelvic surgery, or inflammatory bowel disease—makes this a more likely diagnosis. At least one of these historic factors is present in 50% of women with adhesions (47).

Although nonsurgical methods such as computerized tomography, MRI, or ultrasound may suggest the presence of adhesions, presently the only definitive way to diagnose them is by surgical visualization. Whenever feasible, laparoscopy, not laparotomy, is the gold standard for diagnosing pelvic adhesive disease. Patients suspected of having pain associated with adhesive disease could undergo pain mapping. Laparoscopic pain mapping consists of a laparoscopy performed under local anesthesia, with light sedation to allow an internal visceral examination seeking specific areas of hyperalgesia or allodynia that may account for the patient's underlying CPP. This may determine not only the presence of adhesions but also whether they are likely to be responsible for the pain (48). At the time of diagnostic laparoscopy or pain mapping, it is crucial that the adhesions be fully described in the operative note. This may be important not just in documentation but also in the future care of the patient.

Laparoscopic adhesiolysis for relief of CPP must be approached cautiously with thorough informed consent. Complications may occur in up to 10% of patients, with enterotomies and cystotomies being particularly problematic (44,49). Most patients undergoing laparoscopy for the treatment of adhesions have histories of prior abdominopelvic surgery, so the risk of periumbilical bowel or omental adhesions is significant (50). Because of this, many experts recommend open laparoscopy in such cases. This may not necessarily prevent injury to any bowel adherent at the umbilicus, however (51,52). Because of this, we recommend a left upper quadrant Veres needle and 5-mm trocar placement insertion. This allows insertion of the umbilical trocar under direct vision. One must be certain that the stomach has been aspirated before upper abdominal blind entries. Occasionally, adhesions will have to be cleared from the anterior abdominal wall or alternate insertion sites selected before other trocars can be inserted (53). Several other alternative sites for initial insertions are possible, including mid-abdomen under xiphoid process, paravaginal, left lower quadrant, and suprapubic (54). Additionally, it is possible to safely perform direct trocar insertion at the left upper quadrant and carry out the surgical procedure without placing an umbilical trocar (55).

Adhesiolysis may be accomplished with laser, electrosurgery, or sharp scissors dissection. Preoperative bowel preparation is recommended for all patients. Gentle traction on the bowel is necessary to prevent unintentional enterotomy. Hemostasis should be meticulous with bipolar desiccation. For dense bowel adhesions, scissors dissection should be performed and energy sources avoided, to prevent inadvertent thermal injury. If extensive removal of the parietal peritoneum is necessary, the patient should be watched for subcutaneous emphysema. Retroperitoneal dissection of the pneumoperitoneum might produce compromise of the airway or impaired chest wall excursion postoperatively. Bowel injuries should be immediately repaired. It is important that small bowel injuries be repaired in a transverse closure, not in a longitudinal direction, so as to avoid narrowing of the intestinal lumen. This can safely be performed laparoscopically by surgeons experienced in laparoscopic suturing and stapling techniques. Broad-spectrum antibiotic coverage and conservative diet progression are necessary. Nasogastric suction is no longer considered mandatory postoperatively.

After surgical adhesiolysis, strategies for preventing recurrence should be employed. Although no completely effective method is currently available, consideration may be given to placing barriers in localized areas of tissue injury. Oxidized regenerated cellulose (Interceed, Johnson & Johnson Medical Inc., Arlington, Texas, U.S.), Gore-tex surgical membrane (W.L. Gore Co., Flagstaff, Arizona), and hyaluronic acid–methylcellulose (Seprafilm, Genzyme Corp., Cambridge, Massachusetts) are currently available (56,57). Crystalloid fluid such as Ringer's solution is easy to use laparoscopically, but its effectiveness is limited by rapid absorption. Colloid fluid such as Dextran 70 can cause rapid fluid shifts and anaphylactic reactions. A 4% icodextrin solution (Adept, Baxter Healthcare Corp.) is available, which can be used laparoscopically and appears to decrease adhesions effectively.

ADNEXAL CYSTS

When a woman presents with lateral abdominopelvic pain, it is almost always assumed to be of ovarian origin by patients and physicians alike. The assumption that lateral pelvic pain is usually due to the adnexae frequently leads to an erroneous diagnosis. This assumption also means that the patient's gynecologist is often the first clinician consulted for laterally located pelvic pain. Because of this, it is especially important that gynecologists be familiar with nonreproductive tract sources of pelvic pain.

Ovarian cysts form routinely as part of the reproductive cycle and are not generally responsible for pain. When pain occurs due to an ovarian cyst, it is almost always acute pelvic pain and usually due to some type of pathological change. Ruptured ovarian cyst, endometriosis, and torsion are characteristic reasons for pain due to ovarian cysts.

Nonendometriotic ovarian cysts, even persistent ovarian cysts, usually do not produce chronic pain. Slow distention of the ovary can be completely asymptomatic despite rich visceral innervation. Patients with painlessly advancing ovarian cancer are testimony to this phenomenon. However, anecdotal reports of functional ovarian cysts producing CPP have been published (39,58). Hasson (59), for example, reported laparoscopic treatment of 35 women with CPP attributed to ovarian cysts, with pain resolution in 32 at three months' follow-up. Unfortunately, the definition of CPP, details of the procedures, and histological diagnoses were not reported. Mechanical pressure on adjacent organs and the development of adhesions are more likely to be responsible for any pain associated with adnexal cysts than the cysts themselves. While some clinicians believe that capsular distention from polycystic ovarian syndrome is painful, little evidence for this exists.

Bimanual pelvic examination sometimes establishes the location and size of adnexal cysts. However, the more uncomfortable the examination, the less likely it is to be diagnostic. Colonic stool may obscure the pelvic pathology and also make the diagnosis more difficult. Pelvic ultrasonography is a valuable and cost-effective diagnostic tool if an adnexal cyst is suspected. Location, size, and solid or cystic components may be determined sonographically. Differentiation between an adnexal and a peritoneal cyst can be made with B-mode transvaginal sonography alone, with a specificity of 96% and a sensitivity of 62% (60). Computerized tomography may also be diagnostically helpful in some cases but is more expensive and not always necessary.

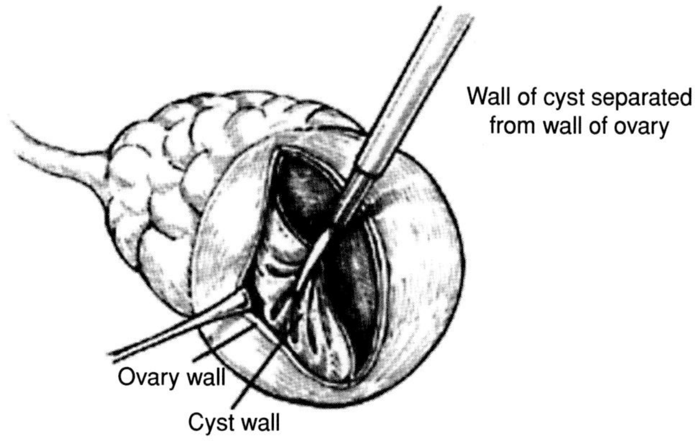

Figure 4 Laparoscopic dissection of ovarian cyst from the ovary.

Long-term hormonal suppression of chronic pelvic cysts is generally unsuccessful. In the uncommon circumstance of cyclical, recurrent pelvic pain associated with functional ovarian cysts, hormonal suppression may be successful (58). Aspiration of adnexal cysts guided by ultrasound is possible, but the recurrence rate may be unacceptable if they are of ovarian origin. One study of 22 patients with simple cysts less than 9 cm and a CA-125 level of less than 35 IU/mL underwent transvaginal aspiration. The recurrence rate was reported as 22.7% over six months (61).

Oophorectomy or cystectomy remains the treatment of choice in most cases. Unless contraindicated by sonographic evidence of malignancy, either procedure may be performed laparoscopically (Figs. 4 and 5). In one series of 683 consecutive patients, younger than 40 years, with adnexal masses, all but 16

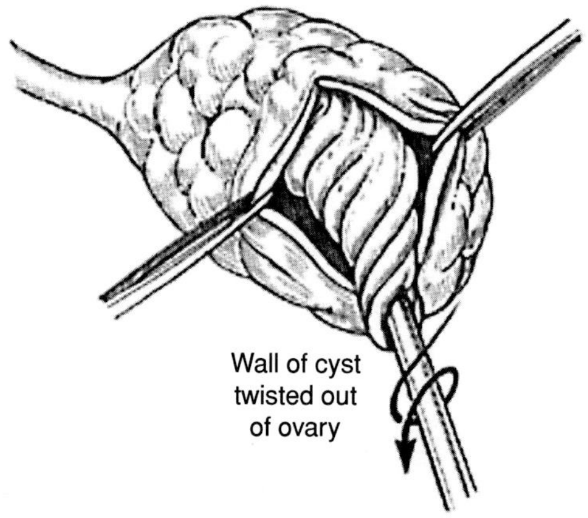

Figure 5 Example of twisting technique for removal of an ovarian cyst laparoscopically.

(2.3%) were managed laparoscopically. The unexpected malignancy rate was only 1.2%, and laparoscopic management did not adversely affect their prognosis (62). Patients who are candidates for laparoscopic treatment of adnexal cysts experience a more rapid recovery, less postoperative pain, and decreased adhesion formation. Laparotomy is appropriate only when laparoscopy is contraindicated (63,64). The surgical management of ovarian cysts and neoplasms is discussed in chapter 10.

ADNEXAL TORSION

Adnexal torsion causes acute or intermittent pelvic pain. Although any component of the adnexae may torse or twist—fallopian tube, paratubal cyst, or ovary—ovarian torsion is by far the most common. Ovarian torsion may occur at any age, although it is most common in women younger than 50 years of age. Most often it occurs with benign cysts or neoplasms. Torsion of ovarian malignancies is uncommon (65). Ovarian torsion often represents a surgical emergency, as torsion may occlude the blood flow of the ovary. Venous flow is more readily interrupted because the thin walls of the veins are more readily compressed than the thicker, more muscular walls of the arteries. When this occurs, continued arterial perfusion with venous obstruction leads to marked ovarian engorgement and enlargement. This may eventually lead to ischemia, necrosis, infarction, and hemorrhage. Although the diagnosis may be suspected based on clinical evidence, definitive diagnosis and treatment of ovarian torsion is surgical.

In the past, surgical treatment was oophorectomy, but it is now clear that detorsion and preservation of the ovary is the preferred approach in almost all cases except malignancies. Even when the ovary appears necrotic, conservation is safe and usually results in normal hormonal function and fertility (66–68). Expedient diagnosis and treatment are advisable to minimize the risk of serious complications such as peritonitis and systemic infection if a necrotic ovary is retained. Oophoropexy can be performed to prevent recurrent torsion, but its role is not clear except in children and adolescents with ovarian torsion (Fig. 6). It is not known if oophoropexy will affect future fertility. If the utero-ovarian ligament appears stretched or longer than normal, surgical shortening of the utero-ovarian ligament has been suggested as a technique to decrease the risk of recurrent torsion (Fig. 7). If there is an identifiable ovarian cyst and cystectomy is feasible, this may also decrease the risk of recurrent torsion. Ovarian cystectomy should be performed at the time of surgery for torsion whenever a cyst is present and if cystectomy is feasible. Occasionally with significant edema and necrosis, ovarian cystectomy is not possible. Surgery for ovarian torsion should be performed laparoscopically, except in cases of suspected malignancy.

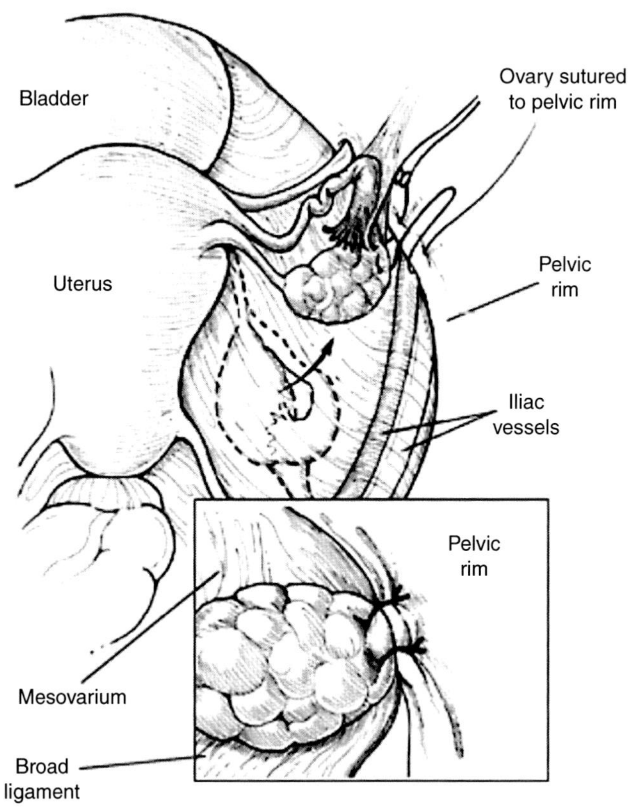

Figure 6 One technique that may be used for oophoropexy for ovarian torsion or recurrent ovarian torsion.

BENIGN CYSTIC MESOTHELIOMA

Benign cystic mesothelioma or multicystic mesothelioma is a rare lesion consisting of multiple mesothelial-lined cysts that affect various parts of the abdominopelvic peritoneal surface (Fig. 8). When present, they are frequently associated with CPP. Benign mesothelial cysts have been reported in men but are much more common in women (69). Although benign mesothelial cysts may occur anywhere in the peritoneum, they are most commonly found in the pelvis. Ultrasonography almost always reveals complex, cystic masses with thin walls and septations. In patients with ovaries, the ovarian fluid may produce cysts around the ovaries if adhesions are present. Of course, this causes the sonographic appearance of a complex adnexal mass.

Observation is an option if symptoms are controlled, and there is no evidence of malignancy. Medical treatments have included case reports with tamoxifen or depot leuprolide.

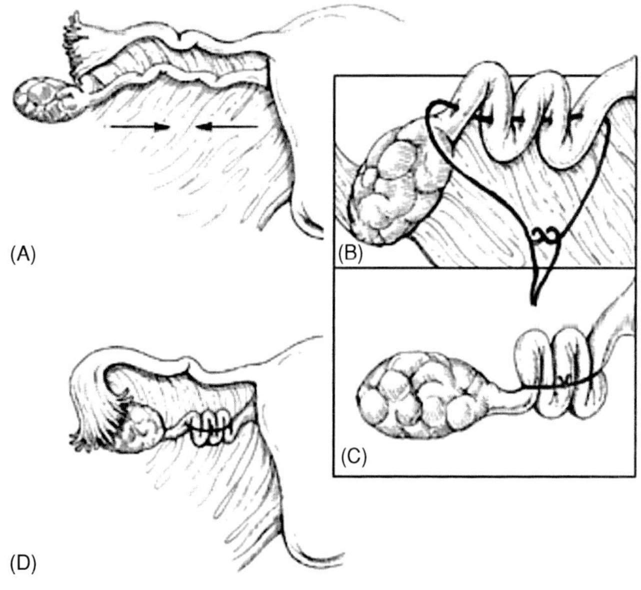

Figure 7 Illustration of a technique to shorten the utero-ovarian ligament to prevent future ovarian torsion.

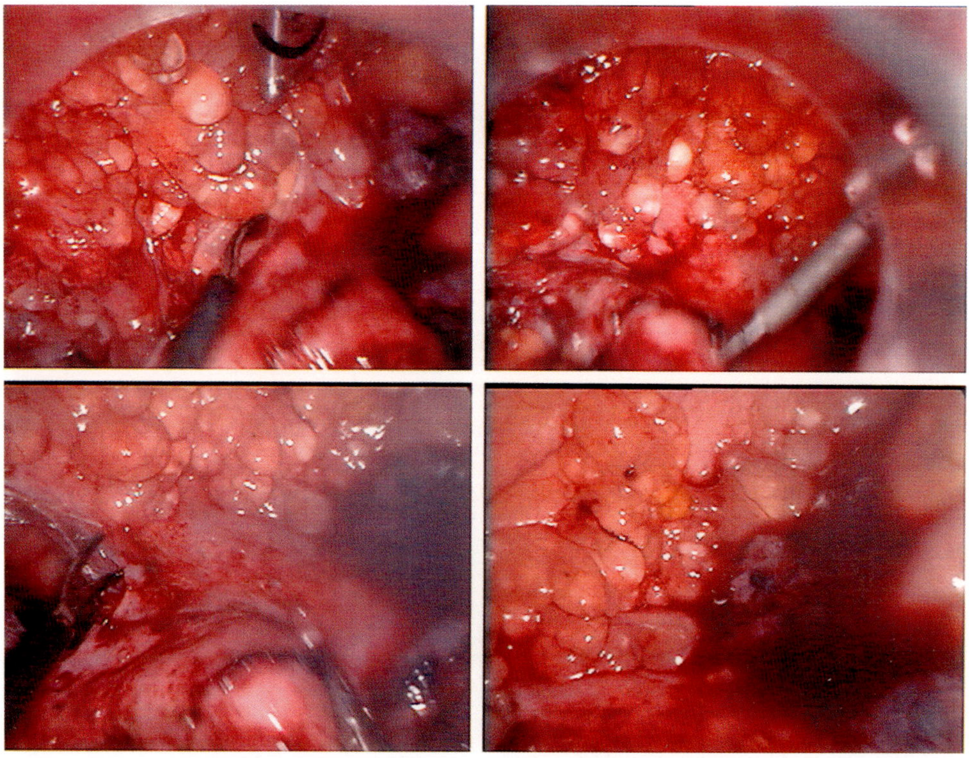

Figure 8 Laparoscopic view of benign cystic mesotheliomas.

Surgical treatment consists of excision and has been reported laparoscopically (70). Such surgery can be tedious and difficult and almost always requires extensive retroperitoneal dissection. Recurrence rates are high (30–50%) after surgical resection (71).

CERVICAL STENOSIS

Cervical stenosis may rarely be a cause of dysmenorrhea but in general is not associated with pelvic pain. It has been suggested that it may correlate with a higher risk of having endometriosis (72). Dilation of the cervical os is generally a sufficient treatment.

ECTOPIC PREGNANCY

Ectopic pregnancy causes acute pelvic pain. Early diagnosis allows medical treatment of ectopic pregnancy with methotrexate in the majority of cases (73). Surgical treatment may be more appropriate if the patient has high β-hCG levels (over 5000 or 10,000 mIU/mL) (74), has a large gestational sac (≥3.5 cm) (75), has fetal cardiac activity, is hemodynamically unstable, is medically noncompliant, has failed methotrexate treatment, or has medical contraindications to methotrexate. In hemodynamically stable patients, surgery should only be performed if an ultrasound shows an adnexal mass suggestive of an ectopic pregnancy. If no mass consistent with an ectopic pregnancy is visible sonographically, it is likely that an ectopic pregnancy will not be visualized or palpated at surgery.

There is clear evidence that laparoscopy is preferable to laparotomy for the treatment of tubal ectopic pregnancies (76–78). Surgical options include salpingostomy and salpingectomy. The choice of surgical procedure depends on the patient's history, her future fertility plans, and the degree of damage to the fallopian tube. When feasible, linear salpingostomy is the preferred technique (Fig. 9). This is performed by making a 10- to 15-mm incision into the antimesenteric tubal segment overlying the ectopic. Many surgeons inject a solution of vasopressin (0.2 IU/mL) into the tube (Figure shows injection into the mesosalpinx this requires caution regarding dilution and total amount injected) prior to making an incision to minimize bleeding at the salpingostomy site. The incision may be made with a laser, monopolar electrosurgical needle, or scissors. Hydrodissection and blunt dissection with a suction irrigator are usually the ideal ways to dislodge the ectopic pregnancy from the tube. After it is mobilized, the products of conception can be grasped and placed in a laparoscopic pouch to minimize any chance of loss of tissue in the abdominal cavity or abdominal wall during the removal from the abdomen. Bleeding from the tube can be controlled with minimal application of bipolar energy, avoiding the tubal endothelium, or by ligation of the mesosalpinx with a fine suture. There appears to be no advantage to closing the tubal incision (79,80).

If salpingectomy is warranted, either a total or a partial salpingectomy can be performed. (Fig. 10) If a total salpingectomy is performed, bipolar electrosurgery or ultrasonic energy is used at or near the tubal cornua to allow hemostatic transaction of the proximal tube. Then the vessels in the mesosalpinx are desiccated and cut to allow removal of the fallopian tube. Care must be taken not to destroy the blood supply of the ovary. A partial or segmental salpingectomy can also be done by desiccating and cutting the tube proximal and distal to the ectopic pregnancy and then desiccating and cutting the mesosalpinx under the ectopic.

The risk of recurrent ectopic pregnancy is 10% to 30%. If the contralateral tube appears pathological, the risk of

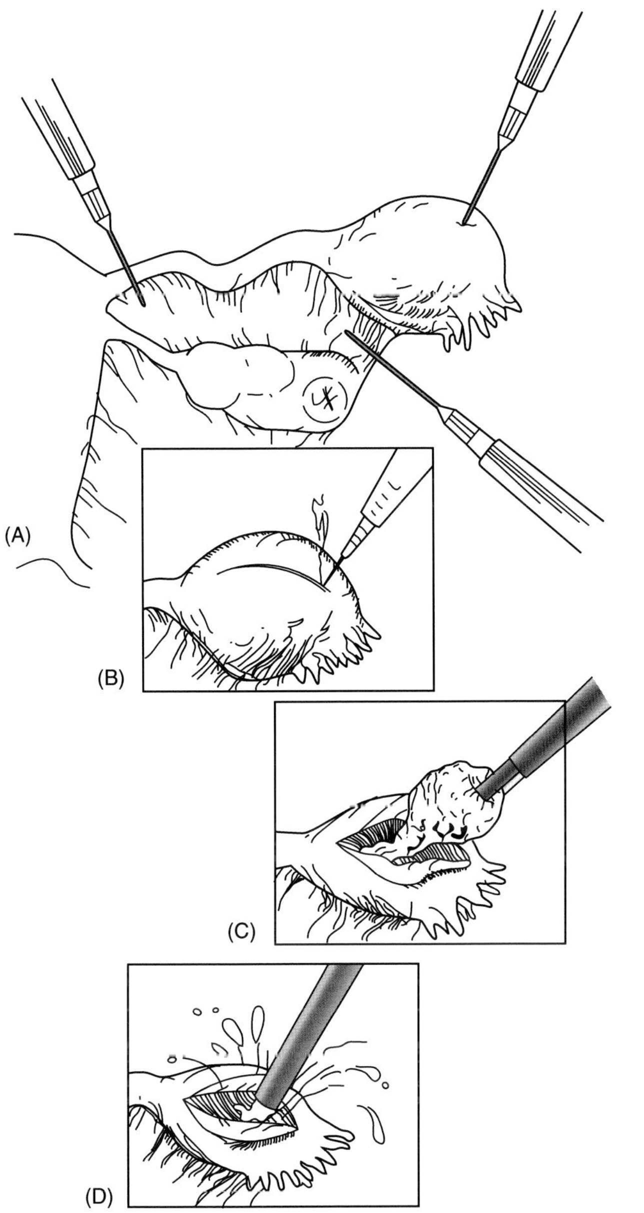

Figure 9 Illustration of technique for linear salpingostomy for tubal ectopic pregnancy. (A) The tube is stabilized and injected with a dilute solution of vasopressin. (B) An incision is made on the antimesenteric border overlying the ectopic. (C) The products of conception are removed using atraumatic forceps. (D) The implantation site is irrigated and hemostasis obtained.

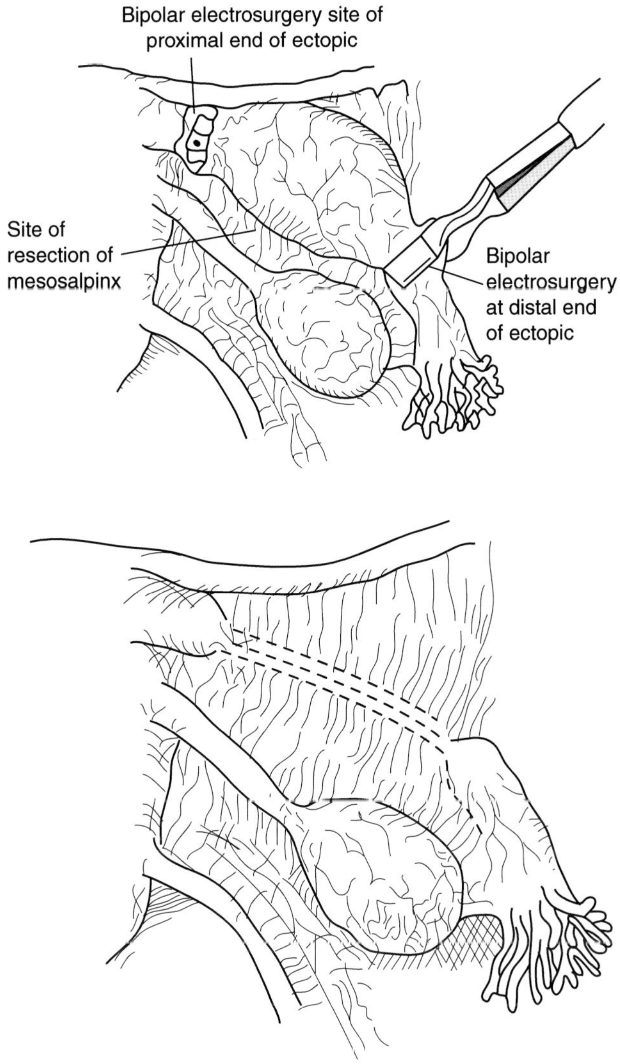

Figure 10 Illustration of the technique for partial salpingectomy for tubal ectopic pregnancy. *Source*: From Nezhat et al. Operative Gynecologic Laparoscopy.

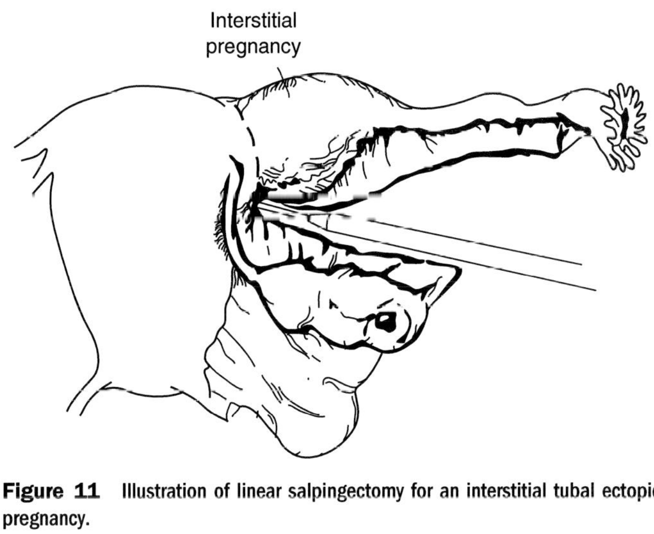

Figure 11 Illustration of linear salpingectomy for an interstitial tubal ectopic pregnancy.

subsequent pregnancy appears to be improved if conservative, rather than radical, surgical treatment is used. Overall data are conflicting regarding the subsequent recurrence rate of ectopic pregnancy, comparing radical to conservation surgical management (81).

Surgical treatment of other types of ectopic pregnancies—cornual, ovarian, cervical, and abdominal—is more problematic. Cornual ectopic pregnancies treated surgically can be challenging, as they usually require wedge resection at the cornua (Fig. 11). Classically this has been done by laparotomy, but it is possible to perform the surgery laparoscopically (82). Hemostasis may be difficult to maintain at the time of laparoscopic cornual wedge resection due to the significant vascularity. Vessel sealing instrumentation can facilitate the wedge resection of the uterus at the cornua, and the ability to perform suturing for hemostasis and repair can be critical to successful laparoscopic treatment (83). Surgical management of ovarian ectopic pregnancies can be challenging, also, as ensuring complete resection without excessive damage to the ovary may be difficult. Attempts at conservative surgical treatment of cervical ectopic pregnancies are ill advised, as hemorrhage is a frequent complication. Hemodynamically stable patients with cervical pregnancy are best treated medically using radiographic embolization, single or multidose methotrexate, and intra-amniotic or intrafetal injection of potassium chloride if fetal cardiac activity is present (84,85). However, experience with this approach is limited (86,87). If heavy vaginal bleeding occurs, then intra-arterial embolization or cervical cerclage is the alternative to hysterectomy to control hemorrhage. If abdominal pregnancy is diagnosed early in its course, then laparoscopic surgical treatment to separate and excise the gestational products from surrounding tissue may be possible (88). If abdominal pregnancy is not diagnosed until the second or third trimester, laparotomy is necessary and is usually complicated by excessive blood loss when the placenta is removed. In many cases, the best approach is to leave the placenta in situ and attempt methotrexate treatment postoperatively. Embolization of the hypogastric, uterine, or other feeding vessels is another option to control the bleeding.

Whenever a conservative surgical treatment of ectopic pregnancy is used, it is important to follow serial β-hCG levels until they are negative. Also, it is important to remember to administer Rh-immune globulin if the patient is Rh negative.

ENDOCERVICAL AND ENDOMETRIAL POLYPS

Cervical and endometrial polyps are common. Cervical polyps are found at the time of annual examination in about 4% of women, and endometrial polyps have been estimated to occur in about 7% of women (89). Endometrial polyps are found in up to 27% of patients who have a cervical polyp. Such polyps are often asymptomatic, although they can cause abnormal vaginal bleeding. The risk of cancer with an endometrial polyp is less than 5% (90). Rarely, women with endocervical polyps present with dysmenorrhea or with intermittent cramping pelvic pain that is speculated to be secondary to cervical obstruction.

Cervical polyps can usually be removed in the office with cervical biopsy forceps or, if large, by placing a clamp approximately 0.5 cm above the origin of the pedicle, tying a surgical ligature between the clamp and the cervix, removing the clamp, and then cutting along the line of the crush. All tissues removed should be sent for pathological review to exclude malignancy. Endometrial polyps can be removed hysteroscopically with a resecting loop or with forceps such as Corson forceps.

ENDOMETRIOSIS

Endometriosis may cause acute pain, intermittent pain, or CPP. The surgical treatment of endometriosis associated pain is discussed in chapters 10 and 11.

ENDOSALPINGIOSIS

Whether endosalpingiosis can cause pelvic pain is unclear. Evidence is anecdotal only. It is most often confused with endometriosis grossly at the time of laparoscopy. Treatment is surgical and is identical to that of endometriosis.

GYNECOLOGICAL MALIGNANCIES

Reproductive tract cancers usually present for longer term may cause acute or intermittent pelvic or abdominal pain, although they may present with either acute or intermittent pain in some cases. Their surgical management is discussed elsewhere in chapters 8 and 26.

LEIOMYOMAS

Leiomyomas may cause significant chronic pressure, discomfort, or pelvic pain. With degeneration, leiomyomas can cause acute pelvic pain. The evaluation and surgical treatment of leiomyomas are discussed in chapter 7.

OVARIAN REMNANT SYNDROME

Ovarian remnant syndrome is the persistence of ovarian tissue inadvertently not removed at the time of intended extirpation of one or both ovaries, with or without hysterectomy. Usually patients with ovarian remnant syndrome present with CPP after a previous bilateral salpingo-oophorectomy and hysterectomy. It may occur in women who still have their uterus and other ovary but is reported less frequently in such patients. Ovarian remnant syndrome probably occurs much more commonly than generally thought (91), because it is often not considered in the patient with pelvic pain who has had a hysterectomy and bilateral oophorectomy (92,93).

Ovarian remnant syndrome most often occurs as a complication of a difficult oophorectomy. The most common predisposing factors are prior PID, adhesive disease from prior surgery, inflammatory bowel disease, and endometriosis. Adhesions, whether from prior abdominopelvic surgery or diseases that cause adhesions, appear to be a quite important etiological factor. The adhesive disease makes the oophorectomy more difficult, increasing the risk of incomplete removal. Using blunt dissection to try to separate the ovary from the peritoneum, rather than removing the adherent peritoneum along with the ovary, may be a major risk factor for subsequent ovarian remnant development. Another surgical technique that may play an etiological role is clamping the ovarian vessels very close to the ovary, with the risk of retaining a portion of ovarian tissue attached to the vessels on the proximal side of the clamp (94). The use of endoloops to ligate the infundibulopelvic ligament without skeletonizing the vessels has also been suggested as a possible cause of ovarian remnant syndrome (95).

A patient with ovarian remnant syndrome may present anytime from a few months to five years or more after her oophorectomy. Symptoms are variable, but the most common presenting symptoms are (1) pelvic pain, (2) dyspareunia, and/or (3) a pelvic mass. More than 90% of women diagnosed with ovarian remnant syndrome present with abdominopelvic pain. The abdominal examination usually reveals multiple surgical scars consistent with a history of prior surgical procedures. Tenderness to deep palpation may be present and is usually on the same side as the remnant. Ovarian remnants are usually too small to be palpated abdominally. At pelvic examination, inspection of the external genitalia and vagina usually reveals signs of estrogen effect, with normal-sized labia and moist, well-cornified vaginal mucosa. Pelvic palpation may reveal tenderness in one or both fornices. Bimanual pelvic examination may reveal a palpable mass, although its absence does not preclude the diagnosis. If a mass is palpable, it is usually tender and small (less than 5 cm) and located on the pelvic sidewall or at the lateral vaginal apex.

Laboratory and imaging studies are important to support the suspicion of an ovarian remnant before these patients are subjected to another surgical procedure. If the patient is not on hormonal replacement therapy, or the therapy is stopped for several weeks, obtaining a follicle-stimulating hormone (FSH) level less than 40 mIU/mL and an estradiol level greater than 30 pg/mL confirms the diagnosis. Premenopausal levels of FSH and estradiol are present in 50% to 75% of women with an ovarian remnant. When ovarian remnant syndrome is suspected and FSH and estradiol levels are in the postmenopausal range, the GnRH agonist (GnRH-a) stimulation test is useful (96,97). GnRH agonists initially stimulate gonadotropin production and, therefore, ovarian estrogen production. This observation is used in the GnRH-a stimulation test, in which a baseline level of estradiol is measured and GnRH agonist (for example, depot leuprolide 3.75 mg intramuscularly once, or leuprolide 1 mg a day for three days subcutaneously) is administered, followed by repeat measurement of estradiol four to seven days later. If hormonally responsive ovarian tissue is present, then a significant rise in estradiol occurs. This test may not be reliable if exogenous hormones are being taken. Imaging studies are important both diagnostically and preoperatively. Vaginal ultrasound shows a pelvic mass in more than 50% of cases (98,99). The diagnostic accuracy of ultrasound may be improved by pretreatment with clomiphene citrate (100). A 5- to 10-day course of clomiphene citrate, 100 mg daily, appears to stimulate follicular formation in up to 90% of cases, and this may permit easier sonographic visualization. Not all ovarian remnants have functional follicles, so this technique is not consistently helpful. Computerized tomography, particularly with intravenous contrast to evaluate the urinary tract (101), can be extremely useful. It is possibly more useful when the remnant is extremely small or is surrounded by dense adhesions and is not cystic. If there is ureteral dilation, hydronephrosis, or ureteral deviation, serum urea nitrogen and creatinine levels should be obtained. In some cases, the diagnosis of ovarian remnant can only be made at the time of surgery and even then it can be difficult. Laparoscopy is an inconsistent diagnostic tool, as dense adhesions frequently hide an ovarian remnant.

Properly performed surgical excision appears to be the optimum treatment for the woman with CPP who has an ovarian remnant (91,92,102,103), in spite of the fact that it is usually a difficult surgery with notable risk of complications and that there is a postoperative recurrence rate of 8% to 15%. Multiple surgeries for remnants are not uncommon (91,102). Alternatives to surgery are medical treatment and radiation therapy (104). Sonographically directed aspiration of cysts has also been suggested as a possible treatment (98).

Surgical treatment may be performed laparoscopically or laparotomically, but laparotomy has generally been preferred (92,103,105). Advocates of laparotomy cite the dense adhesions and anatomic distortion, resulting in extremely difficult surgery in most of the cases, as the reasons for laparoscopy to be inappropriate. There is a significant risk of injury to the ureters, intestines, and major vessels in performing complete resection of ovarian remnants, in addition to the risk of inadvertent injuries due to the dense adhesions and anatomic distortion. There is a legitimate concern that such risks might predispose to less than optimal resection with a laparoscopic approach. In spite of these concerns, there have been reports of laparosocopic treatment of the condition with apparent success (102,106–108). Our unreported success rate with laparoscopic treatment is 95%.

Regardless of the surgical approach, there are preoperative preparations that can optimize outcomes. In cases with small, nonpalpable remnants, the use of clomiphene citrate to stimulate ovarian cyst production, as described previously to help with sonographic evaluation, can also be used to facilitate identification at the time of surgery. Preoperative urinary tract pyelography, computerized tomography, and/or sonography can help identify those at risk of intraoperative ureteral injury. Full bowel preparation is also important, since bowel damage or resection may be necessary.

At surgery, lengthy and tedious adhesiolysis of omentum and bowel is usually required to expose the ovarian remnant. Because of the potential of multiple ipsilateral as well as bilateral remnants, complete restoration of anatomy and exposure of the pelvis are essential. After the remnant is adequately exposed, retroperitoneal dissection is strongly suggested. A retroperitoneal approach allows the safest access to ensure complete excision of an ovarian remnant (Fig. 12). Opening the peritoneum at the pelvic brim and dissecting the entire pelvic course of the ureter allow mobilization and protection of the ureter and permit complete excision of all peritoneum adherent to the remnant. These also permit coagulation or ligation of any vascular supply to the remnant that is identified during the dissection. Dissection along the course of the ureter usually leads to the mass, which in many cases lies on the pelvic sidewall peritoneum at the ovarian fossa or near the angle of the vaginal vault. Dissection of the bladder off the vaginal vault may often be needed. In addition, resection of a portion of the vagina, bladder, colon, or ureter is sometimes unavoidable if the mass is adherent to any of these structures. Ureteral stents may be helpful in avoiding ureteral injury, although there is controversy over their usefulness. Anecdotally, we have found them particularly useful if laparoscopic excision is being attempted. The placement of radio-opaque vascular clips in the area of the removed remnant may be reasonable, as this may help direct radioablative treatment or reoperation in the event of a recurrence. With a 10% recurrence rate, an aggressive approach is mandatory and affords the best opportunity to excise adherent peritoneum and ensure complete resection of the remnant.

OVARIAN RETENTION SYNDROME (RESIDUAL OVARY SYNDROME)

Ovarian retention syndrome (residual ovary syndrome) is the presence of persistent pelvic pain, dyspareunia, or a pelvic mass after intended conservation of one or both ovaries at the time of hysterectomy. The frequency of the syndrome is not certain, but reported frequencies range from 0.9% to 4.9% (109,110). Pelvic adhesions are thought to be a major etiological factor in the development of pain with ovarian retention syndrome, especially if there is encapsulation of the ovary in dense adhesions. There is a high prevalence of adhesive disease in patients with ovarian retention syndrome that often complicates attempts at surgical treatment. A history of pelvic surgery prior to hysterectomy appears to be an etiological factor in ovarian retention syndrome, as this history is present in 35%

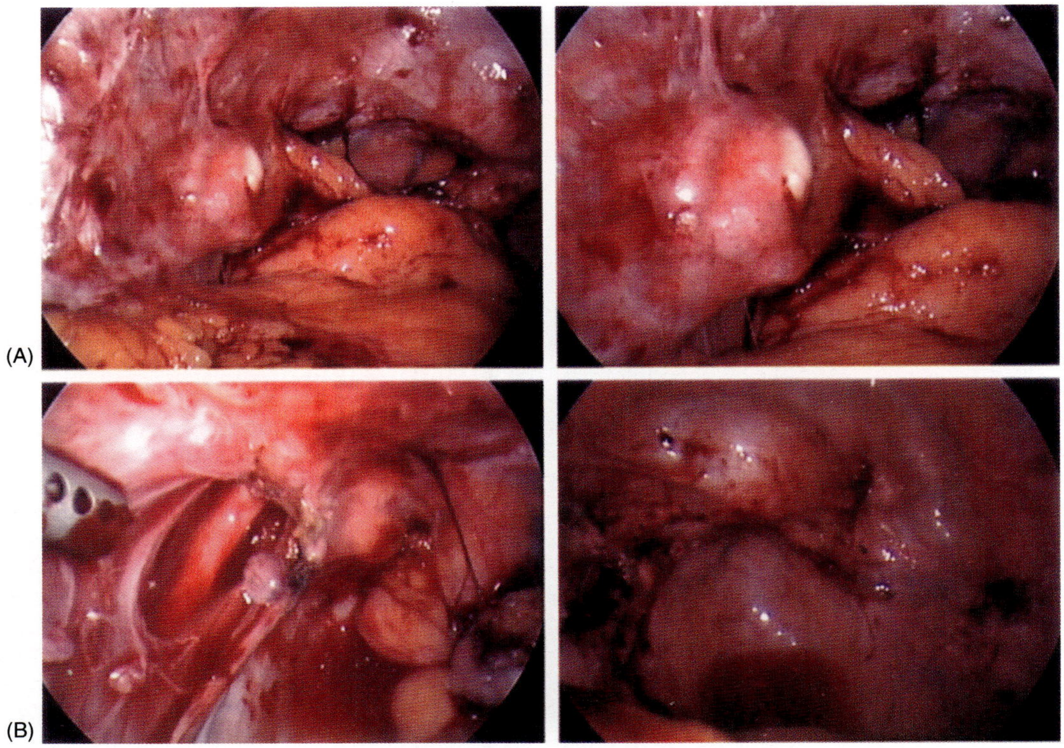

Figure 12 Ovarian remnant syndrome. (A) Ovarian remnant on the left pelvic sidewall. (B) After excision of the ovarian remnant, illustrating the location directly over the left ureter requiring retroperitoneal dissection.

to 79% of cases. Also, many patients with ovarian retention syndrome have histories of pelvic pain prior to hysterectomy. Persistent or recurrent pelvic pain may be due to inadequate treatment of the etiology of pain with a simple hysterectomy, such as may be the case with pelvic congestion syndrome or endometriosis or may be due to the pre-existence of inflammatory or neuropathic pain. The presence of such nociceptive abnormalities may also predispose the patient to pain due to the development of adhesions or persistent functional ovarian cysts.

Ovarian retention syndrome tends to cause intermittent or CPP and is rarely a source of acute pain. If pain is intermittent, it may be cyclical or may occur with coitus. The pelvic examination usually reveals marked tenderness of one or both ovaries, with adherence to the vaginal apex. It may show a tender pelvic mass at the vaginal vault in many patients. Malignancies are not common in ovarian retention syndrome but have been reported in 0.1% to 0.35% of cases, so the potential must be considered in patients with a pelvic mass. Imaging studies are useful both for diagnosing and for evaluating the potential concern of a malignancy. A diagnostic approach using GnRH agonists has been suggested based on the theory that since functional ovaries are an integral part of ovarian retention syndrome, suppressing their function should produce an amelioration of symptoms (97). Laparoscopy may be used both as a diagnostic and as a therapeutic modality.

Medical treatments have been suggested, but published results are scarce. Suggested medical treatments include estrogen replacement therapy, oral contraceptives, GnRH agonists, and progestins such as medroxyprogesterone acetate. Treatment is usually surgical. Oophorectomy is the best way to treat symptomatic ovarian retention syndrome, provided the ovaries are the cause of the pain. The actual surgery differs from case to case but mainly involves salpingo-oophorectomy and extensive adhesiolysis, and in some cases excision or destruction of endometriosis. Almost all reported series have employed an abdominal laparotomy as the surgical approach, but successful surgical treatment using operative laparoscopy has been reported (111). The surgery can be technically demanding because of the preponderance of adhesions found at surgery. Bowel preparation is important, since in some cases bowel resection may be needed and bowel injury during extensive adhesiolysis is not uncommon. Identification of the ureters is crucial due to the adhesions to the pelvic sidewalls. Extensive retroperitoneal dissection of the ureters is often necessary to free the ovaries. Placement of ureteral stents may be helpful in cases where distortion of the anatomy prevents easy visualization of the ureters, especially for laparoscopic procedures.

OVARIAN TUMOR

Benign ovarian tumors do not generally present with pelvic pain. In some cases, especially with rupture or torsion, they may cause acute or intermittent pelvic pain. Their management is not within the prevue of this chapter.

PELVIC CONGESTION SYNDROME

Pelvic congestion syndrome remains a controversial disorder, but substantial research, particularly by Beard and his colleagues, suggests that the syndrome is a legitimate diagnosis and is responsible for pelvic pain in a substantial number of women (112–114). This research suggests that pelvic congestion syndrome is defined most accurately by the triad of pelvic pain, pelvic varicosities, and pelvic venous congestion with delayed emptying of pelvic veins. It is important to recognize that visualizing varicosities does justify a diagnosis of pelvic congestion syndrome and that venography to confirm stasis and congestion is critical to the diagnosis. Using such a definition, Soysal et al. found that pelvic congestion syndrome may be a source of pelvic pain in up to 40%, and potentially the only source in 30%, of women with CPP (115).

Pelvic pain is the essential symptom of pelvic congestion syndrome. The most consistent description is dull, aching pain in the pelvic area, similar to the quality of pain described in the legs of people with symptomatic leg varicosities. Pain is usually brought on or exacerbated by simple acts such as walking or changing posture. It is also most severe premenstrually, which has been termed congestive dysmenorrhea. Congestive dysmenorrhea is present in about 90% of cases of pelvic congestion (114). Occasionally, acute paroxysmal exacerbations of sharp pain may occur, at times severe enough to result in emergency evaluation and lead to mistaken diagnoses such as acute appendicitis or PID. Deep dyspareunia is another consistent symptom of pelvic congestion syndrome, occurring in 70% to 80% of patients. Postcoital pelvic aching, lasting in some cases up to 24 hours, is also typical of pelvic congestion syndrome and occurs in about 65% of cases.

Abdominal palpation reveals tenderness at the ovarian point (Fig. 13), which lies at the junction of the upper and middle thirds of a line drawn from the anterior superior iliac spine to the umbilicus, in about 75% of women with pelvic congestion syndrome (114). Deep abdominal pressure at this point reproduces the pelvic pain complained of by the patient. This is believed to be due to compression of the ovarian vein, leading to back pressure on the plexus of veins at the ovarian hilum. Palpation of the cervix frequently elicits pain and tenderness on movement. Also, the uterosacral ligaments and the parametrium are often tender to palpation. Uterine and adnexal tenderness to palpation are characteristic of pelvic congestion syndrome (114).

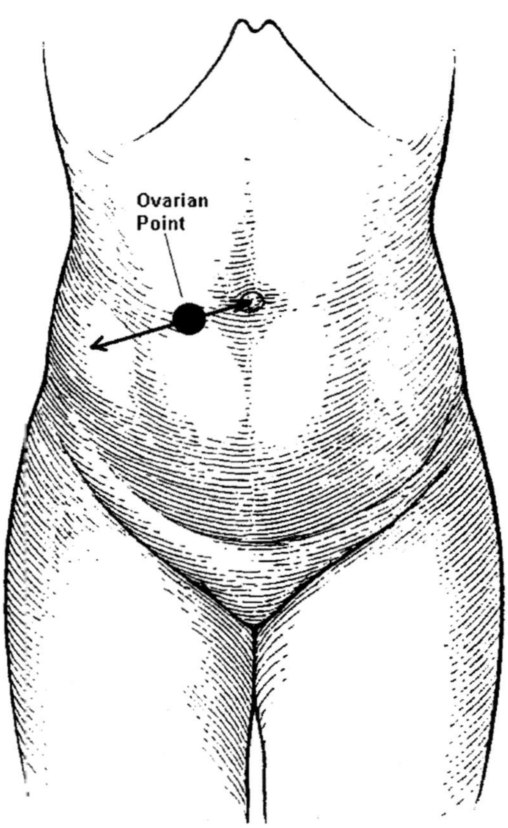

Figure 13 Illustration of the ovarian point on the right lower abdomen. Reproduction of pelvic pain by compression at this point suggests a diagnosis of pelvic congestion syndrome.

Laparoscopy is one of the most common diagnostic studies performed by gynecologists for pelvic pain, but it is not a reliable way to diagnose pelvic congestion syndrome, even though pelvic varicosities can sometimes be visualized (116). The high intra-abdominal pressure and Trendelenburg position used with pelvic laparoscopy, however, promote venous drainage and decrease venous distention and, thus, may obscure pelvic varicosities even when they are present. It is important to realize that neither the identification of varicosities nor the negative findings at the time of laparoscopy are sufficient to make a positive or negative conclusion regarding the diagnosis of pelvic congestion syndrome. If varicosities are noted, then pelvic venography is still needed to confirm the presence of congestion. Similarly, if laparoscopic findings are negative, pelvic venography may be indicated, as Beard et al. found, based on venographic findings, that about 90% of women with pelvic pain and negative laparoscopies had pelvic congestion syndrome (112).

Pelvic venography is the current "gold standard" diagnostic test for pelvic congestion syndrome (112). A variety of techniques have been used, but the most common techniques are selective retrograde ovarian venography and transuterine venography. Transuterine venography is technically easy to perform, is relatively inexpensive, and is the method best validated for accurate diagnosis (112,117,118). Water-soluble contrast medium is introduced into the uterine venous system via injection into the myometrium of the uterine fundus. This is facilitated by using a special single-lumen needle and metal sheath (a reusable system is available from Rocket Needle, Rocket Co., London, U.K.; a disposable system is available from Cook Women's Health, Bloomington, Indiana). The needle is passed through the cervix via a special concentric sheath that covers all but the final 0.5-cm tip of the needle. With the patient on her back and ideally in slight reverse Trendelenburg position, 20 to 30 mL of the contrast medium are injected, with or without abdominal compression. The first image is taken immediately at the end of injection, followed by a second image 20 seconds later, and a third image at 60 seconds (Fig. 14). Transuterine venography is painful and may require heavy sedation and/or general or local anesthesia to perform. Beard and colleagues have described a venogram scoring system based on the maximum diameter of the ovarian veins, time of disappearance of contrast, and the degree of congestion of the ovarian plexus (Table 4) (112). The score can range from 3 to 9, with 3 or 4 being normal and 5 to 9 suggesting increasingly severe pelvic congestion. This method has been validated by others (115).

Selective ovarian venography can either be performed via a jugular venous approach (119) or a transfemoral approach (Fig. 15) (120–122). The technique is performed under local anesthesia, often with sedation, and involves puncturing the common femoral vein and placing a small-diameter introducer sheath. Special Teflon catheters are passed under fluoroscopic guidance into the ovarian veins and nonionic

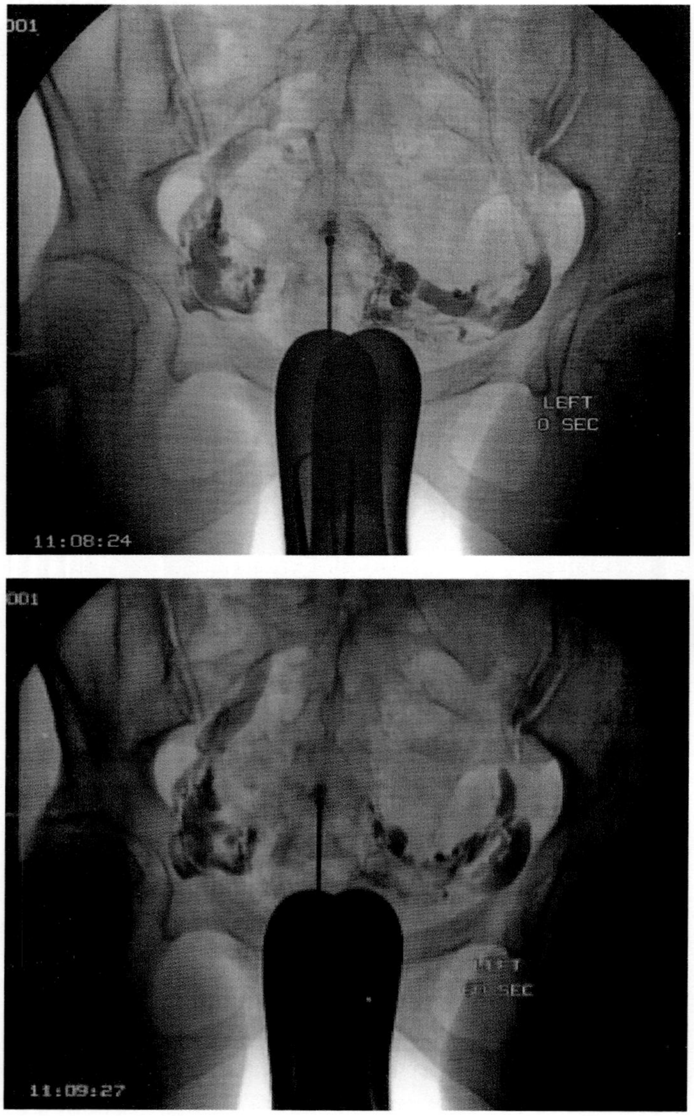

Figure 14 Images from a transcervical antegrade pelvic venogram. Images are at injection and at 60 seconds after injection of contrast.

water-soluble contrast medium injected. Because the right ovarian vein drains directly into the inferior vena cava, it is more difficult to cannulate and usually involves using a catheter of type or size different from the left side. Some consider this invasive technique to be the method of choice for diagnosis of pelvic varicosities. The diagnostic criteria recommended by Kennedy and Hemmingway are maximal ovarian vein diameter of 10 mm, congestion of the ovarian venous plexus, filling of veins across the midline, or filling of vulvar

Table 4 Scoring System for Assessing Transuterine Pelvic Venography

	Score		
	1	2	3
Maximal diameter of ovarian veins (mm)	1–4	5–8	>8
Time to disappearance of contrast medium after end of injection (sec)	0	20	40
Ovarian plexus congestion	Normal	Moderate	Extensive

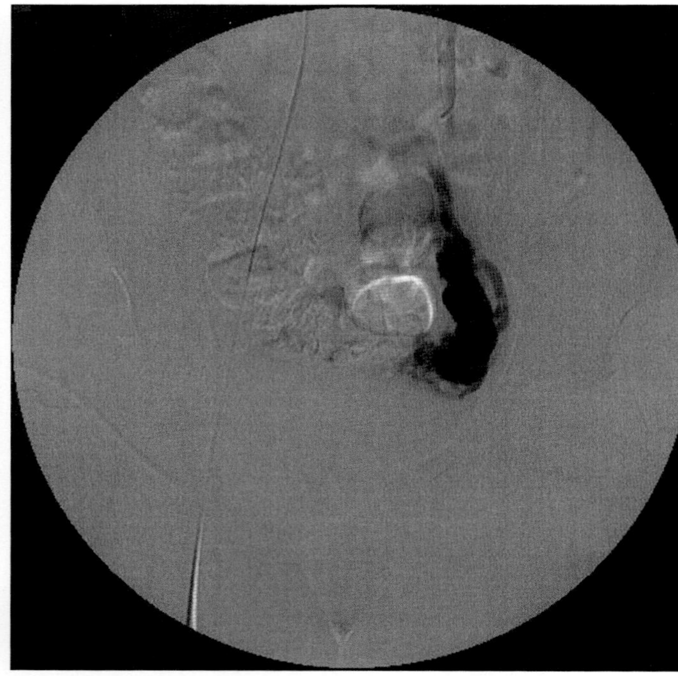

Figure 15 Image from a selective retrograde pelvic venogram.

and thigh varicosities (123). These criteria are not as well validated or standardized as those for transuterine venography.

Medical treatment with medroxyprogesterone acetate, 50 mg/day, has been shown to be effective in a double-blind, randomized, placebo-controlled trial (124). However, when medroxyprogesterone acetate was stopped after four months' treatment, pain levels returned to pretreatment levels rapidly. Psychotherapy was evaluated in this trial also, as solitary therapy was not effective. However, it prolonged the response to medroxyprogesterone acetate. GnRH agonist treatment with goserelin acetate (3.6 mg/mo for six months) has been compared to medroxyprogesterone acetate in another study and shown to be more effective than medroxyprogesterone acetate (115). Recently, transvenous embolization has been used and observational data appear promising (120–122,125–131). There are no published randomized clinical trials of venous embolization therapy as yet.

Surgical treatment has primarily been done by hysterectomy and bilateral salpingo-oophorectomy, although bilateral ovarian venous ligation, performed close to the entry of the right vein into the vena cava and close to the left vein entry into the renal vein, has also been utilized. Observational data suggest that when the diagnosis of pelvic congestion is certain, with venographic confirmation, and there are no other etiologies for pelvic pain, removal of the ovaries and uterus is curative. Beard et al. performed hysterectomy plus bilateral salpingo-oophorectomy on 36 women with pelvic congestion syndrome documented by venography, 33 of whom had failed to obtain relief with long-term medical therapy (132). Their results showed a dramatic improvement in pain scores, a return to normal lifestyles, and a significant increase in frequency of intercourse. The benefits of such surgery must be carefully weighed against the drawbacks of loss of fertility and the necessity of long-term hormonal replacement therapy.

PELVIC INFLAMMATORY DISEASE

Although laparoscopy is considered the gold standard for the diagnosis of PID, the diagnosis is most often made clinically without laparoscopy. Treatment of PID is almost always medical. Surgical treatment is infrequent and done usually only in occasional cases of tubo-ovarian abscess (TOA). When PID is complicated by TOA and medical treatment is insufficient, drainage of the TOA may be necessary. This can be done nonsurgically by placement of a transvaginal or percutaneous drain using ultrasound guidance (133–135). Surgical treatment may be via laparoscopy, laparotomy, or colpotomy. Because laparoscopy and colpotomy are less invasive than laparotomy and appear to give similar outcomes when conservative surgery is performed, they are the preferred approaches (136–138). In some life-threatening cases of TOA, hysterectomy and salpingo-oophorectomy may be necessary.

After PID, up to 30% of women develop CPP. Although this is often called chronic PID, there is no evidence of chronic infection as a cause of the pain (139). There is no clear evidence available to substantiate the effectiveness of any medical or surgical treatments of post-PID CPP, but anecdotal experience suggests that hysterectomy and bilateral salpingo-oophorectomy usually relieve pain.

POSTOPERATIVE PERITONEAL CYSTS

Cysts that develop after pelvic surgery may be peritoneal inclusion cysts or postoperative peritoneal cysts. Peritoneal inclusion cysts are benign adnexal masses that occur secondary to fluid trapped among adhesions surrounding an ovary. Postoperative peritoneal cysts are rare postoperative abdominal or pelvic cysts that are lined by mesothelial cells and are associated with adhesions. Often they present with CPP. Postoperative peritoneal cysts may occur months to years after surgery and occur after a variety of operative procedures. They have been reported only in women (140). Ultrasonography almost always shows one or more large, complex, cystic masses with thin walls and septations.

Treatment can be done sometimes by transvaginal aspiration, but the recurrence rate is about 50% (140). In cases that recur after drainage, drainage followed by ethanol instillation may be an option. Surgical treatment may be excision or simply adhesiolysis. Most often the surgery is difficult and complicated because of prior surgery and significant adhesive disease. It is often not feasible to perform the surgery laparoscopically.

PRIMARY DYSMENORRHEA

Dysmenorrhea is severe, cramping pain in the lower abdomen, lower back, and upper thighs and occurs during menses or may also occur prior to the onset of menses. Dysmenorrhea is a common complaint of both adolescent and adult women and represents a significant individual and public health problem. Some degree of menstrual pain is present in 75% of women, but severe menstrual pain is present in about 15% (141). This leads to significant work absenteeism, with resultant economic and social consequences for the individuals afflicted.

Primary dysmenorrhea refers to severe menstrual pain with no identifiable pelvic pathology that accounts for the pain; thus, it is a diagnosis of exclusion. Primary dysmenorrhea usually begins 6 to 12 months after menarche and coincides with the onset of ovulatory cycles. Many young women, including adolescents, who are thought to have primary dysmenorrhea, in fact, have undiagnosed endometriosis. Primary dysmenorrhea appears to be due principally to prostaglandins F2α and E2 released from the endometrium at menses.

Successful management of severe, primary dysmenorrhea can be challenging. Medical treatment is usually successful with one or more of the following treatments: oral contraceptives, nonsteroidal anti-inflammatory drugs, Cox-2 inhibitors, calcium antagonists such as verapamil or nifedipine, or levonorgestrel-releasing intrauterine contraceptive device insertion. When one or more of these medical treatments are unsuccessful, then surgical evaluation and treatment may be beneficial. In particular, it is important to diagnose and treat endometriosis, which is a frequent cause of dysmenorrhea. When the diagnosis is primary dysmenorrhea, hysterectomy is generally curative, but most women with primary dysmenorrhea are too young to consider this a viable option. The mainstay of conservative surgical treatment has been interruption of neural pathways from the uterus. The afferent sensory innervation of the uterus runs primarily with the autonomic sympathetic nerves (T10–L2) (Fig. 16). Cutting the sympathetic nerves promotes vasodilatation, interrupts sensory input from the uterus, and often relieves the pain of dysmenorrhea. Presacral neurectomy consists of transection of the sympathetic nerves of the superior hypogastric plexus at the sacral promontory (Fig. 16). It has an efficacy of about 75% in relieving midline dysmenorrhea. Uterine nerve ablation, which is performed by transecting the uterosacral ligaments (Fig. 17), may be more easily performed than a presacral neurectomy, but there are less reliable data regarding its efficacy (142). Cervical dilatation has been historically used to relieve dysmenorrhea thought to be secondary to cervical stenosis. Its value is debatable, but it may act by promoting blood flow, disrupting sensory nerves from the cervix, or decreasing intrauterine pressure secondary to obstruction.

Presacral neurectomy for dysmenorrhea was first reported by Jaboulay (143) and Ruggi (144). Black, based on a review of 72 articles published from 1936 to 1963, plus his own cases, estimated that 75% to 85% of women had relief of dysmenorrhea after presacral neurectomy (145). These data, like most regarding presacral neurectomy, were observational. Chen et al. reported a clinical trial of 68 women with primary dysmenorrhea randomized to either presacral neurectomy or uterine nerve ablation, which showed that at 12 months presacral neurectomy had an efficacy of 82% compared to 51% with uterine nerve ablation. Both procedures were performed laparoscopically in this study. The roles of presacral neurectomy and uterine nerve ablation for dysmenorrhea are limited in current practice, but if surgical treatment is thought to be indicated, presacral neurectomy is the preferred procedure.

Technique of Laparoscopic Presacral Neurectomy

Our preferred technique uses three or four ports, depending on the need to retract the sigmoid colon from the prelumbar prominatory. After 5-mm cannulas are placed at the umbilicus and the right and left lower quadrants, the patient is placed in steep Trendelenburg position. Bowel is carefully moved out of the pelvis with an atraumatic laparoscopic instrument to obtain full exposure of the presacral space. If the sigmoid colon still lies over the presacral and prelumbar space, the patient can be tilted to the left. If this still does not provide adequate exposure, then another left-sided 5-mm cannula is inserted superiorly to the left lower quadrant cannula to allow

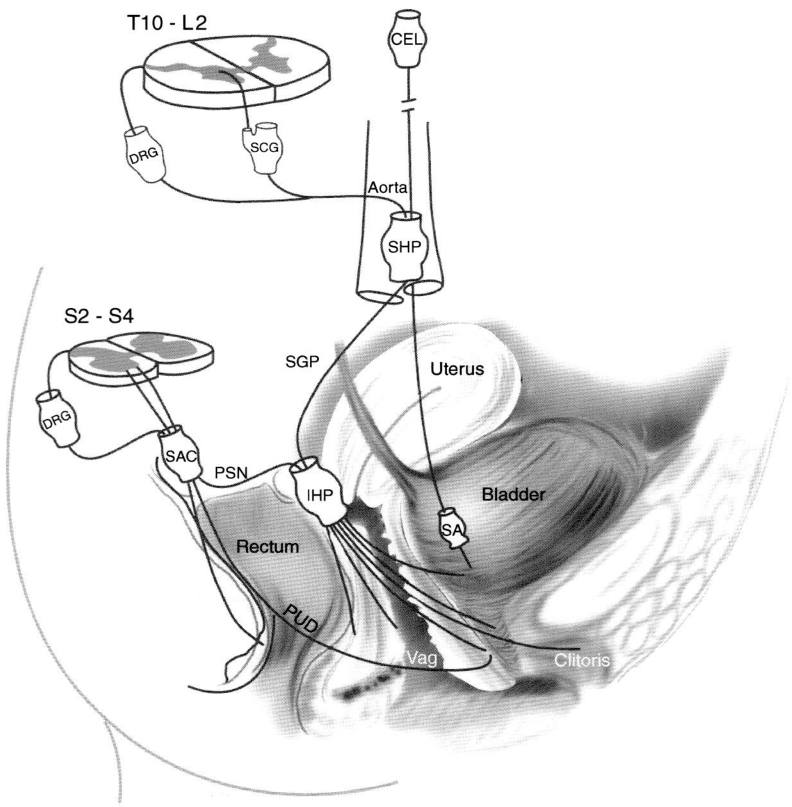

Figure 16 Illustration of the innervation of the pelvis. The superior hypogastric plexus is excised during a presacral neurectomy.

retraction of the sigmoid colon. The peritoneum should be carefully incised to allow visualization of the essential anatomic landmarks. I find that a transverse incision about 5 to 10 cm below the aortic bifurcation, extending from right ureter to left ureter or inferior mesenteric vessels, superior hemorrhoidal artery, and the sigmoid colon provides optimal exposure. (Most often the left ureter is not seen, because it is often covered by the sigmoid colon.) Careful blunt and sharp dissection is performed into the areolar tissue over the presacral and prelumbar spaces. The neural bundles and fibers are grasped, coagulated distally and proximally, and then excised. This is done in the entire presacral space from the left to the right margins of the dissection. The excised tissue is submitted for histological evaluation. The middle sacral vessels are posterior to the superior hypogastric plexus (presacral nerve) and are easily injured during this procedure. This is why I strongly suggest that the specimens should always be proximally and distally coagulated before they are cut. At this level of dissection, the middle sacral vessels can be safely coagulated and cut, but if they are traumatized or cut without ensuring coagulation and hemostasis, then significant hemorrhage can occur and it may be extremely difficult to control. The other vessel that may be easily injured inadvertently is the left common iliac vein. It usually is collapsed due to the pneumoperitoneum, and this may obscure its identification. Obviously, it is important to avoid cutting or coagulating it during the dissection. Although the peritoneal incision can be closed at the completion of the procedure, this is not necessary.

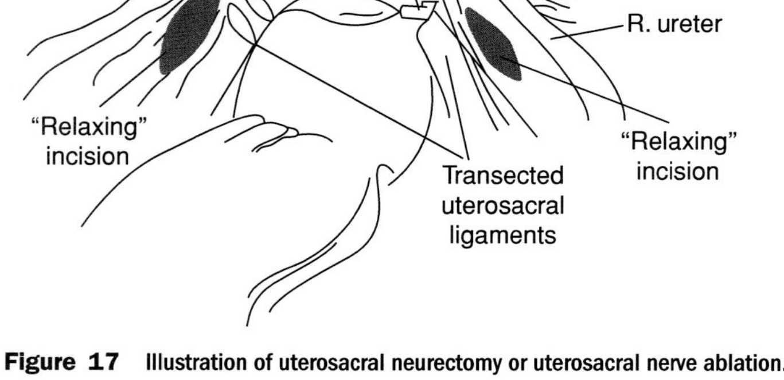

Figure 17 Illustration of uterosacral neurectomy or uterosacral nerve ablation.

Presacral neurectomy has several complications specific to the procedure. As noted already, the anatomic margins of the dissection are the ureters, sigmoid colon, inferior mesenteric and superior hemorrhoidal vessels, and common iliac vessels, so all of these vital structures may be injured with potentially dire consequences. Postoperatively, constipation, painless first stage of labor, urinary urgency, and chylous ascites have all been reported. Constipation appears to be the most significant long-term postoperative complication and has been reported in up to 75% of cases (146), although clinically significant constipation occurs in only 3% to 15% of patients (147).

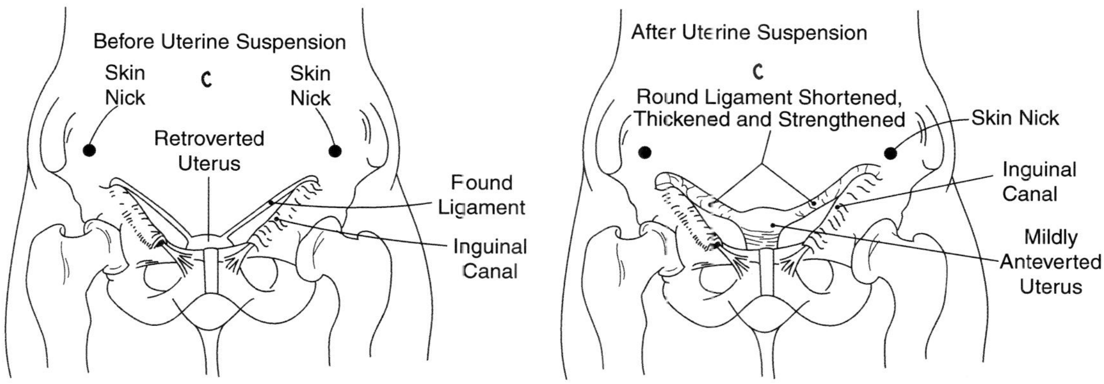

Figure 18 Illustraton of the steps in an uplift uterine suspension procedure.

RESIDUAL ACCESSORY OVARY

Ectopic ovaries may be either accessory or supernumerary. Supernumerary ovary refers to ovarian tissue that is entirely separate from the normally placed ovaries. It is believed to be derived from a separate primordium. Accessory ovary refers to ovarian tissue that is situated near or connected to a normally placed ovary. It is thought to originate from a separated fragment from the developing embryonic ovary. Ectopic ovaries are exceedingly rare. About 30 histologically confirmed cases of supernumerary ovary and about 22 cases of accessory ovaries have been reported since 1891. Ectopic ovaries normally produce no symptoms but can occasionally be associated with CPP, particularly after bilateral salpingo-oophorectomy if the patients undergo cystic or neoplastic transformation (148).

The proper management for symptomatic ectopic ovaries is oophorectomy. Often such ovaries may be retroperitoneal, necessitating retroperitoneal dissection and identification of the ureters and the blood supply to allow safe removal. There are no reports of any trials of medical treatment. Since many of the pelvic ectopic ovaries are retroperitoneal, precautions should be taken to properly identify the major pelvic sidewall vessels and the ureters.

RUPTURED OVARIAN CYSTS

Ruptured ovarian cysts generally cause severe, acute pelvic pain that resolves within 24 to 48 hours and do not need surgical treatment in most cases. Rupture of an ovarian cyst is not an uncommon occurrence in women of reproductive age. Occasionally, significant hemorrhage can occur, especially in women on anticoagulant medications, and surgical intervention is necessary. Surgical intervention may be necessary, also, with rupture of a benign cystic teratoma and spillage of sebaceous material into the abdominal cavity that can cause a marked chemical peritonitis. In other cases, the diagnosis may be uncertain and may require surgical evaluation and treatment. In most cases of ruptured ovarian cysts that require surgical management, the most appropriate procedure is laparoscopic ovarian cystectomy, unless there is a significant concern of malignancy preoperatively or intraoperatively. If malignancy is present, of course, more aggressive surgical debulking and staging are crucial for appropriate surgical management. Even when malignancy is not suspected, it is important to meticulously exclude the diagnosis.

UTERINE RETROVERSION

Uterine retroversion that is not due to pelvic pathology, such as endometriosis or pelvic adhesions, does not generally cause pelvic pain. However, there appears to be a small proportion of women with uterine retroversion who experience persistent deep dyspareunia, which has been termed "collision dyspareunia." Evidence for this syndrome is primarily based on expert opinion. The diagnosis is supported by the reproduction of the patient's pain with digital palpation of the retroverted uterine fundus at the time of physical examination. Relief of pain by a Hodge pessary also supports the diagnosis.

Surgical treatment by uterine ventrosuspension has been reported. One study showed approximately 50% long-term response rate to this procedure (149). A technique for laparoscopic uterine suspension developed by Carter and used to treat patients with deep dyspareunia that appears to be secondary to a retroverted uterus is illustrated in Fig. 18. Reports of case series using this suspension technique suggest a success rate of about 75% in relieving dyspareunia (150,151).

REFERENCES

1. IASP Task Force on Taxonomy. Classification of chronic pain. In: Merskey H, Bogduk N, eds. Seattle: IASP Press, 1994:209–214.
2. Rapkin AJ, Mayer EA. Gastroenterologic causes of chronic pelvic pain. Obstet Gynecol Clin North Am 1993; 20:663–683.
3. Nanda K, Peloggia A, Grimes D, et al. Expectant care versus surgical treatment for miscarriage. Cochrane Database Syst Rev 2006; CD003518.
4. Trinder J, Brocklehurst P, Porter R, et al. Management of miscarriage: Expectant, medical, or surgical? Results of randomised controlled trial (miscarriage treatment (MIST) trial). BMJ 2006; 332:1235–1240.
5. Sawaya GF, Grady D, Kerlikowske K, et al. Antibiotics at the time of induced abortion: The case for universal prophylaxis based on a meta-analysis. Obstet Gynecol 1996; 87:884–890.
6. Prieto JA, Eriksen NL, Blanco JD. A randomized trial of prophylactic doxycycline for curettage in incomplete abortion. Obstet Gynecol 1995; 85:692–696.
7. Bird CC, McElin TW, Manalo-Estrella P. The elusive adenomyosis of the uterus—revisited. Am J Obstet Gynecol 1972; 112:583–593.
8. McElin TW, Bird CC. Adenomyosis of the uterus. Obstet Gynecol Annu 1974; 3:425–441.

9. Guarnaccia MM, Silverberg K, Olive DL. Endometriosis and adenomyosis. In: Copeland LJ, ed. Textbook of Gynecology. Philadelphia, PA: WB Saunders, 2000:687–722.
10. Azziz R. Adenomyosis: Current perspectives. Obstet Gynecol Clin North Am 1989; 16:221–235.
11. Sammour A, Pirwany I, Usubutun A, et al. Correlations between extent and spread of adenomyosis and clinical symptoms. Gynecol Obstet Invest 2002; 54:213–216.
12. Fedele L, Bianchi S, Dorta M, et al. Transvaginal ultrasonography in the diagnosis of diffuse adenomyosis. Fertil Steril 1992; 58:94–97.
13. Fedele L, Bianchi S, Dorta M, et al. Transvaginal ultrasonography in the differential diagnosis of adenomyoma versus leiomyoma. Am J Obstet Gynecol 1992; 167:603–606.
14. Bohlman ME, Ensor RE, Sanders RC. Sonographic findings in adenomyosis of the uterus. AJR Am J Roentgenol 1987; 148:765–766.
15. Mark AS, Hricak H, Heinrichs LW, et al. Adenomyosis and leiomyoma: Differential diagnosis with MR imaging. Radiology 1987; 163:527–529.
16. Togashi K, Ozasa H, Konishi I, et al. Enlarged uterus: Differentiation between adenomyosis and leiomyoma with MR imaging. Radiology 1989; 171:531–534.
17. Atri M, Reinhold C, Mehio AR, et al. Adenomyosis: US features with histologic correlation in an in-vitro study. Radiology 2000; 215:783–790.
18. Bazot M, Darai E, Rouger J, et al. Limitations of transvaginal sonography for the diagnosis of adenomyosis, with histopathological correlation. Ultrasound Obstet Gynecol 2002; 20: 605–611.
19. Fong YF, Singh K. Medical treatment of a grossly enlarged adenomyotic uterus with the levonorgestrel-releasing intrauterine system. Contraception 1999; 60:173–175.
20. Fedele L, Bianchi S, Raffaelli R, et al. Treatment of adenomyosis-associated menorrhagia with a levonorgestrel-releasing intrauterine device. Fertil Steril 1997; 68:426–429.
21. Grow DR, Filer RB. Treatment of adenomyosis with long-term GnRH analogues: A case report. Obstet Gynecol 1991; 78:538–539.
22. Nelson JR, Corson SL. Long-term management of adenomyosis with a gonadotropin-releasing hormone agonist: A case report. Fertil Steril 1993; 59:441–443.
23. Lin J, Sun C, Zheng H. Gonadotropin-releasing hormone agonists and laparoscopy in the treatment of adenomyosis with infertility. Chin Med J (Engl) 2000; 113:442–445.
24. Hirata JD, Moghissi KS, Ginsburg KA. Pregnancy after medical therapy of adenomyosis with a gonadotropin-releasing hormone agonist. Fertil Steril 1993; 59:444–445.
25. McCausland V, McCausland A. The response of adenomyosis to endometrial ablation/resection. Hum Reprod Update 1998; 4:350–359.
26. McCausland AM, McCausland VM. Partial rollerball endometrial ablation: A modification of total ablation to treat menorrhagia without causing complications from intrauterine adhesions. Am J Obstet Gynecol 1999; 180:1512–1521.
27. McCausland AM, McCausland VM. Depth of endometrial penetration in adenomyosis helps determine outcome of rollerball ablation. Am J Obstet Gynecol 1996; 174:1786–1793.
28. Pelage JP, Jacob D, Fazel A, et al. Midterm results of uterine artery embolization for symptomatic adenomyosis: Initial experience. Radiology 2005; 234:948–953.
29. Siskin GP, Tublin ME, Stainken BF, et al. Uterine artery embolization for the treatment of adenomyosis: Clinical response and evaluation with MR imaging. AJR Am J Roentgenol 2001; 177:297–302.
30. Kim MD, Kim S, Kim NK, et al. Long-term results of uterine artery embolization for symptomatic adenomyosis. AJR Am J Roentgenol 2007; 188:176–181.
31. Wang CJ, Yen CF, Lee CL, et al. Laparoscopic uterine artery ligation for treatment of symptomatic adenomyosis. J Am Assoc Gynecol Laparosc 2002; 9:293–296.
32. Vilos GA, Vilos EC, Romano W, et al. Temporary uterine artery occlusion for treatment of menorrhagia and uterine fibroids using an incisionless Doppler-guided transvaginal clamp: Case report. Hum Reprod 2006; 21:269–271.
33. Morita M, Asakawa Y, Nakakuma M, et al. Laparoscopic excision of myometrial adenomyomas in patients with adenomyosis uteri and main symptoms of severe dysmenorrhea and hypermenorrhea. J Am Assoc Gynecol Laparosc 2004; 11:86–89.
34. Ascher-Walsh CJ, Tu JL, Du Y, et al. Location of adenomyosis in total hysterectomy specimens. J Am Assoc Gynecol Laparosc 2003; 10:360–362.
35. Ellis H, Moran BJ, Thompson JN, et al. Adhesion-related hospital readmissions after abdominal and pelvic surgery: A retrospective cohort study [see comment]. Lancet 1999; 353:1476–1480.
36. Miller EM, Winfield JM. Acute intestinal obstruction secondary to postoperative adhesions. AMA Arch Surg 1959; 78: 952–957.
37. Stricker B, Blanco J, Fox HE. The gynecologic contribution to intestinal obstruction in females. J Am Coll Surg 1994; 178:617–620.
38. Drake TS, Grunert GM. The unsuspected pelvic factor in the infertility investigation. Fertil Steril 1980; 34:27–31.
39. Howard FM. The role of laparoscopy in chronic pelvic pain: Promise and pitfalls. Obstet Gynecol Surv 1993; 48:357–387.
40. Swank DJ, Swank-Bordewijk SC, Hop WC, et al. Laparoscopic adhesiolysis in patients with chronic abdominal pain: A blinded randomised controlled multi-centre trial. Lancet 2003; 361:1247–1251.
41. Peters AA, Trimbos-Kemper GC, Admiraal C, et al. A randomized clinical trial on the benefit of adhesiolysis in patients with intraperitoneal adhesions and chronic pelvic pain. Br J Obstet Gynaecol 1992; 99:59–62.
42. Keltz MD, Gera PS, Olive DL. Prospective randomized trial of right-sided paracolic adhesiolysis for chronic pelvic pain. JSLS 2006; 10:443–446.
43. Steege JF, Stout AL. Resolution of chronic pelvic pain after laparoscopic lysis of adhesions. Am J Obstet Gynecol 1991; 165:278–281.
44. Nezhat FR, Crystal RA, Nezhat CH, et al. Laparoscopic adhesiolysis and relief of chronic pelvic pain. JSLS 2000; 4:281–285.
45. Sutton C, MacDonald R. Laser laparoscopic adhesiolysis. J Gynecol Surg 1990; 6:155–159.
46. Fayez JA, Clark RR. Operative laparoscopy for the treatment of localized chronic pelvic-abdominal pain caused by postoperative adhesions. J Gynecol Surg 1994; 10:79–83.
47. Stovall TG, Elder RF, Ling FW. Predictors of pelvic adhesions. J Reprod Med 1989; 34:345–348.
48. Howard FM, El-Minawi AM, Sanchez RA. Conscious pain mapping by laparoscopy in women with chronic pelvic pain. Obstet Gynecol 2000; 96:934–939.
49. Hammoud A, Gago LA, Diamond MP. Adhesions in patients with chronic pelvic pain: A role for adhesiolysis? Fertil Steril 2004; 82:1483–1491.
50. Brill AI, Nezhat F, Nezhat CH, et al. The incidence of adhesions after prior laparotomy: A laparoscopic appraisal. Obstet Gynecol 1995; 85:269–272.
51. Hasson HM. Open laparoscopy vs. closed laparoscopy: A comparison of complication rates. Adv Plan Parent 1978; 13:41–50.
52. Penfield AJ. How to prevent complications of open laparoscopy. J Reprod Med 1985; 30:660–663.
53. Howard FM. Breaking new ground or just digging a hole? An evaluation of gynecologic operative laparoscopy. J Gynecol Surg 1992; 8:143–158.
54. Lee CL, Huang KG, Jain S, et al. A new portal for gynecologic laparoscopy. J Am Assoc Gynecol Laparosc 2001; 8:147–150.
55. Howard FM, El-Minawi AM, DeLoach VE. Direct laparoscopic cannula insertion at the left upper quadrant. J Am Assoc Gynecol Laparosc 1997; 4:595–600.
56. Tarhan OR, Eroglu A, Cetin R, et al. Effects of seprafilm on peritoneal fibrinolytic system. ANZ J Surg 2005; 75:690–692.

57. Inoue M, Uchida K, Miki C, et al. Efficacy of Seprafilm for reducing reoperative risk in pediatric surgical patients undergoing abdominal surgery. J Pediatr Surg 2005; 40:1301–1306.
58. Stone SC, Swartz WJ. A syndrome characterized by recurrent symptomatic functional ovarian cysts in young women. Am J Obstet Gynecol 1979; 134:310–314.
59. Hasson HM. Laparoscopic management of ovarian cysts. J Reprod Med 1990; 35:863–867.
60. Guerriero S, Ajossa S, Mais V, et al. Role of transvaginal sonography in the diagnosis of peritoneal inclusion cysts. J Ultrasound Med 2004; 23:1193–1200.
61. Kocak I, Uzel A, Aytac R. An evaluation of transvaginal ultrasound-guided aspiration of simple adnexal cysts. J Obstet Gynaecol 1998; 18:474–477.
62. Marana R, Muzii L, Catalano GF, et al. Laparoscopic excision of adnexal masses. J Am Assoc Gynecol Laparosc 2004; 11:162–166.
63. Perry CP, Upchurch JC. Pelviscopic adnexectomy. Am J Obstet Gynecol 1990; 162:79–81.
64. Mahdavi A, Berker B, Nezhat C, et al. Laparoscopic management of ovarian cysts. Obstet Gynecol Clin North Am 2004; 31:581–592, ix.
65. Sommerville M, Grimes DA, Koonings PP, et al. Ovarian neoplasms and the risk of adnexal torsion. Am J Obstet Gynecol 1991; 164:577–578.
66. Shalev J, Goldenberg M, Oelsner G, et al. Treatment of twisted ischemic adnexa by simple detorsion. N Engl J Med 1989; 321:546.
67. Shalev E, Bustan M, Yarom I, et al. Recovery of ovarian function after laparoscopic detorsion. Hum Reprod 1995; 10:2965–2966.
68. Zweizig S, Perron J, Grubb D, et al. Conservative management of adnexal torsion. Am J Obstet Gynecol 1993; 168:1791–1795.
69. Weiss SW, Tavassoli FA. Multicystic mesothelioma. An analysis of pathologic findings and biologic behavior in 37 cases. Am J Surg Pathol 1988; 12:737–746.
70. Navarra G, Occhionorelli S, Santini M, et al. Peritoneal cystic mesothelioma treated with minimally invasive approach. Surg Endosc 1996; 10:60–61.
71. Carpenter HA, Lancaster JR, Lee RA. Multiocular cysts of the peritoneum. Mayo Clin Proc 1982; 57:634–638.
72. Barbieri RL. Stenosis of the external cervical os: An association with endometriosis in women with chronic pelvic pain. Fertil Steril 1998; 70:571–573.
73. Stovall TG, Ling FW. Single-dose methotrexate: An expanded clinical trial. Am J Obstet Gynecol 1993; 168:1759–1762.
74. Lipscomb GH, McCord ML, Stovall TG, et al. Predictors of success of methotrexate treatment in women with tubal ectopic pregnancies. N Engl J Med 1999; 341:1974–1978.
75. Gamzu R, Almog B, Levin Y, et al. The ultrasonographic appearance of tubal pregnancy in patients treated with methotrexate. Hum Reprod 2002; 17:2585–2587.
76. Lundorff P, Thorburn J, Hahlin M, et al. Laparoscopic surgery in ectopic pregnancy. A randomized trial versus laparotomy. Acta Obstet Gynecol Scand 1991; 70:343–348.
77. Vermesh M, Silva PD, Rosen GF, et al. Management of unruptured ectopic gestation by linear salpingostomy: A prospective, randomized clinical trial of laparoscopy versus laparotomy. Obstet Gynecol 1989; 73:400–404.
78. Murphy AA, Nager CW, Wujek JJ, et al. Operative laparoscopy versus laparotomy for the management of ectopic pregnancy: A prospective trial. Fertil Steril 1992; 57:1180–1185.
79. Tulandi T, Guralnick M. Treatment of tubal ectopic pregnancy by salpingotomy with or without tubal suturing and salpingectomy. Fertil Steril 1991; 55:53–55.
80. Fujishita A, Masuzaki H, Khan KN, et al. Laparoscopic salpingotomy for tubal pregnancy: Comparison of linear salpingotomy with and without suturing. Hum Reprod 2004; 19:1195–1200.
81. Bouyer J, Job-Spira N, Pouly JL, et al. Fertility following radical, conservative-surgical or medical treatment for tubal pregnancy: A population-based study. BJOG 2000; 107:714–721.
82. Pelosi MA. Successful laparoscopic removal of an interstitial ectopic pregnancy. J Am Assoc Gynecol Laparosc 1994; 1:S28.
83. Tulandi T, Al-Jaroudi D. Interstitial pregnancy: Results generated from the Society of Reproductive Surgeons Registry. Obstet Gynecol 2004; 103:47–50.
84. Martinelli P, Maruotti GM, Oppedisano R, et al. Is uterine artery embolization for cervical ectopic pregnancy always safe? J Minim Invasive Gynecol 2007; 14:758–763.
85. Trambert JJ, Einstein MH, Banks E, et al. Uterine artery embolization in the management of vaginal bleeding from cervical pregnancy: A case series. J Reprod Med 2005; 50: 844–850.
86. Oyer R, Tarakjian D, Lev-Toaff A, et al. Treatment of cervical pregnancy with methotrexate. Obstet Gynecol 1988; 71:469–471.
87. Bakour SH, Thompson PK, Khan KS. Successful conservative management of cervical ectopic pregnancy with combination of methotrexate, mifepristone, surgical evacuation and tamponade using a double balloon three-way catheter. J Obstet Gynaecol 2005; 25:616–618.
88. Dover RW, Powell MC. Management of a primary abdominal pregnancy. Am J Obstet Gynecol 1995; 172:1603–1604.
89. Vilodre LC, Bertat R, Petters R, et al. Cervical polyp as risk factor for hysteroscopically diagnosed endometrial polyps. Gynecol Obstet Invest 1997; 44:191–195.
90. Bakour SH, Khan KS, Gupta JK. The risk of premalignant and malignant pathology in endometrial polyps. Acta Obstet Gynecol Scand 2000; 79:317–320.
91. Steege JF. Ovarian remnant syndrome. Obstet Gynecol 1987; 70:64–67.
92. Webb MJ. Ovarian remnant syndrome. Aust N Z J Obstet Gynaecol 1989; 29:433–435.
93. Nelson DC, Avant GR. Ovarian remnant syndrome. South Med J 1982; 75:757–758.
94. Price FV, Edwards R, Buchsbaum HJ. Ovarian remnant syndrome: Difficulties in diagnosis and management. Obstet Gynecol Surv 1990; 45:151–156.
95. Nezhat CH, Seidman DS, Nezhat FR, et al. Ovarian remnant syndrome after laparoscopic oophorectomy. Fertil Steril 2000; 74:1024–1028.
96. Scott RT, Beatse SN, Illions EH, et al. Use of the GnRH agonist stimulation test in the diagnosis of ovarian remnant syndrome. A report of three cases. J Reprod Med 1995; 40:143–146.
97. Siddall-Allum J, Rae T, Rogers V, et al. Chronic pelvic pain caused by residual ovaries and ovarian remnants. Br J Obstet Gynaecol 1994; 101:979–985.
98. Fleischer AC, Tait D, Mayo J, et al. Sonographic features of ovarian remnants. J Ultrasound Med 1998; 17:551–555.
99. Lafferty HW, Angioli R, Rudolph J, et al. Ovarian remnant syndrome: Experience at Jackson Memorial Hospital, University of Miami, 1985 through 1993. Am J Obstet Gynecol 1996; 174:641–645.
100. Kaminski PF, Sorosky JI, Mandell MJ, et al. Clomiphene citrate stimulation as an adjunct in locating ovarian tissue in ovarian remnant syndrome. Obstet Gynecol 1990; 76:924–926.
101. Koch MO, Coussens D, Burnett L. The ovarian remnant syndrome and ureteral obstruction: Medical management. J Urol 1994; 152:158–160.
102. Nezhat C, Kearney S, Malik S, et al. Laparoscopic management of ovarian remnant. J Minim Invasive Gynecol 2005; 12:459–460.
103. Pettit PD, Lee RA. Ovarian remnant syndrome: Diagnostic dilemma and surgical challenge. Obstet Gynecol 1988; 71:580–583.
104. Thoms WWJ, Hughes LLRJ. Palliation of recurrent endometriosis with radiotherapeutic ablation of ovarian remnants. Fertil Steril 1997; 68:938–940.
105. Symmonds RE, Pettit PD. Ovarian remnant syndrome. Obstet Gynecol 1979; 54:174–177.
106. Rana N, Rotman C, Hasson HM, et al. Ovarian remnant syndrome after laparoscopic hysterectomy and bilateral salpingo-oophorectomy for severe pelvic endometriosis. J Am Assoc Gynecol Laparosc 1996; 3:423–426.
107. Nezhat F, Nezhat C. Operative laparoscopy for the treatment of ovarian remnant syndrome. Fertil Steril 1992; 57:1003–1007.

108. Kamprath S, Possover M, Schneider A. Description of a laparoscopic technique for treating patients with ovarian remnant syndrome. Fertil Steril 1997; 68:663–667.
109. Ranney B, Abu-Ghazaleh S. The future function and fortune of ovarian tissue which is retained in vivo during hysterectomy. Am J Obstet Gynecol 1977; 128:626–634.
110. Grogan RH, Duncan CJ. Ovarian salvage in routine abdominal hysterectomy. Am J Obstet Gynecol 1955; 70:1277–1283.
111. El Minawi AM, Howard FM. Operative laparoscopic treatment of ovarian retention syndrome. J Am Assoc Gynecol Laparosc 1999; 6:297–302.
112. Beard RW, Highman JH, Pearce S, et al. Diagnosis of pelvic varicosities in women with chronic pelvic pain. Lancet 1984; 2:946–949.
113. Reginald PW, Beard RW, Kooner JS, et al. Intravenous dihydroergotamine to relieve pelvic congestion with pain in young women. Lancet 1987; 2:351–353.
114. Beard RW, Reginald PW, Wadsworth J. Clinical features of women with chronic lower abdominal pain and pelvic congestion. Br J Obstet Gynaecol 1988; 95:153–161.
115. Soysal ME, Soysal S, Vicdan K, et al. A randomized controlled trial of goserelin and medroxyprogesterone acetate in the treatment of pelvic congestion. Hum Reprod 2001; 16:931–939.
116. Howard FM. The role of laparoscopy in the evaluation of chronic pelvic pain: Pitfalls with a negative laparoscopy. J Am Assoc Gynecol Laparosc 1996; 4:85–94.
117. Hammen R. The technique of pelvic phlebography. Acta Obstet Gynecol Scand 1965; 44:371–374.
118. Bellina JH, Dougherty CM, Mickal A. Transmyometrial pelvic venography. Obstet Gynecol 1969; 34:194–199.
119. Tarazov PG, Prozorovskij KV, Ryzhkov VK. Pelvic pain syndrome caused by ovarian varices. Treatment by transcatheter embolization. Acta Radiol 1997; 38:1023–1025.
120. Venbrux AC, Lambert DL. Embolization of the ovarian veins as a treatment for patients with chronic pelvic pain caused by pelvic venous incompetence (pelvic congestion syndrome). Curr Opin Obstet Gynecol 1999; 11:395–399.
121. Sichlau MJ, Yao JS, Vogelzang RL. Transcatheter embolotherapy for the treatment of pelvic congestion syndrome. Obstet Gynecol 1994; 83:892–896.
122. Capasso P, Simons C, Trotteur G, et al. Treatment of symptomatic pelvic varices by ovarian vein embolization. Cardiovasc Intervent Radiol 1997; 20:107–111.
123. Kennedy A, Hemingway A. Radiology of ovarian varices. Br J Hosp Med 1990; 44:38–43.
124. Farquhar CM, Rogers V, Franks S, et al. A randomized controlled trial of medroxyprogesterone acetate and psychotherapy for the treatment of pelvic congestion. Br J Obstet Gynaecol 1989; 96:1153–1162.
125. Edwards RD, Robertson IR, MacLean AB, et al. Case report: Pelvic pain syndrome–successful treatment of a case by ovarian vein embolization. Clin Radiol 1993; 47:429–431.
126. Florio F, Balzano S, Nardella M, et al. Ovarian varicocele treated with percutaneous scleroembolization. Description of a case. Radiol Med (Torino) 1993; 85:295–297.
127. Bachar GN, Belenky A, Greif F, et al. Initial experience with ovarian vein embolization for the treatment of chronic pelvic pain syndrome. Isr Med Assoc J 2003; 5:843–846.
128. Maleux G, Stockx L, Wilms G, et al. Ovarian vein embolization for the treatment of pelvic congestion syndrome: Long-term technical and clinical results. J Vasc Interv Radiol 2000; 11:859–864.
129. Cordts PR, Eclavea A, Buckley PJ, et al. Pelvic congestion syndrome: Early clinical results after transcatheter ovarian vein embolization. J Vasc Surg 1998; 28:862–868.
130. Venbrux AC, Chang AH, Kim HS, et al. Pelvic congestion syndrome (pelvic venous incompetence): Impact of ovarian and internal iliac vein embolotherapy on menstrual cycle and chronic pelvic pain. J Vasc Interv Radiol 2002; 13:171–178.
131. Chung MH, Huh CY. Comparison of treatments for pelvic congestion syndrome. Tohoku J Exp Med 2003; 201:131–138.
132. Beard RW, Kennedy RG, Gangar KF, et al. Bilateral oophorectomy and hysterectomy in the treatment of intractable pelvic pain associated with pelvic congestion. Br J Obstet Gynaecol 1991; 98:988–992.
133. Aboulghar MA, Mansour RT, Serour GI. Ultrasonographically guided transvaginal aspiration of tuboovarian abscesses and pyosalpinges: An optional treatment for acute pelvic inflammatory disease. Am J Obstet Gynecol 1995; 172:1501–1503.
134. Gjelland K, Ekerhovd E, Granberg S. Transvaginal ultrasound-guided aspiration for treatment of tubo-ovarian abscess: A study of 302 cases. Am J Obstet Gynecol 2005; 193:1323–1330.
135. Shulman A, Maymon R, Shapiro A, et al. Percutaneous catheter drainage of tubo-ovarian abscesses. Obstet Gynecol 1992; 80:555–557.
136. Henry-Suchet J, Soler A, Loffredo V. Laparoscopic treatment of tuboovarian abscesses. J Reprod Med 1984; 29:579–582.
137. Henry-Suchet J. Laparoscopic treatment of tubo-ovarian abscess: Thirty years' experience. J Am Assoc Gynecol Laparosc 2002; 9:235–237.
138. Reich H, McGlynn F. Laparoscopic treatment of tuboovarian and pelvic abscess. J Reprod Med 1987; 32:747–752.
139. Ness RB, Soper DE, Holley RL, et al. Effectiveness of inpatient and outpatient treatment strategies for women with pelvic inflammatory disease: Results from the Pelvic Inflammatory Disease Evaluation and Clinical Health (PEACH) Randomized Trial. Am J Obstet Gynecol 2002; 186:929–937.
140. Lipitz S, Seidman DS, Schiff E, et al. Treatment of pelvic peritoneal cysts by drainage and ethanol instillation. Obstet Gynecol 1995; 86:297–299.
141. Andersch B, Milsom I. An epidemiologic study of young women with dysmenorrhea. Am J Obstet Gynecol 1982; 144:655–660.
142. Wilson ML, Farquhar CM, Sinclair OJ, et al. Surgical interruption of pelvic nerve pathways for primary and secondary dysmenorrhoea. Cochrane Database Syst Rev 2000;CD001896.
143. Jaboulay M. Le traitment de la nevralgie pelvienne par la paralysie du sympathique sacre. Lyon Med 1899; 90:102–108.
144. Ruggi G. Della Sympatectamia al collo ed ale adome. Policlinico 1899; 193.
145. Black WT Jr. Presacral neurectomy: Report of 70 cases. South Med J 1955; 48:120–126.
146. Chen FP, Soong YK. The efficacy and complications of laparoscopic presacral neurectomy in pelvic pain. Obstet Gynecol 1997; 90:974–977.
147. Zullo F, Palomba S, Zupi E, et al. Long-term effectiveness of presacral neurectomy for the treatment of severe dysmenorrhea due to endometriosis. J Am Assoc Gynecol Laparosc 2004; 11: 23–28.
148. Wharton LR. Two cases of supernumerary ovary and one of accessory ovary, with an analysis of previously reported cases. Am J Obstet Gynecol 1959; 78:1101–1118.
149. Halperin R, Padoa A, Schneider D, et al. Long-term follow-up (5–20 years) after uterine ventrosuspension for chronic pelvic pain and deep dyspareunia. Gynecol Obstet Invest 2003; 55:216–219.
150. Carter JE. Carter-Thomason uterine suspension and positioning by ligament investment, fixation and truncation. J Reprod Med 1999; 44:417–422.
151. Perry CP, Presthus J, Nieves A. Laparoscopic uterine suspension for pain relief: A multicenter study. J Reprod Med 2005; 50:567–570.

14

Surgical treatment of urinary incontinence

Hervé Fernandez and Xavier Deffieux

INTRODUCTION

Urinary incontinence is a prevalent clinical problem throughout the world, which, for many women, remains undeclared to their health care practitioner. Urinary stress incontinence (USI), as recently defined by the International Continence Society (1), is the complaint of involuntary leakage of urine during effort or exertion, or during sneezing or coughing. To date, more than 200 surgical procedures have been described for the treatment of USI. While many of these are simply modifications of the same procedure, no particular method has been universally embraced as the definitive surgical solution for women with this chronic condition. Surgery is customarily recommended after the failure or personal rejection of conservative treatment modalities, which provide short-term cure rates up to 50% from a sustained program of behavior modification combined with pelvic floor therapy (2).

During the past decade, the rationale for surgical treatment of USI has undergone revolutionary changes with the evolution of less invasive techniques that significantly reduce postoperative complications and de novo voiding difficulties, including urinary retention that occurs after traditional colposuspension. Until recently, laparotomic colposuspension (the Burch procedure) has universally been regarded as the gold standard for surgical treatment of USI without intrinsic sphincteric deficiency (3). The laparoscopic approach to colposuspension was introduced in the beginning of the 1990s by Vancaillie and Schuessler (4), who described a new laparoscopic technique for bladder neck suspension. Their original approach underwent a number of modifications including the laparoscopic translation of traditional techniques, the application of a polypropylene mesh with surgical staples (5), and techniques employing entirely extraperitoneal approaches (6). Ankardal et al. (7) conducted a randomized controlled trial (RCT) comparing open Burch colposuspension ($n = 120$) with laparoscopic colposuspension, using polypropylene mesh and staples ($n = 120$). The laparotomic colposuspension group attained higher objective and subjective cure rates one year after the surgery but was associated with greater blood loss, greater risk of urinary retention, and a longer hospital stay. Carey et al. (8) confirmed the absence of difference in objective and subjective measures of cure in patients at three to five years follow-up between laparoscopic ($n = 76$) and open ($n = 88$) Burch colposuspension.

The mid-urethral concept, describing the biomechanical mechanisms of female USI, was developed and presented by Petros and Ulmsten in 1990 (9) (Fig. 1). Based on this new thesis, surgical techniques recreating support and stability between the mid-urethra and the anterior vaginal wall (Fig. 2) have continued to evolve. The tension-free vaginal tape procedure (TVT) Ethicon Womens Health and Urology/Johnson and Johnson (Fig. 3) was the first technical offspring of this construct and has continued to be widely used for the treatment of female USI since 1995 (10). Although TVT has a high long-term success rate, ranging from 85% to 95% (11–13), concerns remain about operative safety including reported injuries to the bowel and major blood vessels, perforation of the bladder and urethra, postoperative urgency, and voiding difficulties (11–13).

With the aim of sparing the retropubic space and thereby reducing associated risks, the transobturator surgical approach (TOT) for the placement of suburethral tape was

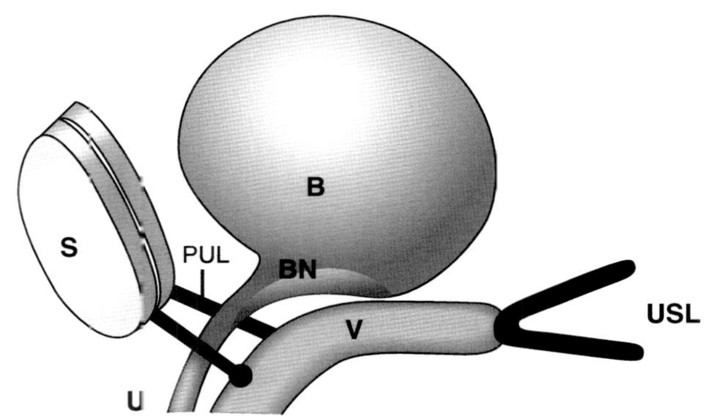

Figure 1 The *midurethral concept* for female urinary incontinence. S, pubic symphysis; U, urethra; PUL, pubourethral ligament; BN, bladder neck; B, bladder; V, vagina; USL, uterosacral ligament.

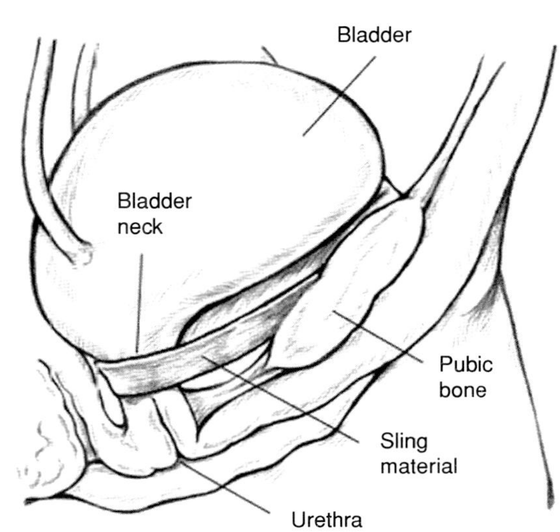

Figure 2 The mid-urethral sling technique.

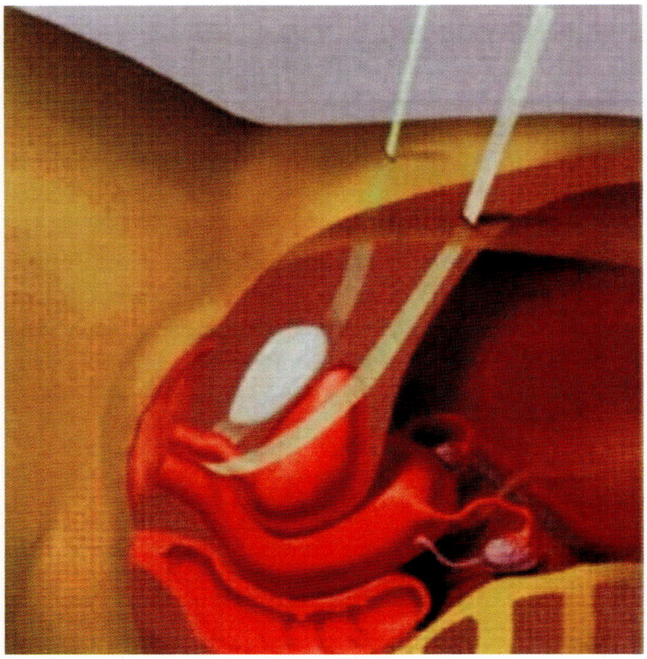

Figure 3 The tension-free vaginal tape procedure (TVT).

developed and then introduced in 2001 (Fig. 4) (14). Clinical results as well as anatomical work using cadaveric dissection have suggested that this approach may be safer than the retropubic route (RPR). In 2003, a modified transobturator approach was described, in which the tape is inserted from a suburethral incision to the skin incisions (TVT-O) (15).

Completely obviating the need for skin incisions by placing a smaller length of polypropylene mesh transvaginally and then directly affixing to the fascial investments of the obturator internus muscle, a mini-sling procedure was released in the United States in late 2006 by Ethicon Womens Health and Urology/Johnson and Johnson® under the name of TVT-Secur™ (Fig. 5). The system has uniquely been designed to

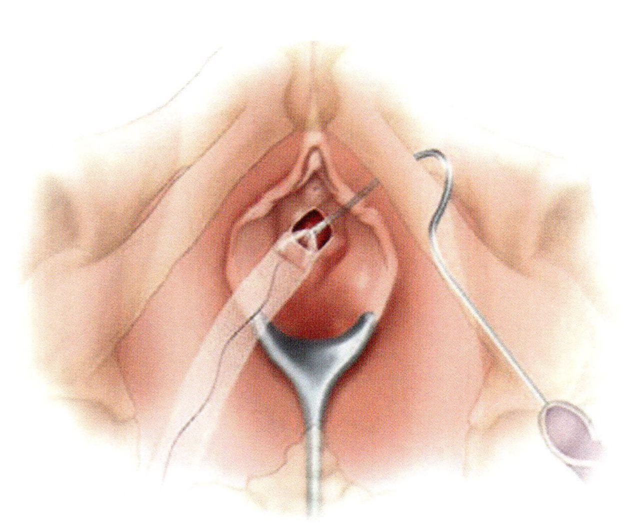

Figure 4 Transobturator surgical approach (TOT) for the placement of suburethral tape.

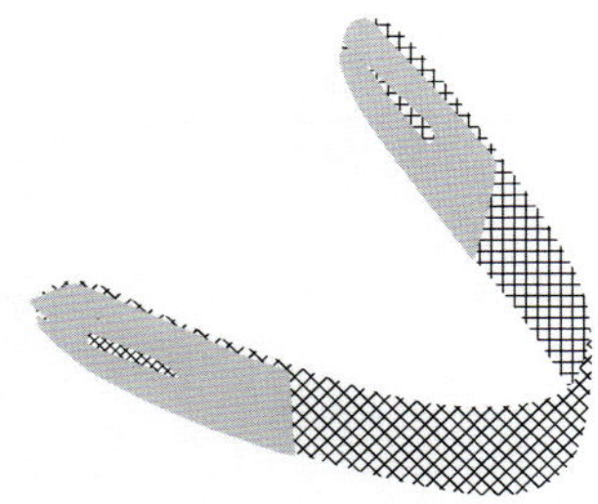

Figure 5 TVT-Secur™ Ethicon Womens Health and Urology/Johnson and Johnson®.

provide sufficient anchoring with less pain and an even faster recovery by eliminating the soft tissue trauma heretofore created by transobturator passage and skin incisions. In March of 2007, AMS® (American Medical Systems, Minneapolis, Minnesota) released a similar mini-sling product to the market named the Mini-Arc™ (Fig. 6), which likewise uses the same fundamental concepts of the tension-free tape mid-urethral slings.

TENSION-FREE VAGINAL TAPE

Background

Able to be performed under local or regional anesthesia and on an outpatient basis, the TVT was introduced in 1995 as

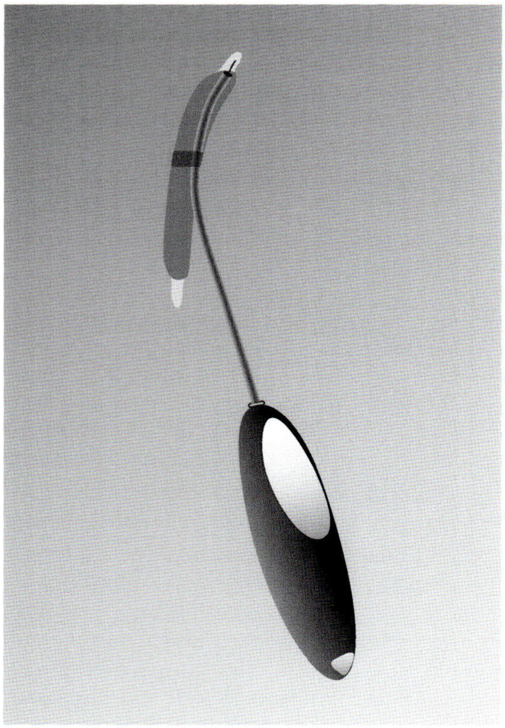

Figure 6 AMS (American Medical Systems)® Mini-Arc™.

a minimally invasive vaginal surgery technique for surgical correction of female genuine stress urinary incontinence. First described in Sweden by Ulmsten and Petros, based on their conception of a novel integral theory to explain the dynamics of female pelvic support (10) (Fig. 3), the TVT retropubic procedure has been used extensively all over the world after clinical trials established its safety and effectiveness.

Although the procedure is based on the concept of the suburethral sling, numerous studies have demonstrated that the TVT procedure is associated with a higher success rate than previous sling procedures and a significantly lower incidence of intra- and postoperative complications (16,17). Quite typically, the learning curve for this procedure is rapid, and outcomes appear to be uniform and independent of surgeon bias. These characteristics make this procedure ideally suited for patients with USI due to urethral hypermobility with or without intrinsic sphincter deficiency (ISD).

Instrumentation

The TVT instrumentation consists of a reusable stainless-steel introducer, a reusable rigid catheter guide, and the TVT device, which is a single-use apparatus composed of a $1 \times 40\ \text{cm}^2$ strip of polypropylene mesh (Prolene®, Ethicon), covered by a plastic sheath and held between two stainless-steel needles. The plastic sheath is designed to cover the synthetic mesh during placement of the sling and thereby reduce the incidence of contamination and postoperative infection resulting in graft rejection and to allow an easy passage of the tape, which is configured to stay fixed in place once the smooth protective cover is removed, before completion of the procedure. The routine use of prophylactic intravenous antibiotics is recommended.

TVT Surgical Technique

The procedure includes the following steps:

1. The patient is placed in the dorsal lithotomy position, with her hips flexed no more than 90° over the abdomen, and the buttocks are positioned flush with the edge of the operating table.
2. Although the TVT procedure can be performed under various types of anesthesia depending on the patient preference and the need for concurrent surgical procedures, some recommend that the procedure be performed under local anesthesia with intravenous sedation so that a cough stress test can be performed intraoperatively. The bladder is filled retrograde with 300 cc, as the level of anesthesia is lightened to facilitate cough on demand. This stress test putatively confirms appropriate adjustment of the tape, maximizes efficacy, and serves to minimize postoperative voiding dysfunction including retention. For the surgeon with insufficient experience to determine ideal sling tension and position with this technique, it can alternatively be performed under spinal or general anesthesia without the use of a cough stress test.
3. The operative field is prepared with a standard antiseptic agent and the patient draped, taking care to keep the arms covered and the suprapubic region in the operative field.
4. The bladder is emptied with a Foley catheter. A rigid guide is inserted into the Foley catheter to facilitate identification of the urethra and the bladder neck during passage of introducers.
5. The desired exit points of the introducers are marked with two 5-mm skin incisions placed 1 cm above the pubic symphysis, and at 2 cm on each side of the midline.
6. A posterior vaginal retractor is inserted into the vagina, to expose the anterior vaginal wall. Using gentle traction on the Foley catheter to identify the location of the bladder neck, 10 mL of local anesthetic or saline (for patients under regional or general anesthesia) is injected into the vaginal epithelium and submucosal tissues in the midline and bilaterally at the level of the mid-urethra, in order to prepare the dissection space. Recommended local anesthesia with intravenous sedation agents includes a solution of 1% Xylocaine® (lidocaine) with epinephrine diluted 1:1 with injectable saline. The vaginal speculum should be inserted to expose the anterior vaginal wall. The local anesthetic solution is injected suburethrally using an 18 gauge needle, starting approximately 1.0 cm from the external urethral meatus and moving proximally. The local anesthetic is injected on each side of the urethra toward the bladder neck and then into the retropubic space. The surgeon should then wait three to four minutes for the anesthesia to take effect. The local anesthetic should also be injected bilaterally via a long spinal needle (25 gauge) into the inferior and posterior aspect of the pubic symphysis. The needle is tunneled through the previously made suburethral vaginal incision. Proper placement of the local anesthesia can be confirmed by careful vaginal finger palpitation to identify the wheal of the local anesthetic solution on the inferior and cephalad aspects of the symphysis.
7. A 10- to 15-mm sagittal incision is made in the midline of the anterior vaginal wall approximately 10 mm below the external urethral meatus. The edges of this incision are grasped using Allis clamps, and minimal dissection is used to free the vaginal wall from the urethra and develop a small paraurethral space bilaterally, using curved scissors. The path of the lateral dissection should be orientated at a 30° angle from the midline sagittal plane, with the tips pointed slightly upward. The dissection is continued toward the inferior edge of the body of the pubic bone, between the pubic symphysis and the inferior pubic ramus. It is not necessary to perforate the endopelvic fascia with the scissors. The dedicated introducers are inserted through the vaginal incision.
8. To minimize the risk of bladder or urethral perforation during this process, the handle of the guide within the Foley catheter is first moved to the ipsilateral side.
9. Before placement of the tape, the introducer is attached to one of the stainless-steel needles and the retractor is removed from the vagina. The shaft of the introducer is grasped, and the tip of the needle is inserted into the previously developed paraurethral space until it reaches the endopelvic fascia. Then, the endopelvic fascia is perforated just behind the inferior surface of the pubic bone. On entry into the retropubic space, the needle is guided up to the abdominal incision, maintaining contact with the back of the pubic bone; this minimizes the risk of vascular or hollow viscous injury. A second layer of resistance is felt as the needle passes through the muscular and fascial layers of the abdominal wall. Passage of the needle is completed once the tip passes through the small abdominal incision on the corresponding side.
10. Before complete extraction of the needle through the suprapubic incision, unintentional bladder perforation must be excluded. The rigid catheter guide is removed and the bladder emptied through the indwelling catheter. The catheter is removed, and a 70° cystoscope is used to confirm bladder integrity. If a bladder perforation is noted, generally on the upper lateral side of the bladder wall, the needle is removed by pulling the introducer, following which the insertion procedure is repeated, making certain that the needle stays *in contact with the back of the pubic bone*

and its direction is not too lateral. Once correct placement has been confirmed by cystoscopy, the needle is detached from the introducer and pulled through the abdominal incision.

11. This technique is repeated in an identical fashion on the contralateral side, making sure that the tape lies flat against the suburethral tissue at the level of the mid-urethra. Then the plastic sheath covering the tape is completely pulled through the skin until the tape appears.
12. The tape is placed into the final position loosely without tension and flat under the urethra. Although the risk for postoperative urinary retention is potentially increased, some advocate performing a cough stress test to determine the final degree of tape tension. For a stress test, once alert enough to be responsive, the patient is asked to cough after the bladder has been filled with 250 cc of fluid. The tape is then tightened to ensure a small amount of urinary leakage on stress.
13. This allows adjustment of the tape so that only a few drops of urine are lost during the coughing process. When the tape is in its final position, the plastic sheathing that covers the tapes is removed. During this step, a blunt instrument (e.g., scissors or forceps) is interposed between the urethra and the tape to prevent the increase of the tension of the tape.
14. The vaginal incision is closed with a delayed absorbable suture, and the ends of the tape are cut bilaterally at their exit points just below the skin. The skin incisions are sutured or closed using a surgical skin adhesive tape or glue.

The indwelling urinary catheter is removed prior to discharge from the operating theatre. Postvoid residuals are checked after full return of consciousness or sensation by intermittent catheterization or via ultrasonographic assessment of the bladder volume. Postoperative analgesia requirements are typically minimal and well managed with oral narcotic congeners and nonsteroidal anti-inflammatory medications. For the minority unable to void or who are unable to have a residual volume of less than 100 cc, adequate bladder drainage is accomplished by recorded intermittent self-catheterization or continuous drainage by Foley catheter with close postoperative follow-up. Prophylactic antibiotics are advisable until catheterization is no longer necessary. Women who are catheterized are seen in 48 hours for removal of the catheter and a repeat voiding trial with measurement of the residual volume. Before discharge, detailed instructions and postoperative precautions are given to the patient, together with a handout containing the same information. Patients are instructed to resume their normal daily activities within one week after the procedure but are cautioned to avoid heavy lifting and strenuous exercise for up to six weeks to allow adequate vaginal healing around the suburethral tape. Patients also are instructed to abstain from sexual intercourse and avoid tampon use during this time. For those able to successfully void before discharge, a routine follow-up appointment occurs in four to six weeks.

Women who continue to have high urine residuals after removal of the indwelling catheter should be offered a choice between (1) immediate surgical reintervention (sling release), (2) management with another indwelling catheter (for at least one week), or (3) continuation or initiation of intermittent self-catheterization. Surgical reintervention should be considered for women who continue to have complete retention more than three days postoperatively, either by surgical section of the sling or by loosening it by progressively dilating the urethra up to 24 F and then placing downward traction on the sling. Women with high urine residuals lasting more than one month postoperatively should undergo surgical section of the sling.

Since its first description by Ulmsten and Petros, many other mid-urethral tapes have been described for the surgical management of genuine stress urinary incontinence (including TVT-O™, UraTape™, ObTape™, IVS™, I-STOP™, Monarc™, and Sparc™); unfortunately, the regulatory approval process permitted their rapid incorporation into the gynecologic marketplace, although unsubstantiated by either scientifically rigorous animal studies and/or controlled clinical trials. Moreover, all of the white papers written to introduce and legitimize these newer devices use short clinical series without adequate statistical analyses, which are handicapped by short follow-up periods. Nevertheless, all monofilament macroporous polypropylene slings gave similar results. It is incumbent upon the gynecologic surgeon to base his or her commitment to use a particular type of suburethral sling on information rigorously collected from studies with sufficient numbers of patients, statistical power, and standardized criteria, with a minimum follow-up of two years.

Clinical Data

More than 500,000 TVT procedures have been performed around the world, confirming the long-term results, reported by Ulmsten and Petros (10), of success in 85%, improvement in 10%, and failure in 5% of cases (11–13). Furthermore, use of the TVT has also been demonstrated to be effective for mixed urinary incontinence (18) and in recurrent USI (19). Nevertheless, the efficacy in patients with ISD is inferior, with a success rate of 75%, and improvement in 10% and failure in 15% of cases (20).

Nilsson et al. (21) has reported the long-term cure rates and late complications rates after seven-year follow-up of the TVT procedure for the treatment of USI. Eighty out of 90 women were available for follow-up. Both objective and subjective cure rates were 81.3%, with de novo urge symptoms in 6.3% of patients. No signs of tape erosion or any tissue reactions indicating tape material rejection were found. This absence of long-term adverse events associated with a high subjective and objective cure rates makes the TVT operation a recommendable surgical treatment for female USI and confirms that TVT is the new gold standard surgery for USI treatment.

Due to these satisfactory outcomes with the TVT procedure, RCTs were performed between TVT and abdominal colposuspension techniques—historically the most popular choice for primary surgery for USI with reported cure rates of up to 96% (22). Ward and Hilton (23) have reported the two-year follow-up of 344 women in an RCT comparing TVT and open Burch colposuspension. The objective cure rates defined as a negative one-hour pad test, ranged from 63% to 85% for the TVT procedure and 51% to 87% for open colposuspension. Subjectively, only 43% of patients in the TVT group and 37% in the open colposuspension group reported cure of their stress leakage. The results are similar to those reported by Black et al. (24), in their large cohort study. The success rate reported in this trial is lower than most published series for USI surgery. However, most studies report success rate based on a poorly defined population with nonvalidated outcome measures.

Another study addressing the same clinical questions has shown similar continence rates between laparoscopic Burch colposuspension and TVT (25), but with advantages for the TVT in terms of reduced operative time and length of

Table 1 TVT/Burch: Results of Randomized Clinical Trial

	Clinical trial					
	Ward et al. (23)	Valpas et al. (27)	Paraiso et al. (28)	Ustun 2003 (29)	Liang 2002 (30)	Liapis 2002 (31)
n TVT	175	70	36	23	23	36
n Burch	169 (open)	51 (laparoscopic)	36 (laparoscopic)	23 (laparoscopic)	22	35
Objective success rate (%) for TVT	63	85.7	96.8	82.6	82.6	84
Objective success rate (%) for Burch	51	56.9	81.2	82.6	77.3	86
Month follow-up	24	12	20.6	3	20	24
95% CI or *P*	<0.01	12.7–43.9	$P < 0.05$	NS	NS	NS

postoperative recovery period. Furthermore, there is no reported risk of posterior compartment prolapse after TVT, as opposed to that with colposuspension (26).

Many RCTs (Table 1) (11,27–31) compared TVT with colposuspension, which has been the gold standard for the treatment of USI. As evident from Table 1, the results of TVT and colposuspension are fairly similar.

Dean et al. (32), in a systematic review, showed that the evidence appears to be in favor of the TVT as the minimal access technique of choice in comparison with Burch colposuspension.

Despite the simplicity, reproducibility, and high long-term success rates associated with the TVT procedure, there are concerns regarding its operative safety. Most of the series have reported a 5% to 10% risk of bladder perforation associated with the placement of the stainless-steel introducer. The other common complication is hematoma of the retropubic space. Reported major operative complications include bowel injuries (33) and major blood vessels injuries (34), their risk resulting in death. Different approaches have been described to avoid the risk of major complications.

In order to avoid the major complications mentioned, one of the approaches suggested is the insertion of the introducer from the suprapubic skin incisions to the suburethral space by abdominal retropubic approach. A randomized comparison with the TVT has shown similar continence rates, but a higher rate of urethral injury using the abdominal approach (4.9% vs. 0%) (35).

Postoperative voiding troubles, such as voiding difficulties and urgency, occur in 5% to 15% of TVT patients (36,37). The rate of voiding difficulties is correlated with the tension applied to the tape. Although preoperative urgency is improved in 60% to 70% of the patients after TVT, there are no preoperative parameters that can predict the outcome.

Segal et al. (38) demonstrated that 57% of patients with preoperative overactive bladder symptoms can expect resolution of these symptoms after a TVT. The proportion of patients in whom de novo overactive bladder (4.3%) and de novo urge incontinence (9.1%) symptoms developed postoperatively is low.

Complications specifically associated with the use of synthetic materials, such as graft rejection/exposure, fistula formation, abscess, or hypersensitivity reactions, have been occasionally reported with the use of monofilament polypropylene tapes such as TVT. However, graft rejection (vaginal erosion/exposure) was reported in up to 9% of cases with the use of a multifilament tape (39).

In response to the concern that the retropubic passage of a trocar carried with it the potential complication of bladder, vascular and urethral injury, Delorme (14) described a modified transobturator tape technique that passed horizontally using an out-to-inside approach passing under the urethra (TOT®, Mentor-Porgès) (Fig. 7).

TRANSOBTURATOR TAPE (TOT)

Background

In 2001, the French Urologist E. Delorme introduced the transobturator approach for the surgical treatment of a tape to correct female stress urinary incontinence (14).

In Delorme's technique, the tunneler is introduced from the skin incisions located 2 cm lateral to the fold of the thigh to the vaginal incision, through the obturator foramen (external

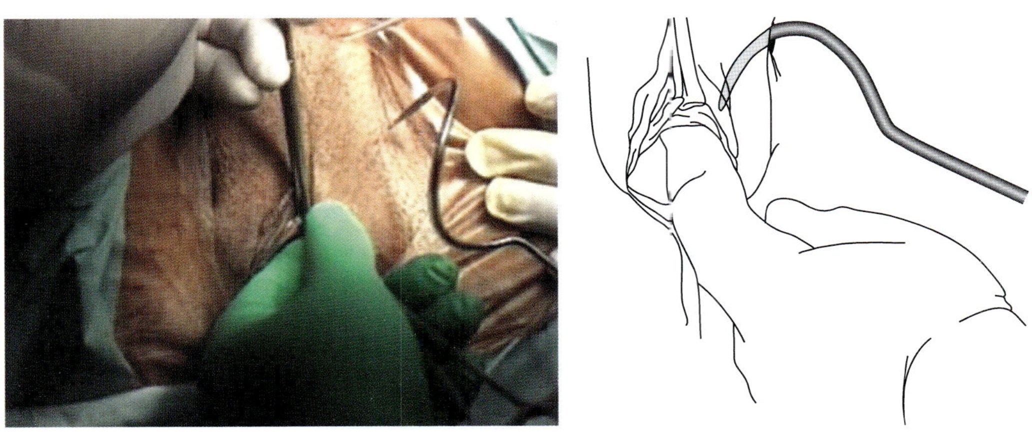

Figure 7 Transobturator tape technique (TOT/Mentor).

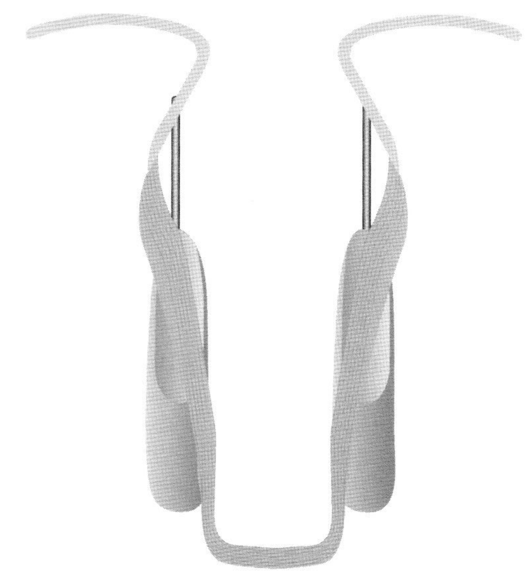

Figure 8 TOT tunneler with needles and introducers.

obturator muscle, obturator membrane, and internal obturator muscle) (Fig. 7). Bladder and urethra are protected by the index finger, which has to be inside the latero-urethral dissection until the obturator internus muscle. The obturator membrane is perforated at 3 cm from the obturator neurovascular bundle. The originality of this technique is its perineal tape position, avoiding the pelvic region and recreating the natural support of the urethra provided by the pubourethral ligaments.

Instrumentation

The "tunneler" is a specially designed curve needle, similar to the Emmet needle. The shape facilitates turning around the ischiopubic bone, from the skin incision to the suburethral incision, and then through the obturator foramen (Fig. 8).

The tape is usually a monofilament of polypropylene, with or without plastic sheath.

TOT Surgical Technique

The procedure includes the following steps:

1. The patient is placed in the dorsal lithotomy position with the hips hyperflexed over the abdomen ($\pm 110°$). The buttocks are positioned flush with the edge of the operating table.
2. The procedure can be carried out under local, regional, or general anesthesia.
3. The operative field is prepared with a standard antiseptic agent and the patient draped, keeping the groin folds exposed.
4. An indwelling urethral catheter is inserted into the bladder which is emptied.
5. A 15-mm sagittal midline incision is made through the vaginal mucosa starting 1 cm below the urethral meatus. This step may be preceded by submucosal infiltration of 5 to 10 mL of saline (or lidocaine for procedures under local anesthesia) to facilitate the dissection.
6. The paraurethral subvaginal dissection is then carried out laterally using pointed and curved scissors, on both sides. The path of the lateral dissection should be orientated at a 45° angle from the midline sagittal plane, with the tips pointed slightly upward, and dissection carried out until the posterior part of the inferior ischiopubic ramus. The channel should be approximately 4 cm deep and wide enough to allow insertion of the index finger, in order to protect the bladder, urethra, and vaginal cuff during the introduction of the tunneler.
7. The obturator region is identified by palpation of the external part of the ischiopubic ramus with the thumb and the index finger of the same hand (left hand of the surgeon for the left side of the patient).
8. A 5-mm incision is made in front of the upper and internal part of the obturator foramen, 15 mm lateral from the ischiopubic ramus, at the level of the clitoris.
9. The curved tunneler is inserted through the skin incision to the obturator foramen. Perforation of the membrane is recognized from the resistance encountered in the process. The index finger is placed into the channel, and the tunneler turned around the ischiopubic ramus, taking care to keep it in contact with the back side of the bone, until the tip of the tunneler reach the finger. The blind part of the procedure, e.g., the distance between the obturator membrane and the finger, is normally less than 15 mm. Before the placement of the tape, the vaginal cuff must be inspected to ensure that there is no perforation. If the blind part is more than 15 mm, or if there is an involuntary vaginal perforation, the tunneler must be pulled back to the level of the back side of the ischiopubic ramus, and the procedure retried.
10. When the tip of the tunneler is in contact with the finger, the tunneler is pushed through the channel until the suburethral space, keeping a permanent contact between the device and the finger. Then, the tip of the tape is attached on to the tunneler, and the tape is pulled outside through the obturator foramen and skin incision. During this process, it may be necessary to grasp the opposite vaginal edge with clamp, in order to stabilize the urethra.
11. The procedure is repeated on the collateral side, making sure that the tape lies flat under the urethra. The tape is positioned loosely (without tension) and flat under the urethra. At this stage, a cough test may be performed. This allows adjustment of the tape so that only a few drops of urine are lost during the cough. To avoid repositioning of the tape due to excessive tension, a blunt instrument (e.g., scissors or forceps) is placed between the urethra and the tape during the adjustment.
12. When the extremities of the tape have been extracted through both skin incisions, the plastic sheaths, when they are present, are removed and the protruding ends are cut just below the skin.
13. Thereafter, the vaginal incision is closed with interrupted absorbable sutures, and the skin incisions are sutured or the edges apposed with surgical skin adhesive.
14. A cystoscopy is not absolutely indicated, e.g., in the absence of operative difficulties. This is obviously dependent on the discretion of the surgeon.
15. The Foley catheter is left in place and removed within the first 24 postoperative hours or immediately after the operation. Thereafter, postvoid residuals are measured by intermittent catheterization or bladder ultrasound. Most patients experience minimal discomfort, and adequate pain control is achieved using oral nonopioid medications. Before discharge, detailed instructions and postoperative precautions are given to the patient, together with a handout containing the same information. Patients usually resume their normal daily activities within one to two weeks but are cautioned to avoid heavy lifting and

strenuous exercise for up to six weeks postoperatively, to allow adequate healing around the tape. Patients also are instructed to abstain from sexual intercourse and avoid tampon use during this time. They are seen for routine follow-up four to six weeks postoperatively.

TRANSOBTURATOR VAGINAL TAPE: INSIDE-OUT (TVT-O)

Background

In 2003, de Leval described a modified transobturator approach, in which the tape is inserted from the suburethral incision to the skin incisions. That modification was named by the author as the inside-out transobturator vaginal tape procedure (TVT-O) (Fig. 9) (15). His main objective was to reduce the risk of bladder and/or urethral injuries, which were occasionally reported with the original TOT technique (38,40–41).

In order to determine the exact anatomical track of the tape and its relationships with the neighboring neurovascular structures and organs, de Leval and colleagues performed cadaver dissections (42). Seven female cadavers aged 65 years or more, with no history of prior pelvic or perineal surgery, were dissected. The positioning of the suburethral tape was carried out in each cadaver according to a standard operative protocol. The anterior perineal and obturator regions were thereafter dissected. The ischiopubic ramus was sectioned and removed to ease the dissection. That dissection studies showed that the tape was inserted according to the following consistent path: penetration from the suburethral space (junction between mid- and distal urethra) into the anterior recess of the ischiorectal fossa, limited medially and cranially by the levator ani muscle, caudally by the deep transverse muscle, and laterally by the obturator internus muscle. Then the tape perforated the obturator membrane and muscles, and exited at the skin level after passing through the adductor muscles and subcutaneous tissues. The tape was at a significant distance from the terminal end of the pudendal nerve (dorsal nerve to the clitoris), which was located much more superficially, below the median perineal aponeurosis, the obturator nerve and vessels, and the femoral vessels. The obturator vascular structures were also carefully dissected. Dissections consistently showed that the anterior branch of the obturator artery lied on the external rim of the ischiopubic ramus and was thus protected by this bony structure from being injured by the passage of the tape (Figs. 10 and 11).

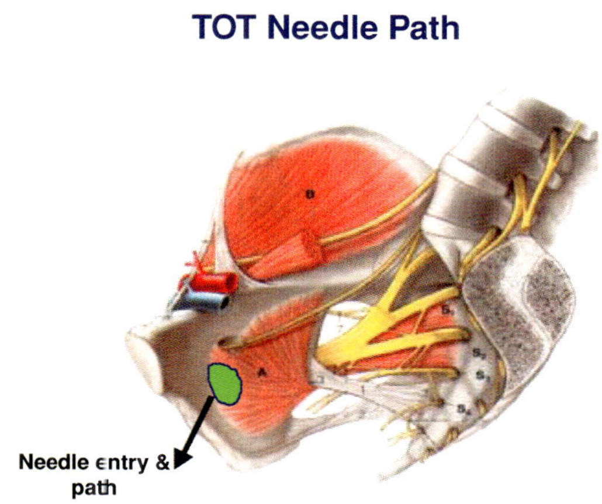

Figure 10 Anatomical route of transobturator tape.

Like the TOT, the TVT-O tape passes from the perineal region through the obturator and thigh regions, without entering the pelvic cavity. The bladder, pudendal nerve, and femoral and obturator neurovascular structures are distant from the tape's dissection track. The urethra and vaginal walls are under direct view.

TVT-O™ Instrumentation

Special instruments have been created to perform this modification of the transobturator procedure. The "helical passers" are a pair of instruments, specific for the left and right sides. They are made of stainless steel comprising a spirally shaped section and a handle. The spiral section has an open circular segment of 3-cm radius, terminated by two linear segments (Fig. 12A). On a horizontal plane perpendicular to the handle's axis, the gap between the extremities of the spiral section is 2 cm. The element supported by the helical passer is a hollow polyethylene "tube." It has a sharp pointed distal end and

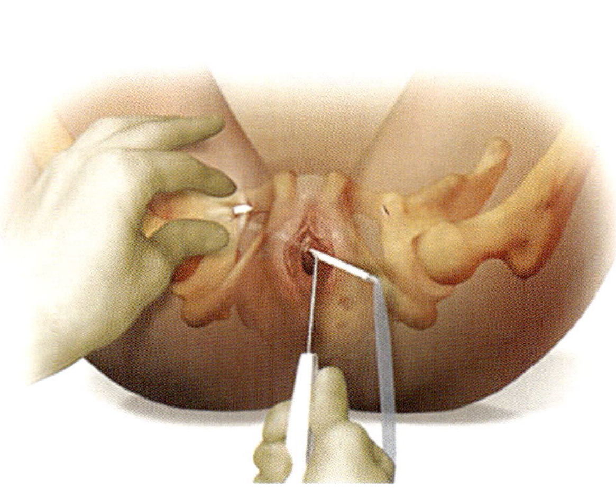

Figure 9 Transobturator vaginal tape: inside-out (TVT-O).

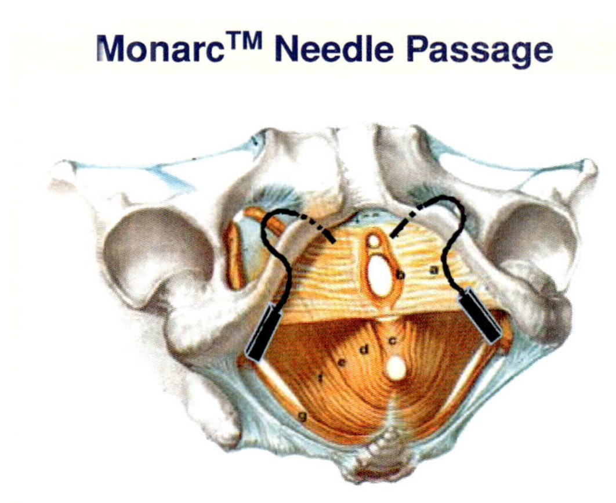

Figure 11 Anatomical route of transobturator tape.

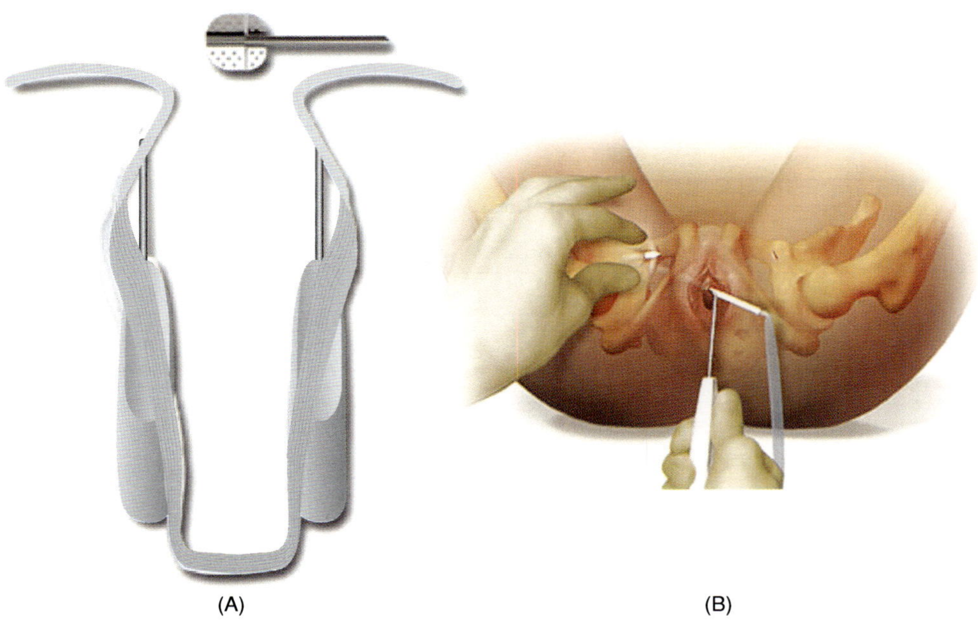

Figure 12 TVT-O™: A. Helical passers with guide. B. Trans-obturator passage of helical guide. (Ethicon Womens Health and Urology/Johnson and Johnson).

a lateral opening, which allows the insertion of the spiral segment of the helical passer into its lumen.

The third instrument is called the "guide." This is a stainless-steel device that comprises a semicircular gutter. The guide acts both as a shoe horn and as a lever arm to ease the slipping in of the passers, introduced alongside the gutter, from the perineal space through the obturator foramens. The guide also plays the role of a barrier, preventing the helical passer to enter the pelvic space. It facilitates a reproducible dissection, which makes finger guidance unnecessary (Fig. 12B).

The TVT-O® tape (Gynecare, Ethicon) is the same non-absorbable polypropylene tape as the one used in the TVT procedure, the only difference being its blue color. The proximal end of the tube is opened and is attached to the tape together with its protective plastic sheath.

TVT-O™ Surgical Technique

The procedure includes the following steps:

1. The patient is placed in the dorsal lithotomy position with the hips hyperflexed over the abdomen ($\pm 110°$). The buttocks are positioned flush with the edge of the operating table.
2. The procedure can be carried out under local, regional, or general anesthesia.
3. The operative field is prepared with a standard antiseptic agent and the patient draped, taking care to keep the groin folds in the operative field.
4. An indwelling catheter is inserted into the bladder that is emptied.
5. The exit points of the plastic tubes are marked with a felt pen, tracing a horizontal line at the level of the urethral meatus. A second line, that is parallel and 2 cm above the first, is traced. It is on this line, 2 cm lateral to femoral genital fold, that the exit points will be located. A 5-mm incision is made at each exit point.
6. Using Allis clamps for traction, a 1-cm midline incision is placed in the vaginal mucosa starting 1 cm below the urethral meatus. Minimal paraurethral subvaginal dissection is then carried out laterally with a blade, over a few millimeters distance, on each side. It is recommended that insertion of the device be completed on one side before beginning the dissection of the contralateral side. Using a "push-spread technique," blunt dissection is carried out, preferably using pointed, curved scissors. The path of the lateral dissection must be orientated at a 45° angle from the midline sagittal plane, with the tips of the scissors pointed slightly upward. Dissection is continued toward the junction between the body of the pubic bone and the inferior pubic ramus. When the "junction" is reached, the tips of the scissors are pointed slightly downward to perforate the obturator membrane. A loss of resistance can be felt when the membrane is perforated. The channel should be approximately 5 to 7 mm in diameter and no deeper than 5 cm. If the bone is not reached after dissecting for 5 cm, it is essential to ascertain that the angle of dissection is correct.
7. The winged "guide" is inserted into the tract created, until it passes the ischiopubic ramus and enters the opening previously made in the obturator membrane. Loss of resistance is felt as the winged guide passes through the obturator membrane. If difficulty is encountered during insertion of the guide, the direction of the tract should be reassessed with the scissors. The open side of the guide must be facing the operator. If necessary (e.g., in obese patients), the bendable tab may be bent to increase the length of the gutter of the guide from 6 to 7 cm.
8. The "helical passer" is inserted into the dissected tract following the channel of the winged guide. The device is pushed inward, traversing, and slightly passing the obturator membrane. At this point, it is important to orient the handle of the device in such a way that the straight tip of the helical passer is aligned with the channel in the winged

guide and remains in that orientation until the tip reaches the obturator foramen.

9. Once in this position, the winged guide is removed and kept sterile for later use on the same patient.
10. Once the guide is removed, the handle of the helical passer is rotated (clockwise for the patient's right side and counterclockwise for the patient's left side) simultaneously as the handle is moved toward the midline. The handle should never be orientated in a horizontal position.
11. The tip of the tube should exit near the previously determined exit points. However, slight skin manipulation may be required. If the skin incision has not been previously made, it is now made where the tip of the helical passer tents the skin.
12. When the tip of the plastic tube appears at the skin opening, it is grasped with a clamp and, while stabilizing the tube near the urethra, the helical passer is removed by reverse rotation of the handle.
13. The plastic tube is pulled completely through the skin incision until the tape appears.
14. The same procedure is repeated on the opposite side ensuring that the tape lies flat under the urethra.
15. When both plastic tubes have been extracted through the skin incisions, the plastic tubes are cut off from the tape and plastic sheaths. The tape is positioned loosely, without tension, and flat under the urethra. At this stage, a cough test may be performed. This allows adjustment of the tape so that only a few drops of urine are lost during the cough. When the tape is in position, the plastic sheath that covers the tape is removed. As for the other procedures, to avoid positioning the tape with excess tension, a blunt instrument (e.g., scissors or forceps) is placed between the urethra and the tape during removal of the plastic sheaths.
16. Thereafter vaginal incisions are closed. The tape ends are cut at the exit points just below the skin. The skin incisions are closed with suture or surgical skin adhesive.
17. A cystoscopy may be performed. If cystoscopy was performed following the first passage, it is necessary to empty the bladder prior to initiating passage of the second side.

Mid-urethral Sling Clinical Data

More than 30,000 transobturator procedures have been performed around the world. The preliminary results from Delorme (14) were confirmed by several series. At one-year follow-up, the success rate is 80% to 90%, improvement 7% to 9%, and failure 0% to 7%.

The mean operative time is about 15 minutes. The risk of intraoperative bladder injury is small (<0.5%). The rates of postoperative voiding dysfunction or de novo urge symptoms are 3.3% and 5%, respectively (43). There have been no reports of vascular, neurological, or bowel injury. Nevertheless, infections were reported with the Uratape® (Mentor-Porgès, Le Plessis-Robinson, France): one infected obturator hematoma and one inguinal abscess. Both infections occurred after a vaginal erosion, but the characteristics of that first TOT (woven and with a silicone patch under the urethra) were probably factors that contributed to this complication.

A French prospective multicenter registry had included 602 patients from November 2001 to September 2004 (44). All patients had clinically demonstrated stress urinary incontinence with a positive preoperative cough stress test. In 508 patients, the TOT was the sole procedure, and 94 patients had associated prolapse repair. The mean age of the patients was 57.3% years (range 29–88). The cohort of patients consisted of a heterogeneous and unselected population since 21.2%, 35%, 11.5%, and 26.9% of the patients enrolled had preoperative urgency, preoperative mixed incontinence, low maximal urethral closure pressure, and a history of previous incontinence treatment or prolapse repair, respectively. The procedure was feasible in all patients. Intraoperative complications were bladder injuries in 5 (0.8%), urethral injuries in 2 (0.3%), hemorrhage in 3 (0.5%), and vaginal perforation in 13 patients (2.2%). There were no gastrointestinal, neurological, or vascular complications. Of the 400 patients followed up for at least 3 months, with a mean follow-up time of 11.7 months, 86.8% were cured, 7.7% improved, and 5.5% failed.

Since March 2002, de Leval et al. have performed more than 375 transobturator inside-out surgical procedures on patients who had clinically demonstrated stress urinary incontinence with a positive preoperative cough stress test. An initial feasibility study had included 113 patients from March 2002 to March 2003 (15). In 77 patients, the TVT-O was the sole procedure and 36 had an associated procedure for prolapse. The mean age of the patients was 62 years (range 29–88 years). The cohort of patients consisted of a heterogeneous and unselected population, since 30%, 10%, 44%, and 15% of the patients enrolled had preoperative urgency, mixed incontinence, low maximal urethral closure pressure, and a history of previous incontinence or prolapse repair, respectively. All patients had a follow-up period of at least 6 months with a mean follow-up of 10 months. One patient was lost to follow-up at the one-month visit, and four additional patients were lost to follow-up at the six-month visit. The procedure was feasible in all patients. All helical passers was passed through the obturator foramen and exited at the skin level exactly where it had been marked and incised. The mean operative time for the TVT-O procedure was 12 minutes (range 6–20 minutes). There were no urethral or bladder injury and no significant bleeding during the procedure. There were no major postoperative complications such as obturator or thigh hematoma, neurological or bowel complications, tape rejection, or fistula.

A prospective study on 250 patients with short-term follow-up has confirmed these initial results (45). There were no urethra, bladder, gastrointestinal, neurological, or vaginal complications. Results showed a complete cure rate of USI of 94%.

There have been few RCTs with these new surgical approaches. Arunkalaivanan and Barrington (46) compared TVT ($n = 68$) with Pelvicol™ sling ($n = 74$) with a 12-month follow-up. The success rates were, respectively, 85 and 89% (NS) respectively.

Neuman (47) compared two anti-incontinence operations: TVT and the TVT-O in two 75-patient groups. In this study, the TVT-obturator group appeared to have less intra- and postoperative surgical complications than the TVT group with similar early failure rates, 1.3% and 2.7% respectively, at one-year follow-up.

Another RCT (48) compared the retropubic (RPR) approach (42 cases) with a transobturator route (TOR) out-inside (46 cases). The immediate functional results were similar. The suburethral sling procedure was less painful by the TOR than by the RPR. Bladder injury, hematomas, and abscesses were observed only in the RPR group, while vaginal injury occurred only in the TOR group.

Other RCTs have been published. Vervest et al. (49) compared TVT-O® ($n = 39$) and Monarc® ($n = 36$), i.e., in-out versus out-in. The effectiveness was similar, and one vaginal perforation occurred with out-in route. Wang et al. (50) compared Monarc versus Sparc®, i.e., out-in transobturator suburethral sling versus suprapubic sling procedure. The out-in route appeared more painful (12.9% vs. 0%) and a trend to vaginal perforation (12.9% vs. 0%).

Liapis et al. (51) observed the same success rate between the classic TVT method and the TVT-O method, with 12-month follow-up. This result is interesting because it tested the same sling using two different routes.

Two recent RCTs (52,53) confirmed that TVT and TVT-O procedures perform equally in terms of objective and subjective cures, in spite of longer hospital stay and more post-operative opiate analgesia in the TVT-O group (52). In the second RCT, RPR and TOR had similar high cure rates and quality-of-life improvement. However, all these comparative or randomized trials have short term follow-up.

In conclusion, suburethral slings have rightfully become the gold standard for surgical treatment for USI, but some questions remain: the choice between retropubic or transobturator approach, and in transobturator approach the choice between out-in and in-out insertions.

The answer requires RCTs with appropriate number of patients, statistics, and suitable subjective and objective outcomes, after minimum follow-up over two years and long-term evaluation of mesh erosion/exposure and postoperative voiding difficulties. Nevertheless, intraoperative diagnostic cystoscopy and bladder catheterization are not mandatory with the transobturator approach. Abdel-Fattah et al. (54) found only four injuries in a consecutive series of 390 TOT insertions using the outside-in technique. Overall, the global trend is toward adoption of this newer approach because it is demonstrably safer, quicker, and easier to learn (55).

TENSION-FREE VAGINAL TAPE SECUR (TVT-SECUR®)

The third-generation of synthetic midurethral slings, TVT-Secur®, was introduced in 2006. This procedure is comparatively less invasive, avoids potentially problematic spaces and organs, needs less dissection requiring only two small paraurethral dissections, requires less anesthesia due to realistic potential to use local anesthesia, and has soft tissue exit points because the sling measures only 8 cm in length. The TVT-Secur essentially eliminates the risks of injury to the bowel, vessels, nerves, and tissues in the pelvis and reduces by postoperative pain by minimal dissection and tissue passage. TVT-Secur utilizes a polypropylene mesh implant that is four times shorter in length than traditional mid-urethral slings. The mesh tape is affixed to the obturator internus fascia using a novel "attach and release" mechanism, which allows for stable and controlled placement. Absorbable fixation tips made of Vicryl® (polyglactin 910) knitted mesh and PDS® (polydioxanone) suture yarn provide mechanical fixation until complete tissue ingrowth occurs, as demonstrated on sheep model. TVT-Secur is directly anchored to the parietal fascia of the obturator internus muscle. The typical procedure takes 10 to 15 minutes to complete under local anesthesia. Tommaselli et al. recently compared TVT-O to TVT-Secur with a RCT in 84 patients, demonstrating no significant differences in cure rate (81.6% vs 83.8%) and fewer complications in the TVT-Secur group (8.1% vs 15.8%) (56).

Instrumentation

The device consists of a one piece blue polypropylene mesh with pieces of fleece made from polyglactin 910 and PDS, that sandwich the end sections of the mesh. The inserters are two curved stainless-steel instruments and are designed to deliver and release the device (Fig. 13).

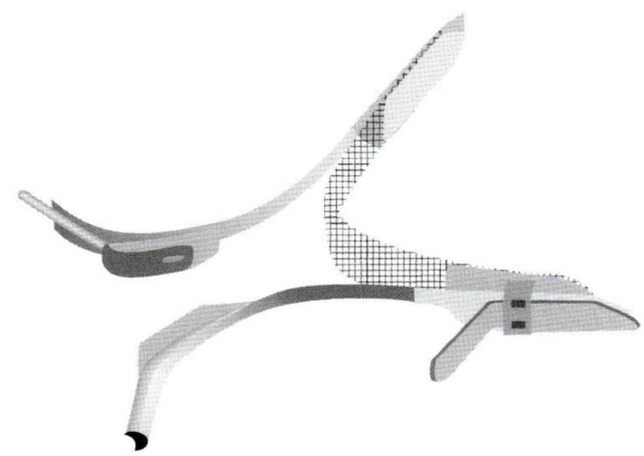

Figure 13 TVT-Secur™ Ethicon Womens Health and Urology (Johnson and Johnson).

TVT-SECUR Surgical Technique

The device may be placed in either a "U" or a "hammock" position under the mid-urethra. Placement orientation is per the surgeon's preference, but in majority the "hammock" position is preferred (Fig. 14).

1. The procedure can be carried out under local, regional, or general anesthesia, with a tendency for local anesthesia.
2. The patient is placed in the dorsal lithotomy position with the hips hyperflexed over the abdomen ($\pm 110°$). The buttocks are positioned flush with the edge of the operating table.
3. An indwelling catheter is inserted into the bladder that is emptied. The Foley catheter guide may be used to position the urethra during *device* placement.
4. Using a small scalpel, a sagittal incision about 1.0 to 1.5 cm long is placed, starting approximately 1.0 cm from the external urethral meatus. Using an Allis clamp, the vaginal wall is grasped at each side of the urethra. After initiating

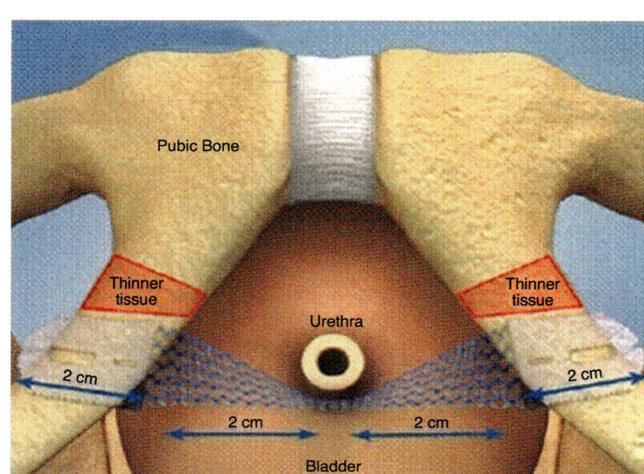

Figure 14 TVT-Secur™ tape placement options.

sharp dissection, two paraurethral dissections of about 1.0 cm are made using a pair of blunt scissors.

5. The internal foil package is removed from the external package and the traceability labels located on the foil package are conserved. Then using aseptic technique, the foil package is opened and the plastic tray containing the Gynecare TVT-Secur System is removed.
6. The plastic tray is than opened and the *inserters* and *device* are removed from the tray.
7. The *inserter* without the protective cover is grasped with a needle driver.
8. Using the needle driver, the *inserter* and *device* are inserted into the previously dissected paraurethral incision. The needle driver/holder and inserter can be held with the index finger on the finger pad. The *inserter* tip is oriented at an angle of 45° from the midline, toward the ischiopubic ramus, while holding the needle driver and *inserter* so that they are parallel to the floor; the *inserter* tip will be in approximately the 9-o'clock position or parallel to the floor.

   The *inserter* is advanced and the inferior edge of the pubic ramus is contacted and then, while maintaining light constant contact with the bone, the *device* is advanced into the obturator internus muscle in a controlled manner.
9. The needle driver is diconnected from the first *inserter.*
10. Than the second *inserter* is grasped with the needle holder and the protective cover removed from the tip before use.
11. Using the needle driver, the *inserter* and *device* are inserted into the previously dissected paraurethral incision, with the index finger on the finger pad.
12. The tip of the inserter is oriented at an angle of 45° from the midline, toward the ischiopubic ramus, while holding the needle driver and *inserter* so that they are parallel to the floor; the *inserter* tip will be in approximately the 3-o'clock position. The *inserter* is advanced to contact the inferior edge of the pubic ramus and then, while maintaining light constant contact with the bone, advance of the *device* is continued into the obturator internus muscle in a controlled manner. The tip of *device* is kept in contact with the bone to minimize the chance of damage to organs, vessels, or other anatomic structures as the *device* is advanced into the obturator internus muscle.
13. The needle driver is than disconnected to assess the tension-free mesh placement under the mid-urethra. Final adjustments as needed are made by reconnecting the needle driver and establishing proper hand position to ensure that the *inserter* tip remains in contact with the bone. The patient's left or right side *inserter* is advanced or retracted, depending on the insertion depth of each *inserter*.
14. The positioning of tension-free tape is assessed (i.e., cough test or other means).
15. Cystoscopy may be performed at the discretion of the surgeon.
16. When satisfied with the final mesh positioning, one of the inserters is released from the *device* by pulling the release wire while stabilizing the *Inserter*.
17. The *inserter* is gently removed from the incision after the release wire hits its "stop." A slight twisting motion of the *inserter* will assist in this maneuver.
18. It is important to ensure final mesh position after removal of the first *inserter*.
19. Step 16 is repeated on the other side. (Stabilize the inserter and pull the release wire.)
20. Followed by step 17.
21. The vaginal incision is closed.

MINI-ARC PROCEDURE

The Mini-Arc™ American Medical Systems (AMS) sling procedure is the most recently introduced minimally invasive treatment for stress urinary incontinence (Fig. 6). As with TVT-Secur, this procedure also reduces the risk of bowel or bladder injury and major bleeding, because it bypasses retropubic or transobturator needle passage altogether. This procedure uses the same concepts of the tension-free tape mid-urethral slings but involves a single vaginal incision (57).

1. The procedure can be carried out under local, regional, or general anesthesia, with a tendency for local anesthesia.
2. The patient is placed in the dorsal lithotomy position with the hips hyperflexed over the abdomen (±110°). The buttocks are positioned flush with the edge of the operating table.
3. A urethral catheter is inserted and the bladder is emptied.
4. The suburethral tissues are infiltrated with a local anesthetic solution, and a 1.5-mm suburethral incision is made (Fig. 15). The incision is identical to the incision made for transobturator slings. The vaginal epithelium is dissected off the underlying suburethral tissues out to the pelvic sidewall, adjacent to the posterior surface of the ischiopubic ramus. This dissection follows the same path as the transobturator slings but is made only slightly larger than the mesh to avoid full dissection. The tunnel that is created should be only large enough to ensure that the mesh lies flat under the urethra and to avoid "button holing" the vagina. The obturator internus fascia and muscle can then be injected with the local anesthetic solution. To aid in the placement of the sling, a mark may be made on the subject's skin just inferior to where the adductor longus tendon meets the pubic ramus.
5. The Mini-Arc blunt needle tip is then inserted into the sling's self-fixating tip to advance the sling into place. The sling/needle assembly is then placed into the dissected tunnel and pushed toward the obturator space into the obturator internus muscle. While advancing, the needle tip should be kept in close proximity to the posterior surface of the ischiopubic ram. This is similar to the "hammock"-type position of the transobturator slings. Once the pelvic sidewall is penetrated, i.e., the obturator fascia and muscle, the needle is advanced until the midpoint of the sling is at or just beyond the mid-urethra. The needle is then easily removed by simply sliding it back out of the fixating tip. Due to the tip's slip-fit design, the sling does not move

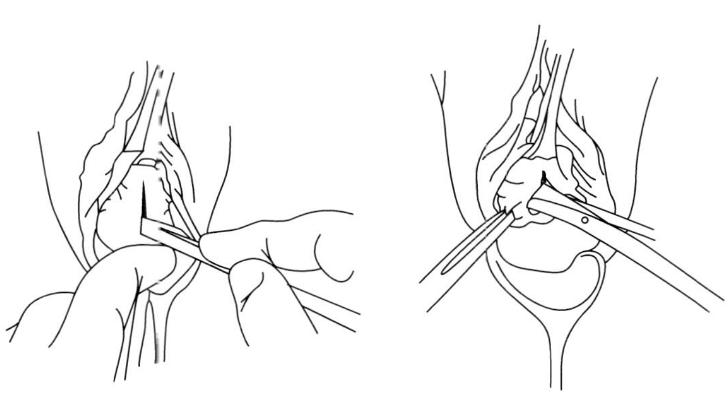

Figure 15 Incision and preparation of sub-urethral tissue.

while disengaging the needle from the sling. The needle is then placed into the other self-fixating tip, and the sling is introduced into the contralateral side. The needle is slowly advanced into the obturator internus muscle until a tension-free adjustment is completed under the mid-urethra. The design of the self-fixating tip and curved needle provides the surgeon with excellent control in advancing the needle to obtain precise tension-free adjustment.

Using a retrospective, dual-center, cohort study comparing the MiniArc to a conventional transobturator sling in one hundred thirty-one consecutive patients at 1 year, 85% of the MiniArc group and 89% of the transobturator group ($p = 0.60$) maintained comparable urinary continence, quality of life and symptom scores. Furthermore, complications were not significantly different between the groups. Either method appeared equally effective in the treatment of stress incontinence at 1 year follow-up (58).

CONCLUSIONS

Four fundamental surgical techniques for synthetic suburethral sling placement are now suitable for the treatment of USI. The TVT™ is a safe and effective, minimally invasive surgical technique with 10-year follow-up and a cure rate comparable to more invasive procedures traditionally accepted as the gold standard. Due to the intra- and postoperative complications associated with this procedure, as outlined in the text, we think that this original technique should be replaced by the TOR™, which is performed equally well by either the out-inside or the inside-out approach. Both of these variants are simple, quick, safe, and without the absolute need to perform cystoscopy. Moreover, the paraurethral and subvaginal dissections are less extensive with the inside-out approach, and the learning curve using this particular method is more intuitive and easier to learn. However, the follow-up and long-term cure rates after the TOR must be systematically collected using rigorous statistical methods, in order to validate our initial conclusions. The last but not the least question concerns the modality of obstetrical delivery after the placement of a mid-urethral tape, regardless of the technique. Indeed, it is likely in the future that more young women will demand treatment prior to completion of childbearing.

REFERENCES

1. Abrams P, Cardozo L, Fall M, et al. Standardisation Sub-committee of the International Continence Society. The standardisation of terminology of lower urinary tract function: report from the Standardisation Sub-committee of the International Continence Society. Neurourol Urodyn 2002; 21(2):167–178.
2. Bo K, Talseth T, Holme I. Single blind, randomised controlled trial of pelvic floor exercises, electrical stimulation, vaginal cones, and no treatment in management of genuine stress incontinence in women. BMJ 1999; 318(7182):487–493.
3. Bidmead J, Cardozo L. Retropubic urethropexy (Burch colposuspension). Int Urogynecol J Pelvic Floor Dysfunct 2001; 12(4):262–265.
4. Vancaillie TG, Schuessler W. Laparoscopic bladderneck suspension. J Laparoendosc Surg 1991; 1(3):169–173.
5. Ou CS, Presthus J, Beadle E. Laparoscopic bladder neck suspension using hernia mesh and surgical staples. J Laparoendosc Surg 1993; 3(6):563–566.
6. O'Shea RT, Seman E. Laparoscopic Burch colposuspension—new approaches. J Am Assoc Gynecol Laparosc 1994; 1(4, Part 2):S26–S27.
7. Ankardal M, Ekerydh A, Crafoord K, et al. A randomised trial comparing open Burch colposuspension using sutures with laparoscopic colposuspension using mesh and staples in women with stress urinary incontinence. Br J Obstet Gynaecol 2004; 111(9):974–981.
8. Carey MP, Goh JT, Rosamilia A, et al. Laparoscopic versus open Burch colposuspension: A randomised controlled trial. Br J Obstet Gynaecol 2006; 113(9):999–1006.
9. Petros PE, Ulmsten UI. An integral theory of female urinary incontinence. Experimental and clinical considerations. Acta Obstet Gynecol Scand Suppl 1990; 153:7–31.
10. Ulmsten U, Petros P. Intravaginal slingplasty: An ambulatory surgical procedure for treatment of female incontinence. Scand J Urol Nephrol 1995; 29:75–82.
11. Ulmsten U, Johnson P, Rezapour M. A three-year follow-up of tension free vaginal tape for surgical treatment of female stress urinary incontinence. Br J Obstet Gynaecol 1999; 106:345–350.
12. Olsson I, Kroon U. A three-year postoperative evaluation of tension-free vaginal tape. Gynecol Obstet Invest 1999; 48:267–269.
13. Nilsson CG, Rezapour M, Falconer C, et al. Seven years follow-up of the tension-free vaginal tape (TVT) procedure. Int Urogynecol J Pelvic Floor Dysfunct 2003; 14(Suppl 1):S35.
14. Delorme E. Transobturator urethral suspension: Mini-invasive procedure in the treatment of stress urinary incontinence in women [in French]. Prog Urol 2001; 11:1306–1313.
15. De Leval J. Novel surgical technique for the treatment of female stress urinary incontinence: Transobturator vaginal tape inside-out. Eur Urol 2003; 44(6):724–730.
16. Chin YK, Stanton SL. A follow up of silastic sling for genuine stress incontinence. Br J Obstet Gynaecol 1995; 102(2):143–147.
17. Weinberger MW, Ostergard DR. Long-term clinical and urodynamic evaluation of the polytetrafluoroethylene suburethral sling for treatment of genuine stress incontinence. Obstet Gynecol 1995; 86(1):92–96.
18. Rezapour M, Ulmsten U. Tension-Free Vaginal Tape in women with mixed urinary incontinence: A long-term follow-up. Int Urogynecol J Pelvic Floor Dysfunct 2001; 12(Suppl 2):S15–S18.
19. Rezapour M, Ulmsten U. Tension-free vaginal tape in women with recurrent stress urinary incontinence: A long-term follow-up. Int Urogynecol J Pelvic Floor Dysfunct 2001; 12(Suppl 2):S9–S11.
20. Rezapour M, Falconer C, Ulmsten U. Tension-free vaginal tape in women with intrinsic sphincter deficiency: A long-term follow-up. Int Urogynecol J Pelvic Floor Dysfunct 2001; 12(Suppl 2): S12–S14.
21. Nilsson CG, Falconer C, Rezapour M. Seven-year follow-up of the tension-free vaginal tape procedure for treatment of urinary incontinence. Obstet Gynecol 2004; 104(6):1259–1262.
22. Jarvis GJ. Surgery for genuine stress incontinence. Br J Obstet Gynaecol 1994; 101(5):371–374.
23. Ward KL, Hilton P, UK and Ireland TVT Trial Group. A prospective multicenter randomized trial of tension-free vaginal tape and colposuspension for primary urodynamic stress incontinence: Two-year follow-up. Am J Obstet Gynecol 2004; 190(2):324–331.
24. Black N, Griffiths J, Pope C, et al. Impact of surgery for stress incontinence on morbidity: Cohort study. BMJ 1997; 315(7121):1493–1498.
25. Maher C, Qatawneh A, Baessler K, et al. Laparoscopic colposuspension or tension-free vaginal tape for recurrent stress urinary incontinence and/or intrinsic sphincter deficiency: A randomised controlled trial [abstract]. Neurourol Urodyn 2004; 23(5/6):433–434.
26. Wiskind AK, Creighton SM, Stanton SL. The incidence of genital prolapse after Burch colposuspension. Am J Obstet Gynecol 1992; 167:399–405.

27. Valpas A, Kivela A, Penttinen J, et al. Tension-free vaginal tape and laparoscopic mesh colposuspension for stress urinary incontinence. Obstet Gynecol 2004; 104(1):42–49.
28. Paraiso MF, Walters MD, Karram MM, et al. Laparoscopic Burch colposuspension versus tension-free vaginal tape: A randomized trial. Obstet Gynecol 2004; 104(6):1249–1258.
29. Ustun Y, Engin-Ustun Y, Gungor M, et al. Tension-free vaginal tape compared with laparoscopic Burch urethropexy. J Am Assoc Gynecol Laparosc 2003; 10(3):386–389. [Erratum in: J Am Assoc Gynecol Laparosc 2003; 10(4):581.]
30. Liang CC, Soong YK. Tension-free vaginal tape versus laparoscopic bladder neck suspension for stress urinary incontinence. Chang Gung Med J 2002; 25(6):360–366.
31. Liapis A, Bakas P, Creatsas G. Burch colposuspension and tension-free vaginal tape in the management of stress urinary incontinence in women. Eur Urol 2002; 41(4):469–473.
32. Dean N, Herbison P, Ellis G, et al. Laparoscopic colposuspension and tension-free vaginal tape: A systematic review. Br J Obstet Gynaecol 2006; 113:1345–1353.
33. Peyrat L, Boutin JM, Bruyere F, et al. Intestinal perforation as a complication of tension-free vaginal tape procedure for urinary incontinence. Eur Urol 2001; 39(5):603–605.
34. Vierhout ME. Severe hemorrhage complicating tension-free vaginal tape: A case report. Int Urogynecol J Pelvic Floor Dysfunct 2001; 12(2):139–140.
35. Lim YN, Rane A, Barry C, et al. The suburethral slingplasty evaluation study in North Queensland (Suspend): A randomized controlled trial [abstract]. Neurourol Urodyn 2004; 23(5/6):495–496.
36. Soulie M, Cuvillier X, Benaissa A, et al. The tension-free transvaginal tape procedure in the treatment of female urinary stress incontinence: A French prospective multicentre study. Eur Urol 2001; 39:709–714.
37. Boustead GB. The Tension-free vaginal tape for treating female stress urinary incontinence. BJU Int 2002; 89:687–693.
38. Segal JL, Vassallo B, Kleeman S, et al. Prevalence of persistent and de novo overactive bladder symptoms after the tension-free vaginal tape. Obstet Gynecol 2004; 104:1263–1269.
39. Pifarotti P, Meschia M, Gattei U, et al. Multicenter randomized trial of TVT and IVS for the treatment of stress urinary incontinence in women [abstract]. Neurourol Urodyn 2004; 23(5/6):494–495.
40. Game X, Mouzin M, Vaessen C, et al. Obturator infected hematoma and urethral erosion following transobturator tape implantation. J Urol 2004; 171(4):1629.
41. Minaglia S, Ozel B, Klutke C, et al. Bladder injury during transobturator sling. Urology 2004; 64:376.
42. Bonnet P, Waltregny D, Reul O, et al. Inside-out transobturator approach for the surgical treatment of female stress urinary incontinence: Anatomical considerations. Presented at the annual meeting of the European Association of Urology, Vienna, 2004.
43. Costa P, Grise P, Droupy S, et al. Surgical treatment of female stress urinary incontinence with a trans-obturator tape (T. O. T.®) Uratape®: Short term results of a prospective multicentric study. Eur Urol 2004; 46(1):102–107.
44. de Tayrac R, Eglin G, Delorme E, et al. TOT multicenter register: Results in specific subgroups (associated prolapse and obese patients). Presented at the Annual Meeting of the International Continence Society & International Urogynecology Association, Paris, 2004.
45. Waltregny D, Reul O, Bonnet P, et al. Inside-out transobturator vaginal tape (TVT-O): Short-term results of a prospective study. Presented at the Annual Meeting of the International Continence Society & International Urogynecology Association, Paris, 2004.
46. Arunkalaivanan AS, Barrington JW. Randomized trial of porcine dermal sling (Pelvicol implant) vs. tension-free vaginal tape (TVT) in the surgical treatment of stress incontinence: A questionnaire-based study. Int Urogynecol J Pelvic Floor Dysfunct 2003; 14(1):17–23; discussion 21–22.
47. Neuman M. TVT and TVT-obturator: Comparison of two operative procedures. Eur J Obstet Gynecol Reprod Biol 2006 Apr 16; [Epub ahead of print].
48. David-Montefiore E, Frobert J-L, Grisard-Anaf M, et al. Peri-operative complications and pain after the suburethral sling procedure for urinary stress incontinence: A French prospective randomised multicentre study comparing the retropubic and transobturator routes. Eur Urol 2006; 49:133–138.
49. Vervest HAM, Bruin JP, Renes-Zeijl CC. Transobturator tape, inside-out or outside-in approaches: Does it matter? Int Urogynecol J Pelvic Floor Dysfunct 2005; 16:S69.
50. Wang AC, Lin YH, Tseng LH, et al. Prospective randomized comparison of transobturator suburethral sling (Monarc) vs suprapubic arc (Sparc) sling procedures for female urodynamic stress incontinence. Int Urogynecol J Pelvic Floor Dysfunct 2006; 17:439–443.
51. Liapis A, Bakas P, Giner M, et al. Tension-free vaginal tape versus tension-free vaginal tape obturator in women with stress urinary incontinence. Gynecol Obstet Invest 2006; 62(3):160–164.
52. Laurikainen E, Valpas A, Kivela A, et al. Retropubic compared with transobturator tape placement in treatment of urinary incontinence: A randomized controlled trial. Obstet Gynecol 2007; 109(1):4–11.
53. Darai E, Frobert JL, Grisard-Anaf M, et al. Functional results after the suburethral sling procedure for urinary stress incontinence: A prospective randomized multicentre study comparing the retropubic and transobturator routes. Eur Urol 2007; 51(3):795–801; discussion 801–802.
54. Abdel-Fattah M, Ramsay I, Pringle S. Lower urinary tract injuries after transobturator tape insertion by different routes: A large retrospective study. BJOG 2006; 113(12):1377–1381.
55. Lim J, Cornish A, Carey MP. Clinical and quality-of-life outcomes in women treated by the TVT-O procedure. BJOG 2006; 113(11):1315–1320.
56. Tommaselli GA, Di Carlo C, Gargano V, et al. Efficacy and safety of TVT-O and TVT-Secur in the treatment of female stress urinary incontinence: 1-year follow-up. Int Urogynecol J Pelvic Floor Dysfunct 2010 May 26. [Epub ahead of print]
57. Moore R, Erickson T, Serels S, et al. "Retrospective review of early experience using the AMS Mini Arc Single Incision Sling System to treat stress urinary incontinence in women." J Minim Invasive Gynecol 2007; (14):S129–S130.
58. De Ridder D, Berkers J, Deprest J, et al. Single incision Mini-sling versus a transobutaror sling: a comparative study on MiniArc and Monarc slings. Int Urogynecol J Pelvic Floor Dysfunct 2010; 21(7):773–778.

The following is a list of references concerning abstracts presented at IUGA Meeting for TVT-SECUR:

Saltz SM, Haff RE, Lucente VR. Short-term assessment of patients undergoing the new tension free vaginal tape: Secur procedure for treatment of stress urinary incontinence. Int Urogynecol J Pelvic Floor Dysfunct 2007; 18(Suppl 1):S25–S105.

Martan A, Masata J, Svabik K. Initial experience with TVT-Secur system procedure and the reason for persistent stress urinary incontinence. Int Urogynecol J Pelvic Floor Dysfunct 2007; 18(Suppl 1):S25–S105.

Albrich S, Naumann G, Skala C,et al. TVT-Secur: A novel approach for the treatment of female genuine stress urinary incontinence. Int Urogynecol J Pelvic Floor Dysfunct 2007; 18(Suppl 1):S25–S105.

Marsh FA, Assassa P. An audit of the introduction of TVT Secure in clinical practice. Int Urogynecol J Pelvic Floor Dysfunct 2007; 18(Suppl 1):S25–S105.

Neumann M. Training TVT Secur: The first 150 teaching operations. Int Urogynecol J Pelvic Floor Dysfunct 2007; 18(Suppl 1):S25–S105.

15

Surgical treatment of pelvic organ prolapse

Geoffrey W. Cundiff and Jean-Bernard Dubuisson

CHOOSING A REPAIR

Careful pelvic examination has shown that virtually all parous women as well as many active nulliparous women have less than perfect pelvic support. Many of these women have few, if any, symptoms associated with their support defects, although 10% to 11% will ultimately undergo surgery for prolapse. Regrettably, up to 30% of women who seek surgical repair return for a subsequent procedure (1). The conscientious surgeon must, therefore, be sure that a patient's symptoms are attributable to her support defects and recognize the limitations of surgical repairs in choosing the most appropriate repair.

The symptoms associated with specific support defects have not been well characterized, as symptoms overlap among different support defects (2). Symptoms such as pelvic pressure and tissue protruding from the vagina occur with anterior, posterior, or apical support defects. Symptoms such as lower abdominal or back pain or pelvic pressure are even less specific and may be altogether unrelated to support defects. Our ability to distinguish clinically significant pelvic organ prolapse (POP) from normal variations in support is impaired by an absence of longitudinal studies that identify symptoms consistently associated with prolapse and insufficient controlled interventional trials that establish cure rates for these symptoms.

SURGICAL LIMITATIONS

Support defects may result from damage to any of the pelvic floor structures, including connective tissues, muscles, or nerves. Recent investigations have helped in characterizing nerve injuries with neurodiagnostic testing, including pudendal and perineal nerve terminal motor latency testing, evaluation of the sacral nerve reflexes, and external anal sphincter electromyography. Neuropathic injury is suspected to predispose women with prolapse to recurrence (3). Ultimately, we may be able to use neurodiagnostic testing in counseling patients regarding the relationship between neuropathic injuries and surgical outcomes. Despite these advances, neurologic injury remains irreversible at present, and we are limited to surgical correction of connective tissue tears and rehabilitation of pelvic floor muscles. Consequently, surgeons are increasingly relying on surgical repairs that use grafts to compensate for patient characteristics, like neuropathy, that increase the risk of surgical failure.

SURGICAL GOALS

The goals of surgical correction are to alleviate the symptoms of pelvic floor support defects, strive for normal anatomical relationships, and maximize bladder, bowel, and coital function. Urinary symptoms can include incontinence, retention, and lower urinary tract symptoms including frequency and urgency. Bowel symptoms can include incontinence, constipation, incomplete emptying, urgency, and dyschezia. Other symptoms include pelvic pressure and tissue protrusion. In correcting any support defect, care must be taken to avoid overcorrection, which can lead to new support problems. This has been well described with the anterior deflection of retropubic urethropexies predisposing to apical prolapse and enterocele formation and with the development of anterior support defects associated with posterior deflection due to sacrospinous ligament fixation.

Successful correction of POP, therefore, must balance the goals and limitations of surgery and address support defects at all levels. A systematic evaluation of the anterior, posterior, and apical compartments must be made prior to the surgery, and any defects identified must be confirmed intraoperatively with careful evaluation at that time as well.

SURGICAL APPROACH

Numerous surgical procedures have been described for each type of support defect. Pelvic reconstructive surgery can be accomplished through a vaginal approach, an open abdominal approach, a laparoscopic abdominal approach, or some combination thereof. Too often, the choice of procedure and the route of approach have been based on the surgeon's biases or preferences rather than on anatomic principles. Improved understanding of normal and abnormal pelvic anatomy and risk factors for recurrent POP now permits a more rational selection of the procedure and the route that can be tailored to the individual patient.

Considerations that impact the choice of procedure include the precise defects responsible for the POP, the etiology of the defects, whether the inciting and promoting events are continuing processes, as well as the patient's desires and expectations. Table 1 lists factors that can contribute to POP and its recurrence.

CATEGORIES OF SURGICAL REPAIR

For the frail patient whose health status precludes prolonged, extensive surgery, an *obliterative* procedure such as colpectomy or colpocleisis can provide symptom relief with minimal morbidity due to shorter operative time and more superficial dissection. Such a procedure is obviously contraindicated, however, for any woman with a desire to maintain vaginal coital function. For women with discrete defects in the fibromuscular layer of endopelvic fascia, an anatomic vaginal repair that simply corrects the defects of the indigenous tissues may be

Table 1 Factors Contributing to Pelvic Organ Prolapse

Genetic variation	Injury to the pelvic floor	Promoting factors	Decompensating factors
Musculoskeletal	Obstetrical injury Connective tissue Pelvic diaphragm Innervation	Obesity	Aging
Connective tissue	Surgical Injury Connective tissue Innervation	Smoking	Hormonal changes of menopause
Neurological		Lung disease	Acquired neuropathy or myopathy
		Constipation	Debilitation
		Recreational or occupational lifting	Medicines

sufficient. Such *restorative* repairs can be accomplished from the vaginal approach. This approach has the advantages of less blood loss and a shorter recovery period than procedures performed through a laparotomy.

There are circumstances such as ongoing occupational or recreational stressors or chronic illness, however, that may compromise the longevity of restorative repairs. Surgeries that use native tissues depend on normal muscular support and function to support the repaired tissue and might be at an increased risk of failure in the presence of neuromuscular compromise of the pelvic diaphragm. Extreme attenuation of native tissues may also compromise the success of these repairs. Women with recurrent POP may require a stronger repair than is provided by an anatomic repair. Under these circumstances, a *compensatory* repair that provides an additional support mechanism is indicated.

Vaginal Procedures

One of the unique aspects of gynecological surgery is the ability to operate through the vaginal approach. The advantages of this approach identified by pioneering gynecological surgeons remain pertinent even today. The vaginal field offers easy access to the pelvic anatomy and can generally be accomplished with less postoperative pain than a laparotomy, resulting in a faster and easier recovery for the patient.

Vaginal Obliterative Repairs

The principal advantages of obliterative procedures are a short operative time and superficial dissection that permits the use of regional or local anesthesia with sedation in place of general anesthesia. These factors significantly decrease perioperative morbidity, making obliterative procedures safer for patients at higher risk of complications due to age or chronic illnesses. Because the dissection is carried out in a superficial plane away from large vessels, blood loss tends to occur more gradually and is more easily controlled than the sudden blood loss that can occur with sacrospinous or sacrocolpopexy procedures. Such gradual blood loss may be better tolerated by patients with chronic illnesses than sudden fluid shifts. The fact that undergoing an obliterative procedure will preclude sexual intercourse must be discussed and must be acceptable to the patient.

Obliterative procedures include partial or total colpocleisis and colpectomy. In the absence of a uterus, either complete colpocleisis or colpectomy can be performed (4). Since obliterative procedures preclude subsequent evaluation of the cervix and uterine cavity, patients with uterine prolapse should be treated either with partial colpocleisis, which leaves lateral drainage channels for cervical secretions, or with concurrent vaginal hysterectomy. If partial colpocleisis is planned, preoperative evaluation should include a Pap smear, a pelvic sonogram, and an endometrial biopsy. While a short operating time is a goal of the obliterative techniques, obtaining optimal results still demands attention to critical support principles. It is important to adequately reduce the enterocele component of the prolapse and to provide preferential support to the urethrovesical junction during colpocleisis if recurrent prolapse and stress incontinence are to be avoided (4). Preoperative evaluation with urodynamics is useful for women with preexisting incontinence or voiding dysfunction. Specific surgical procedures for incontinence, including vaginal procedures such as a transobturator or retropubic midurethral sling, can be easily performed at the time of an obliterative procedure with minimal additional operating time.

Techniques

The most commonly described technique for partial colpocleisis is a variation of the operation originally described by LeFort in 1877. Neugebauer, Langmade, Denehy, and others have described modifications in the procedure (5–7). The prolapsed cervix is grasped with a tenaculum and brought out through the introitus. A surgical marking pen is used to outline an area of vaginal epithelium to be removed on the anterior and posterior vaginal walls. The dimensions are chosen to leave sufficient epithelium for the lateral channels and a 1 to 2 cm dimple at the introitus. The epithelium is incised with a scalpel and sharply dissected off of the underlying tissue using Strully or Metzenbaum scissors. Alternatively, this dissection can be accomplished with needlepoint electrocautery, which minimizes blood loss. This dissection should be superficial to leave the entire rectovaginal and pubocervical fascia. The dissection is continued until the anterior and posterior epithelium is dissected free of underlying tissue.

The closure of the vagina uses delayed absorbable sutures placed in an inverting Lembert fashion, to approximate the proximal edges of the vaginal epithelium over the cervix to begin creating lateral channels on either side for drainage of cervical secretions. The cervix is then further inverted with progressive rows of longitudinal imbricating sutures placed to approximate the pubocervical fascia to the rectovaginal fascia. The successive rows continue in a caudad direction, obliterating the upper portion of the vagina until the bulk of the prolapse has been reduced. The vaginal epithelial edges are then reapproximated with absorbable suture.

The technique for total colpocleisis is similar, with the exception that it is not necessary to leave lateral drainage channels. A circumferential incision is made in the vaginal epithelium just cephalad to the hymenal ring (4). The vagina is then marked into four quadrants and each removed by sharp dissection. The epithelium is dissected sharply off of the underlying fascia and excised. The anterior and posterior fascias are then reapproximated with sequential rows of longitudinal sutures until the lumen of the vagina is obliterated. Alternatively, in a colpectomy, the obliteration of vaginal lumen is accomplished with sequential purse-string sutures.

Plication of the levator ani muscles and perineorrhaphy are frequently added to both techniques. The levator placation provides a firm site of attachment for the obliterating stitches. In either partial or total colpocleisis, once the majority of the prolapse has been reduced, appropriate bladder neck procedures can be performed as needed, prior to completing the colpocleisis. The fixation of the anterior wall to the posterior is usually not carried out all the way to the hymenal ring, as this artificially flattens the posterior vesical neck angle and predisposes patients to incontinence. Finally, the perineorrhaphy provides a narrow introitus (4).

Results

Most recently published evaluations of colpocleisis reveal resolution of symptoms and high patient satisfaction (8,9). DeLancy and Morley reported successful treatment in 32 of 33 women (10). One woman had a recurrence of her vault eversion at one year, and she was treated successfully with a repeat colpocleisis. Average length of follow-up was 35 months. No new cases of stress urinary incontinence (SUI) developed in this group. Earlier papers on the outcome of colpocleisis report similar cure rates of 86% to 100%, although what constitutes a "cure" is generally not defined. In a series reported by Ridley, 50 of 58 patients (86%) had a "satisfactory" outcome at a minimum of one year after the colpocleisis (11). In the same series, 6 of 58 women (10%) required subsequent surgery, 3 patients had surgery for recurrent prolapse, and 3 had surgery for SUI. Fitzgerald and coauthors recently reported a prospective cohort of 153 women treated with colpocleisis (12). At one-year follow-up, 95% of patients reported being either "very satisfied" or "satisfied" with their decision to have vaginal closure for prolapse treatment. All pelvic symptom scores and related problems significantly improved at 3 and 12 months. Anatomic success was 93%. Reported complications following colpocleisis are few, with the most common being the development of SUI. Most series report postoperative incidences of SUI of 1% to 9% (4).

Vaginal Repairs for Apical Prolapse

Regardless of the anchoring site for the vaginal vault suspension, it is essential to re-establish continuity of the anterior and posterior vaginal fascia at the vaginal apex. Failure to approximate these fibromuscular planes can result in an apical enterocele, where the small bowel herniates behind the thin vaginal epithelium without an intervening myofascial layer.

Techniques

There are many techniques for suspending the vaginal apex. For the patient with good pelvic floor muscle strength as assessed by clinical examination and reasonably substantive endopelvic fascia, a vaginal approach using native tissues may be appropriate.

McCall popularized a technique commonly used in New Orleans, now known as the *McCall culdoplasty*, which uses the uterosacral ligaments for suspension of the vaginal vault in conjunction with an extensive posterior culdoplasty (13). The McCall culdoplasty is most commonly done in conjunction with a vaginal hysterectomy but can be used for vaginal vault prolapse as well. Following the opening of the vaginal apex, the uterosacral ligaments are identified and placed under tension. The uterosacral ligaments are then plicated with nonabsorbable sutures placed from one uterosacral ligament to the other, reefing the peritoneum of the posterior cul-de-sac in between. Two to three separate sutures are placed in a progressively cephalad fashion. These initial sutures, or internal stitches, are placed from within the peritoneal cavity. Additional sutures, the external stitches, are then placed from the vaginal side of the incision into the peritoneal cavity, incorporating the vaginal cuff and both uterosacral ligaments. Tying the internal stitches plicates the uterosacral ligaments in the midline, while the external stitches suspend the cuff from the plicated uterosacral ligaments.

The McCall culdoplasty has evolved over the years to the *uterosacral suspension*, which avoids plicating the uterosacrals in the midline. Once the apex has been opened, the patient is placed in Trendelenburg position, and a 6-in. moistened Kerlix is used to pack the bowels up out of the sacral hollow. This greatly aids in visualization of the uterosacral ligaments. A headlamp improves visualization.

Buller and colleagues performed a cadaveric investigation aimed at describing the optimal location for suture placement in the uterosacral suspension (14). The surrounding vasculature and nerves, in conjunction with suture pullout studies, suggested the intermediate segment of the uterosacral ligament as the optimal compromise between strength and safety. The ischial spine was found to be a good marker of this intermediate segment. They also noted that the proximity of the ureter to the anterior border of the fan-shaped uterosacral ligament varies along its length, being closest at the level of the cervix and farthest at the sacrum. Inappropriate suture placement can kink the ureter, causing obstruction. Placing sutures at least 1 cm posterior to the anterior border of the uterosacral ligament minimizes the potential for ureteral injury. Placing the distal uterosacral ligament on tension demonstrates the anterior border of the ligament. A single permanent or delayed absorbable suture is then placed through the uterosacral ligament at approximately the level of the ischial spine, 1 cm posterior to the anterior border. One arm of this suture is brought out through the lateral aspect of the pubocervical fascia, while the other arm is brought out through the lateral aspect of the rectovaginal fascia. A second suture is placed through the contralateral uterosacral ligament and then attached, as previously described, to the pubocervical and rectovaginal fascia. Some authors describe placing additional sutures through each uterosacral ligament in a cephalad fashion and attaching them to progressively more medial aspects of the vaginal cuff.

A horizontal mattress stitch is used to close the intervening cuff medial to the lateral suspension stitches. This stitch reapproximates the anterior and posterior fascia, to prevent subsequent enterocele formation. Tying the uterosacral sutures closes the lateral aspects of the vaginal cuff and anchors them to the uterosacral ligaments in an anatomical configuration. Finally, absorbable sutures are used to close the vaginal mucosa.

No attempt is made to plicate the uterosacral ligaments in the midline, as this is not anatomic and can lead to narrowing of the upper vagina with resultant dyspareunia. It also increases the risk of ureteral obstruction (14). The ureter runs along the distal aspect of the anterior border of the uterosacral ligament and is frequently attached to it by a fibrous band. This leads to a risk of obstruction or injury to the ureter with all procedures that use the uterosacral as an anchorage. The rate of obstruction with uterosacral suspension has been reported to be as high as 11% (15). Should obstruction occur, simply releasing the suture is generally sufficient to restore ureteral flow, although in other cases reimplantation may be necessary. Regardless, postoperative cystoscopy is essential to a safe repair.

In cases where it is not possible to visualize the uterosacral ligaments or when they are extremely attenuated, the fascia of the iliococcygeus muscle, just anterior to ischial spine, can be used to suspend the vaginal vault. The *iliococcygeus suspension* is similar to the description of the uterosacral suspension but uses a different anchorage site. As described by Shull et al., the fascia overlying the iliococcygeus muscle is identified lateral to the rectum and anterior to the ischial spine (16). The bowel is retracted medially, and a suture is placed just anterior to the spine beside the arcus tendineus fascia pelvis and brought out through the pubocervical fascia anteriorly and the rectovaginal fascia posteriorly on the ipsilateral side. Tying the sutures suspends the vagina bilaterally.

The *sacrospinous fixation* is also a widely advocated and used option (17). Both anterior and posterior approaches to the pararectal space have been described. And while fixation is most commonly performed unilaterally, bilateral fixation has also been described (18). Once the pararectal space has been entered, the spine is located and the sacrospinous ligament is identified over its course from the spine to the sacrum. The use of a Miya hook ligature carrier makes placement of the sacrospinous sutures significantly easier. Two nonabsorbable or delayed absorbable sutures are placed through the ligament, the first approximately 2 cm medial and 1 cm cephalad to the spine and the second approximately 1 cm medial to the first. One arm of each suture is then brought through the posterior rectovaginal fascia, and the other is brought through the anterior pubocervical fascia. The sutures are then tied down, directly approximating the vagina to the sacrospinous ligament complex, without a suture bridge.

Each of these procedures for restorative repair of apical prolapse has advantages and disadvantages. The lateral and posterior deflection of the vagina with the typical unilateral sacrospinous ligament fixation is clearly not anatomic due to posterior deflection of the vaginal axis. This exposes the anterior superior vaginal wall to increased force during the increases in abdominal pressure. This may predispose patients to an increase in the incidence of anterior wall prolapse after sacrospinous fixation, although a retrospective study challenges this assumption (19). While the iliococcygeus suspension maintains the normal alignment of the vaginal cylinder, the ischial spines are considerably inferior to the normal position of the vaginal apex, resulting in loss of vaginal length. The origins of the uterosacral ligaments, if sufficiently strong on both sides, allow better vaginal depth with normal alignment. When attenuation of the ligaments mandates plication at the level of the suspension, the resulting midline suspension is not anatomic.

Results

McCall reported no recurrent enteroceles during a three-year follow-up (13), and Given reported a 5% failure rate with an average follow-up of seven years (20). Elkins et al. compared high uterosacral suspension to sacrospinous ligament fixation and found a greater vaginal depth with the former, 10.2 versus 8.3 cm (21).

Although the technique of uterosacral suspension was described four decades ago, most of the data regarding its efficacy are relatively recent. Shull et al. reported on 289 patients with short-term follow-up after a vaginal uterosacral suspension (22). They reported that 87% of patients had optimal anatomical outcomes, with a 1% transfusion rate and 1% ureteral injury rate. Their report was limited to anatomical results, but Barber et al. reported on 46 women followed for a mean of 15 months after a vaginal uterosacral suspension, noting that 90% had both resolution of prolapse symptoms and improvement in the stage of prolapse (15). These results seem to be sustained based on a recent report of five-year outcomes (23). Surgical failure, defined as symptomatic recurrent prolapse of stage II or greater, occurred in 15% of patients, although only 3% had recurrence of apical prolapse greater than stage II. There was also a significant improvement in urinary, bowel, and sexual symptoms, as measured by quality-of-life instruments.

In distinction to the sacrospinous and uterosacral ligaments, the iliococcygeus fascia does not have critical structures such as the pudendal nerve or ureter immediately adjacent to it. Meeks et al. reported a 4% recurrence rate for anterior segment prolapse in 110 women following iliococcygeus suspension (24). This is better than the 19% failure rate in a study of 42 women undergoing iliococcygeal suspension, as reported by Shull et al., although 10 women with recurrence had minimal anterior defects and only 5% had failure of apical support in this series (16). Complications described following sacrospinous fixation include vaginal shortening, sexual dysfunction, pain, and hemorrhage (17,18).

The latter complications are related to the close proximity of pudendal nerves and vessels laterally and gluteal vessels and sacral nerve roots superiorly.

Vaginal Repairs for Anterior Prolapse

Cystoceles have traditionally been repaired by plicating the pubocervical fascia in the midline with a series of horizontal mattress sutures. More recently, interest has turned to a more anatomical repair, the *defect-directed cystocele repair*, which is limited to repair of the precise defect in the pubocervical fascia. Defects in the anterior segment can occur laterally, superiorly, and in the midline. Superior defects are addressed with closure of the cuff, establishing continuity of the anterior and posterior fascia and ensuring adequate apical support. The original description of the repair of lateral defects, the paravaginal repair, used the vaginal approach but can also be performed by laparotomy or laparoscopic approach. Defect-directed repairs are described below.

Techniques

When performed vaginally, the epithelium is incised and dissected from the underlying endopelvic fascia. This dissection is continued beneath the descending pubic rami to the lateral pelvic sidewalls. Placing the contralateral index finger on the ischial spine helps to identify the lateral attachment of the pubocervical fascia to the pelvic sidewall, the arcus tendineus fascia pelvis. The arcus tendineus fascia pelvis runs from the tip of the finger along the medial aspect of the finger to the proximal interphalangeal joint. Lateral defects can be identified by attempting to swing the finger anteriorly or by the identification of retropubic space fat. If a lateral defect is present, permanent or delayed absorbable sutures are placed at 1-cm intervals into the arcus tendineus fascia pelvis from the spine to the pubic bone, while retracting the bladder medially. When all sutures are placed, they are then brought through the lateral aspect of the pubocervical fascia and tied down.

Central defects are most easily accessible from the vaginal approach. Looking for the contrast between the white pubocervical fascia and the ruddy red detrusor muscle, which tends to bleed more easily, identifies the rent. The defect is closed in an interrupted fashion with permanent suture, and the vaginal epithelium is closed.

For patients at risk of recurrent prolapse or those with endopelvic fascia that is too attenuated to repair, an *anterior fascial reinforcement*, using a piece of synthetic mesh or heterologous fascia, can be used. An attempt is made to correct any obvious breaks in the fascia and then the graft is placed over the fascia, in a manner such that a patch would be placed. The graft is secured bilaterally to the arcus tendineus fascia pelvis along its entire course and superiorly to the vaginal cuff.

Following the correction of all fascial defects, support procedures for the urethrovesical junction can be performed as needed for patients with urodynamic stress incontinence or reduces stress incontinence.

Results

Young et al. reported a 98% objective cure rate at one-year follow-up, using a vaginal approach to paravaginal repair, but there are no studies reporting cure rates for the defect-directed approach with all anterior wall defects (25). There is also a paucity of information on the anterior fascial replacement. Julian reported a 66% cure rate for standard vaginal anterior colporrhaphy for recurrent anterior prolapse compared to a 100% cure rate when Marlex mesh was used to substitute for the endopelvic fascia (26). There was, however, a 25% incidence of mesh-related complications. Others have reported a 25% recurrence rate of cystoceles at one year when mesh was used as part of the anterior repair, compared to a 43% recurrence rate with anterior repair alone (27).

Vaginal Repairs for Posterior Prolapse

Repair of rectoceles has traditionally been performed with plication of the levator muscles in the midline, creating a nonanatomic barrier between the vagina and the rectum. This approach has been associated with dyspareunia and constipation postoperatively (28). As with cystocele repairs, recent investigations have advocated the *defect-directed rectocele repair.* The technique for defect-directed repair is described below.

Techniques

The epithelium is incised in a transverse manner, just outside the hymenal ring. This incision is carried out cephalad to the cuff or until the defect has been exposed. The underlying rectovaginal fascia is dissected sharply off the underlying tissue, out laterally to its lateral fascial attachments to the levator ani and obturator fascia. Once the dissection is complete, the rent is identified. Rectoceles occur due to rents in the rectovaginal fascia that occur at various locations. Displacing the anterior rectal wall with a finger in the rectum facilitates identification of discrete fascial tears. The rent is then repaired in an interrupted fashion, burying the knots below the rectovaginal fascia. Careful attention to the attachment of the posterior fascia to the perineal body is essential to prevent recurrent rectocele and to help correct perineal descent. Superior defects are corrected by attachment of the rectovaginal fascia to the pubocervical fascia anteriorly, as well as re-establishing apical support as previously described. Lateral breaks are corrected by reattaching the fascia to the lateral pelvic sidewall in a manner similar to that described above for paravaginal repairs above. As a perineorrhaphy, which artificially enlarges the perineum and superficially constricts the genital hiatus, creates abnormal anatomy with poor functional results (28), perineal reconstruction is limited to reattachment of the rectovaginal fascia to the perineal body, and only if there are discreet breaks in the superficial perineal muscles.

For women with extremely attenuated fascia, *posterior fascial reinforcement* can be considered. It is performed in a manner similar to that described previously for anterior fascial reinforcement, attaching the graft to the arcus tendineus fascia rectovaginalis laterally, the uterosacral ligaments and pubocervical fascia superiorly, and the perineal body inferiorly.

Results

Although traditional posterior colporrhaphy reduces the vaginal bulge effectively in 76% to 96% of cases, relief of associated defecatory and sexual dysfunction symptoms has been much less satisfactory, with dyspareunia in 20% to 50% of cases postoperatively and persistent splinting in 21% to 50% (29,30). One study documenting the cure rate for repair of discrete posterior fascial defects showed improvement in POP quantification (POPQ) stage at six weeks in 67 of 69 women (30). A total of 18% were found to have recurrent rectoceles at one year. Others have reported similar success rates in the range of 81% to 90% with similar follow-up (29). Statistically significant improvement in bowel symptoms such as constipation, splinting, and incontinence and in other symptoms such as dyspareunia has been documented.

In a surgical series of 43 women with advanced posterior vaginal wall prolapse treated with a posterior fascial reinforcement using porcine dermis, Kohli and Miklos reported a 93% surgical cure, defined as <stage II POPQ scores at one year (31). This is a significant improvement over the anatomical cure rates of the defect-directed repair. Nevertheless, in a randomized clinical trial of 98 subjects comparing posterior colporrhaphy, defect-directed repair, or posterior fascial replacement using porcine small intestine submucosa, the perceived benefit of the addition of a graft was not borne out (32). At one-year follow-up, the fascial reinforcement group had a statistically significant lower anatomical cure rate (54%) than the defect-directed repair or posterior colporrhaphy (78% and 86%). In contrast, all intervention groups had significant improvement in prolapse symptoms, including protrusion defecatory function and sexual function, with no difference between groups. While this are level 1 data, it does not necessarily contradict Kohli and Miklos findings, as the two grafts used, porcine small intestine submucosa and porcine dermis, have quite different properties and should not be considered interchangeable. This underlines the need for further studies of the posterior fascial reinforcement.

Total Vaginal Mesh Repairs

Several groups of surgical innovators have developed new vaginal procedures for POP designed to use the surgical concepts of transobturator tapes for incontinence, including reinforcement using mesh and tension-free placement without suture (33). They also advocate mesh placement deep into the endopelvic fascia. These procedures use large pieces of polypropylene mesh with arms that are surgically introduced through muscular tissue using long curved trocars or needles. For example, the anterior mesh has four arms, with the two distal arms brought through the anterior aspect of the obturator fossa membrane and overlying skin, and the two proximal arms brought through the iliococcygeus muscle lateral to the ischial spines, and then through the posterior aspect of the obturator fossa membrane and overlying skin. The posterior mesh has two arms superiorly, which are brought through either the sacrospinous ligament or the iliococcygeus muscle and which exit through skin incisions over the ischiorectal fossa. The distal end of the posterior mesh is attached with delayed absorbable sutures to the perineal body.

There are presently four total vaginal mesh repair kits marketed for prolapse (33). These procedures are advocated as effective for the treatment of all levels of POP, as the proximal mesh arms are felt to provide level 1 support. However, the anterior and posterior meshes can be placed individually for isolated cystoceles or rectoceles.

Results

Reports of efficacy are limited to preliminary results. Fatton and coauthors report three-month follow-up of 106 patients with stage III–IV prolapse treated with anterior (20%), posterior (26%), or both anterior and posterior (54%) Prolift® (Johnson & Johnson, Cincinnati, Ohio) (34). Anatomical success was 95%, with a 5% complication rate due to mesh erosion. Similar results were noted in 41 patients at a median follow-up of seven months, with a 7% anatomical failure rate and 7% mesh erosion rate (35). The Apogee and Perigee systems (American Medical Systems, Minnetonka, Minnesota) have one-year follow-up for 120 patients (36). The anatomical success rate was 93%, and mesh erosions were more common when the anterior mesh was used. Mesh erosion rates from 5% to 11% (33) are consistent among the available studies and raise the question of what rate of surgical complication is reasonable to improve the durability of vaginal repairs without mesh.

LAPAROTOMY PROCEDURES

The historical association of gynecological surgery with a vaginal approach leads some gynecological surgeons to favor this approach for all prolapse surgery, and a strong argument can be made that the advantages in recovery for the patient should make it the default approach, much as it is for hysterectomy. From this perspective, procedures performed via a laparotomy should offer other clear advantages to outweigh the longer recovery compared to vaginal procedures. For prolapse surgery, the perceived advantage is the opportunity to perform compensatory repairs using anchorages for grafts that are not available from the vaginal field.

Laparotomy Repairs for Apical Prolapse

The woman with attenuated fascia, poor pelvic floor muscle strength, or severe ongoing physical stress may benefit from surgical techniques that provide compensatory support. The sacral colpopexy is a well-established compensatory repair for apical prolapse, which reinforces the normal apical support of the cardinal and uterosacral ligaments with a suspensory bridge of either biological or synthetic material between the prolapsed vagina and the anterior sacrum. A variety of synthetic materials, including polyethylene terephthalate, polypropylene, and expanded polytetrafluoroethylene, have been used, as well as xenografts such as porcine dermis or allografts including cadaveric skin or fascia lata. Alternatively, native tissue can be harvested from the rectus fascia or fascia lata of the thigh. The material is then placed in the manner described below.

Techniques

Regardless of the surgical graft material, two straps of tissue measuring 5.5 cm at the base and extending 15 cm in length are cut into a rhomboid shape. Any defect in the rectovaginal or pubocervical fascia is repaired prior to attaching the graft. This is particularly important with rectocele repair to ensure continuity of support from the sacrum all the way down to the perineal body. A large obturator is placed in the vagina to assist in elevating the vaginal cuff. The bladder is dissected off of the vaginal cuff, exposing the superior aspect of the pubocervical fascia to provide a sufficiently broad area to attach the graft. Similarly, the posterior peritoneum is opened at the vaginal apex and the rectovaginal space is dissected until the superior edge of the rectovaginal fascia can be identified.

It is preferable to re-establish the integrity of the pubocervical ring by suturing the superior aspects of the pubocervical fascia and the rectovaginal fascia if they are not already attached. The two straps are attached separately using delayed absorbable sutures, one anteriorly and the other posteriorly, taking care to attach the material over a wide surface area. Most failures occur due to avulsion of the mesh from the vagina. Attaching the graft over a wide surface area, which distributes the force that any one suture has to withstand, minimizes the risk of avulsion. It is also important to avoid bunching of graft material under the sutures and to avoid tying the sutures too tightly, which may predispose patients to necrosis and mesh erosion. After the straps have been attached anteriorly and posteriorly, they are sutured laterally to each other, creating a circumferential attachment around the vaginal cuff.

Many surgeons perform a culdoplasty prior to attaching the mesh to the sacrum, to prevent bowel from slipping behind the mesh. Delayed absorbable or non absorbable suture is used, incorporating the inferior edge of the posterior piece of mesh in the culdoplasty. Failure to obliterate the cul-de-sac has led to reports of enterocele formation behind the posterior mesh (37).

Entering the presacral space requires caution to avoid injury to the retroperitoneal vasculature and presacral nerves. To enter the space, elevate the overlying peritoneum anteriorly and incise the peritoneum and underlying loose areolar tissue using electrocautery. The goal of this dissection is exposure of the anterior sacral ligament without injury to the hypogastric nerves or avulsion to the middle sacral vessels. This is best accomplished by a combination of blunt and sharp dissection with the electrosurgical unit, with all use of the electrocautery directed away from the sacrum. The hypogastric nerves should be identified and avoided. Once the anterior longitudinal sacral ligament has been cleared of loose connective tissue, two 2-0 nonabsorbable sutures are placed through it at the level of the S1–S2 junction. It is helpful to use a needle with a 5/8-inch curve to place these sutures. We encircle the middle sacral vessels so that in the event of bleeding the sutures can be tied, easily controlling the bleeding. Early reports of the procedure described attachment of the suspensory bridge to the sacrum at the S3–S4 level. This site has been associated with an increased risk of hemorrhage, and the anterior ligament is thinner at this location (38). The area from the sacral promontory to the upper third of the sacrum appears to be a preferable site for attachment.

Each suture is passed through both the anterior and the posterior pieces of mesh and then tied down, ensuring that neither strap is under undue tension. The anterior strap is left somewhat longer than the posterior strap, to avoid overelevation of the anterior vaginal wall, which can increase the angle at the posterior urethrovesical junction and lead to incontinence. Following the culdoplasty and attachment of the grafts to the sacral promontory, the peritoneum is closed over the mesh, until all mesh is covered.

Results

There is a considerable difference of opinion among surgeons regarding the relative merit of vaginal and abdominal approaches to surgery for POP. Benson et al. reported the only prospective randomized study comparing vaginal and abdominal approaches for POP (39). This study compared outcomes for all vaginal segments and noted a significantly higher rate of reoperation for recurrent prolapse with surgery from a vaginal approach compared to surgery from an abdominal approach, 33% versus 16%. While this is an appropriate study design for comparing two seemingly equivalent interventions, we believe that these operations are appropriate for different subsets of patients and we would anticipate a higher failure rate with indiscriminate use of a restorative approach. While the authors hypothesized that some of this difference was due to neuropathy caused by the vaginal dissection, some of the difference might also be explained by the use of the sacrospinous ligament suspension and needle urethropexies in the vaginal group. The majority of vaginal failures involved the anterior segment, and sacrospinous fixation has been shown to predispose patients to recurrent anterior wall prolapse, particularly when combined with needle bladder neck suspensions. Other complications described following sacrospinous fixation include vaginal shortening, sexual dysfunction, pain, and hemorrhage (17,18,38). The latter complications are related to the close proximity of pudendal nerves and vessels laterally and gluteal vessels and sacral nerve roots superiorly.

Abdominal sacral colpopexy has a consistent cure rate of over 90% (40,41). It is not without complications, including the risk of rare, but potentially life-threatening, intraoperative hemorrhage (38) and a 3% to 7% incidence of vaginal mesh erosion (41). Erosions can usually be managed with vaginal excision of all visible mesh followed by partial colpocleisis (42). A small subset of patients requires multiple extirpative surgeries for complete removal of eroded mesh.

Repairs for Anterior Prolapse

The vaginal approach to cystocele repair has similar efficacy, with an easier recovery for patients. Consequently, the indication for a cystocele repair via laparotomy is generally the patient's and the surgeon's plan to perform a concurrent sacrocolpopexy. Many surgeons believe that limiting all repairs to a single approach reduces surgical time and potential contamination.

Techniques

The laparotomy approach to the paravaginal repair begins with dissection of the retropubic space to expose several important landmarks, including the arcus tendineus fascia pelvis, running between the posterior aspect of the pubis and the ischial spine, and the more superior and lateral obturator neurovascular bundle. Once landmarks are identified, the endopelvic fascia and lateral vaginal sulcus are sutured to the arcus, with interrupted sutures using delayed absorbable or nonabsorbable sutures.

Opening the vesicouterine peritoneal reflection and mobilizing the bladder after clamping and ligating the bladder pillars, access to the central defect from the abdominal approach can be achieved. Abdominal repair has been reported to be as efficacious as vaginal repair, although there may be an increased risk of bleeding with this approach. Also, although repair of central defects is possible from this approach, we generally avoid it because of the neurologic injury that can occur with ligation of the bladder pillars, as can be seen following radical hysterectomy.

Results

While there are considerable data regarding the efficacy of the abdominal paravaginal defect repair for urodynamic stress incontinence, its efficacy for anterior POP is not as well documented. Richardson et al. reported a cure rate of 95% (43). Shull and Baden also reported a 5% recurrence rate for cystocele but noted a 6% incidence of vault prolapse and a 5% incidence of enterocele (44).

Repairs for Posterior Prolapse

Techniques

The abdominal sacral colpoperineopexy is an abdominal approach to the correction of posterior segment prolapse associated with severe perineal descent and vault prolapse (45). The procedure is similar to the sacral colpopexy, except that the posterior strap is taken all the way down to the perineal body, where it is attached with several interrupted permanent or delayed absorbable sutures. An assistant can perform a rectovaginal examination, elevating the perineal body for easier suture placement. In patients with severe perineal descent due to separation of the rectovaginal fascia from the perineal body, an initial vaginal dissection in conjunction with the dissection via laparotomy ensures correction of the anatomical defect and attachment of the graft to the perineal body. However, the graft should be passed down from above and then sutured in place. A biological graft may be superior to a synthetic graft for vaginal mesh placement, as the synthetic graft has been associated with a high erosion rate, while the biological graft erosions heal spontaneously with minimal drop in the cure rate (46).

Results

Our early experience with abdominal sacral colpoperineopexy demonstrates correction of severe recurrent prolapse to stage 0 in 12 of 19 patients (63%), to stage I in 4 (21%), and to stage II in the remaining 3 (16%) (45). Only one patient (5%) had a recurrent rectocele, and two-thirds of patients had resolution of chronic bowel symptoms. In a retrospective review of 122 patients treated with the sacrocolpoperineopexy, Su and coauthors reported one-year outcomes with good anatomical correction, and 78% of patients stated that they would repeat the procedure (47). Mesh erosion was 7%.

LAPAROSCOPIC PROCEDURES

The progress made in laparoscopic surgery now enables increasingly complex procedures to be carried out laparoscopically. These techniques, adapted from the classical laparotomy techniques, enable all three aspects of POP to be treated less invasively.

Laparoscopic Repairs for Apical Prolapse

The sacrocolpopexy performed by laparotomy is considered by some to be the "gold standard" for the surgical treatment of POP. The laparoscopic approach to the sacrocolpopexy technique was developed based on the procedure performed by laparotomy (48–50). While the anatomical and functional results obtained with this procedure are excellent, it requires advanced laparoscopic skills and has a rate of complications similar to sacrocolpopexy by laparotomy. This has inspired innovative modifications.

Dubuisson et al. described the technique of laparoscopic lateral suspension with mesh in 1998 (51), based on an open abdominal procedure described by Kapandji (52). Originally described with two pieces of mesh, the technique was subsequently modified to use a single mesh placed as a transversal hammock and sutured at its mid portion, inferiorly to the pubocervical fascia and pericervical ring. The lateral ends of the mesh are then attached superiorly to the aponeurosis of the external oblique, ipsilaterally. This is combined with a laparoscopic posterior colporrhaphy to reattach the uterosacral ligaments to the apex of the vaginal vault. This technique is simpler and is believed to minimize the risk of vaginal erosion of the mesh. Further, it enables complete treatment of genital prolapse by laparoscopic access without use of the promontory and need for extensive peritonealization.

For women with good endopelvic fascia and intact pelvic floor muscles, a laparoscopic restorative approach is the laparoscopic uterosacral suspension. Because it is performed without mesh, it eliminates the risk of mesh erosion. This technique is easy to perform and, if combined with laparoscopic anterior and posterior colporrhaphies, will address all support defects.

Techniques

The *laparoscopic uterosacral suspension* begins with dissection of the endopelvic fascia at the vaginal apex. The second assistant stands between the patient's legs and holds a foam swab placed on a long forceps or a long retractor to expose the posterior fornix; this facilitates dissection of the tissues in the lower pelvis. The posterior vaginal wall and the rectovaginal septum are dissected away from the rectum. The extent of the dissection is dependent on the size of the rectocele, as it should continue beyond the lower part of the defect. The upper part of the levator ani muscles is freed bilaterally. During the dissection, the thickness of the sacral segments of the uterosacral ligaments is evaluated; the ureters, above the ligaments, are identified but not dissected. The anterior vaginal wall and the pubocervical fascia are then freed from the bladder, and the dissection is carried down to the lower end of the anterior prolapse. The lateral extent of the dissection is dependent on the size of the anterior prolapse.

For patients with level 2 defects, the laparoscopic anterior and posterior colporrhaphies should be completed as described below, prior to suspending the vaginal vault to the uterosacral ligaments.

The correction of the descent of the uterus or the vaginal vault includes the reattachment of the uterosacral ligaments to the torus uterinum. On each side, the sacral segment of the uterosacral ligaments is sutured to the superior part of the rectovaginal fascia and the torus uterinum with permanent suture, using an extracorporeal technique. The reattachment of the uterosacral ligaments usually corrects the uterine prolapse and reduces the size of the cul-de-sac. The outcome of this part of the procedure is assessed by vaginal and rectal examinations.

The *laparoscopic lateral suspension* (60) begins with the dissection of the endopelvic fascia, as described for the laparoscopic uterosacral suspension (Figs. 1–4). Hysterectomy is then performed when it is required. If the cervix is normal, we prefer to perform a subtotal hysterectomy as opposed to a total hysterectomy. If level 2 defects are present, they should be addressed next by laparoscopic anterior and posterior colporrhaphy, as described below. The lateral suspension of the vaginal vault and the uterus using one mesh, placed as a transverse hammock. A long strip of synthetic mesh of 30-cm length is prepared (Fig. 5). The middle part of this strip may be between 3 and 12 cm wide, depending on the conservation of the uterus, the severity of the anterior prolapse, and the rectocele. The extremities are 3-cm wide. The prepared mesh is introduced in the peritoneal cavity through the midline suprapubic trocar.

After a subtotal (or total) hysterectomy, the posterior flap of the middle part of this strip is fixed bilaterally to the levator ani muscles, using separate interrupted permanent sutures. Then, the posterior flap is applied to the posterior surface of the vagina and the rectovaginal septum using separate interrupted permanent sutures, without transfixing the vagina. In cases with conservation of the uterus, the rectovaginal fascia is reinforced with a rectangular patch of synthetic mesh. The size is adapted to the severity of the rectocele (6–8 cm long and 4–6 cm wide). This patch is first fixed bilaterally to the levator ani muscles using separate interrupted sutures of permanent suture. Then, this patch is applied to the posterior surface of the vagina and the rectovaginal septum using separate interrupted sutures of permanent suture, without transfixing the vagina. In all the cases, the middle part of the mesh and its anterior flap are sutured precisely to the uterine isthmus and the pubocervical fascia with two to five separate permanent sutures, or to the vaginal vault in a patient who had a prior total hysterectomy.

The transverse hammock is placed laterally through fixation of the mesh to the lateral abdominal wall above the iliac crests. This requires the creation of the two lateral retroperitoneal tunnels, one on each side. A small cutaneous incision

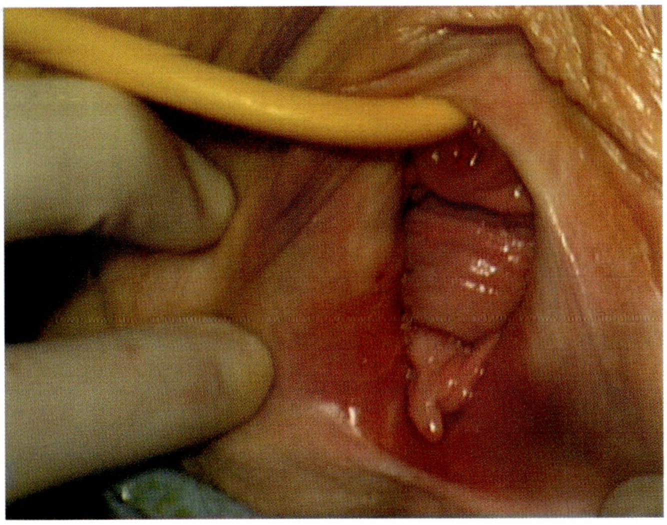

Figure 1 Predominant lateral cystocele.

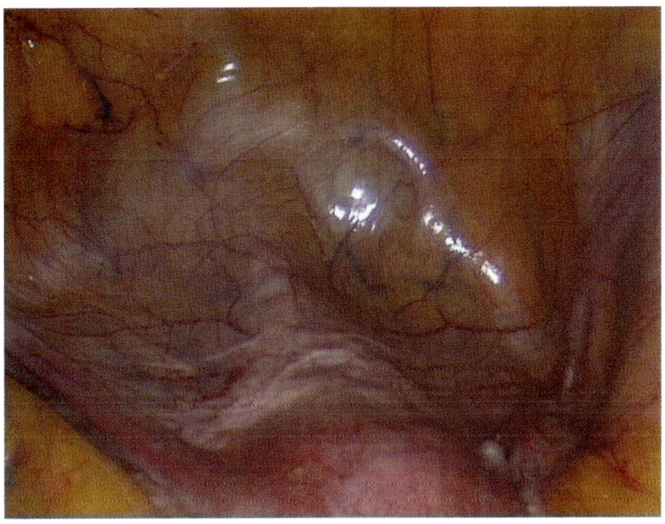

Figure 2 Aspect of the anterior vesico-uterine fornix with the visualization of the lateral descent of the bladder.

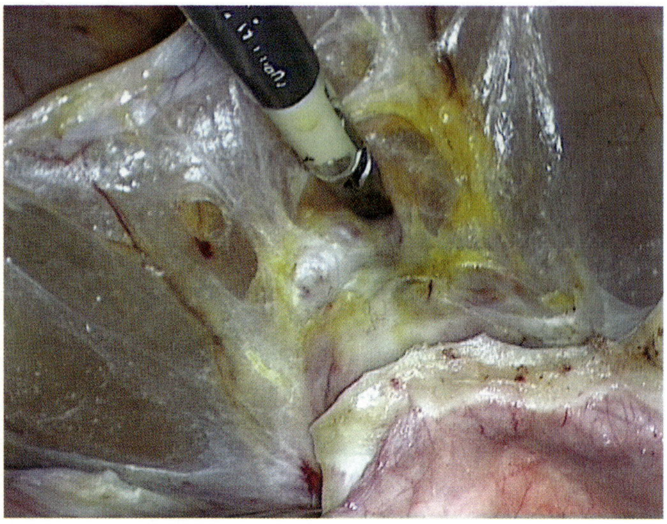

Figure 3 Dissection of the endopelvic fascia.

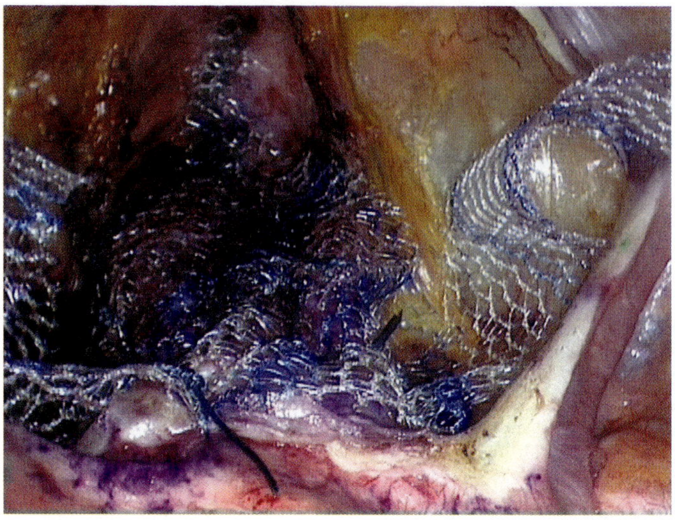

Figure 5 The anterior mesh is placed to treat the cystocele and the uterine descent.

(3 mm) is made 2 cm above and 4 cm lateral to the anterior superior iliac spine (Fig. 6). Through the incision, a laparoscopic atraumatic forceps is introduced, perforating the aponeurosis of the external oblique muscle, and is advanced downward subperitoneally passing under the ipsilateral round ligament and exiting through the supravesical peritoneal incision. This tunneling procedure is performed easily under visual control. On each side, the distal end of the mesh is grasped by the laparoscopic atraumatic forceps and pulled through the cutaneous incision above the iliac crest (Fig. 7). The tension of the hammock is adjusted so that the vaginal vault is suspended at the desired level (Fig. 8). Temporary deflation of the pneumoperitoneum permits proper performance of this important step of the procedure. As in the TVT procedure, the protruding ends of the meshes are maintained in this position until the end of the laparoscopy at the desired level, without suturing. At the end of the operation, the protruding ends are cut 2 mm under the cutaneous incision. Rarely the "tension-free" suspension is not maintained at the desired tension. In these circumstances, the distal mesh ends are sutured to aponeurosis of the external oblique muscles, using a separate interrupted absorbable suture.

The reattachment of the uterosacral ligaments to the torus uterinum is then performed. On each side, the sacral segment of the uterosacral ligaments is sutured to the rectovaginal fascia, under the rectocele, and with the torus uterinum with permanent suture. All the fascia sutures are kept extramucosal to avoid infection and/or erosion. The outcome of this part of the procedure is assessed by vaginal and rectal examinations.

The last step is the reperitonealization of the vesicouterine fornix and the cul-de-sac (or of the vesicorectal space, if

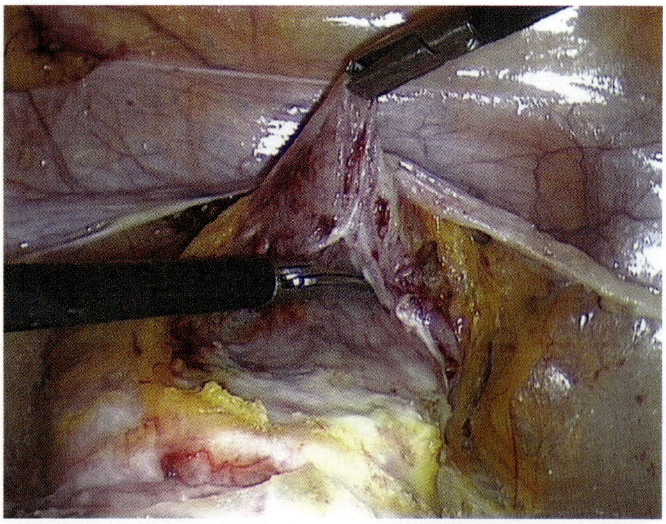

Figure 4 End of the vesico-vaginal cleavage.

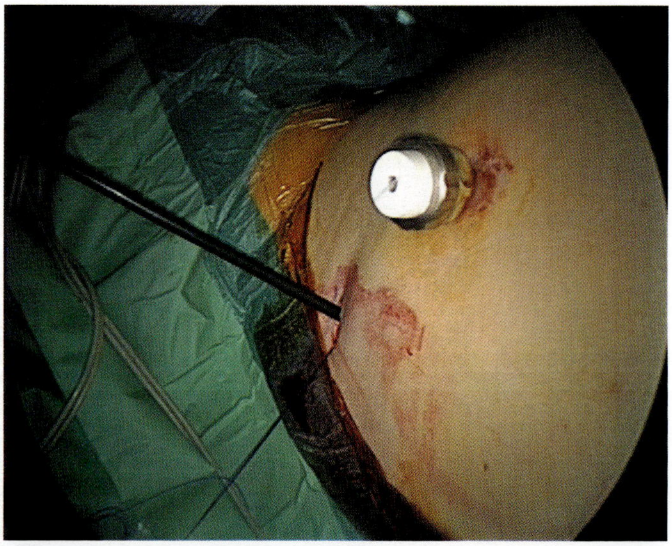

Figure 6 A small cutaneous incision is made 2 cm above and 4 cm lateral to the anterior superior iliac spine.

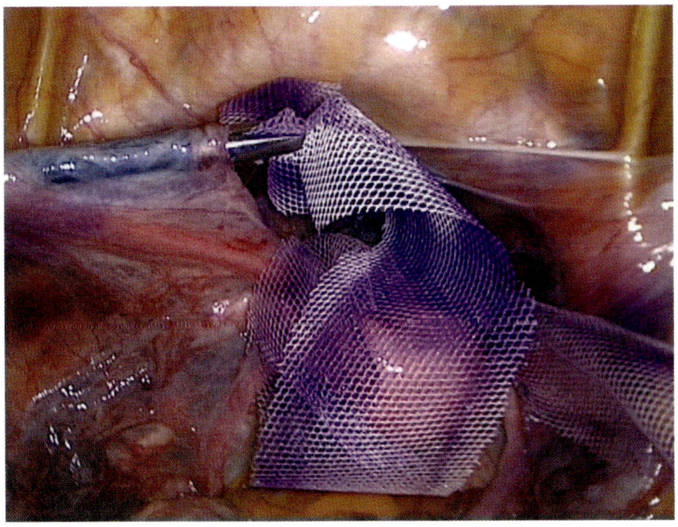

Figure 7 Tunneling procedure under visual control.

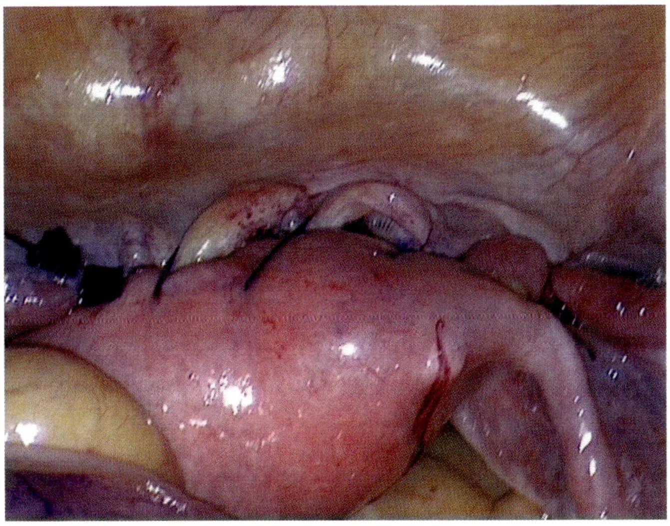

Figure 9 Reperitonealization of the vesico uterine fornix.

the uterus is absent) (Figs. 9 and 10). Reperitonealization is performed using a running absorbable suture. This step is designed to have the mesh completely buried in the retroperitoneal space.

Paraiso and colleagues have described an approach for *laparoscopic sacral colpopexy* (32). A minimum of four ports are placed as follows: a 10/12-mm intraumbilical port; two additional 10/12 ports, one in each lower quadrant; and a 5-mm port in the left mid-abdomen, lateral to the rectus muscles at the level of the umbilicus. An additional 5-mm port may be placed in the right mid-abdomen as needed for retraction. The procedure begins with a similar dissection of the endopelvic fascia as described for the laparoscopic uterosacral suspension. The second step is dissection of the presacral space and preparation of the promontory. The incision of the peritoneum is performed at the level of the sacral promontory, on the right of the sigmoid colon extending longitudinally to the cul-de-sac. The right ureter should be identified to avoid injury prior to beginning the dissection. The presacral vessels should also be identified and can be coagulated to avoid hemorrhage during placement of the sutures for sacrofixation.

The repair continues with attachment of the mesh to the vaginal vault. A strip of synthetic mesh less than 8 cm long (according to the severity of the vaginal vault descent) and 4 to 5 cm wide is prepared. One of the two extremities of the mesh is cut longitudinally to produce two arms. The prepared mesh is introduced in the peritoneal cavity through the midline suprapubic trocar. One of the arms of the mesh is then sutured to the pubocervical fascia corresponding to the anterior prolapse, using separate interrupted permanent sutures. The second arm is sutured to the posterior uterus isthmus or the vaginal vault, the rectovaginal fascia and to the levator ani muscles. The other extremity of the mesh is then

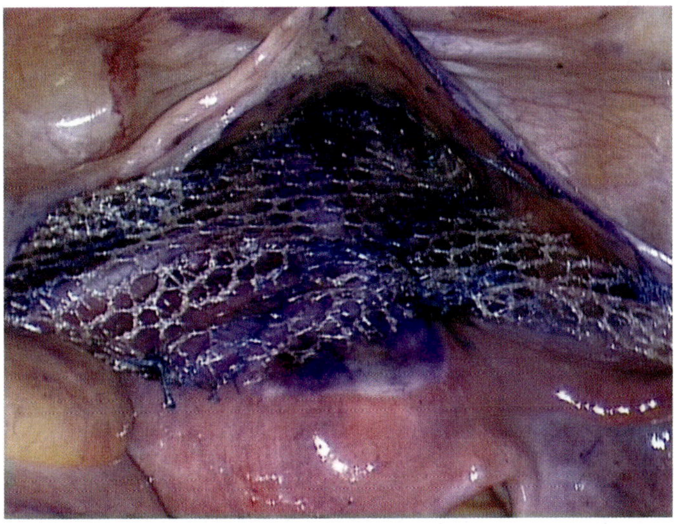

Figure 8 The tension of the hammock is adjusted so that the vaginal vault is suspended at the desired level.

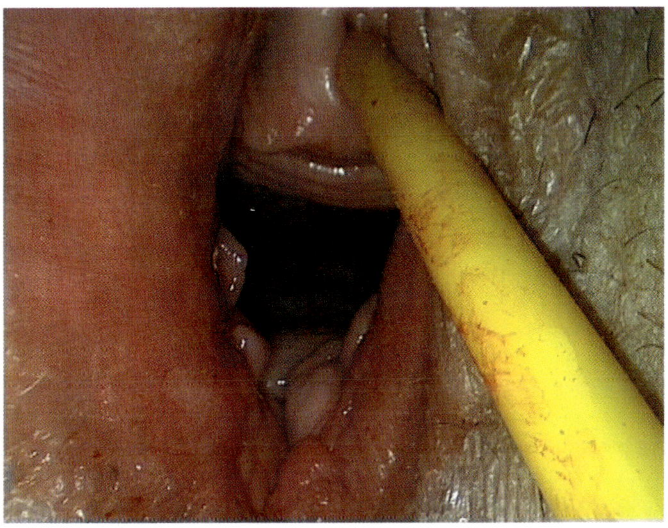

Figure 10 Final aspect with correction of the prolapse.

fixed to the promontory using separate interrupted permanent sutures. The tension of the mesh is adjusted so that the vaginal vault is suspended at the desired level.

The next step is the reperitonealization of the vesicouterine fornix, the cul-de-sac (or of the vesicorectal space, if the uterus is absent), and the promontory. Reperitonealization is performed using running absorbable sutures. This step is designed to have the mesh completely buried in the retroperitoneal space.

Results

Abdominal sacrocolpopexy is considered the reference technique to treat POP. Laparoscopic sacrocolpopexy offers a less invasive alternative that is especially appropriate for sexually active and younger women, as it provides excellent results and may reduce the risk of dyspareunia, due to the absence of vaginal scars (53). Major complications are observed in 2.5% of the cases. In a long-term review of laparoscopic sacrocolpopexy using a mesh of 140 consecutive cases, Higgs et al. noted two cases of bladder perforation, two cases of bowel perforation, and one case of conversion to laparotomy (54). While cure rates for apical prolapse are more than 90%, recurrence at other sites has been reported at 38%, with a reoperation rate of 16% at five years (54).

The laparoscopic lateral attachment procedure, combined with anterior colporrhaphy and reattachment of the uterosacral ligaments to the torus uterinum, re-establishes the pelvic anatomy while correcting the pelvic support defects. This technique that reinforces lateral structures also conforms to the principles of pelvic support as described by DeLancey (55). Level 1 support defects are corrected with this technique by suspension of the vagina and the cervical ring with mesh, and by reattachment of the uterosacral ligaments to the rectovaginal fascia and the torus uterinum. Level 2 defects are also corrected when combined with anterior and posterior colporrhaphy.

In laparoscopic treatment of POP, the use of lateral suspension versus sacral colpopexy is open to debate. With lateral suspension the risk of complications is low at 2%, with no vascular complications reported (51). With sacrocolpopexy, serious complications have been published. Nezhat and coauthors treated 15 patients with laparoscopic sacrocolpopexy (49). One of them had a serious complication that required conversion to laparotomy. In another, a vascular injury occurred during dissection of the sacral promontory. The risk of injury to the vessels located close to the promontory is not specific to the laparoscopic approach. In fact, this complication has been reported with a frequency of 1.6% to 4% during sacrocolpopexy via laparotomy (38). Although no severe infectious complication has been reported to date during laparoscopic sacrocolpopexy, there is a theoretical risk of sacral osteitis. Several investigators have reported such a complication after sacrocolpopexy by laparotomy (56). The laparoscopic lateral suspension may be a preferable alternative for the treatment of POP because it markedly reduces the risk of these two complications. The satisfactory outcomes associated with this approach have been corroborated in several publications (57–59).

Mesh erosion is a complication that is not infrequently observed after laparoscopic sacral colpopexy. Higgs and coauthors observed a mesh erosion rate of 6% with polypropylene (54). We did have such complications with our earlier technique of lateral suspension using meshes (60), but with our current approach we had rare complications related to the mesh.

The technique of lateral suspension has been criticized irrespective of the mode of access whether by laparotomy or by laparoscopy, because it results in an anterior suspension of the uterus, which increases the patient's subsequent risk of developing a rectocele and/or enterocele (57). This was observed with the original "vaginal-isthmic colpopexy" (52). However, this is certainly not the case with the technique we employ, which is a lateral and not an anterior suspension. It is also completely different from the classical round ligament anterior fixation. Furthermore, our technique includes treatment of the posterior compartment by the placement of the posterior flap of the transversal mesh and the reattachment of the uterosacral ligaments with occlusion of the pouch of Douglas. Finally, when necessary, to improve the support of the inferior part of the posterior vaginal wall and reduce the vulvovaginal enlargement, we associate a perineorrhaphy to the procedure that is carried out by the vaginal route.

Although laparoscopic sacrocolpopexy and lateral suspension permit the association of a hysterectomy (total or subtotal), these procedures are particularly indicated for women presenting predominantly with a uterine prolapse and cystocele and who wish to have a conservative surgical treatment. The contraindications of laparoscopic access are severe pelvic and abdominal adhesions, usually secondary to iterative laparotomies for bowel surgery and pelvic peritonitis. Other absolute and/or relative contraindications include obesity, cardiac disease, and respiratory insufficiency. In such cases, procedures that use vaginal access, and when necessary, regional anesthesia would be preferable.

The choice of a laparoscopic technique without using meshes is also a matter of debate. In meshless technique, the main procedure is the reattachment of the uterosacral ligaments. These ligaments are not always a good structure for repairing prolapse. Histological evaluation of the uterosacral ligament has recently been performed by Cole (61). Specimens of uterosacral complexes were dissected in 14 hemipelves from 7 adult female cadavers (6/7 had a hysterectomy). In only three specimens, aligned collagen and interspersed elastin were identified. In conclusion of the study, doubts about the integrity of the uterosacral ligaments as structural supports in pelvic reconstructive surgery were confirmed, particularly in elderly women who have had a hysterectomy. The meshless technique is indicated in patients with quite strong tissues. The low quality of the structural supports in many postmenopausal patients with prolapse justifies the use of meshes. The parameters with high risk of recurrence such as obesity and recurrent prolapse justify the use of mesh.

Laparoscopic Repairs for Anterior Prolapse

Technique

The *laparoscopic paravaginal repair* is similar to the technique via laparotomy. Four laparoscopic ports are placed, as described previously, for laparoscopic apical support procedures, and the bladder is filled in a retrograde fashion to help delineate its boundaries. The peritoneum is grasped in the midline, anterior and superior to the bladder dome, and sharply incised with endoshears. This incision is extended bilaterally until the lateral boundaries of the obliterated median arteries are reached. A combination of blunt and sharp dissection is then used to expose Cooper's ligament. Once the ligament is identified, the dissection of the space of Retzius is continued bluntly posteriorly and inferiorly to the ischial spine, which can be palpated with a blunt probe. Interrupted permanent sutures on a 5/8 needle are then placed, starting with the inferior-most stitch, near the spine, through the arcus and then through the lateral vaginal sulcus until the defect is obliterated.

Laparoscopic anterior colporrhaphy begins with dissection of the vesicovaginal space. The vesicouterine reflection of peritoneum is opened transversely. This is facilitated by elevation of the vault with a sponge on a long forceps or a long retractor. The pubocervical fascia is then freed from the bladder, with the dissection carried out distally to the lower end of the anterior prolapse. The lateral extent of the dissection is dependent on the size of the anterior prolapse.

The plication of the pubocervical fascia is accomplished with two or three separate interrupted permanent sutures. At the end of this step, the repair is assessed by vaginal examination. All the sutures are extramucosal, without transfixing the vagina.

Laparoscopic Repairs for Posterior Prolapse

Technique

Laparoscopic posterior colporrhaphy begins with dissection of the rectovaginal septum. This is facilitated by elevation of the vault with a sponge on a long forceps or a long retractor. The superior cul-de-sac is opened transversely, and the rectum is bluntly separated from the posterior vagina. This dissection is carried out laterally to the levator ani muscles and inferiorly below the defect in the rectovaginal fascia. The reattachment of the rectovaginal fascia to the superior surface of the levator ani muscles occurs bilaterally. This is achieved with one or two separate interrupted permanent sutures on each side. With large rectoceles, additional sutures are used to plicate the rectovaginal septum. All the fascial sutures are kept extramucosal to avoid infection and/or erosion. The sacrocolpoperineopexy is also described from a laparoscopic approach (62).

CONCURRENT PROCEDURES

Concurrent Incontinence Procedure

Approximately half of women with symptomatic POP also have stress incontinence symptoms. In these circumstances, it is reasonable to combine the prolapse repairs with an effective surgical treatment for stress incontinence. This may be a mid-urethral sling, either retropubic or transobturator, or a retropubic urethropexy, either via laparotomy of laparoscopy.

Gynecological surgeons have recognized for many years that some women with symptomatic POP do not have symptoms of stress incontinence but develop the condition after repair of the prolapse. This has led many to advocate urodynamic studies with reduction of the prolapse. This approach was evaluated by the CARE trial, a randomized clinical trial of sacrocolpopexy with and without Burch retropubic urethropexy in 322 women. At the three-month follow-up, there was a significant difference in the primary outcome, of symptoms, signs, or treatment of stress incontinence, with 22% stress incontinence in the Burch group versus 41% in the non-Burch group (63). Despite the difference in the stress incontinence end point, there was no difference in urge incontinence or voiding dysfunction. These differences were maintained at the two-year follow-up. Whether these results can be translated to vaginal and laparoscopic approaches to prolapse repair, and whether a mid-urethral sling is equally effective is yet to be determined.

Concurrent Hysterectomy

Hysterectomy is not required to surgically manage uterine prolapse, and we do not routinely remove the uterus. In the presence of benign uterine pathology associated with the uterine prolapse, a hysterectomy may be indicated. This is discussed preoperatively with the patient. In such a case, if the cervix is normal, we frequently perform a subtotal hysterectomy as opposed to a total hysterectomy. Unless a laparotomy is planned, a vaginal or laparoscopic approach is favored. Available evidence suggests that total hysterectomy increases the risk of infection and secondary erosion of the mesh at the level of the vaginal vault. Recently, Bensinger and coauthors published a retrospective study of 121 patients, comparing three groups treated with abdominal sacral colpopexy using mesh (64). In groups 1 and 2, the procedure was combined respectively with a supracervical hysterectomy and a total abdominal hysterectomy. In group 3, the women had previously undergone total abdominal hysterectomy. All the erosions occurred in group 2 (8.2%; 95% CI: 2.3–19.6; $P = 0.0389$). Patients treated with abdominal sacrofixation at the time of total abdominal hysterectomy had a seven-fold increased risk for mesh erosion compared with patients who underwent sacrofixation with supracervical hysterectomy.

CONCLUSIONS

Today, the surgeon addressing POP has many options to choose from in order to maximize the repair of anatomy, and relief of symptoms, while minimizing complications. The choice of surgical approach and technique, and whether to reinforce the repair with a graft will impact the surgical outcomes and can be tailored to the specific needs of the patient.

REFERENCES

1. Olsen AL, Smith VJ, Bergstrom JO, et al. Epidemiology of surgically managed pelvic organ prolapse and urinary incontinence. Obstet Gynecol 1997; 89:501–506.
2. Ellerkmann RM, Cundiff GW, Melick CF, et al. Correlation of symptoms with location and severity of pelvic organ prolapse. Am J Obstet Gynecol 2001; 185:1332–1338.
3. Welgoss JA, Vogt VY, McClellan EJ, et al. Relationship between surgically induced neuropathy and outcome of pelvic organ prolapse surgery. Int Urogynecol J Pelvic Floor Dysfunct 1999; 10(1):11–14.
4. FitzGerald MP, Richter HE, Siddique S, et al. Ann Weber for the Pelvic Floor Disorders Network. Colpocleisis: A review. Int Urogynecol J Pelvic Floor Dysfunct 2006; 17(3):261–271. Epub June 28, 2005.
5. Goldman J, Ovadia J, Feldverg D. The Neugebauer-Le Fort operation: A review of 118 partial colpocleises. Eur J Obstet Gynecol Reprod Biol 1981; 12(1):31–35.
6. Langmade CF, Oliver JA. Partial colpocleisis. Am J Obstet Gynecol 1986; 154(6):1200–1205.
7. Denehy TR, Choe JY, Gregori CA, et al. Modified Le Fort partial colpocleisis with Kelly urethral plication and posterior colpoperineoplasty in the medically compromised elderly: A comparison with vaginal hysterectomy, anterior colporrhaphy, and posterior colpoperineoplasty. Am J Obstet Gynecol 1995; 173(6):1697–1702.
8. Hullfish KL, Bovbjerg VE, Steers WD. Colpocleisis for pelvic organ prolapse: Patient goals, quality of life, and satisfaction. Obstet Gynecol 2007; 110(2 Pt 1):341–345.
9. Wheeler TL II, Richter HE, Burgio KL, et al. Regret, satisfaction, and symptom improvement: Analysis of the impact of partial

colpocleisis for the management of severe pelvic organ prolapse. Am J Obstet Gynecol 2005; 193(6):2067–2070.
10. DeLancy JO, Morley GW. Total colpocleisis for vaginal eversion. Am J Obstet Gynecol 1997; 176(6):1228–1232.
11. Ridley JH. Evaluation of the colpocleisis operation: A report of fifty-eight cases. Am J Obstet Gynecol 1972: 113:1114–1119.
12. FitzGerald MP, Richter HE, Bradley CS, et al; for the Pelvic Floor Disorders Network. Pelvic support, pelvic symptoms and patient satisfaction after colpocleisis. Int Urogynecol J Pelvic Floor Dysfunct 2008; 19(12):1603–1609.
13. McCall ML. Posterior culdoplasty: Surgical correction of enterocele during vaginal hysterectomy: A preliminary report. Obstet Gynecol 1957; 10:595–602.
14. Buller JL, Thompson JR, Cundiff GW, et al. Uterosacral ligament: Description of anatomic relationships to optimize surgical safety. Obstet Gynecol 2001; 97:873–879.
15. Barber MD, Visco AG, Weidner AC, et al. Bilateral uterosacral ligament vaginal vault suspension with site-specific endopelvic fascia defect repair for treatment of pelvic organ prolapse. Am J Obstet Gynecol 2000; 183:1402–1411.
16. Shull BL, Capen CV, Riggs MW, et al. Bilateral attachment of the vaginal cuff to iliococcygeus fascia: An effective method of cuff suspension. Am J Obstet Gynecol 1993; 168:1764–1771.
17. Nichols DH. Sacrospinous fixation for massive eversion of the vagina. Am J Obstet Gynecol 1982; 142:901–904.
18. Pohl JF, Frattarelli JL. Bilateral transvaginal sacrospinous colpopexy: Preliminary experience. Am J Obstet Gynecol 1997; 177(6):1356–1361.
19. Richter K, Albrich W. Long-term results following fixation of the vagina on the sacrospinal ligament by the vaginal route (vaginaefixatio sacrospinalis vaginalis). Am J Obstet Gynecol 1981; 141:811–816.
20. Given FT. Posterior culdoplasty: Revisited. Am J Obstet Gynecol 1985; 153:135–139.
21. Elkins TE, Hopper JB, Goodfellow K, et al. Initial report of anatomic and clinical comparison of the sacrospinous ligament fixation to the high McCall culdoplasty for vaginal fixation at hysterectomy for uterine prolapse. J Pelvic Surg 1995; 1: 12–17.
22. Shull BL, Bachofen C, Coates KW, et al. A transvaginal approach to repair of apical and other associated sites of pelvic organ prolapse with uterosacral ligaments. Am J Obstet Gynecol 2000; 183:1365–1374.
23. Silva WA, Pauls RN, Segal JL, et al. Uterosacral ligament vault suspension: Five-year outcomes. Obstet Gynecol 2006; 108(2):255–263.
24. Meeks GR, Washburne JF, McGehee RP, et al. Repair of vaginal vault prolapse by suspension of the vagina to iliococcygeus (prespinous) fascia. Am J Obstet Gynecol 1994; 171:1444–1454.
25. Young SB, Daman JJ, Bony LG. Vaginal paravaginal repair: One-year outcome. Am J Obstet Gynecol 2001; 185(6):1360–1366.
26. Julian TM. The efficacy of Marlex mesh in the repair of severe, recurrent vaginal prolapse of the anterior mid-vaginal wall. Am J Obstet Gynecol 1996; 75:1472–1475.
27. Sand PK, Kodure S, Lobel RW, et al. Prospective randomized trial of polyglactin 910 mesh to prevent recurrence of cystoceles and rectoceles. Am J Obstet Gynecol 2001; 184:1357–1364.
28. Kahn MA, Stanton SL. Posterior colporrhaphy: Its effects on bowel and sexual function. Br J Obstet Gynaecol 1997; 104(1):82–86.
29. Porter WE, Steele A, Walsh P, et al. The anatomic and functional outcomes of defect-specific rectocele repairs. Am J Obstet Gynecol 1999; 181:1353–1359.
30. Cundiff GW, Weidner AC, Visco AG, et al. An anatomic and functional assessment of the discrete defect rectocele repair. Am J Obstet Gynecol 1998; 179:1451–1457.
31. Kohli N, Miklos JR. Dermal graft-augmented rectocele repair. Int Urogynecol J Pelvic Floor Dysfunct 2003; 14(2):146–149.
32. Paraiso MF, Barber MD, Muir TW, et al. Rectocele repair: A randomized trial of three surgical techniques including graft augmentation. Am J Obstet Gynecol 2006; 195(6):1762–1771.
33. Debodinance P, Amblard J, Fatton B, et al. The prosthetic kits in the prolapse surgery: Is it a gadget? J Gynecol Obstet Biol Reprod (Paris) 2007; 36(3):267–275.
34. Fatton B, Amblard J, Debodinance P, et al. Transvaginal repair of genital prolapse: Preliminary results of a new tension-free vaginal mesh (Prolift technique)—a case series multicentric study. Int Urogynecol J Pelvic Floor Dysfunct 2007; 18(7):743–752.
35. Solà Dalenz V, Pardo Schanz J, Ricci Arriola P, et al. Prolift system in the correction of female genital prolapse. Actas Urol Esp 2007; 31(8):850–857.
36. Gauruder-Burmester A, Koutouzidou P, Rohne J, et al. Follow-up after polypropylene mesh repair of anterior and posterior compartments in patients with recurrent prolapse. Int Urogynecol J Pelvic Floor Dysfunct 2007; 18(9):1059–1064.
37. Addison WA, Timmons MC, Wall LL, et al. Failed abdominal sacral colpopexy: Observations and recommendations. Obstet Gynecol 1989; 74(3 Pt 2):480–483.
38. Sutton GP, Addison WA, Livengood CH, et al. Life-threatening hemorrhage complicating sacral colpopexy. Am J Obstet Gynecol 1981; 140:836–837.
39. Benson JT, Lucente V, McClellan E. Vaginal versus abdominal reconstructive surgery for the treatment of pelvic support defects: A prospective randomized study with long-term outcome evaluation. Am J Obstet Gynecol 1996; 175:1418–1422.
40. Addison WA, Bump RC, Cundiff GW, et al. Sacral colpopexy is the preferred treatment for vaginal vault prolapse in selected patients. J Gynecol Tech 1996; 2:69–74.
41. Nygaard IE, McCreery R, Brubaker L, et al; Pelvic Floor Disorders Network. Abdominal sacrocolpopexy: A comprehensive review. Obstet Gynecol 2004; 104(4):805–823.
42. Quiroz LH, Gutman RE, Fagan MJ, et al. Partial colpocleisis for the treatment of sacrocolpopexy mesh erosions. Int Urogynecol J Pelvic Floor Dysfunct. Epub ahead of print July 17, 2007.
43. Richardson AC, Lyon JB, Williams NL. A new look at pelvic relaxation. Am J Obstet Gynecol 1976; 568:568–573.
44. Shull BL, Baden WF. A six year experience with paravaginal defect repair for stress urinary incontinence. Am J Obstet Gynecol 1989; 160:1432–1440.
45. Cundiff GW, Harris RL, Coates KW, et al. Abdominal sacral colpoperineopexy: A new approach for correction of posterior compartment defects and perineal descent associated with vaginal vault prolapse. Am J Obstet Gynecol 1997; 177(6):345–355.
46. Visco AG, Weidner AC, Barber MD, et al. Vaginal mesh erosion after abdominal sacral colpopexy. Am J Obstet Gynecol 2001; 184(3):297–302.
47. Su KC, Mutone MF, Terry CL, et al. Abdominovaginal sacral colpoperineopexy: Patient perceptions, anatomical outcomes, and graft erosions. Int Urogynecol J Pelvic Floor Dysfunct 2007; 18(5):503–511.
48. Vancaillie TG. The role of laparoscopy in the management of pelvic floor relaxation. J Am Assoc Gynecol Laparosc 1997; 4(2):147–148.
49. Nezhat CH, Nezhat F, Nezhat C. Laparoscopic sacral colpopexy for vaginal vault prolapse. Obstet Gynecol 1994; 84(5):885–888.
50. Dorsey JH, Cundiff. GW Laparoscopic procedures for incontinence and prolapse [4]. Curr Opin Obstet Gynecol 1994; 6:223–230.
51. Dubuisson JB, Jacob S, Chapron C, et al. Laparoscopic treatment of genital prolapse: Lateral utero-vaginal suspension with 2 meshes. Results of a series of 47 patients. Gynecol Obstet Fertil 2002; 30(2):114–120.
52. Kapandji M. Treatment of urogenital prolapse by colpo-isthmo-cystopexy with transverse strip and crossed, multiple layer, ligamento-peritoneal douglasorrhaphy. Ann Chir 1967; 21(5):321–328.
53. Wattiez A, Boughizane S, Alexandre F, et al. Laparoscopic procedures for stress incontinence and prolapse. Curr Opin Obstet Gynecol 1995; 7(4):317–321.
54. Higgs P, Goh J, Krause H, et al. Abdominal sacral colpopexy: An independent prospective long-term follow-up study. Aust N Z J Obstet Gynaecol 2005; 45(5):430–434.

55. DeLancey JO. Anatomic aspects of vaginal eversion after hysterectomy. Am J Obstet Gynecol 1992; 166(6 Pt 1):1717–1724; discussion 1724–1728.
56. Weidner AC, Cundiff GW, Harris RL, et al. Sacral osteomyelitis: An unusual complication of abdominal sacral colpopexy. Obstet Gynecol 1997; 90:689–691.
57. Hoff J, Manelfe A, Portet R, et al. Promontofixation or suspension with a transverse strip? Comparative study of these 2 techniques in the treatment of genital prolapse [in French]. Ann Chir 1984; 38(5):363–367.
58. Rimailho J, Talbot C, Bernard JD, et al. Anterolateral hysteropexy via abdominal approach. Results and indications. Apropos of a series of 92 patients [in French]. Ann Chir 1993; 47(3): 241–249.
59. Cornier E, Madelenat P. The M. Kapandji hysteropexy: A laparoscopic technique and preliminary results [in French]. J Gynecol Obstet Biol Reprod (Paris) 1994; 23(4):378–385.
60. Dubuisson JB, Yaron M, Wenger JM, et al. Treatment of genital prolapse by laparoscopic lateral suspension using mesh: a series of 73 patients. Journal of Minimally Invasive Gynecology. 2008; 15:49–55.
61. Woodruff AJ, Cole EE, Dmochowski RR, et al. Histopathological evaluation of the uterosacral ligament: Is this a dependable structure for pelvic reconstruction? Urology 2008; 72(1):85–89.
62. Link RE, Su LM, Bhayani SB, et al. Laparoscopic sacral colpoperineopexy for treatment of perineal body descent and vaginal vault prolapse. Urology 2004; 64(1):145–147.
63. Brubaker L, Cundiff GW, Fine P, et al. Pelvic Floor Disorders Network. Abdominal sacrocolpopexy with Burch colposuspension to reduce urinary stress incontinence. N Engl J Med 2006; 354.1557–1566.
64. Bensinger G, Lind L, Lesser M, et al. Abdominal sacral suspensions: Analysis of complications using permanent mesh. Am J Obstet Gynecol 2005; 193(6):2094–2098.

16

Abdominal surgery during pregnancy

Michael Canis, Celine Houlle, Benjamin Cotte, Cécile Rivoire, Kris Jardon, Benoit Rabischong, Revaz Botchorishvili, Jean Luc Pouly, and Gérard Mage

INTRODUCTION

Since all types of gastrointestinal and gynecological surgical disorders may occur during pregnancy, 0.2% to 1% of all pregnant women will have nonobstetrical surgery (1). Although elective intra-abdominal surgery during pregnancy has been discouraged because of the perceived risks of premature birth or miscarriage, the principles of diagnosing and treating a pregnant woman are no different from those used when treating nonpregnant patients. As a general rule, the condition of the mother should be a priority; obviously, adequate management of the mother usually benefits both mother and fetus. Surgery and anesthesia are much less dangerous for mother and fetus than the potential complications from acute conditions such as appendicitis, biliary tract diseases, or adnexal torsion (1–3).

Obviously, when compared to a normal population, the risks of miscarriage and preterm delivery are increased in patients who have to undergo surgery while pregnant. However, these risks are more directly related to the underlying pathological process than to the surgical procedure. There is no evidence that the risk of congenital abnormalities is increased.

Various anatomic and physiologic changes that occur during pregnancy commonly alter the presentation and affect the management of surgical disorders. Adequate supervision of these patients requires sound clinical experience and knowledge of the physiological changes of pregnancy. Moreover, it is essential to understand that the presentation of a surgical disorder is very stressful and anxiety producing for the pregnant patient and her family.

RATIONALE FOR SURGERY

Acute Conditions

When deciding whether or not a pregnant patient should undergo surgical exploration, consultants and gynecologic surgeon alike must remember that the greatest morbidity and mortality for the mother and the fetus are induced by the evolution of the disease process rather than by the anesthesia and/or surgical procedure. For example, most of the maternal and fetal morbidities occurring after surgical treatment of an adnexal mass during pregnancy are generated by complications such as torsion or rupture of a cyst (4). Since the risk of fetal complications including premature delivery or spontaneous abortion are significantly increased by deterioration of the maternal condition, surgery should always proceed without haste once the decision has been made to explore.

Elective Conditions

Although most recent studies suggest that anesthesia and surgery (1,2), including laparoscopic surgery (5), are not dangerous for the pregnant patient or fetus, whenever possible elective surgical procedures should be delayed until after delivery. Since many women will spend the first months closely bonding with their newborn, the surgical procedure will typically be performed up to six months after the delivery.

Intermediate Conditions

The management of an adnexal mass during pregnancy is more challenging and of some controversy, because this is not necessarily an acute condition and delayed surgery may be an appropriate option, However, complications of adnexal masses are unpredictable and may require immediate surgical exploration. Given the risk that affected women may be lost to follow-up after delivery as well, surgical removal of an adnexal mass is warranted if still present at 15 weeks' gestational age. In our experience, as well as others, this plan of management has been demonstrated to be safe and effective (6–9). Moreover, some of these adnexal masses are early-stage malignant tumors for which a delayed diagnosis and treatment may significantly worsen the prognosis (10).

GENERAL ANESTHESIA, FETAL MONITORING, TOCOLYSIS, PNEUMOPERITONEUM, AND TRENDELENBURG

The administration of general anesthesia for surgical exploration of the gravida requires knowledge of the potential effects of all medications exposed to the fetus, as well as the multiple cardiovascular and pulmonary physiologic changes that naturally occur in women during pregnancy. Most analgesics and anesthetics are classified as pregnancy category C; uncertain safety, no human studies, and animal studies show adverse effect (2). Since most teratogenic medications have been shown to have the same effects in humans as in animals, these guidelines should be considered reliable whenever a judgment has to be made whether or not a drug may be used in these circumstances.

During pregnancy, cardiac output, heart rate, total blood volume, and the red blood cell volume are all increased (2). By increasing the intra-abdominal pressure, the enlarged gravid uterus may decrease blood return from the vena cava, potentially accentuating the hemodynamic effects of a pneumoperitoneum coupled with Trendelenburg position, resulting in significant hypotension (5,7).

Although functional residual capacity is decreased, minute ventilation, oxygen consumption, and CO_2 production are increased. All of these changes are accentuated by the increased intra-abdominal pressure from a pneumoperitoneum, which limits diaphragm excursion and thereby increases the alveolar arterial oxygen gradient and intrapleural pressure. All are further magnified by the increased intrathoracic pressure from Trendelenburg position.

Furthermore, the combination of pregnancy and a carbon dioxide pneumoperitoneum increases the risks of hypercapnia and hypoxemia. Both of these physiologic changes may potentially affect fetal well-being. It is unclear if these changes in blood gases require continuous monitoring of arterial blood gases in all pregnant women undergoing laparoscopic surgery. The Society of American Gastrointestinal Surgeons proposed such surveillance after the publication by Leiserowitz et al., who reported four fetal deaths in a series of seven pregnant patients, attributing these complications to prolonged acidosis despite not having recorded blood gas data during these procedures (11). Notwithstanding these original concerns, subsequent series of pregnant women undergoing surgery have demonstrated that noninvasive monitoring, similar to the standard monitoring recommended by the American Society of Anesthesiologists, is sufficient for the safety of the mother and the baby (5,12). The pregnant sheep model has been used to address some of these issues. However, a study in pregnant women demonstrated changes in the $Pa(CO_2)$–$Et(CO_2)$ gradient, which were remarkably different from the results observed in the pregnant sheep model (13). Given the accumulated knowledge to date, as well as the experience from large clinical series of laparoscopic surgery during pregnancy, arterial blood gas monitoring is probably not necessary in otherwise healthy pregnant patients in these circumstances (5,12).

Fetal Monitoring and Tocolysis

The need for continuous fetal monitoring by ultrasound scans has been abandoned because it is too difficult to carry out. For all pregnant women undergoing laparotomic or laparoscopic surgery, pre- and postoperative monitoring of the fetal heart rate and of uterine activity is recommended by all guidelines currently available (1,5). During the first trimester, fetal well-being should be assessed using pre- and postoperative ultrasound scans. The routine use of tocolytic agents for prophylaxis is not indicated but can be appropriate if there is any evidence of sustained uterine activity.

Fetal Effects of Pneumoperitoneum

Animal models used to date to investigate the potentially adverse effects of laparoscopic surgery during pregnancy have not adequately reflected the human pregnancy (13). Therefore, our knowledge about the potential effect of the carbon dioxide pneumoperitoneum is probably not very accurate. Indeed, the worrisome results obtained in the sheep model, including maternal hypercapnia and acidosis, have not been observed in humans (13,14). As yet studies in the human fetus are not possible, so the only approach to understand the effects of a CO_2 pneumoperitoneum would be to design a model in which the ventilation is adjusted to normalize maternal arterial CO_2 before evaluation of the fetal effects.

LAPAROSCOPIC SURGERY

Although the surgical procedures and techniques used to treat pregnant patients are no different from those used in nonpregnant patients, the key is to achieve satisfactory exposure to be able to operate effectively and safely.

Laparoscopy

For the last 30 years, operative laparoscopic procedures have been used increasingly in gynecology and general surgery. This change is also true for the management of pregnant patients. Indeed, during pregnancy the laparoscopic approach has major advantages, including smaller skin incisions, less bowel manipulation, earlier return of gastrointestinal activity, quicker recovery, earlier mobilization, and a decreased risk of thromboembolism and incisional hernia. Furthermore, the decreased postoperative pain and truncated postoperative ileus probably decrease the risk of premature labor as well (15).

Since an accurate preoperative diagnosis of the cause and severity of an acute intra-abdominal condition is more difficult in a pregnant patient (1,2), it is useful to be able to confirm the diagnosis using a laparoscopic evaluation of the peritoneal cavity. This allows the surgeon to avoid inadequate incisions for a laparotomy and to assess the severity of the disease, i.e., the presence of any associated peritonitis. To achieve a complete peritoneal evaluation, the laparoscope may be inserted in different trocars in order to assess peritoneal areas not initially visible, such as behind the gravid uterus.

Peritoneal Access During Laparoscopy

Creation of the Pneumoperitoneum and Insertion of the Primary Trocar

Due to the increased uterine volume and the associated anatomical changes induced by it, insertion of the primary trocar for the laparoscope and of the ancillary trocars is the main challenge for the laparoscopic surgeon during pregnancy.

In a patient without any past history of having undergone abdominal surgery, large retroperitoneal vessel trauma is the main risk related to insertion of the Veress needle and the primary trocar. During pregnancy, the distance between the abdominal wall and large retroperitoneal vessels is increased by the uterine volume. However, uterine vessels are large during pregnancy and the technique used for the initial steps of laparoscopy should prevent any risk of blind trauma to the uterus and/or its large vessels. The technique also depends on the patient's morphology, particularly the distance between the umbilicus and the pubic symphysis. The surgeon should avoid positioning the uterus between the first trocar entry site and the organ that must be treated. For instance, whenever operating on an adnexal cyst the laparoscope should be inserted above the uterine fundus, to allow the surgeon to see behind the uterus.

Laparoscopy During the First Trimester

A closed-entry technique can be safely employed during the first trimester and the beginning of the second trimester (up to 16 weeks) of pregnancy, by inserting the Veress needle in the left upper quadrant. In this area of the abdominal wall, three distinct tissue planes are felt while inserting the needle into the peritoneal cavity. It is essential to insert the needle perpendicular to the abdominal wall, because oblique insertion will increase the risk of uterine trauma. The safety tests after Veress needle insertion should be performed routinely, using a syringe to carry out a three-step safety test. First, the syringe is aspirated to confirm that the needle is not within a significant blood vessel or in the lumen of the bowel. Next, 20 ml of air is injected into the peritoneal cavity and then reaspirated. If the needle is inserted properly within the peritoneal cavity, the reaspiration is negative, as the air injected cannot be aspirated from a previously empty peritoneal cavity. Subsequently, it is essential to attain a satisfactory pneumoperitoneum up to 20 mm Hg before insertion of the primary trocar. The distance between the umbilicus and the gravid uterus depends on the adequacy of the pneumoperitoneum and on the location of the umbilicus. Although it has been suggested that it may be safer to inflate the abdomen to a higher pressure (25–30 mm Hg) before insertion of the first trocar, to provide better proprioceptive feedback and a larger volume, it is not recommended in a pregnant patient because of the physiological changes already induced by the pregnancy itself on the cardiovascular system. If the surgeon judges that insertion of the primary trocar using a closed technique will not be perfectly safe and will risk uterine trauma, he or she should change his or her approach by using an open technique under direct vision. In general, decreasing the force required to penetrate the peritoneal cavity best reduces the risks from the blind insertion of a primary trocar. Reusable trocars should be very sharp to help ensure the reduction of force, and soft tissue dystocia can be averted by ensuring that the skin incision exceeds the outer diameter of the primary cannula. Moreover, the table height should be at or below the surgeon's waist, to avoid any need for the surgeon's arm to be raised during this step. The movement used during insertion should simultaneously use rotation and pressure. For optimum control, both hands should be placed on the trocar: the active hand on the proximal port of the trocar, and the fingers of the passive hand placed between the active hand and the abdominal wall to act as a braking mechanism.

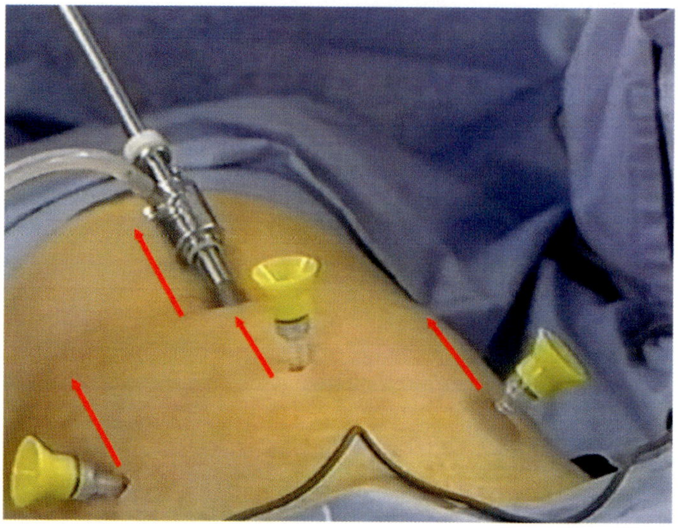

Figure 1 Trocar sites and insertion points during early to mid-pregnancy.

Laparoscopy During the Second and Third Trimesters

During the second half of the second trimester and the third trimester of pregnancy, peritoneal access is most safely accomplished by using an open technique. The site of the first trocar depends on the indication for laparoscopic surgery. Initially, the open technique was described in the umbilicus. Whereas the anatomical site of this approach was motivated by cosmetic reasons, it is possible to use this technique in any area of the abdominal wall, including the left upper quadrant and the epigastric area. To minimize scarring or whenever the best site for initial peritoneal inspection is unclear, a 5-mm laparoscope can be used. During the third trimester, the peritoneal incision should be performed with particular care. It is important to pull firmly enough on the abdominal wall to avoid uterine injury. Since case reports of large vessel trauma have been described during open laparoscopy in nonpregnant patients, there is logically similar risk to the enlarged gravid uterus during dissection of the abdominal wall layers using this technique.

Ancillary Trocars

Ancillary trocars should be inserted in an orderly fashion that assiduously follows a series of simple rules. Whenever possible, the trocar should be inserted perpendicularly into the abdominal wall to avoid unnecessary damage to the fascia, which is weaker in pregnant women and therefore at greater risk of developing a postoperative incisional hernia. Access to the targeted treatment site should not be obstructed or hindered by the gravid uterus, to avoid any risk of uterine laceration during the insertion of ancillary instruments. As a general rule, the minimal distance between ancillary trocar sites on the skin should be 8 cm or more, since the use of parallel instruments is ineffective. Since four hands are always available, three ancillary trocars should be used whenever possible. Ancillary trocars are more effective and ergonomic when the array of trocar entry sites forms a triangle. The surgeon should be able to work comfortably without raising the arms, keeping the upper extremities and shoulders in a natural position.

The trocar entry sites should be adapted to each clinical situation to maximize efficiency and safety. For instance, when treating an acute surgical abdomen during the first trimester of pregnancy, the technique for insertion and the trocar site array are similar to that used for most laparoscopic procedures in nonpregnant women (Fig. 1). On the other hand, it may be necessary to place all the trocars, including the primary cannula, to one side of the uterus when operating on an adnexal mass during the third trimester (Fig. 2) (16). The abdominal distension, which significantly begins during the second half of pregnancy, permits the insertion of all trocars on the same side of the uterus, with adequate distance in between to work effectively. When using this one-sided method, the table is typically tilted to the contralateral side, which shifts the uterus laterally and further frees the operating field.

Uterine Manipulation

For obvious fetal and maternal reasons, uterine manipulation must be performed without the traditional luxury of uterine cannulation. Most commonly, the enlarged gravid uterus

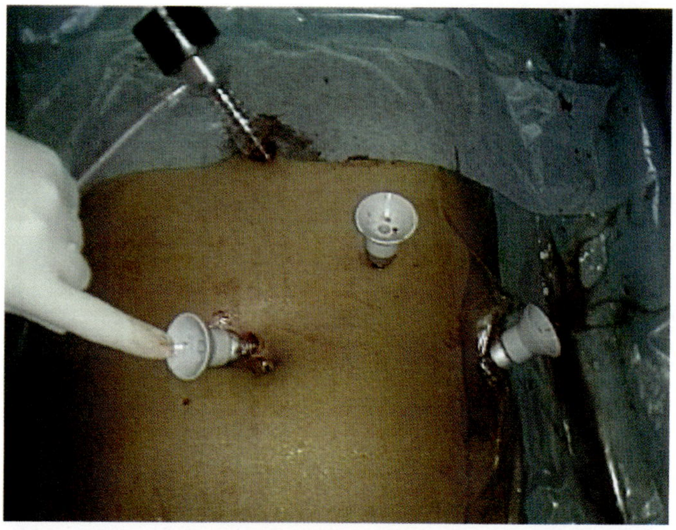

Figure 2 Trocar sites including lateral insertion points during third trimester pregnancy, to treat an adnexal mass.

may be mobilized manually using intraoperative transvaginal manipulation or by lateral inclination of the operating table. Either method can sufficiently mobilize the uterus laterally to allow the surgeon to inspect one of the adnexa. Tilting the table laterally to shift the intra-abdominal position of the uterus is more apt to be effective during the second and even third trimester of pregnancy. Although intraoperative manipulation with blunt instruments may be used for surgical mobilization, it must be performed with great caution to avoid trauma to the gravid uterus.

SURGICAL CONDITIONS

Appendicitis

A higher rate of negative appendectomy is reported and considered acceptable in pregnant patients because of the difficulty of preoperative diagnosis and the potential fetal and maternal complications from perforation (2). Traditionally, surgeons have been taught to move the abdominal incision more laterally and cephalad to the classical McBurney's point as the pregnancy progresses. On the contrary, a recent study demonstrated that the location of the appendix does not move significantly during pregnancy (17). The appendix was found to be more than 2 cm away from the McBurney's point in less than 25% of the cases. During the first two trimesters, a laparoscopic approach is very useful to confirm the diagnosis of appendicitis and to locate the appendix. When the uterus is too large, the conventional recommendation is to incise the abdomen over the location of maximum tenderness; however, a laparoscope may also be inserted in this area using an open technique. Once the primary and ancillary trocars are successfully inserted into their respective positions, the surgical techniques used to treat appendicitis are no different from those used in nonpregnant patients. A recent review showed that appendectomy is associated with a high risk of surgery-induced delivery (4.6%) when compared with other medical conditions (0.8%). This risk is increased when peritonitis is present (17).

Adnexal Mass

Asymptomatic adnexal masses are often detected during routine prenatal ultrasound investigations. Adnexal tumors diagnosed during pregnancy are not rare, but malignant ovarian ones are. A recent population-based study identified 9375 women with a hospital diagnosis of an ovarian mass among 4,846,505 obstetrical deliveries (0.19%) over a nine-year period (10). This result was based on the hospital discharge diagnosis, so that the incidence reported is lower than those reported in studies based on data from routine prenatal ultrasound screening. In this group, 87 patients had ovarian cancers and 115 low malignant potential (LMP) tumors. The incidence of invasive ovarian tumors was 0.93%, and the number of cancers per delivery was 0.0179. If patients with low malignant potential tumors were included, the incidence of malignant ovarian tumors would be 2.15%, similar to that reported in numerous series prior to 1999 (18). It is interesting to note that 65% of invasive ovarian tumors and 81% of the LMP tumors were stage IA or IB.

There is a wide debate about the best method for the management of adnexal masses during pregnancy. Most of these masses are functional cysts, which will resolve spontaneously before the end of the first trimester, so conservative nonsurgical management is the best approach during this period. After this period, there are no randomized controlled trials comparing expectant and surgical management of adnexal masses during pregnancy, but operative laparoscopy seems to be as safe as laparotomy in pregnancy (19,20).

Indication for Surgery

Whatever the term of the pregnancy, surgery is indicated in case of highly suspicious masses and/or in patients with an acute abdomen. MRI, which may safely be performed during pregnancy, is useful in the evaluation of suspicious masses. For instance, if fat tissue is found inside the mass, it is probably a benign teratoma and surgery may be delayed up to the second trimester of the pregnancy. In contrast, if a cancer is confirmed, surgery should be planned as soon as possible.

Low-Suspicious Potential Persistent Adnexal Mass During the Second Trimester

Indications for surgery should be decided according to clinical data, previous surgical history, and the ultrasonographic appearance of the adnexal mass.

The previous surgical history of the patient is important. Reliable surgical evaluation and an effective treatment of adnexal masses fixed to the posterior leaf of the broad ligament are almost impossible during the second trimester of pregnancy, since it is impossible to see the mass behind the uterus. In such a situation, the ovary and the cyst may be freed from the peritoneum using manual ovariolysis by laparotomy. However, even with this approach it is very difficult to perform a complete ovarian cystectomy, as it is often difficult to see whether or not ovariolysis is satisfactory or if part of the cyst remains on the broad ligament. Therefore, in this situation, which is commonly encountered in patients treated for endometriosis with assisted reproductive technologies, the best approach may be conservative management with close ultrasound monitoring until the end of the pregnancy and surgical treatment within two or three months of delivery. Patients with a persistent adnexal mass and no previous surgical history are best operated upon early during the second trimester of pregnancy. This approach seems safe in experienced hands (6–9).

Surgical Treatment of the Adnexal Mass

There are no trials comparing laparoscopic surgery and laparotomy for the treatment of ovarian tumors in pregnancy (20,21). However, as most masses are benign, a laparoscopic approach appears to be the method of choice to manage these young patients. The surgical treatment is similar to that used in nonpregnant patients (22).

As for any adnexal mass, the surgical puncture should not be blind and should be avoided during installation for the laparoscopy. Surgical diagnosis is the initial step. Samples of peritoneal fluid and peritoneal washings are collected for cytologic examination. Then the paracolic gutters, diaphragm, omentum, the entire peritoneal cavity, and ovaries are scrutinized for signs of malignancy. The ovaries may often be inspected before mobilization of the adnexal mass, because when the laparoscope is inserted above the uterine fundus, it is often possible to inspect the pelvic peritoneum without uterine cannulation and manipulation. The laparoscope is slowly moved behind the uterus, and there is often some space laterally between the adnexa and the pelvic sidewall, making it possible to inspect the peritoneum and part of the ovarian surface. The use of a 30-degree optic may facilitate inspection behind the uterus and along the lateral pelvic sidewall.

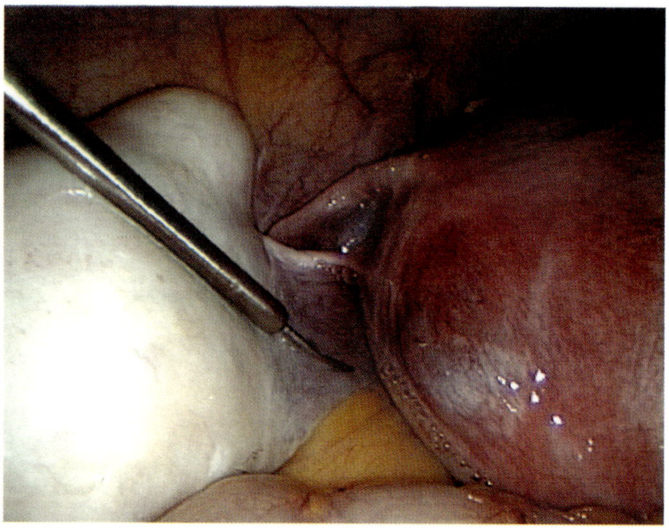

Figure 3 Adnexal mass above pregnant uterus.

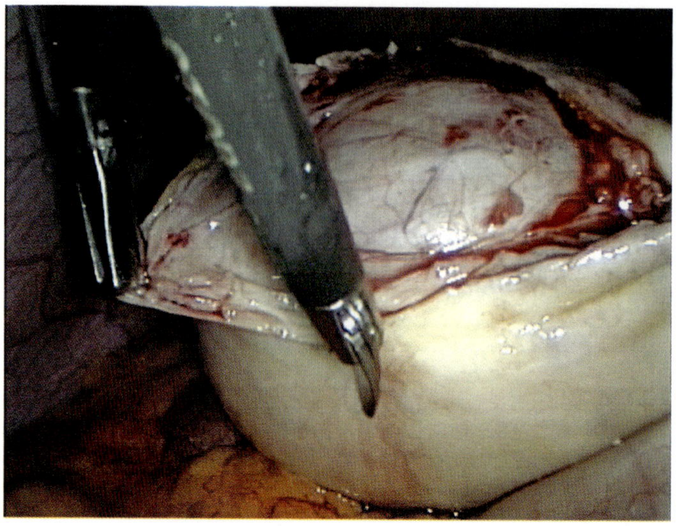

Figure 4 Incision of the ovarian cortex.

Mobilization of the Adnexal Mass

Two situations may be encountered: the adnexal mass is immediately visible because the adnexa is above the uterus (Fig. 3), or the adnexal mass is located in the posterior cul-de-sac and is hidden behind the uterus. In the first situation, it is important to grasp the adnexa before puncture of the cyst to avoid the mass "disappearing" after drainage into the posterior cul-de-sac. In the second situation, the mass should first be lifted into the abdomen using probes and graspers. The mass should be pulled slowly to avoid trauma of the ovarian ligaments. This may be facilitated by using a lateral tilt of the table toward the opposite side, which will shift the uterus to the opposite side and free some space, making it easier to mobilize the adnexa. Simultaneous vaginal examination may also be helpful to push the adnexal mass towards the abdomen. In most cases, it is possible to avoid blind vaginal rupture of the adnexal mass.

When the mass cannot be seen, a laparotomy is probably the best choice because access to the mass will not be easy. In our experience, it was possible to see and treat the mass using a laparoscopic approach, except in patients with severe pelvic adhesions.

Treatment of the Mass

When the mass is visible, the surgical management is similar to that used in nonpregnant patients. The key point is to always grasp the adnexa to avoid it falling back behind the uterus again before the end of the procedure. Indeed, mobilization of the adnexa is the most traumatic part of the procedure for both the adnexa and the uterus, and it is essential to do it only once. Techniques used for laparoscopic ovarian cystectomy by the authors have been described previously (22) and is summarized below under the heading "Other benigh adnexal cysts".

Ovarian Dermoid Cyst

The ovary is grasped on the antimesenteric surface with an atraumatic forceps. A small superficial incision of the ovarian cortex is made with scissors (Fig. 4). Then hydrodissection is used through this small incision, which is enlarged carefully. The plane is identified with atraumatic grasping forceps, scissors, or further hydrodissection. The best cleavage plane is to be found when the surface of the cyst is white or yellow without any red tissue. Most cases of rupture occur while enlarging the incision. Inadvertent rupture of the cyst and its consequences can be reduced by placing the adnexa in a bag before the cystectomy, performing the dissection without grasping or pushing the cyst, avoiding the use of instruments perpendicularly to the surface of the cyst, keeping the active instruments as parallel as possible to the surface of the cyst, always moving the instruments away from the cyst, careful dissection and manipulation especially at the end of the procedure, and aspirating any cyst contents immediately and effectively.

In our department, cystectomy without puncture has been successful in about 50% of the cases whatever the experience of the surgeon. This technique is not used for cysts of more than 7 cm in diameter. To treat large teratomas (>8 cm), a careful puncture performed inside an endobag with a 10-mm aspiration device should be preferred. If spillage occurs, aspiration and extensive lavage should be performed as quickly as possible.

Very large teratomas should be treated using a transparietal or extra-abdominal cystectomy. "Transparietal cystectomy" is a cystectomy performed by minilaparotomy after laparoscopic diagnosis and puncture (22,23). After puncture and drainage of the cyst with a 5- and/or a 10-mm aspirating device, a 3-cm abdominal incision is made. The fascia and the muscles are opened using a classic surgical technique. Then the cyst and the ovary are grasped through the peritoneum, which is incised while pulling the ovary against the abdominal wall, thus facilitating extraction of the ovary. The cyst and the ovary should be grasped close to the puncture site to minimize spillage. Thereafter, drainage of the cyst is completed using the 3-cm incision, and the ovary is extracted through the abdominal wall. The cystectomy is performed using a classic surgical technique. The ovary is released in the peritoneal cavity without any suture, and the abdominal wall is closed.

During pregnancy, this technique should be used cautiously. Because of the uterine volume, the distance between the origin of the ovarian vessels and the abdominal incision is often increased. Therefore, this method should be reserved for very large masses, which are generally accompanied by very long ligaments. The site of the minilaparotomy should be decided in each case to take account of the length of the ligament. If the traction applied on the ligament is too strong, the adnexal vessels may be torn away; a laparotomy may be necessary to prevent this complication.

Other Benign Adnexal Cysts

Benign ovarian cysts are generally punctured using a 5-mm laparoscopic needle if they are less than 6 cm in diameter, or a 5-mm laparoscopic conical trocar and an aspiration-lavage device if larger. The ovary is then opened with scissors, and the internal cyst wall inspected. Careful inspection of the ovarian incision will allow identification of the cleavage plane, and the cystectomy is performed using efficient grasping forceps. During pregnancy, three efficient grasping forceps should be available, since one is always used to prevent the ovary from falling behind the uterus. The procedure should be performed under permanent visual control. The cleavage plane should always be exposed as perfectly as possible by coupling meticulous technique with proactive hemostasis. When pulling the forceps in opposite directions, short and slow movements must be used and the position of the forceps on the cyst wall and on the remaining ovarian tissue adjusted often enough to obtain perfect exposure of the plane. Hemostasis should be performed during dissection, firstly because bleeding may obscure the cleavage plane and secondly because hemostasis is often more difficult at the end of the procedure when the ovarian tissue has retracted.

To avoid ovarian damage, the "best" cleavage plane should be followed. This plane is identified when the outside surface of the cyst wall is white. If red tissue is seen on the cyst wall, however, this is an indication that this is not the best plane and the procedure is probably removing some healthy ovarian tissue.

Adnexal Torsion

It is essential to stress, particularly for general practitioners, that treatment of adnexal torsion is a surgical emergency (24), even if the acute pelvic pain may be effectively relieved using medications. A late diagnosis will increase the risk of adnexal necrosis, spontaneous abortion, and/or premature labor (4).

The management of adnexal torsion during pregnancy is similar to that used in nonpregnant patients. Adnexal ischemia is assessed according to the initial appearance of the adnexa and the recovery after it was untwisted. Gangrenous adnexa are removed; adnexa with mild or severe ischemia (immediate complete or partial recovery) are preserved whenever possible, depending on the treatment of the etiology. To untwist the fragile ischemic adnexa, it is essential to use an atraumatic technique. The surgeon should use a 5-mm probe or a closed atraumatic forceps and should avoid grasping the ischemic tissue. Untwisting is generally easy, observing that the adnexa typically turn toward the center of the pelvis in a clockwise fashion on the left side and in a counterclockwise fashion on the right. Occasionally, the adnexa cannot be untwisted until an associated cyst is decompressed or periadnexal adhesions are lysed.

Generally speaking, oophoropexy is not routinely indicated as an adjunctive procedure. However, we do advocate it whenever there is an early recurrence of torsion associated with an ovarian ligament that is abnormally long and a very short mesovarium. However, in cases of adnexal torsion induced by an adnexal mass, it is difficult to reliably judge whether the length of the utero-ovarian ligament is normal, as the forces created by the weight of the enlarged adnexa naturally increase it. Therefore, the decision to perform an oophoropexy should be based on the comparative assessment of the contralateral adnexa. If the contralateral utero-ovarian ligament is not shorter than the ligament of the twisted adnexa, one may hypothesize that the ligament was not lengthened by the weight of the cyst and that an ovariopexy should be performed. When indicated, the ovariopexy should be bilateral. Moreover, it should be routinely performed in any patient with a solitary adnexa and in those with bilateral torsion. To perform an ovariopexy, a nonabsorbable suture is used to shorten the utero-ovarian ligament (Fig. 5), by fixing the antimesenteric surface of the ovarian cortex to the posterior surface of the broad ligament in the ovarian fossa, which also serves to reduce the risk of adhesion formation between the tube and the ovary. Since it is impossible to suture the ovary to the broad ligament during the second and the third trimesters of pregnancy, a second-look laparoscopy may be warranted after return to a normalized nongravid state.

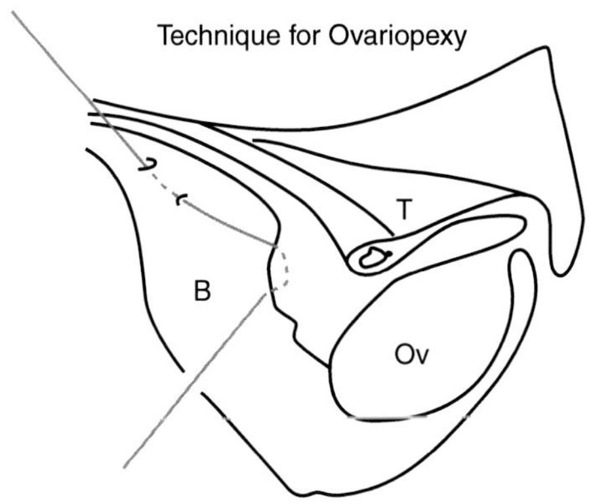

T = tube, B: Peritoneum of the broad ligament, Ov: ovary

Figure 5 Ovariopexy as adjunctive treatment for ovarian torsion.

REFERENCES

1. Parangi S, Levine D, Henry A, et al. Surgical gastrointestinal disorders during pregnancy. Am J Surg 2007; 193:223–232.
2. Melnick DM, Wahl WL, Dalton VK. Management of general surgical problems in the pregnant patient. Am J Surg 2004; 187:170–180.
3. Fatum M, Rojansky N. Laparoscopic surgery during pregnancy. Obstet Gynecol Surv 2001; 56:50–59.
4. Hess LW, Peaceman A, O'Brien WF, et al. Adnexal mass occurring with intrauterine pregnancy: Report of fifty-four patients requiring laparotomy for definitive management. Am J Obstet Gynecol 1988; 158:1029–1034.
5. O'Rourke N, Kodali BS. Laparoscopic surgery during pregnancy. Curr Opin Anaesthesiol 2006; 19:254–259.
6. Moreno-Sanz C, Pascual-Pedrono A, Picazo-Yeste J, et al. Laparoscopic appendectomy during pregnancy: Between personal experiences and scientific evidence J Am Coll Surg 2007; 205:37–42.
7. Lenglet Y, Roman H, Rabishong B, et al. Laparoscopic management of ovarian cysts during pregnancy. Gynecol Obstet Fertil 2006; 34:101–106.
8. Colomb S, Bonnin M, Bolandard F, et al. Pregnant woman anaesthetic management in gynaecologic laparoscopic surgery at the maternity hospital of Clermont-Ferrand. Ann Fr Anesth Reanim 2006; 25:11–16.
9. Yuen PM, Ng PS, Leung PL, et al. Outcome in laparoscopic management of persistent adnexal mass during the second trimester of pregnancy. Surg Endosc 2004; 18:1354–1357.

10. Yuen PM, Chang AM. Laparoscopic management of adnexal mass during pregnancy. Acta Obstet Gynecol Scand 1997; 76:173–176.
11. Leiserowitz GS, Xing G, Cress R, et al. Adnexal masses in pregnancy: How often are they malignant? Gynecol Oncol 2006; 101:315–321.
12. Amos JD, Schorr SJ, Norman PF, et al. Laparoscopic surgery during pregnancy. Am J Surg 1996; 171:435–437.
13. Bhavani-Shankar K, Steinbrook RA, Brooks DC, et al. Arterial to end-tidal carbon dioxide pressure difference during laparoscopic surgery in pregnancy. Anesthesiology 2000; 93:370–373.
14. Camann W, Kodali BS. Maternal insufflation during the second trimester equivalent produces hypercapnia, acidosis, and prolonged hypoxia in fetal sheep. Obstet Anesth Digest 2005; 25(2):68–69.
15. Al-Fozan H, Tulandi T. Safety and risks of laparoscopy in pregnancy. Curr Opin Obstet Gynecol 2002; 14:375–379.
16. Hodjati H, Kazerooni T. Location of the appendix in the gravid patient: A re-evaluation of the established concept. Int J Gynaecol Obstet 2003; 81:245–247.
17. Cohen-Kerem R, Railton C, Oren D, et al. Pregnancy outcome following non obstetrics surgical intervention. Am J Surg 2005; 190:467–473.
18. Whitecar MP, Turner S, Higby MK. Adnexal masses in pregnancy: A review of 130 cases undergoing surgical management. Am J Obstet Gynecol 1999; 181:19–24.
19. Bunyavejchevin S, Phupong V. Laparoscopic surgery for presumed benign ovarian tumor during pregnancy. Cochrane Database Syst Rev 2006; 18(4):CD005459.
20. Oelsner G, Stockheim D, Soriano D, et al. Pregnancy outcome after laparoscopy or laparotomy in pregnancy. J Am Assoc Gynecol Laparosc 2003; 10(2):200–204.
21. Soriano D, Yefet Y, Seidman DS, et al. Laparoscopy versus laparotomy in the management of adnexal masses during pregnancy. Fertil Steril 1999; 71:955–960.
22. Canis M, Botchorishvili R, Manhes H, et al. Management of adnexal masses: Role and risk of laparoscopy. Semin Surg Oncol 2000; 19:28–35.
23. Roman H, Accoceberry M, Bolandard F, et al. Laparoscopic management of a ruptured benign dermoid cyst during advanced pregnancy. J Minim Invasive Gynecol 2005; 12:377–378.
24. Mage G, Canis M, Manhes H, et al. Laparoscopic management of adnexal torsion. A review of 35 cases. J Reprod Med 1989; 34:520–524.

Congenital anomalies of the female reproductive tract

Leila V. Adamyan and Geoffrey W. Cundiff

INTRODUCTION

Congenital malformations of female reproductive tract comprise approximately 4% of all congenital anomalies. Due, in part, to this rarity as well as difficult diagnosis, misunderstanding of malformations of uterus and vagina can lead to mismanagement, ranging from incorrect diagnosis to counterproductive treatments, including unsuccessful or disfiguring surgery. The proper management begins with a clear understanding of the normal embryology of the female reproductive tract and the physical manifestations of abnormal organogenesis. With proper diagnosis, the surgeon can intelligently address the patient's limitations that result from a given congenital anomaly.

In this chapter, we bring experience in treating more than 1500 female patients affected by congenital anomalies of the reproductive tract. We will address the application of modern imaging techniques and endoscopy, in the diagnosis of congenital anomalies, as well as surgical treatment and rehabilitation, including our own original methods of minimally invasive reconstructive plastic surgery.

EMBRYOLOGY

The structures of the upper female reproductive tract derive from the paramesonephric ducts, two tubular structures that form in the sixth week lateral to the mesonephric duct. At this stage, the embryo is undifferentiated, but in the absence of testosterone and müllerian inhibiting substance produced by the testes, the mesonephric ducts regress and the paramesonephric ducts develop into the müllerian system. Initially, three parts can be seen: (*i*) a cranial vertical portion opening into the coelomic cavity, (*ii*) a horizontal portion that crosses the mesonephric ducts, and (*iii*) a caudal vertical portion that fuses with the contralateral paramesonephric duct (Fig. 1). As the ovary descends, the fused paramesonephric ducts give rise to the corpus and cervix of the uterus. They are surrounded by a layer of mesenchyme that differentiates into the myometrium. When the paramesonephric ducts reach the urogenital sinus, the sinovaginal bulbs form. Further proliferation occurs in the cranial direction, followed by canalization (Fig. 2). This forms the four-fifths of the vagina, while the lower one-fifth derives from the urogenital sinus rather than from the

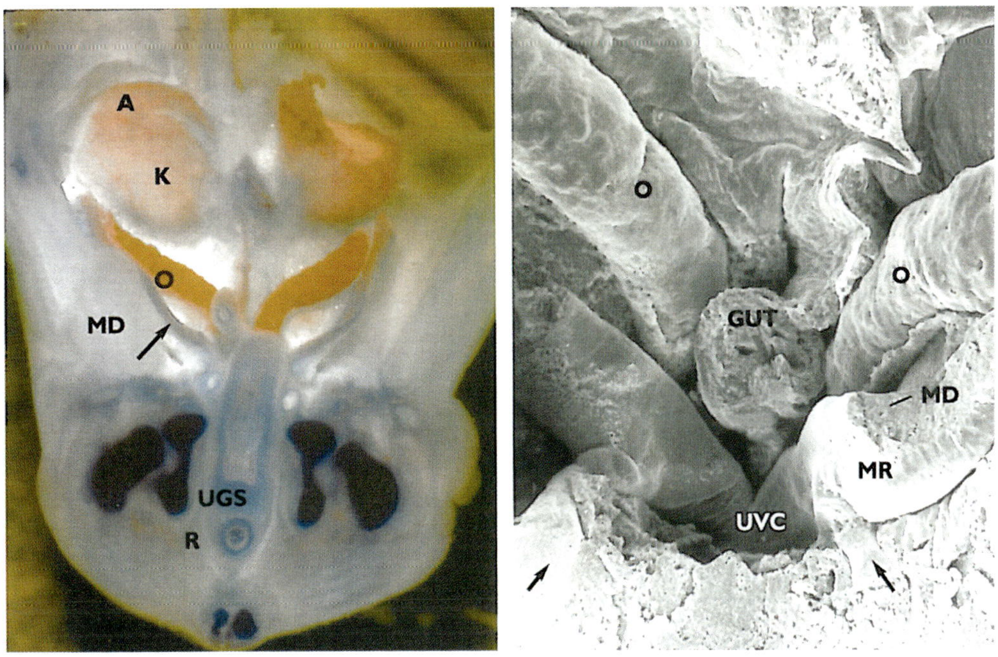

(A) (B)

Figure 1 (A) Pelvic dissection at eight weeks showing ovaries (O), mullerian ducts (MD), urogential sinus (UGS), Kidneys (K), adrenals (A), and rectum (R). The upper portion of the mullerian ducts contribute to the fallopian tubes; the lower portions fuse to a single uterovaginal primordium, which gives rise to the uterus and upper four-fifths of the vagina. (B) The ducts are fusing at the midline into the uterovaginal canal (UVC). *Source*: From Ref. 37.

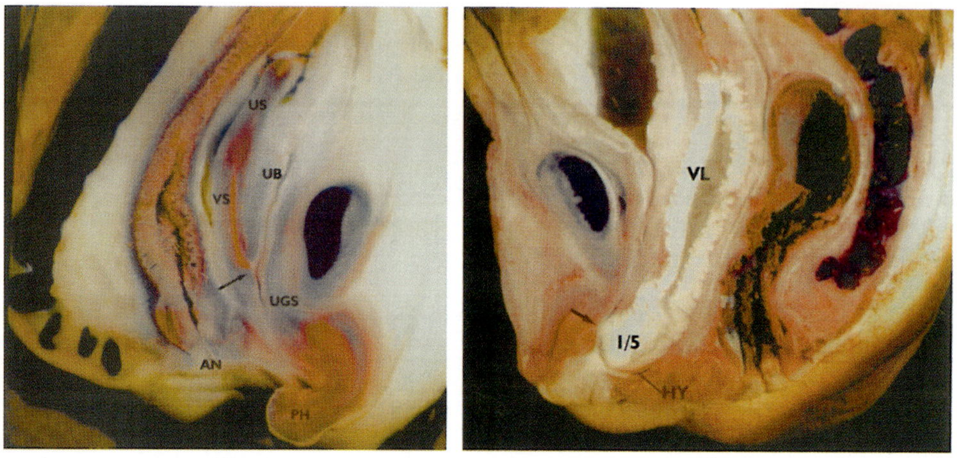

(A) (B)

Figure 2 (A) Midline sagittal section of the pelvic organs. The uterovaginal canal consists of a uterine segment (US) and a vaginal segment (VS). The tip of the fused mullerian ducts fuses with the pelvic portion of the urogenital sinus (arrow). (B) As the epithelium of the mullerian ducts regresses, the vagina becomes lumenized. The mullerian tubercle gives rise to the hymen (HY). *Source*: From Ref. 37.

müllerian origin. The ovaries are not of müllerian origin either, as they develop from germ cells that migrate from the primitive yolk sac into the mesenchyme of the peritoneal cavity and subsequently develop into ova and supporting cells.

Complete formation and differentiation of the müllerian ducts into the segments of the female reproductive tract occurs in three stages. Both paramesonephric (müllerian) ducts migrate inferiorly and medially. As they meet in the midline, they fuse together inferiorly in a process referred to as longitudinal or lateral fusion. The medial walls then reabsorb to create the uterine cavity, while the unfused superior portions become the fallopian tubes. The descending müllerian system (upper one-third of the vagina) then fuses with the ascending sinovaginal bulb (lower two-thirds) to complete the vaginal patency. This is referred to as transverse or vertical fusion.

Abnormal progression of each of these stages results in different anomalies. If one müllerian duct does not develop fully, the patient will have a unicornuate uterus. If neither müllerian duct forms, then uterine agenesis or hypoplasia results. Abnormalities in longitudinal fusion of the two müllerian ducts result in different uterine anomalies, which vary based on the degree of fusion, including bicornuate or didelphis uterus. Failure of septal reabsorption results in a septate uterus. Incomplete vertical fusion results in a transverse vaginal septum or imperforate hymen.

Aplasia of the vagina and uterus (Mayer–Rokitanski–Kuster–Hauser syndrome) is a malformation characterized by congenital absence of uterus and vagina in the presence of normally functioning ovaries (Figs. 3 and 4). Affected patients have a normal female phenotype and karyotype (46XX), although they frequently have other congenital anomalies, including skeletal, urinary tract, and digestive tract abnormalities. It represents abnormalities of both longitudinal and transverse fusion, and consequently these patients frequently have lateral remnants of the mullerian system noted as two muscular rudiments, or less commonly asymmetric muscular embankments or complete absence of rudiments.

Mayer–Rokitanski–Kuster–Hauser syndrome has a prevalence of 1/4000 to 1/1000 live-born females. The absence of a vagina is frequently noted in puberty. The dramatic nature of this finding usually leads to an early referral, which is why almost a half of patients referred to our clinic with different anomalies of genital tract have Mayer–Rokitanski–Kuster–Hauser syndrome.

CLASSIFICATION OF CONGENITAL ANOMALIES

The most accepted method to classify congenital anomalies of the female reproductive tract is the American Fertility Society (AFS) Classification Scheme (1). This system has seven classifications (Table 1).

DIAGNOSIS

While congenital anomalies of the female reproductive tract are present at birth, they are frequently not diagnosed until after puberty. As the ovaries are not part of the müllerian

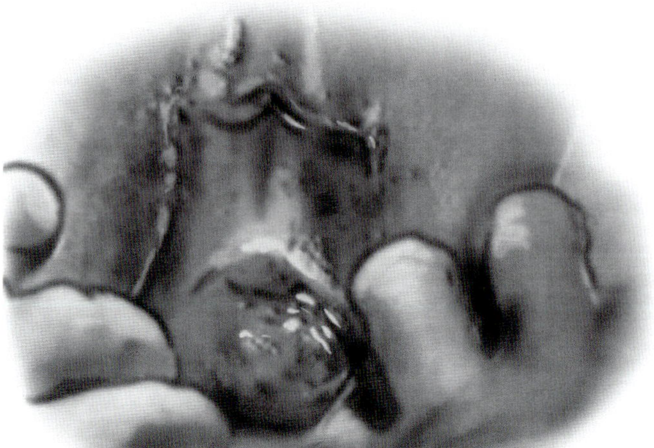

Figure 3 Aplasia of vagina.

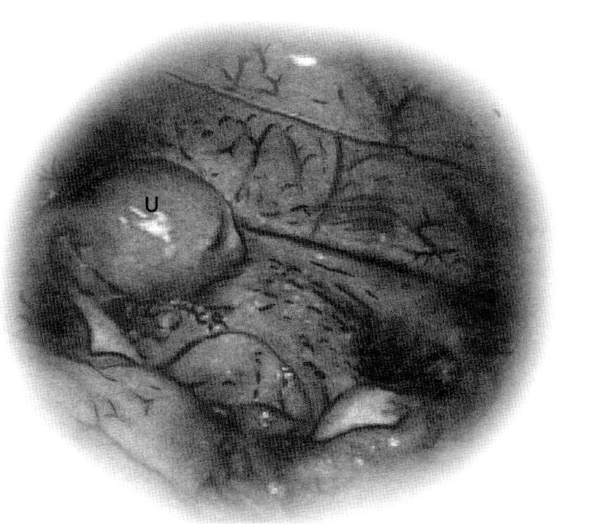

Figure 4 Transperitoneal view of aplasia of vagina and uterus with rudimentary left uterine horn visible (U).

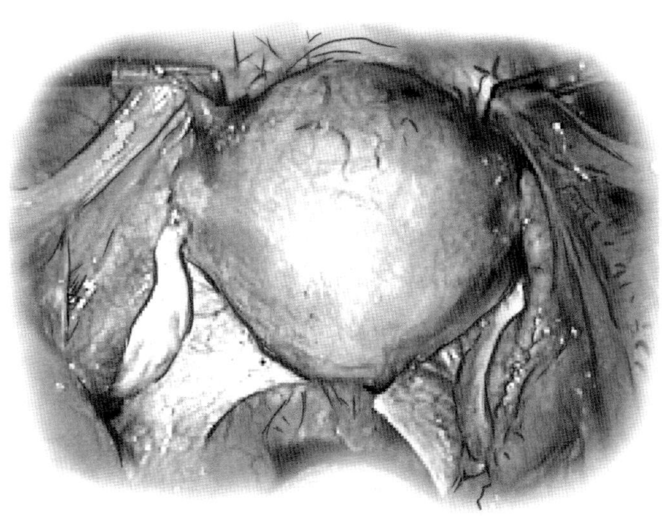

Figure 5 Laparoscopic view of functional uterus with cervical and vaginal aplasia.

system, they are usually unaffected, so hormonally mediated changes of puberty, such as thelarche and adrenarche proceed at a normal pace. Menarche, however, does not proceed normally. If the uterus is completely absent, patients usually present in the later teens with primary amenorrhea. If rudimentary uterine horns are present, in addition to primary amenorrhea, patients may develop cyclical pelvic pain from hematocolpos or hematometra. They generally present earlier, and, if untreated, this can progress to chronic pelvic pain resulting from endometriosis due to retrograde menstruation or infection resulting in pyometra or pyocolpos.

The diagnostic requirements of congenital anomalies of the female genital tract usually follow from the presentation. Disorders of lateral fusion usually present as infertility or inability to carry a pregnancy to full gestation. Useful diagnostic modalities include hysterosalpingography, hysterosonography, and endoscopic techniques including hysteroscopy and diagnostic laparoscopy, which provide a means to define morphology and patency of the uterus and tubes. The management of these disorders is discussed elsewhere in the text.

Table 1 American Fertility Society (AFS) Classification Scheme for Female Congenital Anomalies (1)

Class I: This class includes uterine/cervical agenesis or hypoplasia, of which the most common form is the Mayer-Rokitanski-Kuster-Hauser syndrome that includes agenesis of the uterus, cervix, and upper portion of the vagina.
Class II: Complete, or almost complete, arrest of development of one müllerian duct, resulting in a unicornuate uterus. The majority of these patients (90%) have incomplete arrest, resulting in a rudimentary horn with or without functioning endometrium.
Class III: This anomaly results from complete nonfusion of both müllerian ducts resulting in didelphis uterus, with two individual horns and two cervices. A longitudinal or transverse vaginal septum may be noted as well.
Class IV: Partial nonfusion of the müllerian ducts results in a bicornuate.
Class V: A septate uterus results from failure of resorption of the septum between the two uterine horns. The septum can be partial or complete, in which case it extends to the internal cervical os. Histologically, the septum may be composed of myometrium or fibrous tissue. The uterine fundus is typically convex but may be flat or slightly concave (<1-cm fundal cleft).
Class VI: An arcuate uterus has a single uterine cavity with a convex or flat uterine fundus, the endometrial cavity, which demonstrates a small fundal cleft or impression.
Class VII: Anomalies resulting from in uterine exposure to diethylstilbestrol, an estrogen analog with teratogenic effects on the reproductive tracts female.

Disorders of transverse fusion frequently present at a younger age. The main clinical features of uterine and vaginal aplasia are the absence of menstruation and inability to pursue successful sexual intercourse. Uterine rudiments may also be affected by adenomyosis, resulting in pelvic pain. The diagnosis is based on the patient's complaints and physical examination, confirmed by imaging. Karyotyping is useful to rule out disorders with similar presentation, such as testicular feminization. Ultrasonography provides important data but is wisely augmented by other imaging modalities, such as computed tomography or magnetic resonance imaging (MRI), which provide further information about pelvic soft tissues. These modalities also provide important information about coexisting anomalies of the skeleton, and lower urinary and digestive tracts. Given the proximity of the lower urinary tract, many surgeons will pursue an intravenous pyelogram to clearly define the surrounding anatomy prior to pursuing surgery.

Aplasia of the vagina associated with functional normal or functional rudimentary uterus is a very rare malformation (Fig. 5). The main clinical features are the absence of menstruation, cyclical or permanent pelvic pain beginning at menarche, and inability to have successful sexual intercourse. In addition, most affected patients have hematometra and/or pyometra, chronic endometritis and perimetritis, and hematosalpinx and pyosalpinx, and patients with partial vaginal aplasia have hematocolpos and/or pyocolpos. Computed tomography or MRI can be very helpful in sorting out the anatomical consequences.

MANAGEMENT

This chapter focuses on the management of disorders of transverse fusion and vaginal aplasia, which generally involves the creation of a neovagina. The timing of intervention for creation of a neovagina and the management of the emotional impact of the condition are important therapeutic considerations. Most patients with congenital anomalies have some degree of negative body image related to their condition. We generally initiate sexual counseling following diagnosis and certainly prior to contemplating surgery. We also try to postpone surgery until the patient has a sexual partner. From a practical standpoint, this helps to maximize vaginal patency as they can initiate coitus shortly after surgery, but it also helps to set patient expectations. We continue this counseling in the postoperative period.

Creation of a Neovagina

Surgical correction of the Mayer–Rokitanski–Kuster–Hauser syndrome is substantiated not by general health issues but by the desire of the patient to pursue sexual activity and fertility. Given the limited success and associated morbidity of early surgical techniques, the ethics and advisability of creating an artificial vagina have been historically controversial. The efforts have focused on the search for a technique that balances safety with reliable results for a functional vagina (2,3). In an effort to avoid surgical misadventures, some authors have advocated different methods of gradual vaginal dilation or colpoelongation (4,5). These techniques use vaginal dilators to gradually transform the perineal dimple between the urethra and anus into a functional invagination. While these techniques are minimally invasive and reasonable results are published, they require considerable time and patient compliance and are not always effective.

The Vechietti operation was developed to expedite vaginal dilation by replacing the intermittent pressure from below with constant traction on the vesicorectal space from above via a surgically implanted mobile button or dummy (6). This pressure is provided by ventral traction on sutures, which are placed through the dummy and then traverse the subperitoneal space, exiting through the abdominal wall. The dummy is removed after adequate vaginal length is achieved, which usually takes approximately one week. Maintaining vaginal patency requires use of a vaginal dilator for eight hours a day for a minimum of one month. The operation can also be accomplished from a laparoscopic approach (7). A recent series reported 98% anatomical success with minimal complications and one-year sexual outcomes based on validated measures, comparable to normal controls (8).

The most commonly used surgical techniques for creation of a neovagina involve a perineal approach to the creation of a canal between the urinary bladder and rectum and its subsequent tamponade and dilatation with prosthetic appliances (9). McIndoe and Banister popularized this approach, advocating the use of a partial-thickness skin graft harvested from the buttocks (10). The skin graft is held in apposition to the vaginal canal by a vaginal stent, which is left in place for a minimum of one week, followed by daily vaginal dilation to prevent stenosis. Others have advocated replacing the partial-thickness skin graft with full-thickness grafts harvested from the inguinal region (11). This provides a more cosmetic outcome and has been reported to minimize stenosis, although the rate of graft rejection may be higher. In smaller patients, it may be difficult to obtain an adequate full-thickness graft from the groins. In these circumstances, we have used tissue expanders to maximize the size of the harvested graft and resultant vaginal length, while optimizing cosmesis (12) (Fig. 6). Others have described techniques using flaps developed from the vulva and perineum, although this may not provide adequate tissue to create a normal vaginal caliber or length (13,14). Okada et al. recommended perineal tissue expanders to overcome this limitation (15). Other innovators have attempted to overcome the limitations of skin grafts or flaps through the use of buccal mucosa (16), amnion (17,18), artificial dermis (19), surgical adhesion barriers (20,21), and fibrin glue (22).

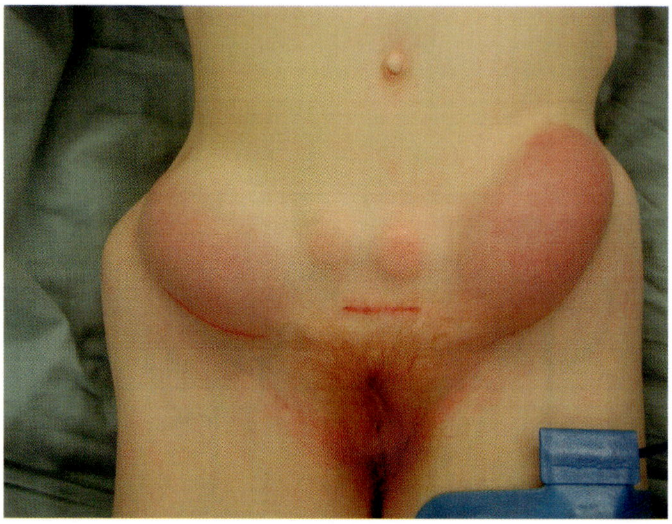

Figure 6 View of the abdomen with bilateral tissue expanders in place.

Creation of a neovagina, or colpopoiesis, with the use of skin flaps is rather simple and safe, with a relatively low rate of stenosis. The disadvantages of the method, besides the cosmetic issues, are possibility of flap rejection, and scarring and further skin tissue functioning. Moreover, the long-term use of the prosthesis may cause pathologic wound healing resulting in scarring. Further development of this surgical technique comprised lining of the canal between urinary bladder and rectum with segments of bowel (23–25). The use of a segment of bowel, with its own vascular pedicle in place of the graft, promised immediate results without subsequent dilation. Unfortunately, the surgical development of the intestinal segment has been proved to be very complex and traumatic, often followed by fistula formation, prolapse of neovagina, and excessive secretion of intestinal mucus. Synthetic materials, although promising, have minimal outcome data at this point and have not gained widespread use so far, but possibly will develop into a new treatment option.

In 1969, Davydov reported a technique for colpopoiesis using pelvic peritoneum (26). The operation comprised creation of a canal between the rectum and the urinary bladder and laparotomy to permit mobilization of pelvic peritoneum to line the canal. The technique for one-stage transperineal colpopoiesis from pelvic peritoneum was published almost simultaneously in the Russian literature by Davydov and by Kurbanova and Kravkova in 1972 (27–29). This modification eliminated the necessity of laparotomy and offered excellent results in terms of rapid epithelialization, and sufficient capacity and depth of the neovagina. However, the elimination of the laparotomy made the mobilization of peritoneum risky. To increase safety while maintaining a minimally invasive approach, we introduced a laparoscopic method of colpopoiesis using pelvic peritoneum in 1993 (30,31).

The technique begins with diagnostic laparoscopy to specify the character of the malformation, including the number and location of muscular rudiments. Enlarged uterine rudiments frequently cause pelvic pain, in which case they should be removed before proceeding. The mobility of the pelvic peritoneum of cystorectal reflection is accessed prior to beginning the perineal dissection. The laparoscope in the

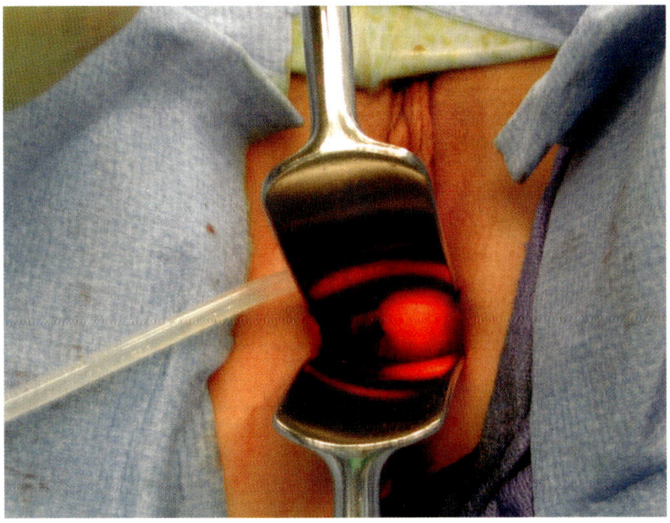

Figure 7 Perineal view of the trans-illuminated cystorectal reflection.

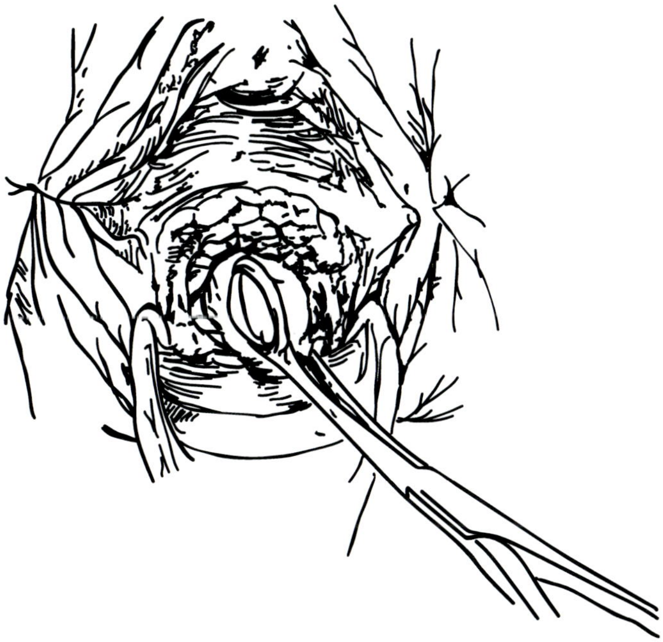

Figure 9 Blunt dissection between rectum and bladder.

peritoneal cavity permits transillumination of the incision site during the perineal dissection which helps to prevent inadvertent injury to the bladder and rectum. The perineal dissection begins with 3 to 3.5 cm transverse incision in the dimple between the external urethral meatus and the rectum at the level of lower border of labia minora (Figs. 7 and 8). Following initial sharp dissection, blunt dissection in a transverse direction between the urinary bladder and rectum creates a canal up to the pelvic peritoneum (Figs. 9 and 10). The risk of injury to the bladder or the rectum may be increased in cases of atypical (posteriorly) located urethra or in the presence of scarring from prior courses of colpoelongation or perineal surgery that may create a false route directed toward the rectum.

The most mobile part of the peritoneum between the bladder and the rectum is identified using laparoscope (Fig. 11). This is often the transverse fold between two muscular rudiments. Using an atraumatic laparoscopic instrument, the mobilized peritoneum is brought down into the created canal (Figs. 12 and 13). The peritoneal fold is incised transversely and the edges of peritoneum are sutured to the edges of

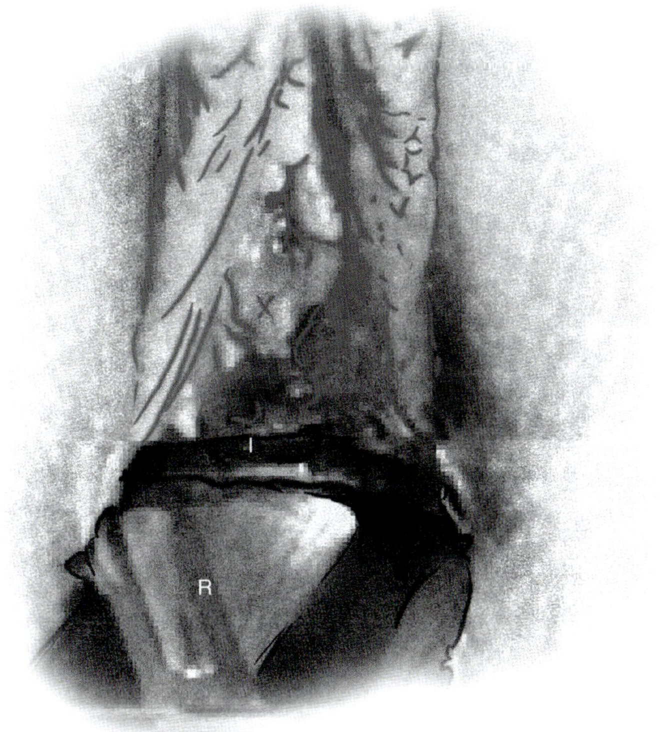

Figure 8 Transverse incision of perineal skin at the level of lower border of labia minora. I, incision; R, retractor.

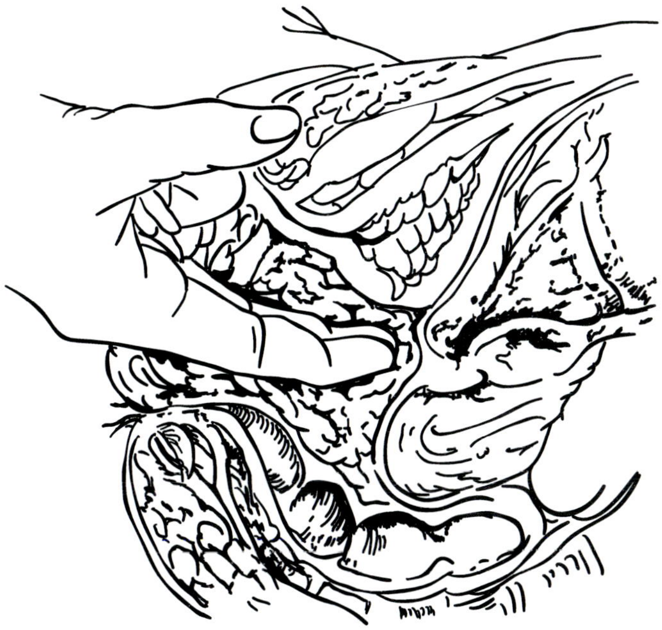

Figure 10 Blunt dissection between rectum and bladder.

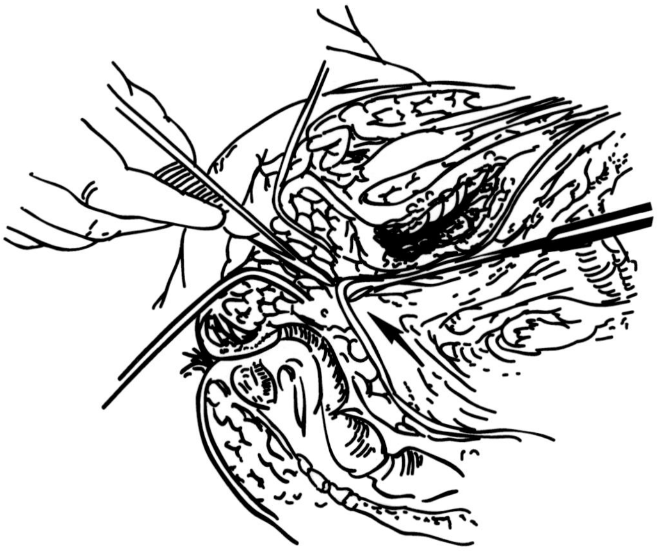

Figure 11 Identification of most mobile part of pelvic peritoneum and its bringing down to the canal.

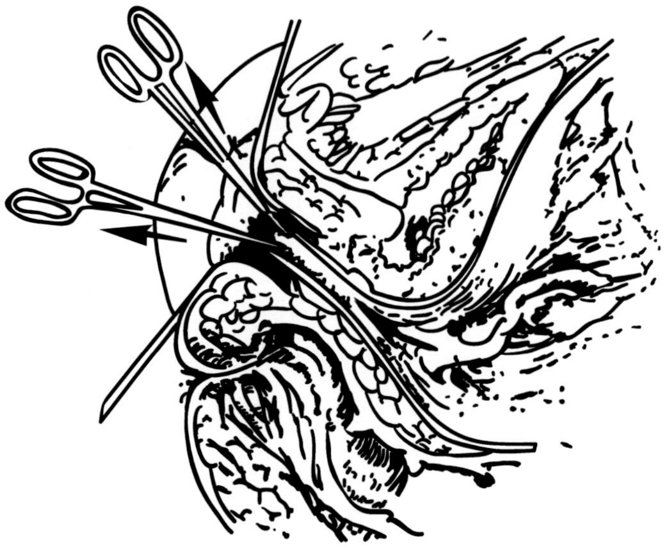

Figure 13 Bringing the peritoneum down and suturing to the edges of perineal skin incision.

skin incision with interrupted stitches of a delayed absorbable suture, forming the introitus (Figs. 14 and 15). The neovaginal vault is created laparoscopically through the placement of a purse-string, semi–purse-string, or interrupted sutures that incorporate the bladder peritoneum, muscular rudiments, and peritoneum lining the pelvic sidewalls and sigmoid colon (Figs. 16 and 17). We generally use extracorporeal suturing to accomplish this step. Typically, the laparoscopically assisted colpopoiesis requires 25 to 45 minutes, with minimal blood loss. We use antibiotic prophylaxis, bladder drainage, and a vaginal pack. The patients are mobilized five to six hours after surgery. Gynecologic examination is performed at one week to assess the tissue ingrowth. Most patients initiate sexual activity by four weeks.

The anatomical results at three to four months after operation include an absence of the border between the introitus and neovagina itself, and vaginal length of 11 to 12 cm, with adequate breadth (Figs. 18 and 19). The walls are moderately rugated and produce some mucus. Morphologically, the neovaginal epithelium is similar to the stratified squamous epithelium of normal vagina, due to metaplasia. Functionally, most patients appear to be absolutely satisfied with their sexual life, which significantly contributes to their psychoemotional and social adaptation.

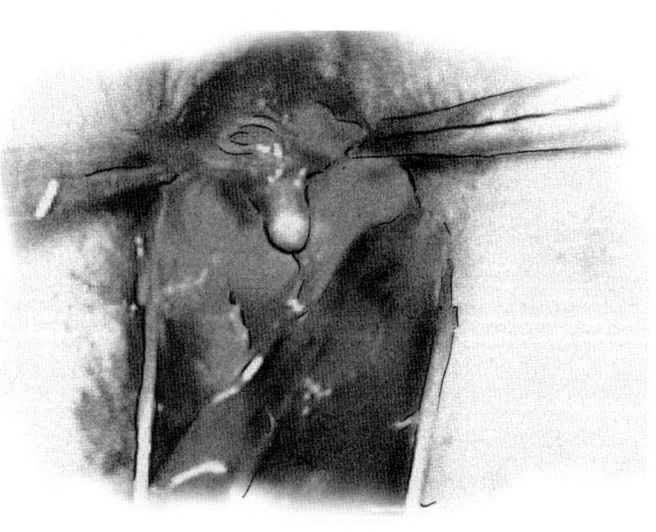

Figure 12 Grasping of pelvic peritoneum in the rectovesical canal.

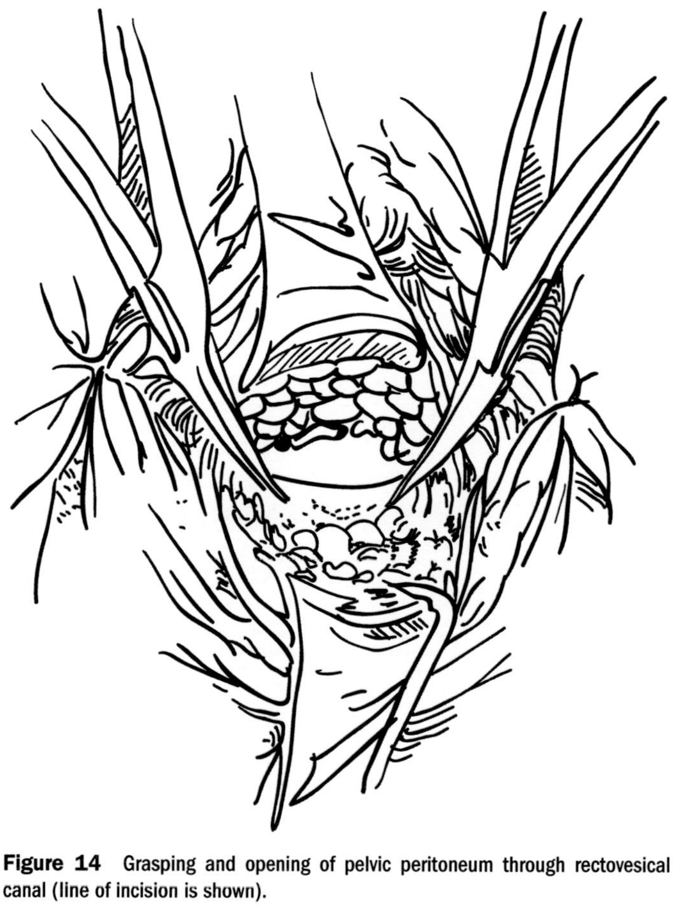

Figure 14 Grasping and opening of pelvic peritoneum through rectovesical canal (line of incision is shown).

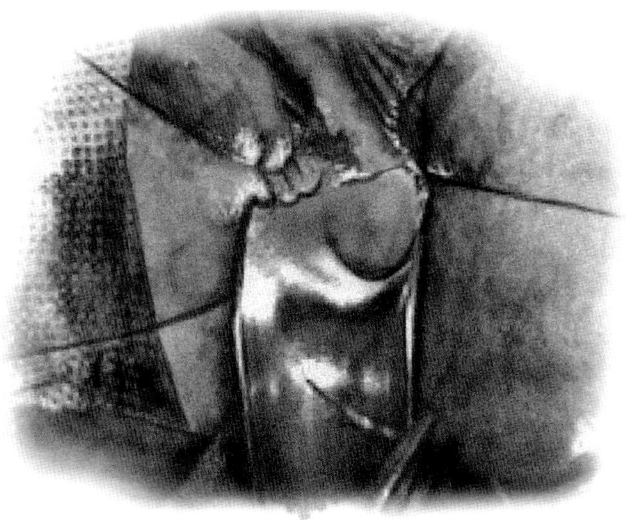

Figure 15 Suturing of peritoneal lining to the edges of perineal skin incision.

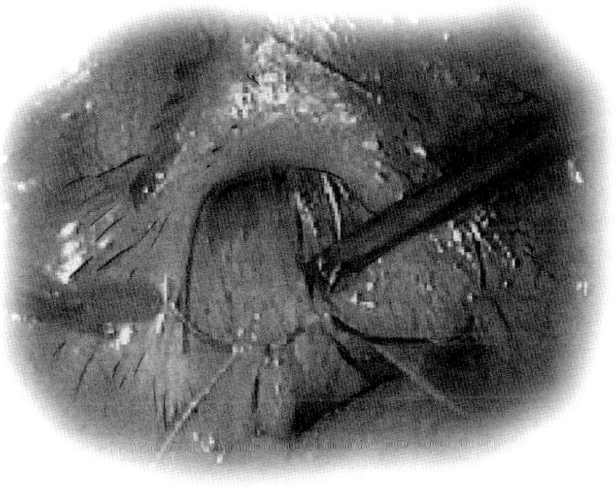

Figure 16 Formation of neovaginal vault by laparoscopic suturing with extracorporeal knot tying.

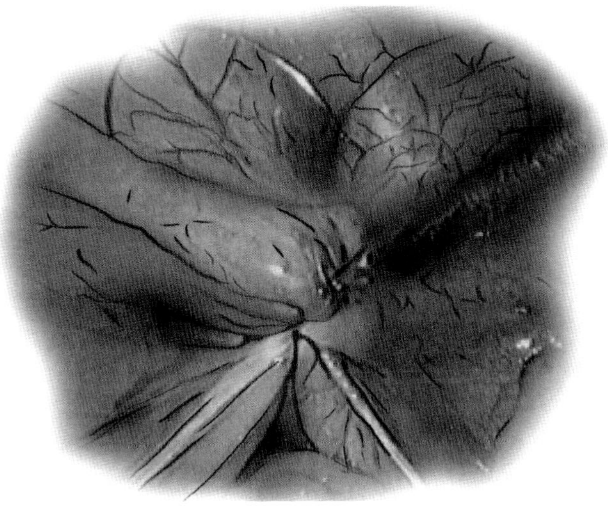

Figure 17 Neovaginal vault is formed with one purse-string suture.

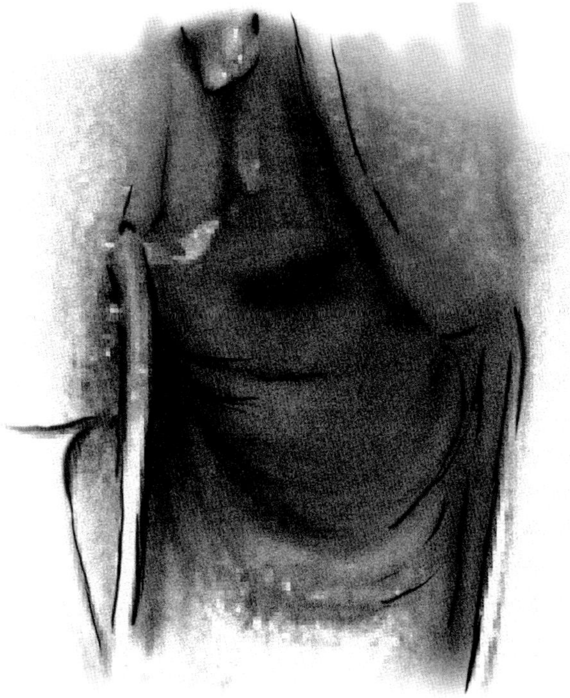

Figure 18 Final view of neovagina.

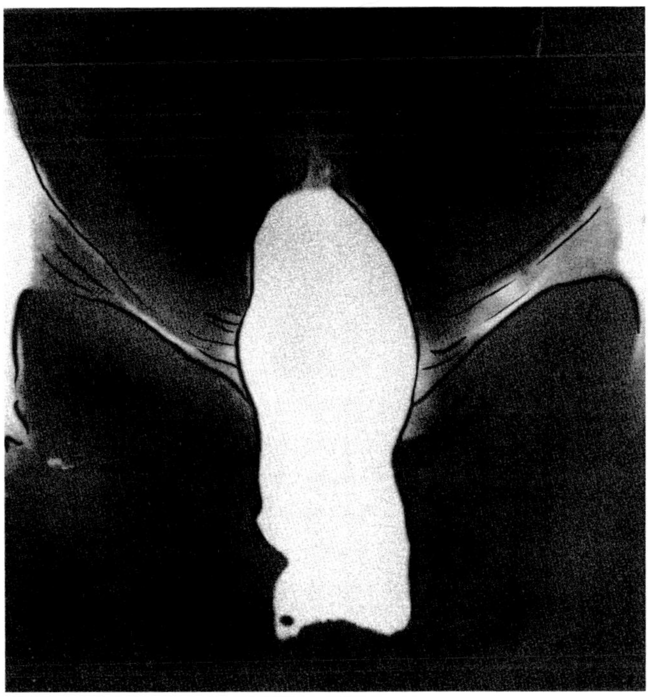

Figure 19 Long-term result. Contrast roentgenogram of neovagina.

Management of Disorders of Transverse Fusion

Aplasia of vagina associated with functional normal or functional rudimentary uterus is more challenging. In the first place, most patients have associated hematometra or hematocolpos shortly after menarche, with associated pelvic pain and at times pyometra or pyocolpos. This compromises preoperative counseling and optimal surgical timing, as surgical correction cannot be postponed, and should be undertaken as soon as the diagnosis is established. In patients with complete aplasia of the vagina with a functional uterus, the crucial aspect to be determined for choice of surgical modality is absence or presence of a cervical canal. For this purpose, we have introduced the method of retrograde hysteroscopy via the laparoscopic approach (32). After establishing laparoscopic access, a small hysterotomy is created in the uterine fundus and an endoscope, with sheath, is introduced into the uterus (Fig. 20) Following copious irrigation of the uterine cavity, the endoscope can evaluate the uterine cavity and determine whether a cervical canal is present. The endoscope also provides transillumination, which makes dissection of the transverse vaginal septum safer. Surgical correction, which may be attempted to preserve the functional uterus in patients with cervical and vaginal aplasia, is creation of a tunnel between the uterus and neovagina (33,34). Preoperative MRI to predict the thickness of the septum is very helpful in planning this step. Once the canal is created, the peritoneum of rectouterine pouch is opened laparoscopically to mobilize the peritoneal incision edges, which are then sutured to the introital skin or top of the vaginal epithelium.

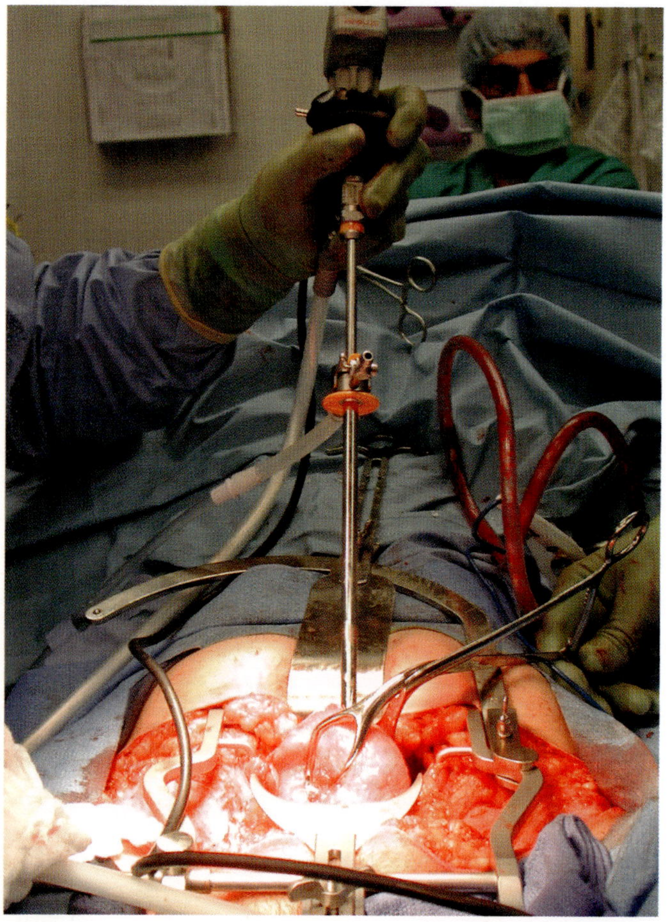

Figure 20 Retrograde hysteroscopy through a fundal puncture, during a laparotomy.

If retrograde hysteroscopy fails to identify a cervical canal, it may be possible to create a neocervix by tunneling between the uterine cavity and neovagina. In this circumstance, the new cervical canal must be stented, bringing the stent into the neovagina, with fixation of the uterus at the tunnel. We have successfully created patent cervices using this technique, although it may require further hysteroscopic surgery to maintain patency. If such correction appears impossible or ineffective, resulting in atresia of a previously created tunnel, a total laparoscopic hysterectomy may be preferable prior to proceeding with laparoscopically assisted colpopoiesis from pelvic peritoneum (30,35,36).

CONCLUSIONS

All of the available methods of colpopoiesis have potential advantages, and limitations, disadvantages, or complications. The technique of laparoscopically assisted colpopoiesis using pelvic peritoneum offers a good balance between the risks of surgery and the results achieved, as pelvic peritoneum provides a physiological lining of the canal that promotes epithelialization without the need for retrieval of other tissues. It is also a technique that is relatively simple, relying on skill in gynecologic laparoscopy, but not in general or plastic surgery. The laparoscopic access also allows the surgeon to address associated pelvic pathology. As with all pelvic surgery, specific patient's needs and pathology may warrant a different technique, which is why the surgeon treating congenital anomalies should have a broad understanding of the different techniques available and their relative merits and limitations. Optimal outcomes for the surgical management of congenital anomalies also demand that the surgeon carefully considers the impact of the condition on the patient's overall health, including emotional well-being. Perioperative counseling is therefore essential.

REFERENCES

1. American Fertility Society. The American Fertility Society classifications of Mullerian anomalies and intrauterine adhesions. Fertil Steril 1989; 51:199–201.
2. Buttram VC. Mullerian anomalies and their management. Fertil Steril 1983; 40:159–163.
3. Karim RB, Hage JJ, Dekker JJ, et al. Evolution of the methods of neovaginoplasty for vaginal aplasia. Eur J Obstet Gynecol Reprod Biol 1995; 58:19–27.
4. Frank RT. The formation of artificial vagina without operation. Am J Obstet Gynecol 1938; 35:1053–1055.
5. Ingram JM. The bicycle seat stool in the treatment of vaginal agenesis and stenosis: A preliminary report. Am J Obstet Gynecol 1981; 140:867–873.
6. Vecchietti G. Neovagina nella sindrome di Rokitansky–Kuster–Hauser. Attual Ostet Ginecol 1965; 11:131–147.
7. Fedele L, Buscca M, Candani M, et al. Laparoscopic creation of a neovagina in Meyer–Rokitansky–Kuster–Hauser syndrome by modification of Vecchietti's operation. Am J Obstet Gynecol 1994; 171:268–269.
8. Fedele L, Bianchi S, Frontino G, et al. The laparoscopic Vecchietti's modified technique in Rokitansly syndrome: Anatomic, functional, and sexual long-term results. Am J Obstet Gynecol 2008; 198:377.
9. Wharton LR. A simple method of constructing a vagina; report of four cases. Ann Surg 1938; 107:842–852.

10. McIndoe AH, Banister JB. An operation for the cure of congenital absence of the vagina. J Obstet Gynaecol 1938; 45:490–494.
11. Akn S. Experience with neovaginal construction using the full-thickness skin graft in vaginal agenesis. Ann Plast Surg 2004; 52(4):391–396.
12. Loveless M, Gutman R, Cundiff GW. Tissue Expanders Optimize Harvesting of Full-thickness Skin Grafts in Select Patients Undergoing McIndoe Neovagina. J Pelvic Med Surg 2008; 14(3):185–190.
13. Giraldo F, Gaspar D, Gonzales C, et al. Treatment of vaginal agenesis with vulvoperineal fasciocutaneous flaps. Plast Reconstr Surg 1994; 93:131–138.
14. Hwang WY, Chang TS, Sun P, et al. Vaginal reconstruction using labia minora flaps in congenital total absence. Ann Plast Surg 1985; 15:534–537.
15. Okada E, Iwahira Y, Maruyama Y. Treatment of vaginal agenesis with an expanded vulval flap. Plast Reconstr Surg 1996; 98:530–533.
16. Lin WC, Chang CY, Shen YY, et al. Use of autologous buccal mucosa for vaginoplasty: A study of eight cases. Hum Reprod 2003; 18:604–607.
17. Ashworth MF, Morton KE, Dewhurst J, et al. Vaginoplasty using amnion. Obstet Gynecol 1986; 67:443–446.
18. Nisolle M, Donnez J. Vaginoplasty using amniotic membranes in cases of vaginal agenesis or after vaginectomy. J Gynecol Surg 1992; 8:25–30.
19. Noguchi S, Nakatsuka M, Sugiuama Y, et al. Use of artificial dermis and recombinant basic fibroblast growth factor for creating a neovagina in a patient with Mayer–Rokitansky–Kuster–Hauser syndrome. Hum Reprod 2004; 19(7):1629–1632.
20. Jackson ND, Rosenblatt PL. Use of Interceed absorbable adhesion barrier for vaginoplasty. Obstet Gynecol 1994; 84:1048–1050.
21. Motoyama S, Laoag-Fernandez JB, Mochizuki S, et al. Vaginoplasty with interceed absorbable adhesion barrier for complete squamous epithelialization in vaginal agenesis. Am J Obstet Gynecol 2003; 188(5):1260–1264.
22. Tercan M, Balat O, Bekerecioglu M, et al. The use of fibrin glue in the McIndoe technique of vaginoplasty. Plast Reconstr Surg 2002; 109(2):706–709.
23. Emiroglu M, Gultan SM, Adanali G, et al. Vaginal reconstruction with free jejunal flap. Ann Plast Surg 1996; 36:316–320.
24. Ota H, Tanaka J, Murakami M, et al. Laparoscopy-assisted Ruge procedure for the creation of a neovagina in a patient with Mayer–Rokitansky–Kuster–Hauser syndrome. Fertil Steril 2000; 73:641–644.
25. Parsons JK, Gearhart SL, Gearhart JP. Vaginal reconstruction utilizing sigmoid colon: Complication and long-term results. J Pediatr Surg 2002; 37:629–633.
26. Davydov SN. Colpopoiesis from the peritoneum of the uterorectal space. Obstet Gynecol 1969; 12:55–57.
27. Davydov SN. Modification of colpopoiesis from peritoneum of the rectoenterouterine recess. Akush Ginekol (Mosk) 1972; 48(2):56–57.
28. Kurbanova AG, Krakova EV. Single stage method of colpopoiesis from peritoneum. Akush Ginekol (Mosk) 1972; 48(2):55–56.
29. Davydov SN, Zhvitiashvili OD. Formation of vagina (colpopoiesis) from peritoneum of Douglas pouch. Acta Chir Plast 1974; 16:35–41.
30. Adamyan LV. Laparoscopic management of vaginal aplasia with or without functional noncommunicating uterus. In: Arregui ME, et al. eds. Principles of Laparoscopic Surgery: Basic and Advanced Techniques. Springer-Verlag, 1995:652–671.
31. Adamyan LV. Therapeutic and endoscopic perspectives: Colpopoiesis in vaginal and uterine aplasias. In: Nichols D, ed. Gynecologic and Obstetric Surgery. Mosby, 1999:187–195.
32. Loveless MB, Cundiff GW. Retrograde hysteroscopy: A technique for repair of vaginal obstruction and noncommunicating mullerian anomalies. J Pelvic Med Surg 2006; 12(5):269–272.
33. Chakravarty B, Konar H, Chowdhury NN. Pregnancies after reconstructive surgery for congenital cervicovaginal atresia. Am J Obstet Gynecol 2000; 83(2):421–423.
34. Bugmann Ph, Amaudruz M, Hanquinet S, et al. Uterocervicoplasty with a bladder mucosa layer for the treatment of complete cervical agenesis. Fertil Steril 2002; 77(4):831–835.
35. Rock JA, Schlaff WD, Zacur HA, et al. The clinical management of congenital absence of the uterine cervix. Int J Gynaecol Obstet 1984; 22(3):231–235.
36. Adamyan LV. Laparoscopy in surgical treatment of vaginal aplasia: Laparoscopy assisted colpopoiesis and perineal hysterectomy with colpopoiesis. Int J Fertil 1996; 41(1):40–45.
37. Jirasek JE. An Atlas of Human Prenatal Developmental Mechanics. London: Taylor & Francis; 2004.

18

Intractable neural pelvic pain

Marc Possover

INTRODUCTION

The pelvis contains not only different organs such as the bladder, rectum, or genital organs but also blood vessels and nerves. Different specialties have focused on the pathologies of all these different anatomical structures. Gynecology deals with diseases of the urogenital organs in women and urology with the urogenital organs in men, while diseases of the gastrointestinal tract are the domain of general surgeons, but no specialty deals electively with the pathologies of the pelvic nerves! This is even more astounding that, after the central nervous system and the spinal cord, no other part of the body contains so many and such important nerves: pelvic nerves are not only involved in sexuality, voiding, storage functions of the bladder and the rectum, standing up, and walking but also in the transport of all sensitive information coming from the lower limbs and the pelvis, including the proprioception involved in equilibrium. One kind of such information being transported by the pelvic nerves to the central nervous system is the information of pain, pelvic pain, and/or pain from the lower extremities.

"NEUROLOGIC" DEFINITION OF PAIN

Chronic pelvic pain is a commonly encountered problem for GPs and gynecologists in daily practice. It is estimated that 12% of all women around the world suffer from chronic pelvic pain (1). As gynecologists, one of the first steps in pelvic pain management is to find an etiology to be treated; thus, laparoscopy has become the standard for diagnosis and treatment of classical etiologies such as adhesions, endometriosis, or inflammatory pelvic disease. However, we have to keep in mind that "pain" is physically simply an electrical information transmitted by nerves to the central nervous system. Therefore, the fact that endometriosis or adhesions are painful does not mean that these lesions are in themselves painful but that they involve, in some form, nerves that create and transport this electrical information of "pain" to the central nervous system: trauma to the somatic pelvic nerves during surgery involving the lateral pelvic wall can lead to "somatic pelvic pain," while trauma to sympathetic nerves, especially those contained in the inferior hypogastric plexus (IHP), during radical pelvic surgery or nonradical procedures such as simple hysterectomies or prolapse surgery can induce chronic "visceral pelvic pain" (2,3).

Injury to nerves, which are predominantly composed of sensory fibers, yield three types of pain:

Neuroma pain: Pain that is triggered by pressure, irritation, or stimulation of the nerve at the site where it has been injured or divided. The stimulus causes an electrical current–like pain, which is localized by the patient in the distal zone of distribution of the injured nerve. This type of pain commences approximately six weeks after the nerve's injury, during which the neuroma develops. Consequently, the neuroma pain starts slowly and reaches a plateau weeks later.

Neuropathic pain: Pain that includes "hyperpathic pain" and "allodynia." Hyperpathic pain is a pain of unbearable intensity, which is felt on the skin or the anatomical structures (i.e., vagina and rectum) located in the distal distribution area of the injured nerve, when it is repeatedly stimulated, for example, as may be experienced during defecation or sexual intercourse.

Allodynia pain: Pain that is permanently present as a burning sensation, and that can be aggravated by an innocuous stimulus of the most distal region innervated by the injured nerve. For example, subsequent to the injury of the obturator nerve, during a lymphadenectomy, the patient may experience a burning sensation in the inner aspect of the thigh, which may become very severe by the simple rubbing of the two thighs.

This emphasizes the importance of obtaining a detailed history from the patient.

PRINCIPLES OF TREATING NEURAL PAIN

It is beyond discussion that the first step for the treatment of neural pain is not the symptomatic treatment but the etiologic treatment. For example, in cases of apparition of a neural somatic pain following a surgical procedure, the suspicion of a surgical lesion of the nerve justifies a surgical revision to remove, for example, a fibrosis, clip, suture, or mesh tying the suspected nerve responsible for the pain. This makes even more sense, as the earlier the treatment is carried out, the better the chances of success. It is well known that in nearly all cases of neural pain, the pain becomes chronic over a period of time and becomes memorized and encrusted in the central nervous system. Consequently, a "pain scar" develops in the brain, which then is extremely difficult to treat, and even more so when further factors such as pension application, invalidity application, or compensation for pain in the form of a judicial action intensifies the situation. However, even when the pain has become chronic, an etiologic therapy still makes sense. The aim is the complete disparition of the pain, but even a reduction in the pain, which results in the reduction of pain medication and therefore a reduction in the side effects, is of benefit to the patient.

From a neurosurgical perspective, three possibilities exist for the operative therapy of neuropathic neurotomy, neurolysis, and the neuromodulation. All of these techniques need the use of a microscope, or the magnification provided by the endoscope, to enable the gentle handling of nerve tissues, to avoid damaging them further. Nerves with loss of continuity or untreatable intraneural fibrosis will need to be reconstructed if possible.

Neurotomy—the transection of the nerve proximal to the primary nerve lesion—is in fact not a therapeutic option, as the majority of the pelvic somatic nerves are mixed nerves and therefore also have a motoric function. Furthermore, when a nerve is transected, additional to the sensory loss, the pain is initially gone, but through the formation of a recurrent neuroma, this pain inevitably returns after a few weeks or months. Neurolysis and interfascicular neurolysis—the releasing of the nerves—is in contrast a very effective method, especially when external factors such as fibrosis, endometriosis, sutures/clips, etc. aggravate the nerve. This option is the method of choice in the therapy of neural pain.

In axonal lesions, simple nerve decompression or neurolysis cannot improve the pain. A well-known method to control neural pain is then the use of electricity: neuromodulation. Neuromodulation refers to the stimulation of large afferent A-fibers of the peripheral nerves, which rapidly transport the low-energy electrical stimulus to the brain, reducing the impact of the pain input conveyed via the small unmyelinated and thinly myelinated C-fibers. Because the conduction velocity of A-fibers is much faster than that of the C-fibers, this process has the capacity to "gate out" pain stimuli from being transmitted to the cortex (4). The surgical procedure is designed to implant an electrode in contact to the injured nerve, which is connected to a pacemaker that produces continuous low-level electrical current. Such procedures require the precision afforded by the use of endoscopic access.

Until now, neuromodulation to control pelvic neuralgia has been limited to the implantation of a single electrode at a much higher level—at the level of either the spinal cord or the root of the sacral nerve by percutaneous, transforaminal implantation.

We developed the technique of laparoscopic implantation of neuroprothesis—LION procedure—to enable us to implant microelectrodes on the injured nerves immediately above the level of injury for selective neuromodulation (5). Laparoscopy is the only surgical access mode that enables the implantation of electrodes on all pelvic nerves and plexi, even on those placed deep in the pelvis and thus inaccessible with the use of classical techniques of implantation.

LAPAROSCOPIC ACCESS TO THE PELVIC NERVES

The most probable reason for the omission of the pelvic nerves in the field of the neurosurgery, but also in the field of the pelvic surgery, may be associated with the anatomy of the pelvic nervous system, which is difficult to understand, and the limitation of open surgery, which is inadequate to dissect pelvic nerves that are hidden deep in the retroperitoneal space behind the pelvic vessels. Thus, it is not at all surprising that the field of pelvic neurosurgery is not well developed. This limitation was overcome with the introduction of laparoscopy into the field of pelvic surgery, together with the development of videoendoscopy and microsurgical instruments, enabling good access to all areas of the retroperitoneal pelvic space, providing the necessary visibility and the possibility to work with appropriate instruments. This, in turn, has permitted a unique and reproducible surgical approach to all pelvic nerves that could never be achieved by classical open surgery (6). Due to the magnification offered by the laparoscope and the possibility of a bloodless dissection even in the deepest areas of the pelvis, laparoscopic surgery in the retroperitoneum is becoming one of the most useful and important instruments for learning the pelvic retroperitoneal anatomy. Laparoscopic surgery does not just incite the surgeon to learn pelvic anatomy but obliges him/her to do so: The combination of a good knowledge of pelvic neuroanatomy with the optimal magnification of the structures with the endoscope provides us the same quality of dissection as on cadaver, but we require less time as the tissues are fresh and all the structures have their natural aspect and color.

However, since a lot of nerves are located in the pelvis, confusion of the different nerves, especially at the level of the sacral plexus, can occur. To gain intraoperative information in regard to the motor function of the exposed nerves, we developed the new concept, the laparoscopic neuronavigation—LANN technique (7). During surgery, while exposed, the nerves are stimulated with a laparoscopic bipolar forceps, giving a current with a square-wave pulse duration of 250 microseconds, a pulse frequency of 35 Hz, and an electric potential varying between 1 and 12 V. For a successful intraoperative electrostimulation; myorelaxants must not be used as part of the general anesthesia. The stimulation of the pelvic somatic nerves induces motor muscle reactions, mostly visible to the naked eye.

The autonomous pelvic motor nerves—the pelvic splanchnic nerves—which are involved in visceral pelvic function originate from S2, S3, and S4/5; identification of these sacral nerve roots is of importance (Figs. 1 and 2). Stimulation of S3 nerves is confirmed visually by a deepening and flattening of the buttock groove, as well as a plantar flexion of the large toe and to a lesser extent of the smaller toes. Stimulation of S2 produces an outward rotation of the leg and plantar flexion of the foot, as well as a clamp-like squeeze of the anal sphincter from anterior to posterior (8). Neurostimulation of the splanchnic pelvic nerves is performed with the same bipolar forceps and the same current as for the stimulation of the sacral roots (Fig. 3): electrostimulation of the vesical nerves induces a contraction of the detrusor with a rise in the intrav esical pressure, while stimulation of the rectal parasympathetic nerves induce a contraction of the terminal rectosigmoid with an isolated rise in the intrarectal pressure (9). Stimulation of S2

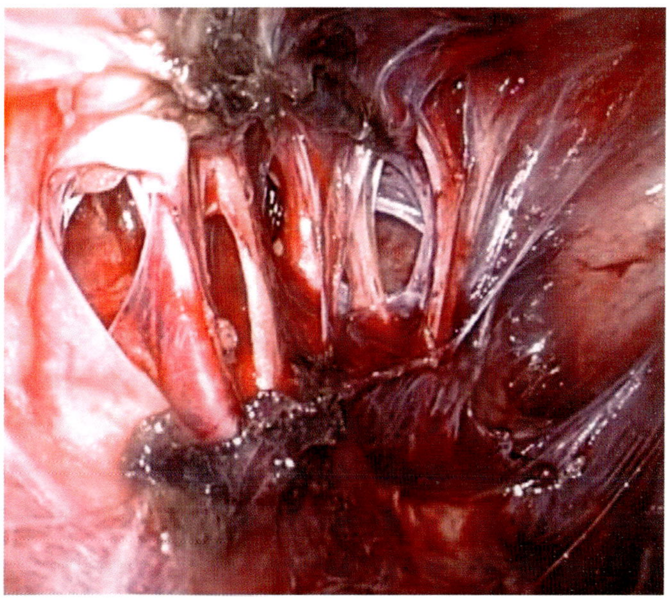

Figure 1 Laparoscopic exposure of the left sacral plexus (sacral nerve roots S1 to S4).

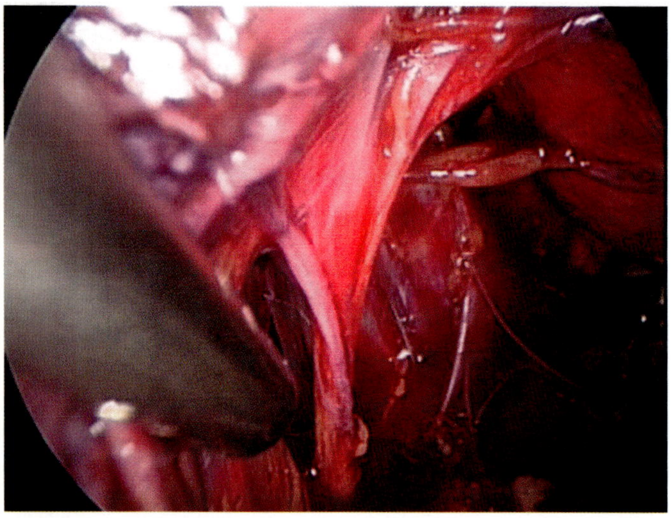

Figure 2 Laparoscopic exposure of the left sacral nerve root S4; the difference in color between the afferent and efferent fibers can be observed.

also induces a contraction of the gluteal muscles and, in men, an erection.

SOMATIC PELVIC PAIN

Symptoms

Somatic pelvic pain is pain due to damage to the pelvic somatic nerves, which are responsible for the innervation of the red muscles. In the pelvis, the somatic nerves are the sacral nerve roots, the sciatic nerve and its endopelvic branches (inferior and superior gluteal nerves), the pudendal nerve, and the obturatoric nerve. The management of lesions of these nerves responsible for neuropathic pelvic pain is frequently confusing for both patient and physician alike: gynecologists are not trained either in clinical and diagnostic neurology or in the techniques of neurosurgical procedures; on the other side, neurosurgeons and neurotraumatologists are not trained in pelvic surgery, especially in laparoscopic pelvic surgery, and are not acquainted with gynecologic diseases. Patients with neural pelvic pain frequently end up being referred from one specialist to another and subjected to a variety of different, but usually ineffective, treatments.

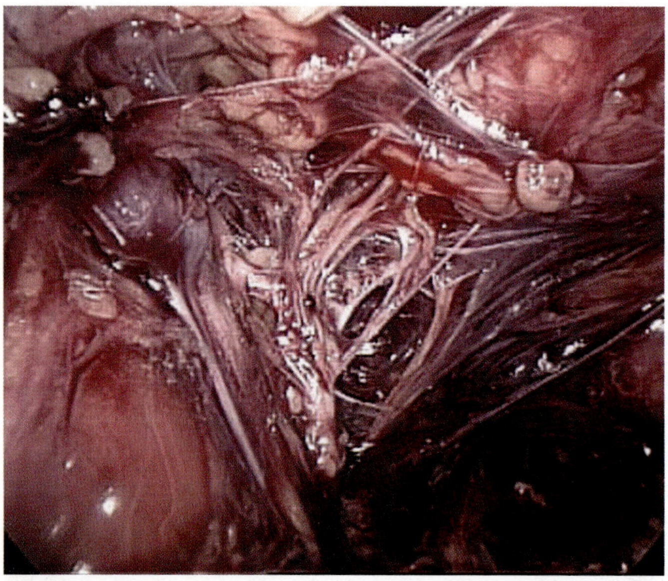

Figure 3 Laparoscopic exposure of the pelvic splanchnic nerve from S3 and S4 on the left side.

"Somatic pelvic pain" is a classical neuropathic pain and is described as a clearly located pain in a specific area of the pelvis with clearly defined irradiation in the perineal and/or perianal regions, or in the lower limb, according to the different well-known skin metameres. In the case of surgical damage, this pain usually appears directly after the procedure if a direct trauma of a nerve has occurred, but a lapse of six weeks is not unusual as postsurgical fibrosis can also lead to such pain.

The most frequent somatic pelvic pain is sciatica: this pain can be due to the irritation of the sciatic nerve itself or its roots (sacral radiculopathy), which causes a pain that starts low in the pelvis and shoots down the buttock and the leg. The second most frequent somatic pelvic pain is pudendal neuralgia: this pain is typically located in the genitoanal region; the intensity of the pain usually increases when the patient is sitting or riding a bicycle. The well-recognized Alcock's canal syndrome is also one of these entities (10). Lesions of the endopelvic portion of the pudendal nerve or a sacral radiculopathy, especially from S2 and S3, can also cause such perineal or perianal pain similar to a pudendal neuralgia, but without an increase in the pain in the sitting position (11).

Pelvic radiculopathy is usually combined with a different pain, depending on the anatomic level of the lesion: a radiculopathy of S2 is usually combined with perianal/perineal pain and with sciatica and/or pain in the teritorium of the posterior cutaneous nerve (as this nerve is a branch of the inferior gluteal nerve, its afferent fibers pass through S2). A radiculopathy of S3 and S4 also produces perianal/perineal pain but mostly combines disorders of the sensation of the bladder (similar to an interstitial cystitis) and sometimes difficulties of emptying the bladder and the rectum (constipation). The combination of different neuropathies is a strong argument in favor of lesions in the pelvis or above at the spinal cord. Bilateral pain is a strong argument for a lesion at the spinal cord but does not exclude a pelvic lesion.

Etiologies

In the largest series of somatic pelvic pain to date, we reported that endometriosis of the pelvic retroperitoneal space (12,13) and the postsurgical pelvic nerve damages (14) are the two most frequent causes of somatic pelvic pain, followed by vascular entrapment of the sacral nerve roots.

The most frequent etiology for somatic pelvic pain is surgical damage to the nerves during pelvic surgery. The most frequent injured somatic nerve after pelvic surgery is the second sacral nerve root, especially on the right side following anterior rectopexy and colposacro/promontofixation and on the left side following pexy of the sacrouterine ligaments. The second most frequent injury involves the sciatic nerve (left more frequently than right), especially after pelvic lymphadenectomy and surgical procedures for genital prolapse. The lesions of the sciatic nerve are mostly on its caudal border in the infrapyriform space, so that the pain is due to radiculopathy of S3 and S4, with the clinical combination of a partial sciatica, perianal and/or perineal pain, and occasionally neuralgia of the inferior gluteal nerve (S2). Motoric disorders are nearly always absent. Lesions of the inferior gluteal nerve are generally accompanied by lesions of the homolateral pudendal nerve and/or the sciatic nerve, while lesions of the superior gluteal nerve are mostly associated with lesions of the lumbosacral trunk and sometimes S1.

Since we started to report in meetings and in the international literature about the absolutely new option of laparoscopic management of pelvic nerve injuries, we have had increasing numbers of patients with "nongynecologic" indications such as pelvico-abdominal neuralgias secondary to radical prostatectomy, rectum surgery, prolapse and incontinence surgery, pelvic traumas, or pelvic radiotherapy referred to us for laparoscopic management. The significant increase in the number of such cases is certainly not due to the increase of their incidence but rather the increased awareness of the physicians about the existence of this condition and the potential of operative laparoscopy for its treatment.

The second most frequent etiology for pelvic somatic neuropathies is endometriosis. Endometriosis is able to infiltrate the parametrias until the pelvic sidewall and the infiltrate as well the sacral nerve roots and the sciatic nerve itself (Fig. 4). In this last situation, involvement of the sciatic nerve is mostly accompanied by a concomitant lesion of the obturator nerves, both gluteal nerves (especially the superior gluteal nerve), and occasionally the pudendal nerve. We also reported on isolated infiltrative endometriosis of the sciatic nerve without any further intra or retroperitoneal manifestation of endometriosis (Fig. 5): In women at a reproduction age, cyclical sciatica or other pelvic somatic neuropathia can be due to endometriosis even when CT scan/MRI of the pelvis are normal, and gynecologic examination and laparoscopic exploration of the pelvis do not show any endometriosis. Thus, in cyclical pelvic somatic pain, a laparoscopic retroperitoneal exposure of the suspected nerves is mandatory (13).

Other, less frequent conditions can also induce pelvic somatic neuropathia: vascular entrapment (Fig. 6), retroperitoneal fibrosis (idiopathic or secondary), but also axonal lesions such that are known to exist in patients with multiple sclerosis or other neurogenic neuropathies.

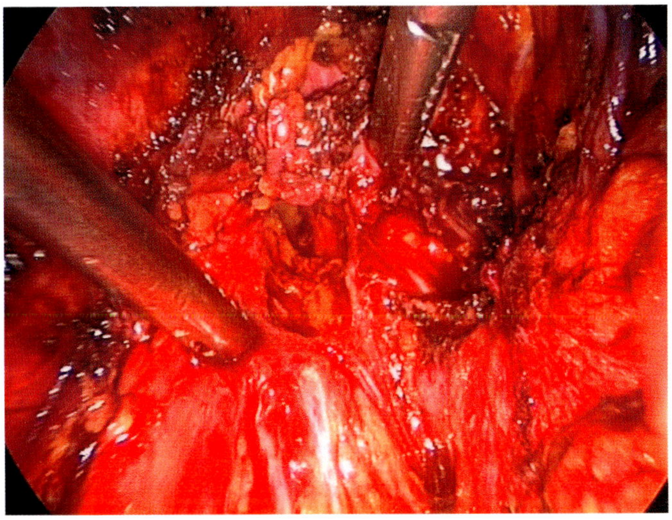

Figure 5 Laparoscopic resection of an isolated endometrioma in the middle of the sciatic nerve.

Treatments

In patients with such "somatic pelvic pain," operative laparoscopy is an effective approach to both the diagnosis and the treatment of the condition. Classic neurosurgical techniques of nerve decompression or intrafascicular neurolysis can be performed by laparoscopic access (15). If during laparoscopic exposure of the suspected nerve no pathology to the somatic nerves can be determined, a neural electrode is placed on the nerve for postoperative neuromodulation (Fig. 7).

By far more difficult procedures are the neurolysis of the sacral nerve roots after sacro-/promontopexy procedures with mesh material. In laparoscopic management of these, it is imperative to preoperatively estimate the potential location of the lesion, in order to orient the surgical dissection and

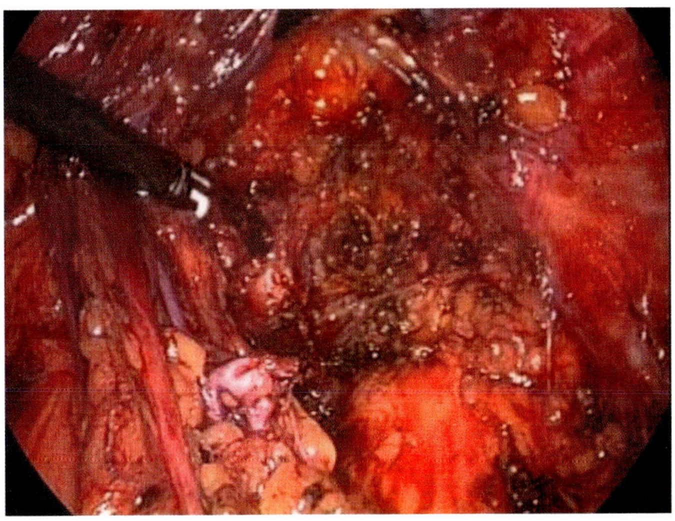

Figure 4 End result after neurolysis of the right sciatic nerve and resection of the entire obturator muscle and partial resection of the pyriform muscle.

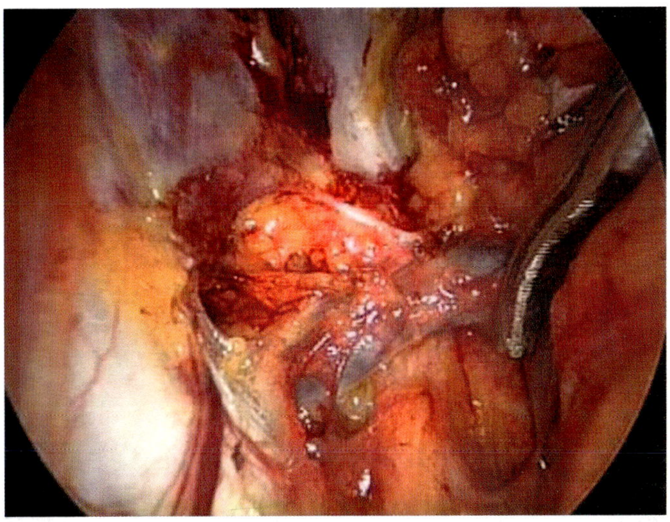

Figure 6 A young women suffering from a sciatica on the left side: laparoscopic exposure of the sciatic nerve shows an atypical superior gluteal vein, which was crossing over the sciatic nerve, and causing pressure on it. After bipolar coagulation and transection of the vein, pain was relieved completely.

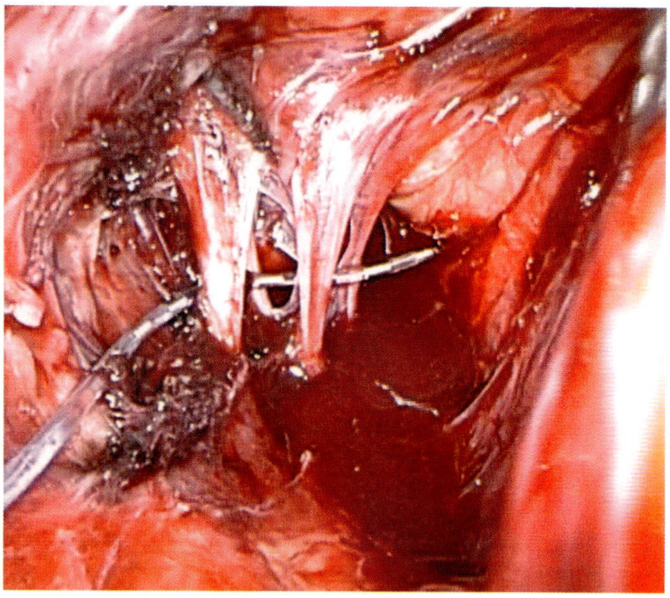

Figure 7 A multiple channel electrode is placed on the sacral nerves roots.

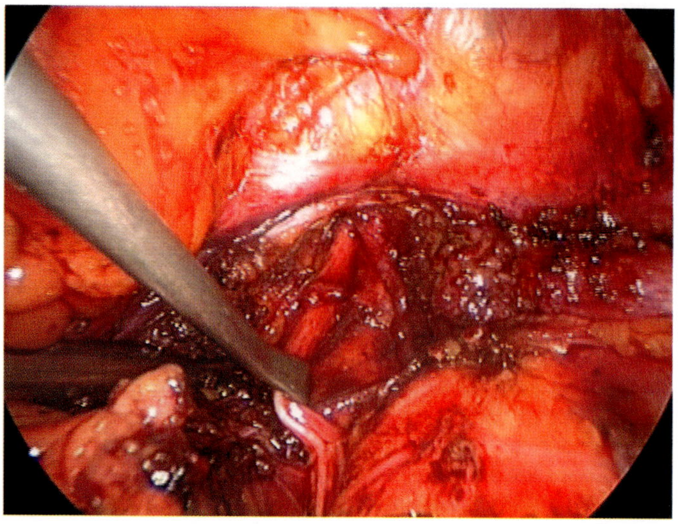

Figure 8 Laparoscopic transperitoneal neurolysis of the right pudendal nerve until the Alcock's canal.

avoid unnecessary exposure of the pelvic nerves not involved in the pathology. Patients are generally able to describe a precise location of the pain, but it is not evident that the stimulus that produces the pain is located where the patient describes it. An absolute knowledge of clinical neurology is mandatory to establish a clear neurologic diagnosis of which kind of neuralgia the patient is suffering from. An absolute knowledge of pelvic surgery is also essential in order to know which nerves in which areas of the pelvis could be injured during which surgery. Only the synthesis of all these considerations permits an optimal diagnosis of the neural lesion. All our laparoscopic approaches to pelvic somatic neuralgia secondary to pelvic surgery is based on this principle, and the combination of different neuralgias makes the neurologic diagnosis even more difficult but permits a more precise estimation of the exact location of the neural lesion.

In a series of 134 consecutive patients of laparoscopic management of pudendal pain (experienced in the perineal and perianal regions) who underwent laparoscopic approach to the sacral plexus (radiculopathy as the etiology) and/or to the pudendal nerve (Alcock's canal syndrome and other pudendal neuralgia) (11), neurosurgical procedures, such as decompression of nerves or implantation of electrodes to the sacral plexus for neuromodulation—"sacral LION procedure," were performed in all patients by laparoscopic transperitoneal approach. In 18 patients with Alcock's canal syndrome, subsequent to sacrospinal fixation for vaginal prolapse, laparoscopic decompression with transposition of the nerve resulted in disappearance of pain in 15 [mean follow-up was 21 months ($\pm$7.04, range 6–34 months)] (Fig. 8). Of the three patients who had no improvement, one had a subsequent LION procedure that produced significant improvement. The other 109 patients had endopelvic lesions, which also affected the root of the sacral nerve. Laparoscopic neurolysis of the sacral nerve root was performed in addition to the surgical excision of the diseased tissues. Fifty-three of these had postsurgical nerve damage. A reduction of pain of at least 50% was obtained [visual analog scale (VAS) score] in 62% of the patients (follow-up mean 17 months, range 3–39 months) (Fig. 9). Fifty had endometriosis. A reduction of pain of at least 50% was obtained (VAS score) in 78% of the patients (mean follow-up 21 months, range 2–42 months). All six patients with vascular entrapment were cured. The remaining seven had a LION procedure for pain resulting from various etiologies. In six patients, the outcome was satisfactory (11).

In a series of 113 patients with neural pain resulting from surgical trauma to various pelvic somatic nerves, significant improvement was obtained in 65.5% of them subsequent to neurolysis ($n = 98$) and LION's procedure ($n = 15$) (14). Therefore, in somatic pelvic pain secondary to pelvic surgery, we strongly believe that laparoscopy must be considered in the first-line management before medical treatment and as soon as possible after the surgical procedure before memory of pain is incrusted on the central nervous system.

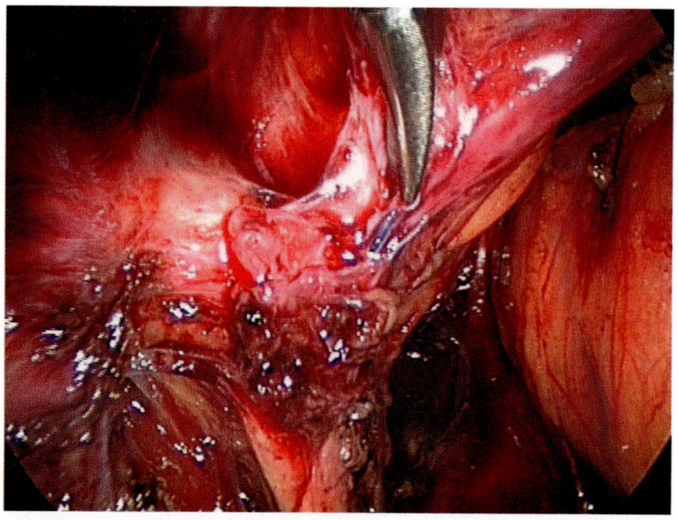

Figure 9 Laparoscopic exposure of S2 in the patient with a pudendal pain: a suture to S2 could be found and removed.

VISCERAL PELVIC PAIN

Symptoms

"Visceral pelvic pain" is due to a lesion of the IHP. This pain is usually located in the entire lower abdomen and is described as vague, poorly localized, and dull in nature—a sensation of pressure rather than real pain, usually with a symptom-free interval after the surgical procedure. This pain is very often associated with vegetative symptoms such as nausea, vomiting, pallor, diaphoresis, and tachycardia. Thus, visceral pelvic pain is similar to the usual pelvic pain well known in endometriosis patients; however, it is quite permanent during the cycle, with paroxysm during menstrual bleeding but without any improvement either by hormonal therapy or by resection of the pelvic adhesions or endometriosis. It also frequent that, in such pain, laparoscopic inspection of the pelvis does not permit identification of any pathology able to explain the pain. Typical for neuralgia of the IHP, the patients presented with apparition from one minute to the next of a well-located unilateral perianal pain described as an "electrical pain" (sometimes with irradiation to the gluteal region of the dorsal aspect of the thigh), mostly with a sensation of strong anal cramps. The patients are then not able to either sit or walk because of this pain, and pressure on the point of the pain can sometime improve the pain. This pain usually disappears after few minutes, sometimes hours. Usual painkillers such as nonsteroidal anti-inflammatory medications do not improve this pain.

Treatment

In this "visceral pelvic pain," our therapy concept is based on the blockade of the sympathetic afferent pathways coming from the IHP using neuromodulation. If during laparoscopic exploration of the pelvis, any "nonpostoperative" pathology of the nerves such as endometriosis or adhesions is found, surgical treatment of these lesions is performed. In patients where no etiology can be found, laparoscopic full exposure of the superior hypogastric plexus (SHP) between the level of the inferior mesenteric artery and the aortic bifurcation is performed and then a multiple channel electrode is placed surrounding the entire SHP (Fig. 10). The electrode used is a multiple-channel electrode, and systematic fixation is performed with a nonresorbable suture 5.0, while the cable is passed extraperitoneally under the descending colon avoiding any contact with the left ureter before connecting it to an external test stimulator. The decision to implant a permanent stimulator is made after a test phase of external electrostimulation over several days, with alternative switching "off" and "on," to gain objective efficacy or not of the neuromodulation.

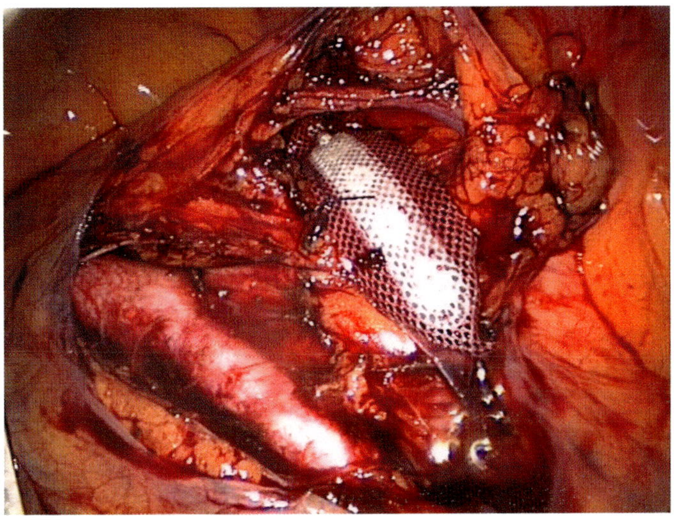

Figure 10 Electrode placed on the superior hypogastric plexus in place.

In visceral pelvic pain secondary to (radical) hysterectomy or excisional surgery of the parametria, the pain occurred from lesions of the IHP, which can be considered as "pelvic phantom pain" and may be due to the development of neuromas of the IHP comparable with phantom stump pain following lower extremity amputation. However, in order to try to surgically find pelvic neuromas in the IHP even by laparoscopy is utopic; destruction of this plexus is not an option as it is involved in the important pelvic visceral reflexes (16), and blockade of all afferent pathways is also very difficult as there are five major autonomic pathways that can transmit nociceptive information (17). Information may also not necessarily follow just one pathway, and high stimuli may result in the activation of neighboring unmyelinated fibers originating from a different site so that a blockade of just one particular pathway is most unlikely to provide complete pain relief. Thus, the aim of the blockade is to try to block the most possible amount of pathways involved in pain transmission. As the IHP is composed of three different functional levels as we have previously demonstrated (7), the kind of injured afferent sympathetic fibers and consequently the site of the blockade of afferent pathways could depend on the level of the lesion on the plexus: in lesions of the first segment (upper third)—as in simple hysterectomy—the injury will affect the majority of the afferent fibers passing through both inferior hypogastric nerves and thereafter the SHP. In lesions affecting the second segment of the IHP, injuries of the sympathetic fibers contained in the first segment will be associated with lesions of the sympathetic fibers joining the sympathetic trunks, so that pain is generally associated with a sensation of fullness of the rectum or the bladder. A lesion of the lower third of the IHP, as in a radical hysterectomy or deep anterior rectum resection, will affect the pelvic splanchnic nerves. These nerves are branches from the anterior rami of the sacral nerve roots S2, S3, and S4/5 and contain the pelvic parasympathetic nerves so that their bilateral destruction induces systematic atonia of the bladder and of the rectum (18,19). Thus, in patients with suspected elective lesions of the first and/or the second segments of the plexus as in a simple hysterectomy, plastic or resection of the sacrouterine ligaments, we electively blocked the SHP: different surgical (20) and chemical (21) blockades of the SHP have been reported in literature, but all these techniques are destructive and irreversible. We opted for a more expensive but reversible and nondestructive method, the LION procedure for neuromodulation to the SHP. This laparoscopic technique does not require extensive dissection, and the entire plexus can be covered with just one multiple-channel electrode.

In the previously mentioned publication (14), we reported on seven patients with visceral pelvic pain who underwent a LION procedure to the SHP for visceral pelvic pain after previous pelvic surgery. Four of them reported a significant reduction in the symptoms under neuromodulation of the SHP.

In more caudal lesions of the parametrias involving the lower third of the IHP, blockade of the pelvic splanchnic nerves can be obtained by a LION procedure to the sacral nerve roots

S2, S3, and S4/5 directly after their emergence out of the sacral foramens with just one multiple channel.

In conclusion, laparoscopy is a unique method for diagnosis and therapeutic management of surgically damaged nerves and must be considered as a first-line option in the treatment of pelvic somatic pain, while, in regard to the management of pelvic visceral pain, medical treatment remains the first-line treatment.

NEUROPATHY/NEURALGIA OF THE PELVIC AND ABDOMINAL NERVES (ILIOINGUINAL/GENITOFEMORAL/LATERAL CUTANEOFEMORAL NERVES)

Lesions of the ilioinguinal, iliohypogastric, genitofemoral, or lateral cutaneofemoral nerves can occasionally occur; the classical lesion is that of the genitofemoral nerve during lymphadenectomy. The most frequent lesions occur within the pelvic and abdominal wall: lesions of the genitofemoral nerve and/or of the ilioinguinal nerve occur in 2% of the surgeries for inguinal hernias. A further classical situation causing a lesion of this nerve is during laparoscopy, when the lower abdominal trocars are introduced laterally, too distant from the epigastric vessels.

Techniques for neurolysis of the nerves within the pelvico-abdominal wall does not provide good results, as their exposure inside the wall is extremely difficult and, in cases of axonal lesion of the nerve, simple neurolysis does not improve the pain. Neuromodulation is also an alternative, but the implantation of an electrode onto these nerves in the abdominal cavity requires extensive dissection. For this reason, less invasive percutaneous or subcutaneous implant techniques were developed, but the electrodes are placed bluntly and result in unspecific implantation (22). When pain relief is not obtained, it is uncertain whether this is due to the nerve not responding to electromodulation or a nonstimulation of the nerve because of wrong placement of the electrode.

Laparoscopy offers an optimal minimal invasive approach to all these nerves without requiring extensive dissection. Before hiding in the pelvico-abdominal wall, all these nerves run into the abdominal cavity (extraperitoneally) on the surface of deeply placed muscles (iliopsoas muscle). Laparoscopy permits the placement of electrodes for neuromodulation at exactly this level in direct contact with the nerves and consequently proximal to the level of the neural lesion—a condition necessary for successful neuromodulation in painful neuralgia (Figs. 11–13) (5).

The advantages of the LION procedure in comparison to the classical alternative, which is a neurotomy, are the following: (1) there is no additional sensory loss and (2) there is no risk of inducing a neuropathic pain or increasing the level of the pre-existing pain.

To date, we have performed the LION procedure in 14 consecutive patients. The VAS was reduced more than 80% in 11 of the patients, and the other 3 had a pain reduction between 50% and 80%. The follow-up period varied between three months and three years (23).

FURTHER APPLICATIONS OF THE LAPAROSCOPIC APPROACH TO THE PELVIC NERVES

"Laparoscopic Nerve-Sparing Pelvic Surgery"

Based on our findings using this LANN technique during laparoscopic radical pelvic surgery for gynecologic cancer or for deep infiltrating endometriosis of the retroperitoneal space, we elaborated a functional cartography of the IHP. We demonstrated that this plexus is not an anarchic patchwork of sympathetic and parasympathetic neural fibers, as it is always reported in literature, and that, in fact, it has three distinct functional levels (5). The upper part is constituted of sympathetic fibers coming from both inferior hypogastric nerves, which are responsible for the wetness of the vagina and the different feeling to the cervix and the vagina (pain/sexuality). More caudally of these fibers, the anastomoses sprouting out of both sympathetic trunks anastomose with the plexus and are responsible for the sensation of fullness of the bladder and the rectum. Sprouting much deeper from the sacral nerve roots S2 and mainly from S3 and S4/5, the parasympathetic nerves (autonomous motor fibers destined for the bladder, rectum, and sexual organs) lie upward to the pelvic plexus and anastomose to it just caudally and laterally of the precedent sympathetic nerves (Fig. 14).

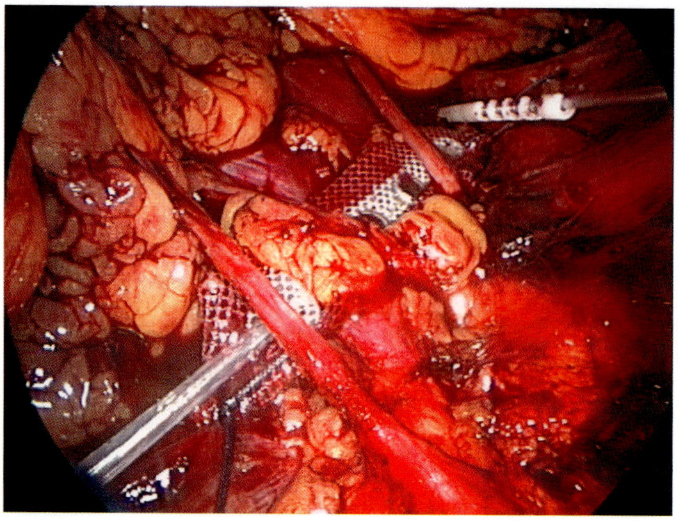

Figure 11 Electrode placed on the ilioinguinal and iliohypogastric nerves.

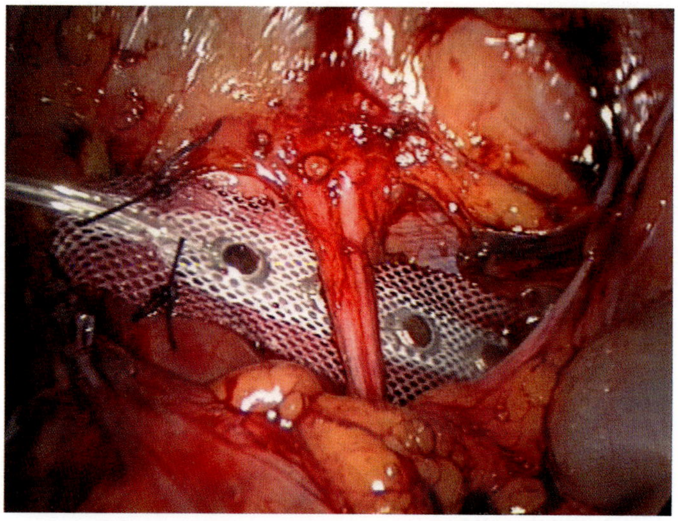

Figure 12 Electrode placed on the right genitofemoral nerve.

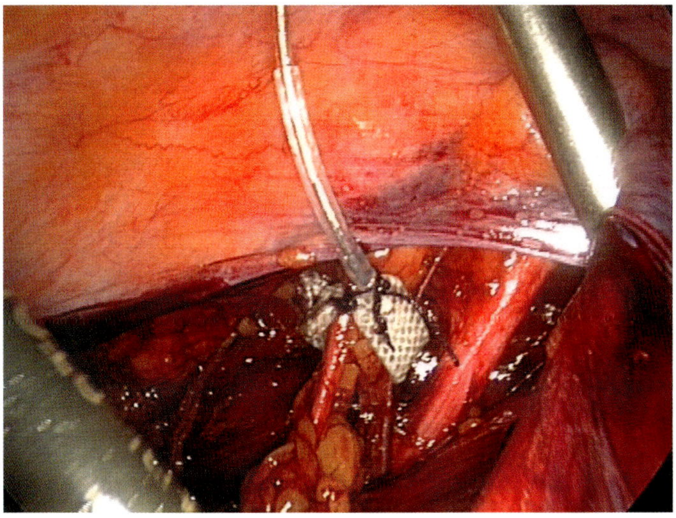

Figure 13 Electrode in place on the left lateral femoral cutaneous nerve.

Based on these findings about the functional pelvic neuroanatomy, we have developed the technique of "laparoscopic splanchnic nerves sparing radical pelvic surgery." This technique is not based on the sparing of the ligaments or pelvic compartments that contain the motor autonomic pelvic nerves, but on the elective exposure of the pelvic parasympathetic nerves, starting at their emergence out of the sacral nerve roots S2, S3, and S4/5 to their anastomosis in the IHP, and not during but before the transection or resection of the parametria is performed. In a prospective series of 163 consecutive patients who underwent a laparoscopic-assisted vaginal radical hysterectomy (Piver 3 radicality) for cervical cancer and 91 further consecutive patients who had a laparoscopic deep anterior rectum resection/anastomosis for deep infiltrating endometriosis of the rectum, we reported a very significant reduction in the rate of postoperative bladder dysfunction—to less than 1% (24) compared to a rate of up to 40% reported in the literature (25).

Therefore, the classical functional morbidities of radical pelvic surgery can no longer be accepted as common side effects of the procedure, and appropriate knowledge of the neurofunctional anatomy of the pelvis must become mandatory for all surgeons involved in radical pelvic surgery (rectum resection, radical prostectomy, etc.)

The LION Procedure to Control or Restore Pelvic Nerve Functions

The LION procedure has been used to control or recover neurologic pelvic functions (5). The technique of sacral nerve root neuromodulation to treat sphincter dysfunction is well established, but the LION procedure is the only one that permits the implantation of a single electrode, placed tangentially to the entire sacral plexus, and the neuromodulation of all sacral nerves roots together or separately (Fig. 15). Thus, this has opened a new approach to the control of bladder atonia or incontinence (after radical pelvic surgery such as radical rectum resection or radical prostatectomy, surgery for cauda equine). It has also been applied successfully to detrusor hyperactivity or detrusor-urethral-sphincter dyssynergy in patients with interstitial cystitis, diabetic cystopathy, multiple sclerosis, Parkinson disease, and spina bifida and in completely paralyzed patients following spinal cord injury (26).

Our group has performed the first reported laparoscopic implantation of a Finetech–Brindley bladder controller onto the endopelvic sacral nerve roots in a Th8 completely paralyzed woman for recovery of bladder and rectum function (Fig. 16) (27). Since then, the LION procedure to the pelvic nerves has enabled control of the bladder overactivity, without requiring a dorsal deafferentation and the severing of any nerves in paralyzed patients, but also electrical-induced micturition, defecation, erection, and ejaculation. The laparoscopic approach to the pelvic nerves has clear advantages in paralyzed patients, as it avoids the classical laminectomy with risk of meningitis, encephalitis, and/or liquor leakage.

This approach represents the only option for implantation of electrodes to control bladder function in children with spina bifida, as the dorsal approach is generally not feasible. Laparoscopy also offers a selective approach to all pelvic

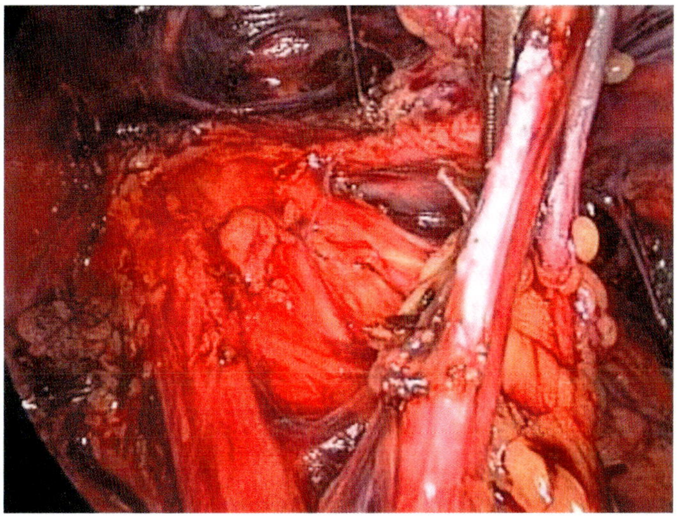

Figure 14 The sacral plexus.

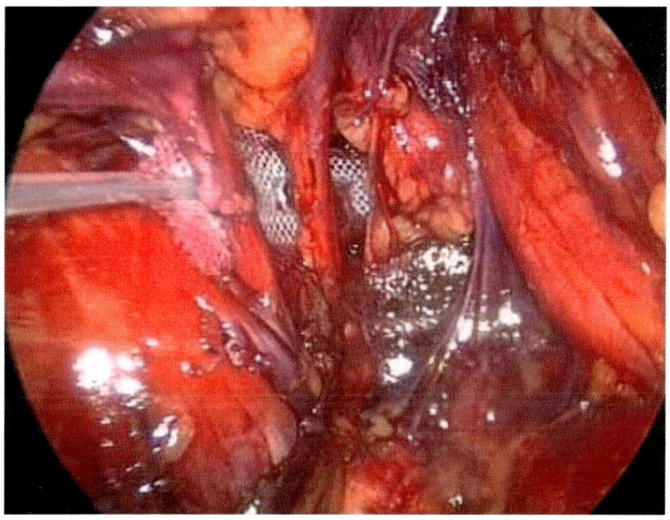

Figure 15 Electrode placed perpendicularly to the sacral nerve roots S2 to S4/5.

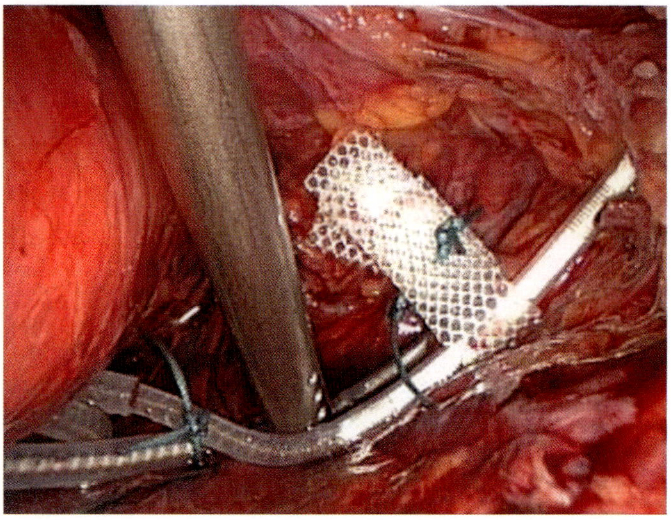

Figure 16 Brindley electrode in place to the right sacral nerve root S2.

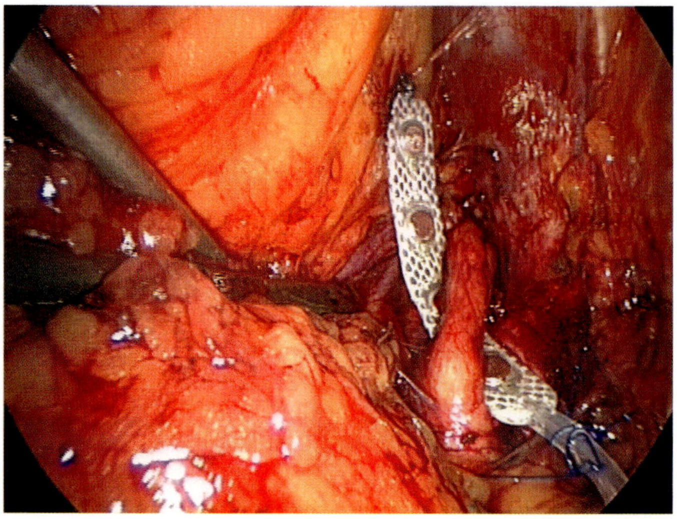

Figure 17 Electrode placed on the right sciatic nerve.

somatic nerves involved in the motion of the lower extremities; options for selective laparoscopic implantation of neural electrodes to these nerves can/will open new paths to recover locomotion in paralyzed patients.

Other Applications

The LION procedure has been successfully employed in nongynecologic applications such as treatment of stump residual pain and phantom pain after amputation of the lower limb(s).

Phantom limb pain following surgical amputation of a limb may be associated with a sensation that the amputated limb is still attached to the body. Phantom pain in a limb that no longer exists is common following amputation and affects 50% to 80% of all amputees (28).

The LION procedure now offers a new therapeutic option, the option of elective neuromodulation of the entire sciatic nerve: We reported on our technique of LION procedure to the sciatic nerve for the treatment of stump residual pain and phantom pain in 14 consecutive patients; significant reduction in pain in about 70% of patients was obtained, with follow-up varying between three years and few months (Fig. 17) (29).

The LION procedure has also been used in the treatment of polyneuropathy of the lower limbs. Polyneuropathy is the deterioration, degeneration, or breakdown of multiple nerves. There are many causes for painful polyneuropathies. The most common cause is diabetes; other causes include intoxication from chemotherapy, drugs, alcohol abuse, and AIDS. However, in up to one-third of patients, no underlying cause can be found.

We have had the opportunity to perform the procedure in four patients, with variable results depending strongly on the origin of the polyneuropathy.

CONCLUSION

The neuropelveology is a branch of medicine specializing in the disorders of the nerves of the pelvis and/or in the pelvic disorders that involve and/or disturb the pelvic nerves. Thus, this new specialty deals with pelvic diseases such as endometriosis, tumors, trauma resulting from surgery or radiotherapy, other conditions that disturb the pelvic nerves in their function and/or induce neural pain, and pathologic conditions of the nerves themselves such as multiple sclerosis, spinal cord injury, or spina bifida.

The aims of surgical treatment are (1) to spare the nerves during the intervention in order to preserve sexuality, bladder and intestinal functions, etc., (2) microsurgical neurolysis and reanastomosis of transected nerves, and (3) precise application of microelectrodes for neuromodulation in order to control neural pain, neurogenic visceral dysfunction such as bladder and bowel dysfunction associated with multiple sclerosis, and recovery of function as in paralyzed subjects.

It is evident that this field encroaches upon several medical specialties and requires those who practice it to acquire the necessary anatomical, clinical, and surgical expertise.

REFERENCES

1. Walker EA, Katon WJ. The prevalence of chronic pain and irritable bowel syndrome in two university clinics. J Psychosom Obstet Gynaecol 1991; 12:66.
2. Lowenstein L, Dooley Y, Kenton K, et al. Neural pain after uterosacral ligament vaginal suspension. Int Urogynecol J Pelvic Floor Dysfunct 2007; 18:109–110.
3. Brandsborg B, Nikolajsen L, Hansen CT, et al. Risk factors for chronic pain after hysterectomy: A nationwide questionnaire and database study. Anesthesiology 2007; 106:1003–1012.
4. Melzack R, Wall P. Pain mechanisms: A new theory. Science 1965; 150:971–979.
5. Possover M, Baekelandt J, Chianteras V. The laparoscopic implantation of neuroprothesis – LION technique – to control intractable abdomino-pelvic neuralgia. Neuromodulation 2007; 10:18–23.
6. Possover M. Laparoscopic exposure and electrostimulation of the somatic and autonomous pelvic nerves: A new method for implantation of neuroprothesis in paralysed patients? J Gynecol Surg Endosc Imaging Allied Tech 2004; 1:87–90.
7. Possover M, Rhiem K, Chiantera V. The "laparoscopic neuro-navigation" – LANN: From a functional cartography of the pelvic autonomous neurosystem to a new field of laparoscopic surgery. Minim Invasive Ther Allied Technol 2004; 13:362–367.

8. Brindley GS, Polkey CE, Rushton DN, et al. Sacral anterior root stimulators for bladder control in paraplegia: The first 50 cases. J Neurol Neurosurg Psychiatry 1986; 49:1104–1114.
9. Possover M, Chiantera V, Baekelandt J. Anatomy of the sacral roots and the pelvic splanchnic nerves in women using the LANN technique. Surg Laparosc Endosc Percutan Tech 2007; 17(6):508–510.
10. Amarenco G, Savatosky I, Budet C, et al. Nevralgies perineales et syndrome du canal éAlcock. Ann Urol (Paris) 1989; 6:488–492.
11. Possover M. Laparoscopic management of endopelvic etiologies of pudendal pain in 134 consecutive patients. J Urol 2009; 181:1732–1736.
12. Possover M, Baekelandt J, Flaskamp C, et al. Laparoscopic neurolysis of the sacral plexus and the sciatic nerve for extensive endometriosis of the pelvic wall. Minim Invasive Neurosurg 2007; 50(1):33–36.
13. Possover M, Chiantera V. Isolated infiltrative endometriosis of the sciatic nerve: About three cases. Fertil Steril 2007; 87(2):417–419.
14. Possover M. Laparoscopic management of neural pelvic pain in women secondary to pelvic surgery. Fertil Steril 2009; 91:2720–2725.
15. Possover M, Baekelandt J, Chiantera V. The laparoscopic approach to control intractable pelvic neuralgia: From laparoscopic pelvic neurosurgery to the LION technique. Clin J Pain 2007; 36–45.
16. Cervero F. Sensory innervation of the viscera: Peripheral basis of visceral pain. Physiol Rev 1994; 74:95.
17. Bosscher H. Blockade of the superior hypogastric plexus block for visceral pelvic pain. Pain Pract 2001; 2:162–170.
18. Low JA, Mauger GM, Carmichael JA. The effect of Wertheim hysterectomy upon bladder and urethral function. Am J Obstet Gynecol 1981; 139:826–834.
19. Barnes W, Waggoner S, Delgado G, et al. Manometric characterization of rectal dysfunction following radical hysterectomy. Gynecol Oncol 1998; 42:116–119.
20. Soysal ME, Soysal S, Gurses E, et al. Laparoscopic presacral neurolysis for endometriosis-related pelvic pain. Hum Reprod 2003; 18:588–592.
21. Gamal G, Helaly M, Labib YM. Superior hypogastric block: Transdiscal versus classic posterior approach in pelvic pain. Clin J Pain 2006; 22:544–547.
22. Lawrence W, Stinson LW, Roderer GT, et al. Peripheral subcutaneous electrostimulation for control of intractable post-operative inguinal pain: A case report series. Neuromodulation 2001; 3:99–104.
23. Possover M. The LION procedure for treatment postsurgical damages of the iliohypogastric nerve, the ilioinguinal nerve, the lateral cutaneous nerve and of the genitofemoral nerve. Am J Neurosurg, in press.
24. Possover M, Quakernack J, Chiantera V. The "LANN-technique" to reduce the postoperative functional morbidity in laparoscopic radical pelvic surgery. J Am Coll Surg 2005; 6:913–917.
25. Junginger T, Kneist W, Heintz A. Influence of identification and preservation of pelvic autonomic nerves in rectal cancer surgery on bladder dysfunction after total mesorectal excision. Dis Colon Rectum 2003; 46:621–628.
26. Possover M. The laparoscopic implantation of neuroprothesis to the sacral plexus for therapy of neurogenic bladder dysfunctions after failure of percutaneous sacral nerve stimulation. Neuromodulation, in press.
27. Possover M, Baekelandt J, Kaufmann A, et al. Laparoscopic endopelvic sacral implantation of a Brindley controller for recovery of bladder function in a paralyzed patient. Spinal Cord 2008; 46(1):70–73.
28. Postone N. Phantom limb pain: A review. Int J Psychiatry Med 1987; 17:57–70.
29. Possover M. The laparoscopic implantation of neuroprothesis to the sciatic nerve to control residual stump pain and phantom pain after lower limb amputation. J Neurol Urodynamics, in press.

19

Leiomyoma and infertility

Elizabeth L. Taylor, Elizabeth A. Pritts, William H. Parker, and David L. Olive

HISTORY

Uterine fibroids or leiomyomas are a common, benign disease of the uterus. The earliest accurate description of uterine fibroids was provided by Reinier De Graff (1641–1673). He described uterine fibroids as sharply circumscribed, firm, white tumors that can vary in size from tiny nodules to large tumors that fill the pelvis. The average affected uterus exhibits six to seven fibroids, which can range in size from 10 mm to over 20 cm (1). Fibroids can be found protruding into the uterine cavity (submucosal), within the uterine wall (intramural), beneath the uterine serosa (subserosal), and in rare instances attached to abdominopelvic structures (parasitic).

Uterine fibroids can cause considerable symptoms: menorrhagia, dysmenorrhea, pelvic pressure, bowel and bladder symptoms, and infertility. Historically, symptomatic fibroids were treated with hysterectomy. The first hysterectomy for the management of uterine fibroids occurred in 1843. Charles Clay (1801–1893) of Manchester, United Kingdom, started what he expected to be his fifth successful oophorectomy. After he had opened the abdomen, the patient coughed and a large fibroid uterus was extruded through the incision, which he was unable to replace. He was forced to perform the first subtotal abdominal hysterectomy, in the midst of "great hemorrhage," and the patient succumbed shortly after the operation (2). The first planned hysterectomy for uterine fibroids was carried out by John Bellinger (1804–1860) of South Carolina, United States, in 1846. Unfortunately, the patient died of sepsis on the fifth postoperative day (3).

Since the 19th century, numerous refinements in anesthesia and surgery have permitted women with fibroids to be managed such that their fertility may be preserved. This chapter summarizes the anatomic features, clinical presentation, and management options of uterine fibroids, focusing on the infertile woman.

PATHOLOGY

On histological examination, the fibroid is composed of well-differentiated whorled bundles of smooth muscle cells that resemble normal myometrium. Characteristically, the individual smooth muscle cells are uniform in shape and size and have a long, slender, spindle-like cytoplasmic process. The nuclei are elongated with tapered ends. Mitotic figures are infrequent (Fig. 1) (4).

Several molecular techniques have demonstrated that fibroids are a proliferation of a single clone of smooth muscle cells. Each one of the multiple fibroids in a particular uterus appears to be a distinct clone (5–7). Approximately 40% of fibroids have chromosomal abnormalities detectable by conventional cytogenetic analysis (8). The other 60% of fibroids are chromosomally normal, suggesting that genetic aberrations may be subchromosomal for these tumors. The most prevalent types of chromosomal rearrangements include the translocation t(12;14)(q14–q15;q23–q24), rearrangement of 6p21, and the deletion del (q22q32) (7). The variety of these aberrations implies that multiple genetic mechanisms may exist in fibroid development (9). The relevance of cytogenetic abnormalities to fibroid diagnosis or treatment remains to be determined.

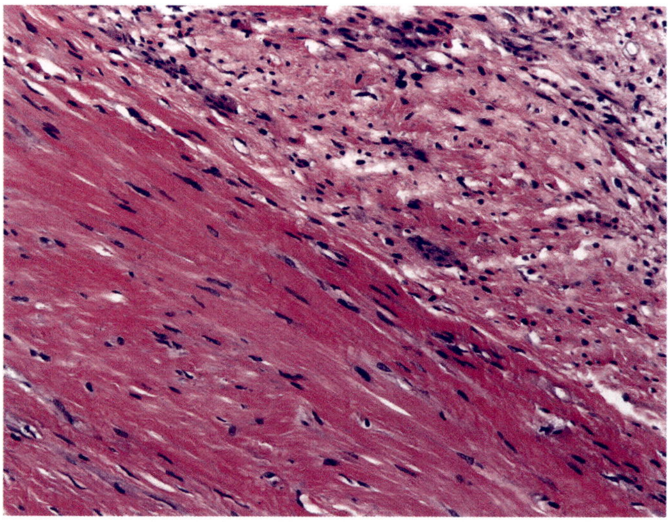

Figure 1 H&E stain of uterine myoma.

Fibroids grow under the influence of local growth factors: cytokines and sex hormones, including estrogen and progesterone (10,11). Originally, estrogen was the major sex steroid hormone held responsible for fibroid growth; however, newer data suggest that progesterone may also play a role (12). During the follicular phase of the menstrual cycle, estrogen is known to increase expression of genes associated with fibroid growth, but in the luteal phase of the cycle, progesterone has been shown to increase the mitotic activity of fibroids, particularly in premenopausal women (13,14). In addition, both selective estrogen and selective progesterone receptor modulators decrease the growth of uterine fibroids (15). It appears that estrogen and progesterone act in conjunction to promote fibroid growth.

EPIDEMIOLOGY

The prevalence of uterine fibroids varies with age, race, and diagnostic modality. In a random sample of U.S. women, aged 35 to 49 years, the cumulative incidence of fibroids by the age of 50 years was >80% for black women and approaching 70% for white women, as diagnosed by a review of surgical specimens and/or ultrasonography (16). Further, African-American women have been shown to have an earlier age of fibroid diagnosis, larger and more abundant tumors, higher hysterectomy rate for fibroids, and more severe symptoms (16–19).

In three European cohort studies, there was a lower prevalence of fibroids than in those examining U.S. populations. A German cohort study found 10.7% of women of mean age 40 years reported being diagnosed with a fibroid (20). An Italian cohort study found 21.4% of women, aged 30 to 60 years, with a uterus had ultrasonographically detectable fibroids (21), while a Swedish study found only 7.8% of women, between 33 and 40 years of age, had ultrasonographically detectable fibroids (22).

In a controlled study of 1585 women undergoing laparoscopic tubal ligation, the prevalence of fibroids observed at the time of surgery was 9% in Caucasian women and 16% in African-American women. Several risk factors for the presence of fibroids include age 40 to 44 years, more than 4 years since last delivery, menstrual cycle length of >30 days, and menstrual bleeding for more than 5 days (23).

Several other risk factors for the development and growth of fibroids have been identified (24,25). They are more commonly seen in women with earlier age of menarche, and postmenopausal women have a 70% to 90% reduction in risk.

Fibroids have been shown to cluster within families, suggesting a genetic basis of disease development. Familial aggregation studies have observed that first-degree relatives are more likely to develop fibroids (26). A U.S. study observed that first-degree relatives of women with fibroids are 2.5 times more at risk of developing fibroids as compared with women without affected relatives. This risk increases to 5.7 for women with an affected first-degree relative of less than 45 years old (25). A Russian study also observed this familial aggregation (26).

Twin studies have also suggested a genetic predisposition for fibroids when hysterectomy data are analyzed. Monozygotic twins have been shown to have two times the correlation for hysterectomy than dizygotic twins, concordant with the degree of their genetic relationship (27).

Studies addressing exogenous steroid hormones as a risk factor for fibroids are conflicting. While looking at oral contraceptive use, studies show increased, decreased, and no association with fibroids; similar conflicting evidence is seen with medroxyprogesterone contraception (19,28–32). Postmenopausal estrogen administration appears to increase the risk two- to six-fold with long-term use (33,34).

Other factors have been examined for fibroid risk with varying results. The effect of increased weight is unclear, with some evidence suggesting higher risk with increased body mass and weight gain in adulthood (35). Cigarette smoking reduces the risk of fibroids by 20% to 50% (23). Physical activity may reduce the incidence of fibroids (36). Diet may also influence the risk: red meat produces a twofold increase, whereas green vegetables reduce the risk by 50% (37).

However, all the above epidemiological data should be viewed with caution. A large proportion of women with fibroids never consult a physician for fibroid-related problems. Only 10% to 30% ever have fibroids removed, thus making histological confirmation impossible in most. In addition, most studies are performed in homogeneous, Caucasian female populations. Furthermore, due to a lack of universal screening through imaging, the ability to define cases and controls for such studies is hampered. There exists a strong need for a prospective, longitudinal study of a wide cross-section of women to more precisely define risk factors for fibroid development.

CLINICAL PRESENTATION

Most commonly, fibroids are asymptomatic masses detected on clinical examination or diagnostic imaging. In a study examining the prevalence of fibroids observed at the time of laparoscopic tubal ligation, just one-third of the women who had fibroids diagnosed during the procedure had previously been given a diagnosis of fibroids, indicating that either fibroids had not been detected on previous examinations or the women had not reported sufficient symptoms to have been diagnosed (23). This emphasizes the largely asymptomatic nature of uterine fibroids.

When fibroids do cause symptoms, those most commonly seen are menorrhagia, dysmenorrhea, pelvic pressure, bowel and bladder symptoms, and infertility (38). While some women with fibroids have heavy and prolonged menses, this is far from universal. Suggested mechanisms include mechanical venous compression and excessive vasoactive growth factor production. Pain is an unusual symptom and is more commonly acute (due to ischemia) rather than chronic. Finally, the mass effect of large fibroids on the bladder may produce urinary frequency, while rectal compression may result in constipation.

DO FIBROIDS CAUSE INFERTILITY?

Approximately 5% to 10% of infertile women have one or more fibroids, and it is the sole abnormal finding in 1% to 2.4% of infertile women (39). There are various potential mechanisms by which fibroids could cause infertility. These include interference with sperm or oocyte transport, chronic endometrial inflammation, abnormal vascularization, increased uterine contractility, and abnormal local endocrine patterns (39–41).

However, the question that must be considered is whether or not fibroids act to decrease fertility. Existing studies have had substantial methodological shortcomings, including poor and widely varying diagnostic methods; suboptimal techniques for determining location, size, and number of fibroids; lack of correction for known or possible risk factors for fibroid development; and low statistical power.

To help clarify the relationship, we performed a systematic review and meta-analysis on the topic of fibroids and infertility in 2001 (42), and this was updated with additional studies in 2008 (43). In the latter analysis, 18 studies were included, and data were evaluated for the rates of clinical pregnancy, implantation, live birth or ongoing pregnancy (beyond the first trimester), preterm labor, and spontaneous abortion.

When evaluating the outcomes of women with fibroids in any location, the relative risk of clinical pregnancy, implantation, ongoing pregnancy, and live birth were all significantly lower in women with fibroids than in women in the control group. In addition, the spontaneous abortion rate was significantly higher in women with fibroids. No significant difference in the preterm delivery rates was observed (Table 1).

In an attempt to determine which types of fibroids might be related to these effects, data were broken down by fibroid location. In the analysis, women were classified by the fibroid closest to the uterine cavity. For example, in women with more than one fibroid in which one involved the uterine cavity, the location was classified as submucous. Similarly, if no submucous fibroids were present but at least one was intramural, the location was classified as intramural.

The results for women with fibroids classified as "submucous" were consistent with traditional dogma. When compared to infertile women without fibroids, those with submucous fibroids demonstrated a significantly lower clinical

Table 1 Effect of Fibroids on Fertility: All Locations

Outcome	Number of studies/ substudies	Relative risk	95% Confidence interval	Significance
Clinical pregnancy rate	18	0.849	0.734–0.983	$P = 0.029$
Implantation rate	14	0.821	0.722–0.932	$P = 0.002$
Ongoing/live birth rate	17	0.697	0.589–0.826	$P < 0.001$
Spontanous abortion rate	18	1.678	1.373–2.051	$P < 0.001$
Preterm delivery rate	3	1.357	0.607–3.036	Not significant

Table 3 Effect of Fibroids on Fertility: Subserosal Fibroids

Outcome	Number of studies/ substudies	Relative risk	95% Confidence interval	Significance
Clinical pregnancy rate	6	0.901	0.707–1.149	Not significant
Implantation rate	2	1.028	0.701–1.508	Not significant
Ongoing/live birth rate	2	1.028	0.679–1.558	Not significant
Spontanous abortion rate	2	1.197	0.465–.3.086	Not significant
Preterm delivery rate	0	–	–	–

Table 2 Effect of Fibroids on Fertility: Submucous Fibroids

Outcome	Number of studies/ substudies	Relative risk	95% Confidence interval	Significance
Clinical pregnancy rate	4	0.363	0.179–0.737	$P = 0.005$
Implantation rate	2	0.283	0.123–0.649	$P = 0.003$
Ongoing/live birth rate	2	0.318	0.199–0.850	$P < 0.001$
Spontanous abortion rate	2	1.678	1.373–2.051	$P = 0.022$
Preterm delivery rate	0	–	–	–

pregnancy rate, implantation rate, ongoing/live birth rate, and a significantly higher spontaneous abortion rate. No difference was seen in rate of preterm delivery. Thus, submucous fibroids lower fertility (Table 2).

When women with only subserous fibroids were examined in comparison to women without fibroids, no difference was observed for any outcome measure; it thus appears that when only subserous fibroids are present, there is no evidence that fertility is impaired (Table 3).

The importance of intramural fibroids on fertility status has long been debated. In our original meta-analysis, no effect was observed (42). However, in our recent work, we observed that intramural fibroids produced significantly lower clinical pregnancy rates, implantation rates, and ongoing/live birth rates and significantly higher spontaneous abortion rates (Fig. 2). No difference was seen in the rate of preterm delivery (Table 4). When the analysis was restricted to prospective studies, only the clinical pregnancy rate lost statistical significance; all other effects remain unchanged. When the analysis was limited to those studies using a high-quality method to assess the uterine cavity in all subjects, only implantation rate maintained statistical significance. No changes in results are seen by elimination of studies involving subjects with prior surgery or restricting inclusion to assisted reproduction studies. Thus, it appears likely that intramural fibroids do indeed adversely affect fertility, although the finding is at best tenuous, based upon the limited quality of the data.

Most investigators have not included size of fibroids as a variable when attempting to determine the influence of fibroids on fertility. Five investigators have reported fibroid size and stratified their analysis accordingly. No studies identified a significant effect on fertility when infertile women with one or more fibroids were compared to infertile women

Study name	Subgroup within study	Outcome	Risk ratio	Lower limit	Upper limit	p-Value	Events / total: Fibroid	Events / total: Control	Relative weight
Bernard, 2000	IM	Clinical Pregnancy	0.536	0.196	1.466	0.224	4 / 16	7 / 15	2.05
Bulletti, 1999	IM	Clinical Pregnancy	0.215	0.054	0.855	0.029	2 / 34	29 / 106	1.14
Check, 2002	IM	Clinical Pregnancy	0.724	0.469	1.119	0.146	21 / 61	29 / 61	8.07
Dietterich, 2000	IM	Clinical Pregnancy	0.873	0.418	1.822	0.717	5 / 9	7 / 11	3.58
Eldar-Geva, 1998	IM	Clinical Pregnancy	0.531	0.286	0.987	0.045	9 / 55	98 / 318	4.77
Gianaroli, 2005	IM	Clinical Pregnancy	0.849	0.621	1.162	0.306	45 / 129	53 / 129	11.94
Hart, 2001	IM	Clinical Pregnancy	0.690	0.475	1.004	0.053	25 / 106	110 / 322	9.77
Klatsky, 2006	IM	Clinical Pregnancy	0.629	0.461	0.858	0.003	30 / 88	149 / 275	12.07
Oliveira, 2004	IM	Clinical Pregnancy	1.038	0.838	1.288	0.731	76 / 163	110 / 245	16.45
Surrey, 2001	IM	Clinical Pregnancy	0.868	0.680	1.108	0.255	37 / 73	191 / 327	15.00
Wang, 2001	IM	Clinical Pregnancy	1.219	0.762	1.949	0.409	10 / 19	57 / 132	7.27
Yarali, 2002	IM	Clinical Pregnancy	0.909	0.584	1.415	0.673	16 / 53	90 / 271	7.88
			0.810	0.696	0.941	0.006			

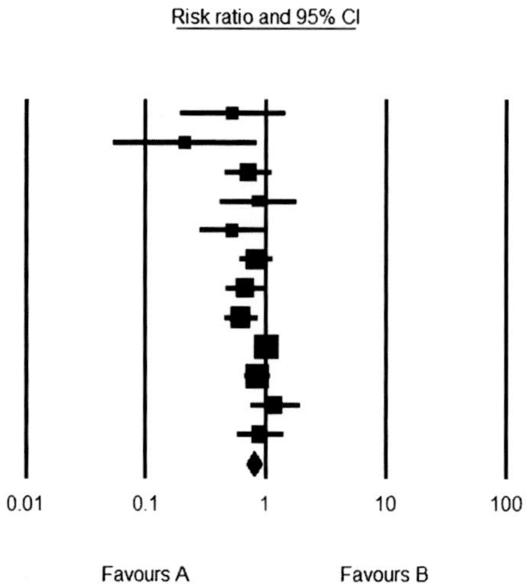

Figure 2 Meta-analysis of all nontreatment studies examining clinical pregnancy rate in women with intramural fibroids versus those with no fibroids.

Table 4 Effect of Fibroids on Fertility: Intramural Fibroids

Outcome	Number of studies/substudies	Relative risk	95% Confidence interval	Significance
All studies				
Clinical pregnancy rate	12	0.810	0.696–0.941	$P = 0.006$
Implantation rate	7	0.684	0.587–0.796	$P < 0.001$
Ongoing/live birth rate	8	0.703	0.583–0.848	$P < 0.001$
Spontanous abortion rate	8	1.747	1.226–2.489	$P = 0.002$
Preterm delivery rate	1	6.000	0.309–116.606	Not significant
Propective studies				
Clinical pregnancy rate	3	0.708	0.437–1.146	Not significant
Implantation rate	2	0.552	0.391–0.781	$P = 0.001$
Ongoing/live birth rate	2	0.465	0.291–0.744	$P = 0.019$
Spontaneous abortion rate	2	2.384	1.110–5.122	$P = 0.002$
Preterm delivery rate	0	–	–	–

without fibroids. The influence of fibroid size and volume on fertility is unclear, and further study is warranted (43).

CONSERVATIVE TREATMENT OPTIONS FOR UTERINE FIBROIDS

Medical Management

Gonadotropin-releasing hormone agonists (GnRH-a) induce a hypoestrogenic state and therefore can reduce fibroid volume up to 40%, with improvement in symptoms in most women (44–46). GnRH-a therapy reduces fibroid volume by 30% (47). The reduction in fibroid volume occurs mostly within the first three months of therapy (44,48–50).

Unfortunately, GnRH-a use is limited by side effects and decrease in bone density. It is estimated that up to 6% of bone mineral density might be lost in the first six months of GnRH-a therapy. However, the bone loss is restored almost completely two years after stopping treatment (51). On the other hand, irreversible loss of bone with pathological consequences may occur with prolonged (>6 months) treatment (49). The use of estrogen and progestin or raloxifene add-back may mitigate the negative effect of GnRH agonists on bone density (52,53).

After discontinuation of GnRH-a, menses return in four to eight weeks, and uterine size returns to pretreatment levels within four to six months. However, 64% of women remained asymptomatic 8 to 12 months after treatment (54).

Other medical therapies have also been utilized in an attempt to reduce fibroid volume. Danazol, mifepristone, raloxifene, letrozole, and fadrozole have all been demonstrated to temporarily decrease the size of fibroids, although studies are of varying size and quality. As all medical therapies studied to date have a negative effect on fertility, most commonly by inhibition of ovulation, or are contraindicated during the periconception period, medical management is not indicated for the management of uterine fibroids in women hoping to conceive.

While considerable effort is underway to develop medical therapies for the treatment of uterine fibroids, it is unclear how such options will improve fertility. It may be possible to medically treat fibroids with a specifically targeted drug that does not affect follicular development, ovulation, implantation, and embryo development, but no such medication currently exists.

Uterine Artery Embolization

Uterine artery embolization (UAE) involves injection of a sclerosing substance or mechanical plug into one or both uterine arteries to embolize the fibroids blood supply (Fig. 3). This has been shown to decrease the size of fibroids and to reduce symptomatology (55). However, this procedure is not without risk.

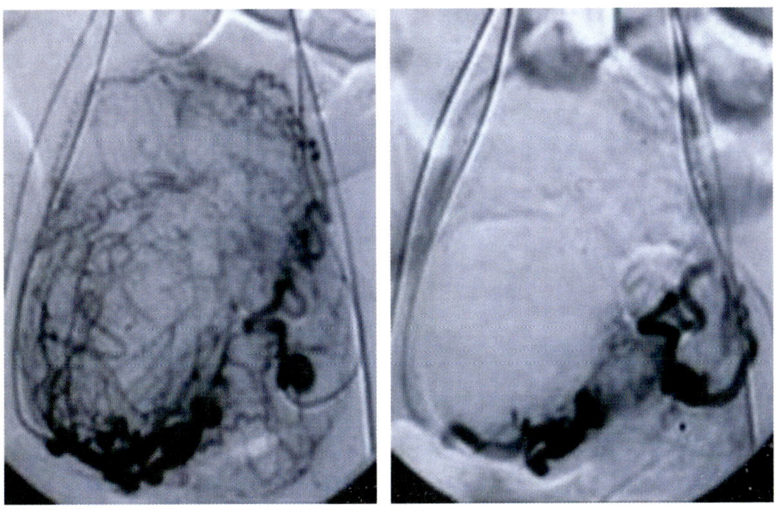

(A) (B)

Figure 3 Angiography of uterine fibroid vasculature (**A**) before and (**B**) after uterine artery embolization.

The acute degenerative procedure can be painful, and pelvic infection can occur, in 1% to 2% of procedures. Hysterectomy is necessary after UAE in 1% of women for hemorrhage or severe tissue necrosis (56). Endometrial adhesions have also been reported, as well as uterine cavity to fibroid fistulas.

Future fertility is uncertain and may be compromised by inadvertent interference with the ovarian blood supply. In young women, this rate of postprocedure ovarian failure is approximately 5%; however, in women older than 45 years, the risk is as high as 40% (55,57). Nevertheless, pregnancies have been reported after UAE. Of 34 pregnancies achieved after UAE, 32% ended in a spontaneous abortion (58). In a report of 164 women desiring future fertility before UAE, during 24 months of follow-up, 21 women achieved pregnancy, 4 (24%) had a spontaneous abortion, 2 had elective terminations, and 18 had live births (59). However, in those women who had live births, the complications included postpartum hemorrhage, preterm delivery, abnormal placentation, and fetal malpresentation. These were seen at an increased rate when compared with the general population and in comparison with women undergoing UAE for reasons other than the treatment of uterine fibroids (58–63). In two of the reported cases of postpartum hemorrhage, an emergent cesarean hysterectomy was necessary and uterine rupture has also been reported. For these reasons, UAE is not currently recommended for the treatment of fibroids in women wishing to preserve or enhance their fertility.

CONSERVATIVE SURGERY

Uterine Artery Occlusion

Distal occlusion of the uterine arteries induces ischemia in the uterine myometrium and associated fibroids. Revascularization of the myometrium occurs via ovarian artery anastomoses and retrograde flow though the middle hemorrhoidal artery (64); however, fibroids are not adequately revascularized and eventually necrosis occurs. This principal is exploited by UAE, and more recently through laparoscopic uterine artery occlusion and transvaginal uterine artery occlusion.

Laparoscopic uterine artery occlusion is performed by first incising the peritoneum overlying the external iliac artery between the round ligament and the infundibulopelvic ligament. The iliac vessels are identified, and the retroperitoneal space is developed. The uterine artery is occluded, most commonly with a clip, at the level of the internal iliac artery. This technique has only recently been described and data are preliminary. The only randomized trial to date compared laparoscopic uterine artery occlusion to UAE and observed similar clinical outcomes in both groups (65).

Transvaginal occlusion is performed by placing a specially designed clamp in the vaginal fornices and, guided by Doppler ultrasound auditory signals, positioning it to occlude the uterine arteries. The clamp is left in place for six hours and then removed. This was first described in 2004 and has had some documented success in reducing fibroid size (66); two other reports (67,68) have documented success in reducing fibroid size. This technique may become an alternative, noninvasive means to manage fibroids; however, the effect on fertility is unknown.

Myolysis

Myolysis refers to the technique where an attempt is made to disrupt or abolish the blood supply to the fibroid and cause shrinkage using radiofrequency electricity, supercooled cryoprobes, or focused ultrasound (69). The procedure is rarely performed and is not recommended for women who wish to get pregnant, since there is a significant risk of uterine rupture (70,71).

Myomectomy

The most commonly utilized treatment for fibroids, when future fertility is to be preserved or enhanced, is surgical myomectomy. There are a number of different techniques to achieve surgical access for this procedure, depending upon size, number, and location of the fibroids as well as the surgeon's skill and experience.

Abdominal Myomectomy

Myomectomy by laparotomy or minilaparotomy incision (abdominal myomectomy) is the technique of choice for women with multiple fibroids or a significantly enlarged uterus (72). After a laparotomy is performed and access to the peritoneal cavity is achieved, the surgeon should evaluate the size, location, and number of fibroids present. Conservation of uterine blood supply and minimization of blood loss are priorities. Methods to minimize blood loss are discussed below but cannot replace good surgical technique. A minimal number of incisions in the uterus are made. An incision is made linearly sagittally, ideally over the largest fibroid where the overlying myometrium is thinnest and more than one fibroid can be removed. The incision is carried down through the overlying myometrium onto the fibroid. The fibroid is grasped with a tenaculum, and traction is applied. Using a combination of sharp and blunt dissection, the fibroid is enucleated from its bed. Morcellation of fibroids during removal may reduce the size of both the uterine and the skin incisions required. As many fibroids as possible should be removed through each uterine incision. Closure of the defect left by the fibroid is performed in multiple layers, if necessary, to achieve hemostasis. Particular care must be taken near the endometrium to ensure that no suture material is placed within the endometrial cavity that may impede healing of the endometrium in the event the cavity is broached. The serosal edge is carefully approximated using a small gage, absorbable suture.

Complications of abdominal myomectomy can occur intra- or postoperatively. Intraoperative complications include injury to the bowel or urinary tract and excessive blood loss. The volume of blood lost during abdominal myomectomy varies with the size and location of fibroids. Fibroids are often surrounded by large supporting blood vessels that originate in the surrounding myometrium. These vessels should be secured prior to fibroid enucleation, as blood loss from these vessels can be significant and can necessitate conversion to hysterectomy. An average blood loss of 540 cc was reported in a review of abdominal myomectomy for uterine sizes exceeding 14 weeks (73). A number of methods have been used to minimize blood loss during surgery. Mechanical techniques including tourniquets and clamps to occlude the uterine and ovarian arteries have been shown to be effective. A randomized trial of 28 women, which evaluated the use of triple tourniquets applied to both the ovarian and the uterine arteries during abdominal myomectomy, found significantly less blood loss in the tourniquet group compared with the control group with no tourniquets (difference of 1870 mL; 95% CI: 1159–2580; $P < 0.0001$) (74). However, the pressure exerted by such tourniquets can damage the uterine artery or its branches as well as mask inadequate hemostasis that becomes apparent once the tourniquet is removed. Laparoscopic uterine artery occlusion prior to myomectomy has also been associated with a reduction in intraoperative blood loss; however, the effect on fertility is unknown (75).

Nonmechanical techniques to reduce blood loss during abdominal myomectomy were the subject of a recent Cochrane Library review (76). The review highlights the paucity of randomized data on the use of such techniques. Eight randomized control trials were included: two addressing intramyometrial vasopressin and analogs, and one each focused upon vaginal misoprostol, IV oxytocin, pericervical tourniquet, chemical dissection with mesna, intramyometrial bupivacaine plus epinephrine, and the enucleation of the fibroid by morcellation while it is attached to the uterus. A significant reduction in blood loss was observed with misoprostol (−149.00 mL; 95% CI: −229.24 to −68.76), vasopressin and analogs (−298.72 mL; 95% CI: −593.10 to −4.34), bupivacaine plus epinephrine (−68.60 mL; 95% CI: −93.69 to −43.51), and pericervical tourniquet (−1870.00 mL, 95% CI −2547.16 to −1192.84). There was no evidence of effect upon blood loss with fibroid enucleation by morcellation or with the use of oxytocin.

GnRH agonists have been used to minimize blood loss by reducing uterine volume preoperatively. A number of controlled and uncontrolled studies of women with uterine fibroids have documented a reduction in uterine volume after treatment with a GnRH agonist. The reported reduction in volume varied between 35% and 65% (77). A Cochrane Library review evaluated the role of pretreatment with GnRH agonists before hysterectomy or myomectomy for uterine fibroids (78). The review included 20 randomized, controlled trials that compared GnRH agonists to no pretreatment or placebo. Pre- and postoperative hemoglobin and hematocrit were significantly improved by GnRH analog therapy prior to surgery. Uterine volume, uterine gestational size, fibroid volume, intraoperative blood loss, and the rate of vertical incisions were all reduced, suggesting that pretreatment for three to four months with a GnRH agonist prior to myomectomy is beneficial. No difference in surgical time was noted.

Despite the use of one or more of these techniques, 31% of U.K. gynecologists report the regular need for blood transfusions, with rates varying from less than 10% to more than 30% (79).

Pelvic adhesions occur commonly after myomectomy and may decrease future fertility. Such adhesions occur in more than 90% of women following the procedure and may be found at the uterine incision site and/or in the adnexa. Careful surgical technique with minimization of tissue damage is important, but adhesions are frequent even following surgery by the most meticulous of surgeons. The use of adhesion-prevention adjuvants has been advocated to reduce adhesion formation, and indeed several have been shown to be effective. Adhesion prevention is reviewed elsewhere (chap. 2). There is no evidence that the use of any adhesion-prevention barriers improves fertility (80).

Laparoscopic Myomectomy

Laparoscopic myomectomy requires the same thoughtful approach as abdominal myomectomy (Fig. 4A–F). Conservation of uterine blood supply and minimization of blood loss are priorities, and a minimal number of incisions to remove the fibroids should be made.

The technique of laparoscopic myomectomy is detailed elsewhere (chap. 7).

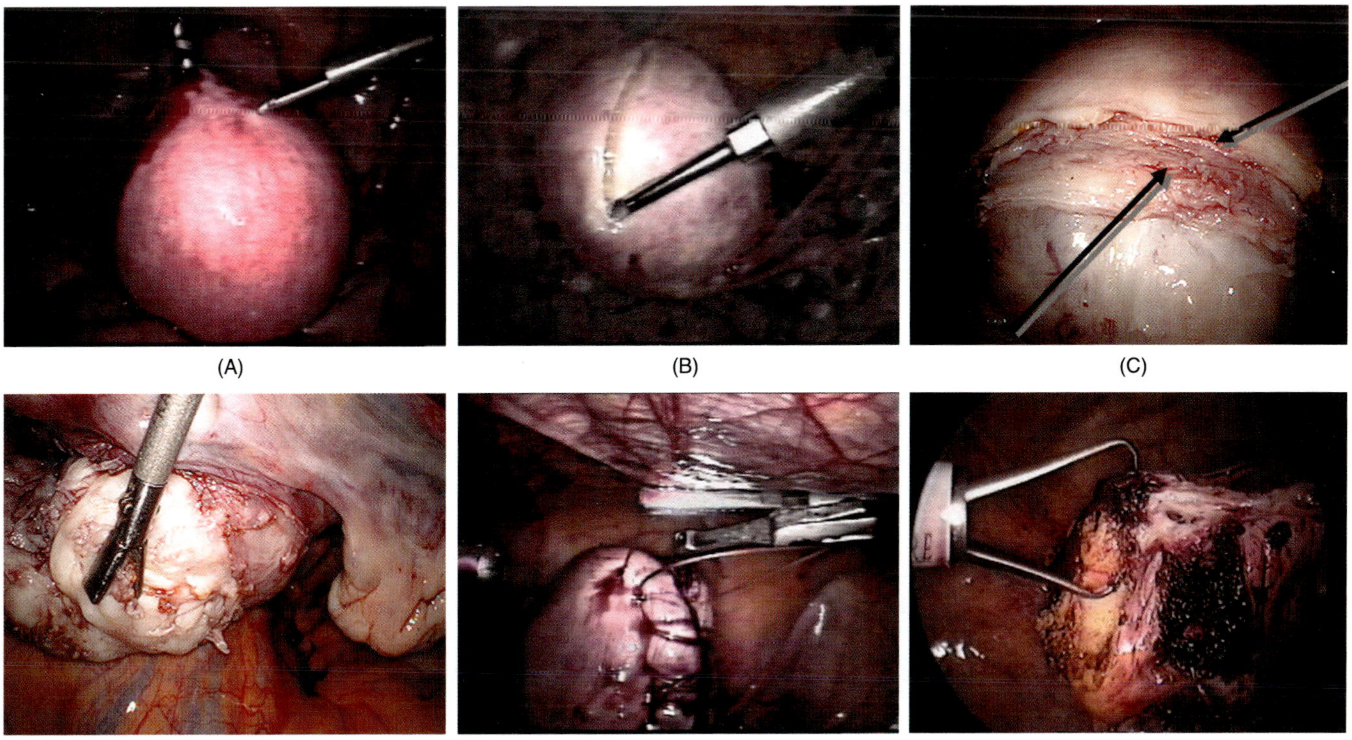

(A) (B) (C) (D) (E) (F)

Figure 4 Laparoscopic myomectomy. **(A)** Injection of the myoma with pitressin; **(B)** use of the harmonic scalpel (with hook tip) to incise the uterine serosa; **(C)** identification of the fibroid pseudocapsule; **(D)** Enucleation of the fibroid from the surrounding myometrium; **(E)** Use of the Endostitch® (U. S. Surgical Corp.) to close the uterine defect in multiple layers; and **(F)** Use of the mechanical morcellator to remove fibroid from the abdomen.

Abdominal Versus Laparoscopic Myomectomy

The first randomized controlled trial comparing abdominal and laparoscopic myomectomy was published in 1996 (81) and found less postoperative pain, shorter hospitalization, and shorter recovery time after laparoscopic surgery—known advantages of laparoscopic access. Two case–control studies also found laparoscopic myomectomy to be associated with less postoperative pain and shorter hospitalization; however operative time was significantly longer in the laparoscopic myomectomy groups and in one report was associated with greater blood loss (82,83).

The only randomized comparison of abdominal versus laparoscopic myomectomy for fertility (84) found no significant difference in reproductive outcomes between groups. One hundred and thirty-one women were randomized and followed for an average of 32.4 months. Both groups had similar rates of pregnancy, abortion, preterm delivery, and cesarean section. There were no reports of uterine rupture with pregnancy in either group. Nonrandomized comparisons have also reported similar pregnancy rates following laparotomy compared to laparoscopic myomectomy (85,86).

While the recurrence rate of fibroids is difficult to assess precisely, it is estimated that 10% of women will have a clinically significant recurrence 10 years after abdominal myomectomy (87). There appears to be no difference in the rate of recurrent fibroids observed by ultrasound at 40 months after laparoscopic or laparotomic myomectomy (88).

Laparoscopic myomectomy has advantages over abdominal myomectomy with respect to postoperative pain, duration of hospitalization, and cosmesis. Laparoscopic myomectomy is associated with fewer postoperative adhesions than abdominal myomectomy. Postoperative adhesions, present at the site of uterine incision and in the adnexae, as documented by second-look laparoscopy, are present in 51.1% of women after laparoscopic myomectomy and in 89.6% after laparotomy (89), but the impact of such adhesions on pregnancy rates is unknown. Laparoscopic surgery may offer less traumatic manipulation of tissue and minimized peritoneal contamination. However, laparoscopic myomectomy is not without limitation. Laparoscopic myomectomy is associated with a longer operative time and requires advanced endoscopic skills, including laparoscopic suturing ability. Further, laparoscopic removal of large fibroids (>8 cm) increases the risk of hemorrhage, the risk of conversion to laparotomy, and operative time.

Uterine rupture is a concern of surgeons undertaking laparoscopic myomectomy. However, there are no adequate comparisons of rates of rupture with laparoscopy versus laparotomy. It appears, however, that rupture is rare regardless of the technique. Several large prospective studies have observed no or few cases (90–92) of uterine rupture (93).

Hysteroscopic Myomectomy

Hysteroscopic myomectomy is a minimally invasive approach to fibroid excision and is ideal for submucous or intramural fibroids with an intracavity component.

Once the decision has been made to proceed with hysteroscopic myomectomy, preoperative administration of a GnRH agonist may be considered. GnRH agonists have been shown to reduce preoperative anemia and decrease the size of submucous fibroids (78,94,95). Preoperative treatment with a GnRH agonist may also reduce surgical time, bleeding, and the volume of distension fluid required, although conflicting results have been reported (96,97). However, a GnRH agonist should not be used unless the largest diameter of the fibroid is within the uterine cavity; if the largest diameter is within the myometrium, shrinkage may cause a loss of access to the fibroid hysteroscopically. Preoperative intravaginal misprostol improves cervical dilation and reduces the risk of cervical laceration (98).

The technique of hysteroscopic myomectomy is detailed elsewhere (chap. 6).

The complication rate of hysteroscopic myomectomy increases with increasing size and number of fibroids. While a wide range of complication rates has been reported (0.8–12%), this likely reflects differences in what is considered a complication. Complications of hysteroscopic myomectomy include uterine perforation, fluid overload, hemorrhage, cervical laceration, and infection. In the largest series reported to date, the complication rate after 789 hysteroscopic myomectomies was 0.8%. Uterine perforation was the most common complication, occurring in 0.76% of cases. The rate of fluid overload was 0.5% (99). In another series ($n = 128$), the most common complication of hysteroscopic myomectomy was fluid overload (4.7%), followed by hyponatremia (2.3%) and infection (1.5%) (100). This rate of postoperative infection is consistent with other series that report rates of approximately 1% (101–103). Perioperative hemorrhage is an uncommon complication, occurring in less than 1% of procedures, but can necessitate abandoning the procedure or even hysterectomy (101–103).

Standard electrosurgical operative hysteroscopy mandates the use of an electrolyte-free, low-viscosity solution. These solutions, if absorbed in excessive amounts, lead to hypo-osmolality and hyponatremia. Long-term morbidity and even death have been reported, making prevention critical. Fluid intravasation increases as the intrauterine pressure increases; therefore, the minimum pressure needed to maintain safe visualization should be maintained. If a monopolar electrode is used for fibroid resection, the use of electrolyte-free fluids is mandatory to reduce potentially dangerous electrical dispersion. Electrolyte-free solutions include 1.5% glycine, 3% D-sorbitol, 5% mannitol, and cystosol. Electrolyte-rich solutions, such as normal saline, can be used if a bipolar electrode is employed (e.g., Versapoint®). Recording and termination of the procedure when the fluid loss exceeds 1000 to 1500 mL should be adopted to minimize fluid-related complications.

The treatment of submucous fibroids with deep intramural extension is more difficult, and multiple procedures may be necessary for complete resection. As many as 22% will require a second procedure for incomplete resection or symptom recurrence (104), and fibroids recur, as seen by ultrasound, in 6% of women at 24 months postoperative (97).

There is a case report of a uterine rupture during a pregnancy subsequent to a hysteroscopic myomectomy. In this single report, a uterine perforation occurred during the procedure, which was sutured during a concomitant laparotomy (105).

Fertility Enhancement with Myomectomy

While it is clear that fertility can be maintained following myomectomy, a critical issue to the gynecologist is the role of myomectomy in enhancing fertility in the subfertile woman. As shown earlier, submucous and possibly intramural fibroids exert a detrimental effect upon fertility. However, before surgery can be advocated for fertility enhancement, it must be shown that myomectomy improves reproductive outcome in such women. A published meta-analysis has analyzed this issue (43).

To investigate this question, two types of trials exist: those whose control groups include women with a fibroid

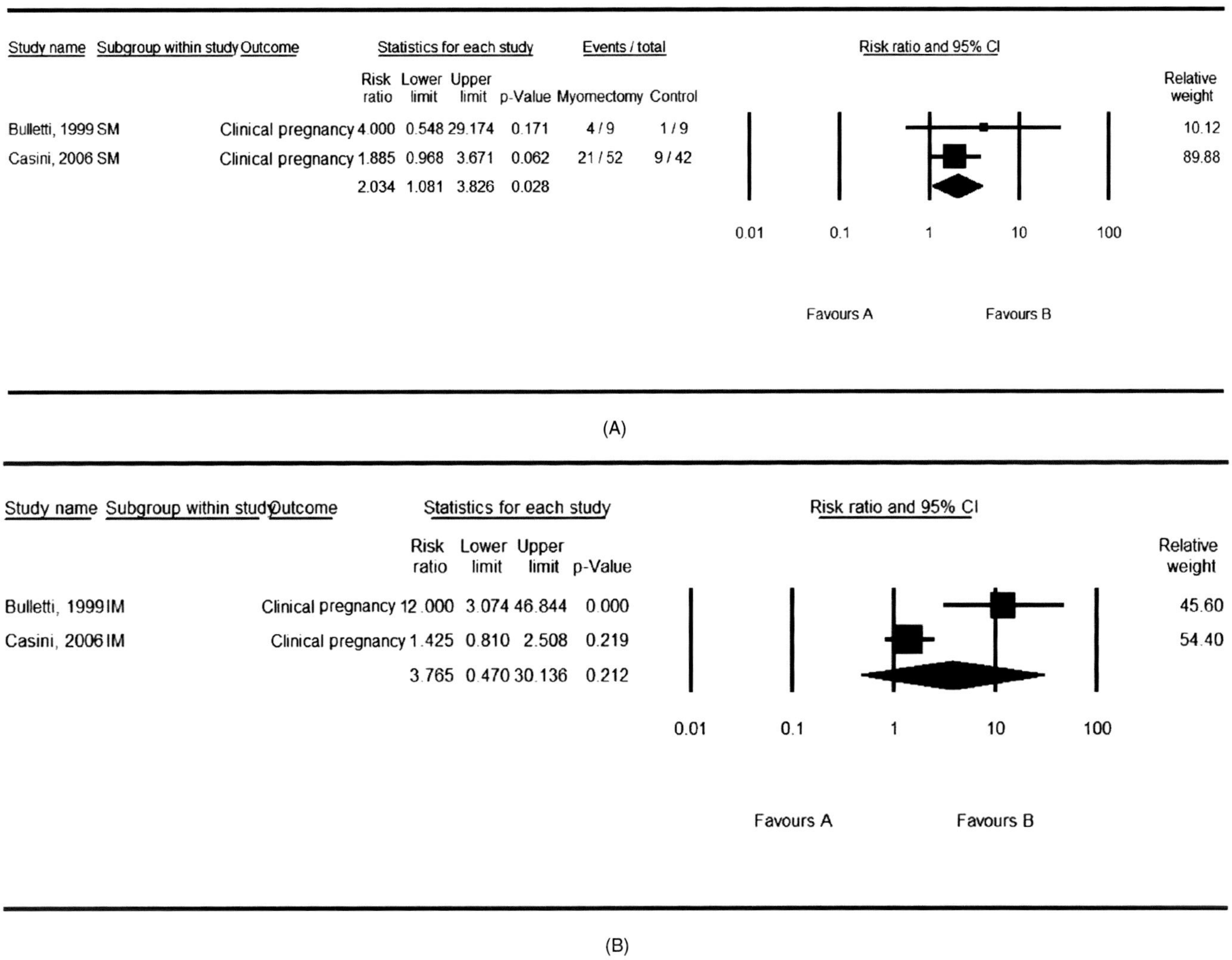

Figure 5 Meta-analysis of all treatment trials examining clinical pregnancy rate in women with intramural fibroids undergoing myomectomy. (**A**) Submucous fibroids undergoing myomectomy versus submucous fibroids in situ. (**B**) Intramural fibroids undergoing myomectomy versus intramural fibroids in situ.

in situ and those whose control group includes women without a fibroid. In the studies thus far, many of the women have multiple etiologies for their infertility, including uterine fibroids. If fibroid removal is beneficial, women undergoing myomectomy would be expected to have a higher pregnancy rate and lower abortion rate than those with fibroids in situ. In those with submucous fibroids, clinical pregnancy rate is indeed higher in the myomectomy group (Fig. 5), but ongoing/live birth rate fails to reach a statistically significant difference. The spontaneous abortion rate appears unchanged (Table 5). In women with intramural fibroids, no significant differences are seen (Table 6). In both cases, studies are sparse.

When the control group is infertile women with no fibroids, myomectomy might be expected (if beneficial) to

Table 5 Effect of Myomectomy on Fertility: Submucosal Fibroids

Outcome	Number of studies/substudies	Relative risk	95% Confidence interval	Significance
Controls fibroids in situ (no myomectomy)				
Clinical pregnancy rate	2	2.034	1.081–3.826	$P = 0.028$
Implantation rate	0	–	–	–
Ongoing/live birth rate	1	2.654	0.920–7.658	Not significant
Spontaneous abortion rate	1	0.771	0.359–1.658	Not significant
Preterm delivery rate	0	–	–	–
Controls infertile women with no fibroids				
Clinical pregnancy rate	2	1.545	0.998–2.391	Not significant
Implantation rate	2	1.116	0.906–1.373	Not significant
Ongoing/live birth rate	3	1.128	0.959–1.326	Not significant
Spontaneous abortion rate	2	1.241	0.475–3.242	Not significant
Preterm delivery rate	0	–	–	–

Table 6 Effect of Myomectomy on Fertility: Intramural Fibroids (Fibroids In Situ Controls)

Outcome	Number of studies/substudies	Relative risk	95% Confidence interval	Significance
Clinical pregnancy rate	2	3.765	0.470–30.136	Not significant
Implantation rate	0	–	–	–
Ongoing/live birth rate	1	1.671	0.750–3.723	Not significant
Spontaneous abortion rate	1	0.758	0.296–1.943	Not significant
Preterm delivery rate	0	–	–	–

normalize the rates compared to controls. This is indeed seen in women having submucous fibroids, as clinical pregnancy rate (Fig. 5), ongoing/live birth rate, and spontaneous abortion rate are all statistically similar to controls (Table 5). This question has not been studied for women with intramural fibroids.

It thus appears that myomectomy is likely to prove beneficial in the treatment of infertile women with submucous fibroids. However, there is no clear evidence, at this time, that myomectomy for intramural fibroids improves fertility, despite the presence of a randomized clinical trial. However, given the magnitude of the risk ratio and the small number of studies and participants, it certainly deserves much further study. It would appear that investigation of removal of intramural fibroids would head the priority list of issues for contemporary clinical fibroid research. Ancillary issues in need of being addressed are the number of intramural fibroids that necessitate removal, the size of intramural fibroids that affect fertility, and whether or not proximity to the endometrium is of clinical importance. Hopefully, these will be topics carefully and thoroughly addressed by future investigators.

CONCLUSIONS

Uterine fibroids are common benign tumors of women. They cause a variety of clinical problems and have been associated with infertility. In the woman with fibroids wishing to preserve her fertility, there are medical, radiological, and surgical approaches to treatment that retain the uterus in situ. However, the only technique, to date, shown to be both safe and effective for the woman desiring future fertility is myomectomy.

For the infertile woman with uterine fibroids, there is evidence that submucous fibroids and perhaps intramural fibroids may be causative factors. Limited treatment data suggest that removal of submucous fibroids and intramural fibroids that distort the endometrial cavity will enhance fertility. Currently, there is no evidence that excision of an intramural fibroid that does not distort the endometrial cavity is beneficial. The influence of fibroid size, location, and the degree of cavity distortion is unknown and should be the subject of future investigation.

REFERENCES

1. Cramer SF, Patel A. The frequency of uterine leiomyomas. Am J Clin Pathol 1990; 94:435–438.
2. Clay C. Observations on ovariotomy, statistical and practical. Also, a successful case of entire removal of the uterus, and its appendages. Trans Obstet Soc Lond 1863; 5:58–74.
3. Bellinger J. J South Med Pharm 1847; 2:241.
4. Zaloudek C, Hendrickson M. Mesenchymal tumors of the uterus. In: Kurman RJ, ed. Blaustein's Pathology of the Female Genital Tract. New York, NY: Springer-Verlag, 2002: 564–583.
5. Townsend DE, Sparkes RS, Baluda MC, et al. Unicellular histogenesis of uterine leiomyomas as determined by electrophoresis by glucose-6-phosphate dehydrogenase. Am J Obstet Gynecol 1970; 107:1168–1173.
6. Mashal RD, Fejzo ML, Friedman AJ, et al. Analysis of androgen receptor DNA reveals the independent clonal origins of uterine leiomyomata and the secondary nature of cytogenetic aberrations in the development of leiomyomata. Genes Chromosomes Cancer 1994; 11:1–6.
7. Hashimoto K, Azuma C, Kamiura S, et al. Clonal determination of uterine leiomyomas by analyzing differential inactivation of the X-chromosome-linked phosphoglycerokinase gene. Gynecol Obstet Invest 1995; 40:204–208.
8. Rein MS, Friedman AJ, Barbieri RL, et al. Cytogenetic abnormalities in uterine leiomyomata. Obstet Gynecol 1991; 77: 923–926.
9. Morton CC. Genetic approaches to the study of uterine leiomyomata. Environ Health Perspect 2000; 108(Suppl 5):775–778.
10. Sozen I, Arici A. Interactions of cytokines, growth factors, and the extracellular matrix in the cellular biology of uterine leiomyomata. Fertil Steril 2002; 78:1–12.
11. Cook JD, Walker CL. Treatment strategies for uterine leiomyoma: The role of hormonal modulation. Semin Reprod Med 2004; 22:105–111.
12. Mauro T, Matsuo H, Samoto T, et al. Effects of progesterone on uterine leiomyoma growth and apoptosis. Steroids 2000; 65:585–592.
13. Anderson J. Factors in fibroid growth. Bailleres Clin Obstet Gynaecol 1998; 12(2):225–243.
14. Rein MS. Advances in uterine leiomyoma research: The progesterone hypothesis. Environ Health Perspect 2000; 108(Suppl 5):791–793.
15. Ohara N. Selective estrogen receptor modulator and selective progesterone receptor modulator: Therapeutic efficacy in the treatment of uterine leiomyoma. Clin Exp Obstet Gynecol 2005; 32:9–11.
16. Baird D, Dunson D, Hill M, et al. High cumulative incidence of uterine leiomyoma in black and white women: Ultrasound evidence. Am J Obstet Gynecol 2003; 188:100–107.
17. Kjerulft KH, Guzinski GM, Langenberg PW, et al. Hysterectomy and race. Obstet Gynecol 1993; 82:757–764.
18. Marshall LM, Spiegelman D, Barbieri RL, et al. Variation in the incidence of uterine leiomyoma among premenopausal women by age and race. Obstet Gynecol 1997; 90:967–973.
19. Faerstein E, Szklo M, Rosenshein N. Risk factors for uterine leiomyoma: A practice-based case-control study. I. African-American heritage, reproductive history, body size, and smoking. Am J Epidemiol 2001; 153:1–10.
20. Heinemann K, Thiel C, Mohner S, et al. Benign gynecologic tumors: Estimated incidence results of the German Cohort Study on Women's Health. Eur J Obstet Gynecol Reprod Biol 2003; 107:78–80.
21. Marino J, Eskenazi B, Warner M, et al. Uterine leiomyoma and menstrual cycle characteristics in population based cohort study. Hum Reprod 2004; 19:2350–2355.
22. Borgfeldt C, Andolf E. Transvaginal ultrasonographic findings in the uterus and endometrium: Low prevalence of leiomyoma in a random sample of women age 25–40 years. Acta Obstet Gynecol Scand 2000; 79:202–207.
23. Chen C, Buck G, Courey N, et al. Risk factors for uterine fibroids among women undergoing tubal sterilization. Am J Epidemiol 2001; 153:20–26.

24. Schwartz SM, Marshall LM, Baird DD. Epidemiologic contributions to understanding the etiology of uterine leiomyomata. Environ Health Perspect 2000; 108(Suppl):821–827.
25. Schwartz S. Epidemiology of uterine leiomyomata. Clin Obstet Gynecol 2001; 44:316–326.
26. Vikhlyaeva EM, Khodzhaeva ZS, Fantschenko ND. Familial predisposition to uterine leiomyomas. Int J Gynaecol Obstet 1995; 51:127–131.
27. Treloar SA, Martin NG, Dennerstein L, et al. Pathways to hysterectomy: Insights from longitudinal twin research. Am J Obstet Gynecol 1992; 167:82–88.
28. Wise LA, Palmer JR, Harlow BL, et al. Reproductive factors, hormonal contraception, and risk of uterine leiomyomata in African-American women: A prospective study. Am J Epidemiol 2004; 159:113–123.
29. Chiaffarino F, Parazzini F, La Vecchia C, et al. Use of oral contraceptives and uterine fibroids: Results from a case-control study. Br J Obstet Gynaecol 1999; 106(8):857–860.
30. Marshall LM, Spiegelman D, Goldman MB, et al. A prospective study of reproductive factors and oral contraceptive use in relation to the risk of uterine leiomyomata. Fertil Steril 1998; 70:432–439.
31. Barbieri RL. Reduction in the size of a uterine leiomyoma following discontinuation of an estrogen-progestin contraceptive. Gynecol Obstet Invest 1997; 43(4):276–277.
32. Friedman AJ, Thomas PP. Does low-dose combination oral contraceptive use affect uterine size or menstrual flow in premenopausal women with leiomyomas? Obstet Gynecol 1995; 85(4):631–635.
33. Ramcharan S, Pelligrin FA, Ray R, et al. The Walnut Creek Contraceptive Drug Study. A prospective study of the side effects of oral contraceptives. NIH Pub. No. 81–564. Center Popul Res Monogr 1981; 3:69–74.
34. Romieu I, Walker AM, Jick S. Determinants of uterine fibroids. Post Market Surveill 1991; 5:119–133.
35. Terry KL, De Vivo I, Hankinson SE, et al. Anthropometric characteristics and risk of uterine leiomyoma. Epidemiology 2007; 18:758–763.
36. Baird DD, Dunson DB, Hill MC, et al. Association of physical activity with development of uterine leiomyoma. Am J Epidemiol 2007; 165:157–163.
37. Chiaffarino F, Parazzini F, La Vecchia C, et al. Diet and uterine myomas. Obstet Gynecol 1999; 94:395–398.
38. Parker WH. Etiology, symptomatology, and diagnosis of uterine myomas. Fertil Steril 2007; 87:725–736.
39. Donnez J, Jadoul P. What are the implications of myomas on fertility? A need for a debate? Hum Reprod 2002; 17:1424–1430.
40. Hunt JE, Wallach EE. Uterine factors in infertility–an overview. Clin Obstet Gynecol 1974; 17:44–64.
41. Buttram VC Jr, Reiter RC. Uterine leiomyomata: Etiology, symptomatology, and management. Fertil Steril. 1981; 36:433–445.
42. Pritts EA. Fibroids and infertility: A systematic review of the evidence. Obstet Gynecol Surv 2001; 56:483–491.
43. Pritts EA, Parker WH, Olive DL. Fibroids and infertility: An updated systematic review of the evidence. Fertil Steril 91(4):1216–1223.
44. Friedman AJ, Hoffman DI, Comite F, et al. Treatment of leiomyomata uteri with leuprolide acetate depot: A doubleblind, placebo-controlled, multicenter study. The Leuprolide Study Group. Obstet Gynecol 1991; 77:720–725.
45. Friedman AJ, Daly M, Juneau-Norcross M, et al. Long-term medical therapy for leiomyomata uteri: A prospective, randomized study of leuprolide acetate depot plus either oestrogen-progestin or progestin 'add-back' for 2 years. Hum Reprod 1994; 9:1618–1625.
46. Vercellini P, Crosignani PG, Mangioni C, et al. Treatment with a gonadotrophin releasing hormone agonist before hysterectomy for leiomyomas: Results of a multicentre, randomized controlled trial. BJOG 1998; 105:1148–1154.
47. Schlaff WD, Zerhouni EA, Huth JA, et al. A placebo-controlled trial of a depot gonadotropin-releasing hormone analogue (leuprolide) in the treatment of uterine leiomyomata. Obstet Gynecol 1989; 74:856–862.
48. Broekmans FJ. GnRH agonists and uterine leiomyomas. Hum Reprod 1996; 11(Suppl 3):3–25.
49. Costantini S, Anserini P, Valenzano M, et al. Luteinizing hormone-releasing hormone analog therapy of uterine fibroid: Analysis of results obtained with buserelin administered intranasally and goserelin administered subcutaneously as a monthly depot. Eur J Obstet Gynecol Reprod Biol 1990; 37: 63–69.
50. Palomba S, Affinito P, Di Carlo C, et al. Long-term administration of tibolone plus gonadotropin-releasing hormone agonist for the treatment of uterine leiomyomas: Effectiveness and effects on vasomotor symptoms, bone mass, and lipid profiles. Fertil Steril 1999; 72:889–895.
51. Paoletti AM, Serra GG, Cagnacci A, et al. Spontaneous reversibility of bone loss induced by gonadotropin releasing hormone analog treatment. Fertil Steril 1996; 65:707–710.
52. Pickersgill A. GnRH agonists and add-back therapy: Is there a perfect combination? Br J Obstet Gynaecol 1998; 105:475–485.
53. Palomba S, Orio F Jr, Russo T, et al. Long-term effectiveness and safety of GnRH agonist plus raloxifene administration in women with uterine leiomyomas. Hum Reprod 2004; 19:1308–1314.
54. Letterie GS, Coddington CC, Winkel CA, et al. Efficacy of a gonadotropin-releasing hormone agonist in the treatment of uterine leiomyomata: Long-term follow-up. Fertil Steril 1989; 51:951–956.
55. Lumsden MA. Embolization versus myomectomy versus hysterectomy: Which is best, when? Hum Reprod 2002; 17:253–259.
56. Marshburn PB, Matthews ML, Hurst BS. Uterine artery embolization as a treatment option for uterine myomas. Obstet Gynecol Clin North Am 2006; 33:125–144.
57. Pron G, Bennett J, Common A, et al. The Ontario Uterine Fibroid Embolization Trial. Part 2. Uterine fibroid reduction and symptom relief after uterine artery embolization for fibroids. Fertil Steril 2003; 79:120–127.
58. Goldberg J, Pereira L, Berghella V, et al. Pregnancy outcomes after treatment for fibromyomata: Uterine artery embolization versus laparoscopic myomectomy. Am J Obstet Gynecol 2004; 191:18–21.
59. Pron G, Mocarski E, Bennett J, et al. Ontario UFE Collaborative Group. Pregnancy after uterine artery embolization for leiomyomata: The Ontario multicenter trial. Obstet Gynecol 2005; 105:67–76.
60. McLucas B, Goodwin S, Adler L, et al. Pregnancy following uterine fibroid embolization. Int J Gynaecol Obstet 2001; 74: 1–7.
61. Goldberg J, Pereira L, Berghella V. Pregnancy after uterine artery embolization. Obstet Gynecol 2002; 100(5 Pt 1):869–872.
62. Carpenter TT, Walker WJ. Pregnancy following uterine artery embolisation for symptomatic fibroids: A series of 26 complicated pregnancies. BJOG 2005; 112(3):321–325.
63. D'Angelo A, Amso NN, Wood A. Spontaneous multiple pregnancy after uterine artery embolization for uterine fibroid: Case report. Eur J Obstet Gynecol Reprod Biol 2003; 110(2): 245–246.
64. Istre O. Management of symptomatic fibroids: Conservative surgical treatment modalities other than hysterectomy and abdominal or laparoscopic myomectomy, Best Pract Res Clin Obstet Gynaecol, 2008; 22(4):735–747.
65. Hald K, Kløw NE, Qvigstad E, et al. Laparoscopic occlusion compared with embolization of uterine vessels: A randomized controlled trial. Obstet Gynecol 2007; 109:20–27.
66. Istre O, Hald K, Qvigstad E. Multiple myomas treated with a temporary, noninvasive, Doppler-directed, transvaginal uterine artery clamp. J Am Assoc Gynecol Laparosc 2004; 11:273–276.
67. Dickner SK, Cooper JM, Diaz D. A nonincisional, Doppler-guided transvaginal approach to uterine artery identification and control of uterine perfusion. J Am Assoc Gynecol Laparosc 2004; 11:55–58.

68. Vilos GA, Vilos EC, Romano W, et al. Temporary uterine artery occlusion for treatment of menorrhagia and uterine fibroids using an incisionless Doppler-guided transvaginal clamp: Case report. Hum Reprod 2006; 21:269–271.
69. Zupi E, Sbracia M, Marconi D, et al. Myolysis of uterine fibroids: Is there a role? Clin Obstet Gynecol 2006; 49:821–833.
70. Arcangeli S, Pasquarette MM. Gravid uterine rupture after myolysis. Obstet Gynecol 1997; 89:857:29.
71. Vilos GA, Daly LJ, Tse BM. Pregnancy outcome after laparoscopic electromyolysis. J Am Assoc Gynecol Laparosc 1998; 5:289–292.
72. Hillis SD, Marchbanks PA, Peterson HB. Uterine size and the risk of complications among women undergoing abdominal hysterectomy for leiomyomas. Obstet Gynecol 1996; 87: 415–419.
73. West S, Ruiz R, Parker WH. Abdominal myomectomy in women with very large uterine size. Fertil Steril 2006; 85:36–39.
74. Taylor A, Sharma M, Tsirkas P, et al. Reducing blood loss at open myomectomy using triple tourniquets: A randomised controlled trial. BJOG 2005; 112:340–345.
75. Liu WM, Wang PH, Chou CS, et al. Efficacy of combined laparoscopic uterine artery occlusion and myomectomy via minilaparotomy in the treatment of recurrent uterine myomas. Fertil Steril 2007; 87:356–361.
76. Kongnyuy E, Wiysonge C. Interventions to reduce haemorrhage during myomectomy for fibroids. Cochrane Database Syst Rev 2007; (1):CD005355.
77. Gutmann JN, Corson SL. GnRH agonist therapy before myomectomy or hysterectomy. J Minim Invasive Gynecol 2005; 12:529–537.
78. Lethaby A, Vollenhoven B, Sowter M. Pre-operative GnRH analogue therapy before hysterectomy or myomectomy for uterine fibroids. Cochrane Database Syst Rev 2001; (2): CD000547.
79. Taylor A, Sharma A, Tsirkas P, et al. Surgical and radiological management of uterine fibroids: A UK survey of current consultant practice. Acta Obstet Gynecol Scand 2005; 84: 478–482.
80. Practice Committee of the American Society for Reproductive Medicine. Pathogenesis, consequences, and control of peritoneal adhesions in gynecologic surgery. Fertil Steril 2007; 88:21–26.
81. Mais V, Ajossa S, Guerriero S, et al. Laparoscopic versus abdominal myomectomy: A prospective, randomized trial to evaluate benefits in early outcome. Am J Obstet Gynecol 1996; 175: 654–658.
82. Silva BA, Falcone T, Bradley L, et al. Case-controlled study of laparoscopic versus abdominal myomectomy. J Laparoendosc Adv Surg Tech A 2000; 10:191–197.
83. Stringer NH, Walker JC, Meyer PM. Comparison of 49 laparoscopic myomectomies with 49 open myomectomies. J Am Assoc Gynecol Laparosc 1997; 4:457–464.
84. Seracchioli R, Rossi S, Govoni F, et al. Fertility and obstetric outcome after laparoscopic myomectomy of large myomata: A randomized comparison with abdominal myomectomy. Hum Reprod 2000; 15:2663–2668.
85. Campo S, Campo V, Gambadauro P. Reproductive outcome before and after laparoscopic or abdominal myomectomy for subserous or intramural myomas. Eur J Obstet Gynecol Reprod Biol 2003; 110:215–219.
86. Soriano D, Dessolle L, Poncelet C, et al. Pregnancy outcome after laparoscopic and laparoconverted myomectomy. Eur J Obstet Gynecol Reprod Biol 2003; 108:194–198.
87. Fauconnier A, Chapron C, Babaki-Fard K, et al. Recurrence of leiomyomata after myomectomy. Hum Reprod Update 2000; 6:595–602.
88. Rossetti A, Sizzi O, Soranna L, et al. Long-term results of laparoscopic myomectomy: Recurrence rate in comparison with abdominal myomectomy. Hum Reprod 2001; 16:770–774.
89. Dubuisson JB, Fauconnier A, Babaki-Fard K, et al. Laparoscopic myomectomy: A current view. Hum Reprod Update 2000; 6:588–594.
90. Altgassen C, Kuss S, Berger U, et al. Complications in laparoscopic myomectomy. Surg Endosc 2006; 20:614–618.
91. Paul PG, Koshy AK, Thomas T. Pregnancy outcomes following laparoscopic myomectomy and single-layer myometrial closure. Hum Reprod 2006; 21:3278.
92. Seracchioli R, Manuzzi L, Vianello F, et al. Obstetric and delivery outcome of pregnancies achieved after laparoscopic myomectomy. Fertil Steril 2006; 86:159–165.
93. Dubuisson J, Fauconnier A, Deffarges J, et al. Pregnancy outcome and deliveries following laparoscopic myomectomy. Hum Reprod 2000; 15,869–873.
94. Mencaglia L, Tantini C. GnRH agonist analogs and hysteroscopic resection of myomas. Int J Gynaecol Obstet 1993; 43: 285–288.
95. Donnez J, Schrurs B, Gillerot S, et al. Treatment of uterine fibroids with implants of gonadotropin-releasing hormone agonist: Assessment by hysterography. Fertil Steril 1989; 51:947–950.
96. Perino A, Chianchiano N, Petronio M, et al. Role of leuprolide acetate depot in hysteroscopic surgery: A controlled study. Fertil Steril 1993; 59:507–510.
97. Campo S, Campo V, Gambadauro P. Short-term and long-term results of resectoscopic myomectomy with and without pretreatment with GnRH analogs in premenopausal women. Acta Obstet Gynecol Scand 2005; 84:756–760.
98. Crane JM, Healey S. Use of misoprostol before hysteroscopy: A systematic review. J Obstet Gynaecol Can 2006; 28: 373–379.
99. Jansen FW, Vredevoogd CB, van Ulzen K, et al. Complications of hysteroscopy: A prospective, multicenter study. Obstet Gynecol 2000; 96:266–270.
100. Propst AM, Liberman RF, Harlow BL, et al. Complications of hysteroscopic surgery: Predicting patients at risk. Obstet Gynecol 2000; 96:517–520.
101. Scottish Hysteroscopy Audit Group. A Scottish audit of hysteroscopic surgery for menorrhagia: Complications and follow up. Br J Obstet Gynaecol 1995; 102:249–254.
102. Aydeniz B, Gruber IV, Schauf B, et al. A multicenter survey of complications associated with 21,676 operative hysteroscopies. Eur J Obstet Gynecol Reprod Biol 2002; 104:160–164.
103. Shveiky D, Rojansky N, Revel A, et al. Complications of hysteroscopic surgery: "Beyond the learning curve". J Minim Invasive Gynecol 2007; 14:218–222.
104. Batra N, Khunda A, O'Donovan PJ. Hysteroscopic myomectomy. Obstet Gynecol Clin North Am 2004; 31:669–685.
105. Yaron Y, Shenhav M, Jaffa AJ, et al. Uterine rupture at 33 weeks gestation subsequent to hysteroscopic uterine perforation. Am J Obstet Gynecol 1994; 170:786–787.

20

Polycystic ovarian syndrome and ovarian drilling

Saad A. K. Amer and Tin Chiu Li

INTRODUCTION

Polycystic ovarian syndrome (PCOS) is a common endocrine disorder affecting 6% to 8% of women of reproductive age (1) and the most common cause (~75%) of anovulatory infertility (2). According to the 2003 ESHRE/ASRM (Rotterdam) criteria, PCOS is defined as a syndrome of ovarian dysfunction along with the cardinal features of hyperandrogenism and polycystic ovary morphology (3). It is characterized by a varied combination of clinical (oligo/amenorrhea, hirsutism, and obesity), biochemical (increased serum levels of luteinizing hormone (LH) and androgens), and sonographic (enlarged polycystic ovaries) features. PCOS is also associated with insulin resistance and compensatory hyperinsulinemia (4).

In women presenting with anovulation associated with PCOS, clomiphene citrate (CC) is the standard first-line treatment for induction of ovulation. Patients, who either remain anovulatory (CC resistance) or fail to conceive despite ovulation on CC, can be offered laparoscopic ovarian drilling (LOD), gonadotrophin ovarian stimulation, or metformin. Whilst the efficacy of LOD and gonadotrophin in inducing ovulation in women with PCOS has been well established (5,6), the efficacy of metformin in these cases has recently been questioned (7,8) LOD offers several advantages over gonadotrophin therapy and may therefore be recommended as the preferred second-line treatment for ovulation induction after CC.

This chapter will present an overview of PCOS and the current role of LOD in its management. The chapter will also discuss the techniques, clinical outcomes, possible mechanisms of action, complications, and predictors of success of LOD.

HISTORICAL BACKGROUND

Early in the 20th century, Stein and Leventhal were the first to define the association of polycystic ovaries with amenorrhea, hirsutism, and obesity (9). The diagnosis of PCOS was based on the clinical and histological features (10). In the 1970s, after the development of immunoassays of androgens and gonadotrophins, the diagnosis of PCOS was based more on biochemical features. Increased LH (11) and augmented androgen levels (12) were the main diagnostic features of this condition. In the late 1970s, improvement in ultrasound technology provided a noninvasive technique for assessment of ovarian morphology. Swanson and coworkers were the first to describe the ultrasound findings (enlarged ovaries containing an increased number of small follicles encircling the ovarian cortex) associated with PCOS (13). Ultimately, the advent of the high-resolution transvaginal ultrasonography permitted a more precise means of assessment of the internal morphological features of the polycystic ovaries and has gained an increasing importance in the diagnosis of PCOS.

Before 1930, there was no mention in the literature of any treatment for infertility associated with this PCOS. Stein and Leventhal first reported the success of ovarian wedge resection in inducing ovulation in PCOS women (9). Ovarian wedge resection was then accepted as the standard treatment for PCOS and remained the only available method of ovulation induction in women with this syndrome. In the 1960s, with the introduction of medical ovulation induction, ovarian wedge resection was largely abandoned due to its associated morbidity (14). Instead, CC became the standard treatment in anovulatory PCOS (15). In the late 1960s, with the development of operative laparoscopy, there was a renewed interest in the surgical treatment of PCOS carried out laparoscopically. The laparoscopic approach has been claimed to reduce the likelihood of postoperative adhesions compared with laparotomy. Several operative techniques were introduced for ovulation induction in CC-resistant PCOS, including ovarian biopsy, ovarian electrocautery, and ovarian laser treatment. Electrocautery and laser treatment result in thermal injury to the ovary via a number of punctures, hence the term "*ovarian drilling*" was used. In Table 1, the evolution of the different laparoscopic techniques is summarized.

ETIOLOGY AND PATHOGENESIS

Excess of Ovarian Androgen Production

The exact underlying etiology of PCOS remains largely unexplained. An increasing body of evidence suggests that an excess of ovarian androgen production remains central in the pathogenesis of PCOS. Three possible mechanisms for this androgen hypersecretion have been postulated, including (*i*) a genetically determined thecal cell functional defect, namely thecal cell hypertrophy; (*ii*) pituitary LH hypersecretion resulting in excessive thecal cell stimulation; or (*iii*) hyperinsulinemia resulting from insulin resistance, which stimulates thecal cell androgen production possibly through direct stimulatory effects on 17α-hydroxylase/17,20-lyase or indirectly by enhancing GnRH-stimulated LH release (19). Furthermore, hyperinsulinemia decreases the production of sex hormone–binding globulin (SHBG) by the liver, resulting in an increased serum concentration of free androgens (4,20).

Table 1 History of Important Development in the Treatment of Anovulation Associated with PCOS

Year	Treatment
1930	Bilateral ovarian wedge resection (9)
1961	Clomiphene citrate (15)
1967	Laparoscopic ovarian biopsies (16)
1978	Laparoscopic ovarian drilling (diathermy) (17)
1988	Laparoscopic ovarian drilling (laser) (18)

The excess ovarian androgen secretion results in an increased availability of precursors for estrogen production in granulosa cells. The granulosa cells of small antral follicles in PCOS acquire LH receptors prematurely (at follicular diameter of 4 mm), possibly due to hyperinsulinemia. This results in LH-induced aromatase activity in the small antral follicles, resulting in enhanced estrogen production. The resulting increased levels of circulating estrogens result in an increased positive feedback on LH and a negative feedback on follicle-stimulating hormone (FSH) secretion, thus causing disordered folliculogenesis.

Disordered Folliculogenesis

Despite a normal stock of primordial follicles and a normal early FSH-independent follicular development in polycystic ovaries, the follicular growth becomes arrested at the small antral phase with failure of dominance and escape from the natural process of atresia. This results in an increased number of primary, secondary, and small antral follicles (2–8 mm in diameter). The mechanism of this disturbed folliculogenesis in PCOS remains largely unknown. Several theories have been postulated, including relative FSH deficiency, abnormal LH stimulus, deficiency of certain local growth factors, or abnormal ovarian steroidogenesis.

Overweight/Obesity and PCOS

PCOS is typically associated with upper-body obesity, which promotes insulin resistance. The abdominal adipose tissue is highly lipolytic in nature, and testosterone further enhances its lipolysis. Increased lipolysis results in elevated plasma-free fatty acids that impair insulin-mediated glucose uptake (21). Obesity, therefore, exacerbates the biochemical and clinical features of PCOS through insulin resistance.

FEATURES OF PCOS

Clinical Features

Clinically, PCOS is associated with short- and long-term consequences. The short-term consequences include three groups of disorders, namely hyperandrogenic, reproductive (chronic oligo-/anovulation), and metabolic disorders. The manifestations of these disorders coexist in variable combinations in different women with PCOS. The long-term sequelae include diabetes mellitus, dyslipidemia, hypertension, cardiovascular disease, and endometrial carcinoma. These will not be discussed in this chapter.

Anovulatory Symptoms

Chronic anovulation is very common in women with PCOS and is often associated with menstrual irregularities, which characteristically date from the time of the menarche (22). The majority of PCOS women present with oligo- or amenorrhea, although other menstrual disorders such as polymenorrhea and irregular bleeding can be seen in ~10% of women with PCOS. About 15% to 20% of women with PCOS have regular menstrual cycles, and some women with menstrual abnormalities may resume regular ovulatory cycles for prolonged periods of time.

Hyperandrogenic Symptoms

Hyperandrogenic symptoms are common in women with PCOS and are typically mild to moderate. These include hirsutism, acne, and alopecia, which have been described in ~70%, 30%, and 8% of women with PCOS, respectively (23,24). Hirsutism typically starts in the decade between 15 and 25 years and progresses slowly to become noticeable one year after its onset. Virilization (e.g., clitoromegaly, temporal baldness, deepening of voice, or increase in muscle mass) is rare in PCOS and should be investigated to exclude other causes (24,25).

Metabolic Symptoms

Overweight/obesity (BMI > 25 kg/m^2) affects ~50% of women with PCOS (25) and is typically characterized by an upper-body obesity, which is defined as a ratio of waist-to-hip circumference exceeding 0.85 (26). This type of distribution, which is associated with increased insulin resistance, is detected even in nonobese PCOS women (27).

Acanthosis nigricans is a nonspecific cutaneous marker of moderate to severe insulin resistance, which is found in some cases of PCOS and is more common among obese patients (26). It is characterized by patchy, velvety, hyperpigmented skin changes affecting the neck, axillae, underneath the breasts, body folds, extensor surfaces of the joints, and vulva (28).

Ultrasound Features of PCOS

According to the ESHRE/ASRM Rotterdam consensus (2003), the criteria with sufficient specificity and sensitivity to define PCO include the presence of 12 or more follicles in each ovary measuring 2 to 9 mm in diameter, and/or increased ovarian volume (>10 mL) (29). A peripheral follicular distribution is no longer essential for the definition of PCO. This definition does not apply to women taking the oral contraceptive pill, since its use modifies ovarian morphology in normal women and putatively in women with PCO (30). Only one ovary fitting this definition is sufficient to define PCO (Fig. 1).

Endocrinological Features of PCOS

The most frequently found endocrine abnormalities in PCOS are summarized in Table 2 and include hyperandrogenism, elevated serum concentration of LH, LH:FSH ratio ≥2, and hyperinsulinemia.

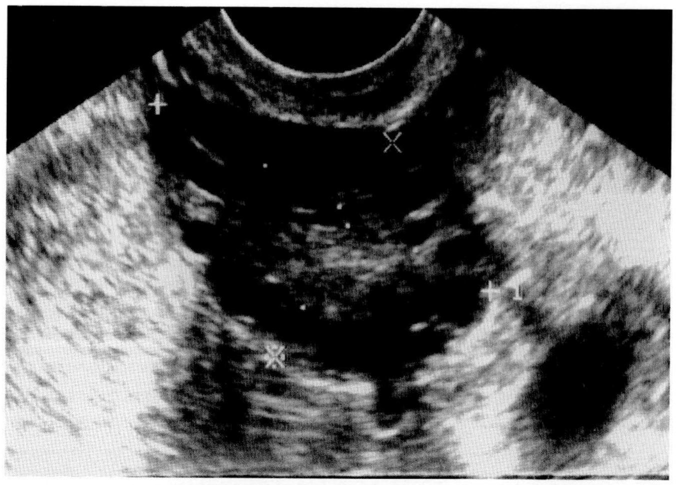

Figure 1 Appearance of the polycystic ovary on transvaginal ultrasound PCO is defined when the ovary contains 12 or more follicles measuring 2 to 9 mm in diameter and/or when its volume is increased (>10 mL).

Table 2 Endocrinological Features of PCOS

Hormone	Feature in PCOS	% Patients
LH	↑ >10 IU/L	60
LH/FSH ratio	↑ >2	95
Testosterone	↑ >2.5 nmol/L	70
Androstenedione	↑ >10 nmol/L	50
SHBG	↓	50
FAI	↑ >4.5	75
Prolactin	↑	30
Insulin	↑	50

Luteinizing Hormone

The serum concentrations of LH (above the 95th percentile of normal) are chronically elevated in ~60% of women with PCOS (31). This is due to increased amplitude and frequency of LH pulses (32). An elevated LH/FSH ratio is also a characteristic feature of PCOS and is observed in up to 95% of subjects (31). Although not included in the ESHRE/ASRM (Rotterdam) revised criteria of PCOS, an elevated serum LH level and/or elevated LH/FSH ratio has been considered useful secondary parameters in the definition of this syndrome (3).

Androgens

In most women with PCOS, serum concentrations of testosterone and androstenedione are modestly elevated, and in some cases dehydroepiandrosterone, dehydroepiandrosterone sulfate, and 17α-hydroxyprogesterone are also elevated. The most frequently detected biochemical marker in PCOS is an increased serum testosterone concentration, which occurs in ~70% of cases (33). Suppression of the SHBG serum level occurs in ~50% of PCOS women, resulting in an increase in free androgen index (FAI) (34). The latter has been shown to be more sensitive than total androgen concentrations in assessing hyperandrogenemia and is therefore considered a useful marker for PCOS (35).

Hyperinsulinemia

Peripheral insulin resistance occurs in about 50% of PCOS cases and is further aggravated by obesity (26). It is seldom necessary to measure the serum insulin concentration, as this will not affect the management of the patient. However, glucose intolerance develops in ~50% and diabetes in ~20% of obese women with PCOS (36). Assessment of glucose tolerance is therefore important in obese women. Hyperinsulinemia resulting from insulin resistance also has a principal role in the development of cardiovascular risk factors (26).

DIAGNOSIS OF PCOS

Until recently, the diagnostic criteria of PCOS have been the subject of much debate, with no universally agreed definition of this common syndrome. There have been two main schools for the diagnosis of PCOS; in Europe, the diagnosis of PCOS was primarily based on ovarian ultrasound morphology and to some extent on serum LH level and/or LH:FSH ratio (24,33), whereas in North America, the diagnosis was based on the 1991 NIH consensus, which emphasized on chronic anovulation and hyperandrogenism without necessarily finding PCO on ultrasound scan (37,38). In May 2003, experts from both sides of the Atlantic gathered in a PCOS consensus workshop in Rotterdam to revise the diagnostic criteria of this syndrome. The workshop concluded that the diagnosis of PCOS should be based on the presence of at least two of three criteria, including (*i*) oligo-/anovulation, (*ii*) hyperandrogenemia (clinical and/or biochemical), and (*iii*) polycystic ovaries on ultrasound scan (3).

The significance of a single finding of PCO on ultrasound scan in apparently normal (non-PCOS) women is controversial. While some believe that it may represent a normal variation (39), others consider it a silent form of the syndrome, which may develop into full-blown PCOS in the future (38).

MANAGEMENT OPTIONS FOR PCOS

Management of PCOS includes a symptom-orientated approach to the presenting problem and a preventive strategy for the associated long-term morbidity. A general approach to tackle both the short- and the long-term consequences of PCOS is to encourage weight loss in all overweight/obese patients. It is well established that weight reduction improves all PCOS symptoms and corrects the endocrine profile. Menstrual irregularity can be treated with the combined oral contraceptive pill or cyclical progestogen therapy. Hyperandrogenic skin symptoms may be treated with the contraceptive pill containing cyproterone acetate or with antiandrogen therapy. Anovulatory infertility in PCOS women can be treated with insulin sensitizing measures (such as weight reduction and metformin), CC, laparoscopic ovarian diathermy (LOD), and FSH ovarian stimulation.

LAPAROSCOPIC TREATMENT OF PCOS

Current Role of LOD in Women with PCOS

Currently, all overweight and obese PCOS women should first be encouraged to lose weight through lifestyle measures before any medical treatment. While CC remains the standard first-line treatment in anovulatory PCOS women, the second-line treatment has been the subject of much debate, with competition between LOD, gonadotrophin, and metformin to be the preferred choice (Fig. 2). Perhaps, with the increasing awareness of the predictors of success/failure of each of these treatments, it may now be possible to apply an individually tailored treatment according to each patient's pretreatment characteristics. The initial reports on the efficacy of metformin in ovulation induction in PCOS were encouraging (40,41). However, more recent data from large randomized trials showed metformin not to be as effective as initially it was thought to be (7,8). On the other hand, LOD and gonadotrophins have been shown to be equally effective in inducing ovulation and producing high pregnancy and live birth rates in women with PCOS (Table 3) (5,6). While some reproductive specialists advocate gonadotrophin ovulation induction for CC-resistant PCOS, others (including the authors of this chapter) are in favor of LOD. LOD may be seen as a preferred choice for ovulation induction after CC resistance/failure, as it offers several advantages over gonadotrophin therapy (Table 4). Importantly, in contrast to gonadotrophin therapy, LOD results in mono-ovulation, with no risk of ovarian hyperstimulation syndrome (OHSS) and with an incidence of multiple pregnancies no higher than background rates (5,6). Moreover, LOD is less costly and does not require complex monitoring. The cost per term pregnancy has been estimated to be €14,489 for gonadotrophin and €11,301 for LOD (22% lower) (42). In addition, with LOD, a single treatment leads to repeated physiological ovulatory cycles and potentially repeated pregnancies

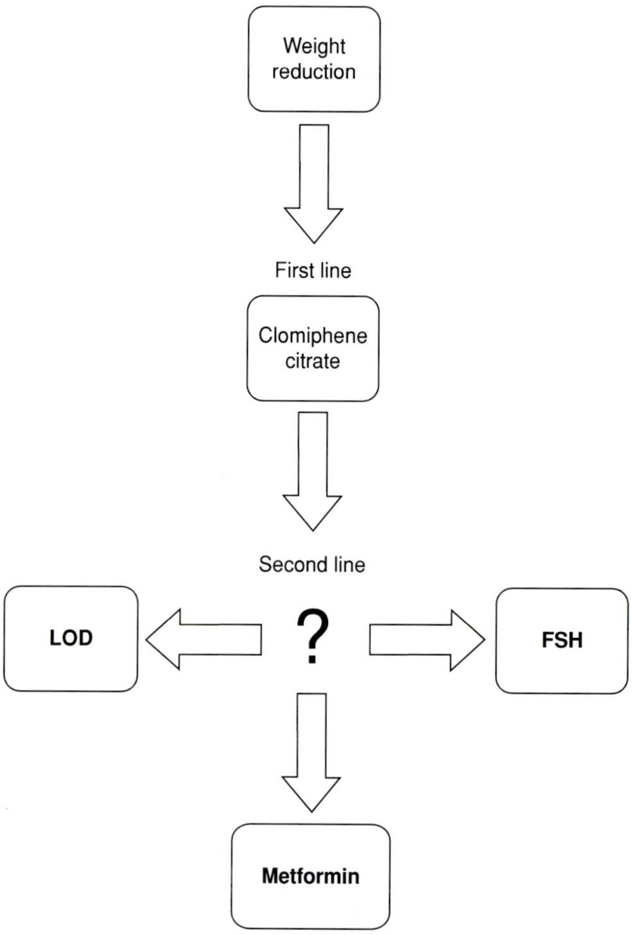

Figure 2 Management options for anovulatory infertility associated with PCOS. Weight reduction should be considered before any medical induction of ovulation in all overweight/obese PCOS women. Clomifene citrate (CC) is the standard first-line medical ovulation induction in nonobese PCOS women. The second-line treatment after CC resistance/failure is still uncertain, with competition between LOD, gonadotrophin, and metformin to be the preferred choice.

without the need for repeated courses of medical treatment. The main drawback of LOD is the need for general anesthetic and surgery. Other complications such as iatrogenic adhesion formation and premature ovarian failure are rare and appear to be of little clinical significance.

Table 3 LOD Versus rFSH in Clomiphene Citrate-Resistant Women with PCOS

	LOD strategy[b] ($n = 83$) (%)	rFSH[c] ($n = 85$)
Ovulation (per cycles)	70%	69%
Conception at 12/12	63 (76%)	64 (75%)
Multiple pregnancies	1[d] (<2%)	9 (14%)
Miscarriage rate	7 (11%)	7 (11%)
Live birth rate	51 (64%)	53 (60%)

[a]RCT by Bayram and coworkers (5).
[b]LOD strategy:
LOD alone ($n = 36$) → 31/83 pregnancies (37%),
LOD followed by CC and/or rFSH ($n = 47$) as follows:
LOD followed by CC only ($n = 24$) → 14/83 pregnancies (17%),
LOD followed by CC then rFSH ($n = 21$),
LOD followed by rFSH directly ($n = 2$) → 18/83 pregnancies (22%).
[c]rFSH: chronic low-dose step-up protocol.
[d]One patient had quintuplets after rFSH. A successful embryo reduction led to the live birth of twins.

Table 4 Advantages and Disadvantages of LOD Compared to FSH

Advantages
At least as effective as gonadotrophin treatment
Less costly
Avoids intensive, inconvenient, and complex monitoring
Single treatment produces repeated ovulatory cycles and potentially repeated pregnancies
Avoids OHSS
No increase in muliple pregnancies

Disadvantages
The need for surgery under general anesthetic
Iatrogenic adhesion formation
Theoretical risk of premature ovarian failure

Techniques of LOD

Several techniques of laparoscopic ovarian surgery to induce ovulation in PCOS have been described in the literature. Most of the techniques involve either taking ovarian biopsies or making multiple punctures on the surface of the ovary using electrosurgery or laser. More recently, there have been several attempts to use a transvaginal route to perform the ovarian surgery using either a fertiloscopy- or an ultrasound-guided approach. Currently, the most widely used technique for ovarian surgery is LOD using electrosurgery due to its simplicity, effectiveness, relative safety, and low cost. This technique will be described in details in this section.

LOD Using Electrosurgery

Three-puncture laparoscopy is established and the pelvis is thoroughly inspected for any pathology, and the ovaries are examined for the features of PCO. The utero-ovarian ligament is grasped with a pair of atraumatic grasping forceps, and the ovary is lifted up and stabilized in position away from the bowel (Fig. 3). This is essential to avoid direct or indirect thermal injury to the bowel. A specially designed monopolar electrosurgical probe (the Rockett of London ovarian diathermy needle, Fig. 4) is used to penetrate the ovarian capsule at a number of points. The probe has a distal stainless-steel

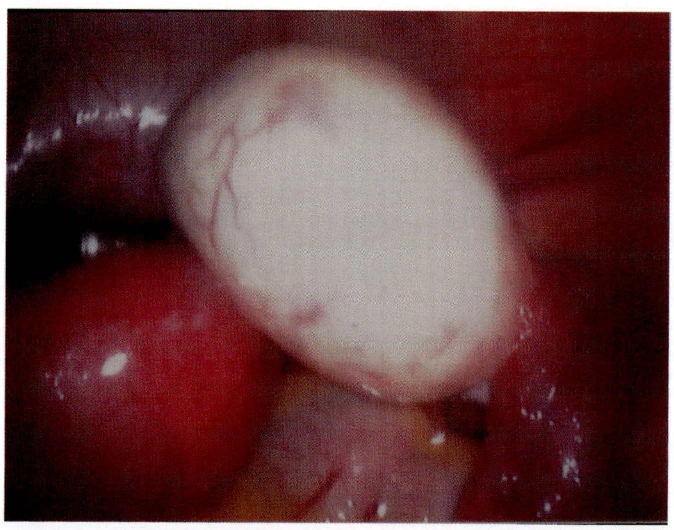

Figure 3 Stabilizing the ovary for LOD. The utero-ovarian ligament is grasped with atraumatic grasping forceps, and the ovary is lifted up away from the bowel.

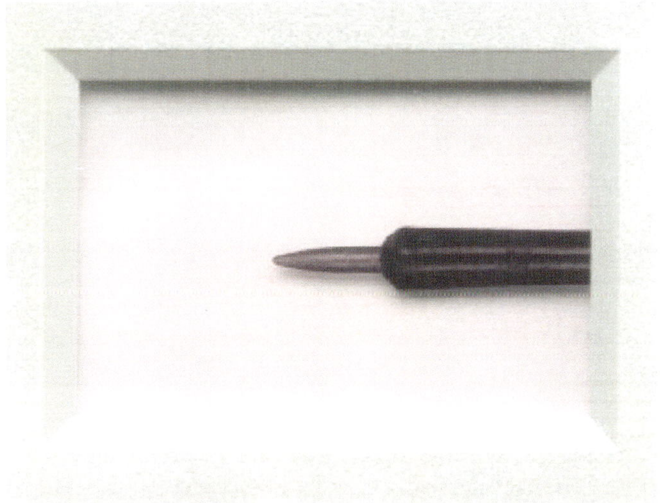

Figure 4 The Rockett of London ovarian diathermy needle probe. The distal stainless-steel needle measures 8 mm in length and 2 mm in diameter and projects from an insulated solid cone of 6 mm maximum diameter.

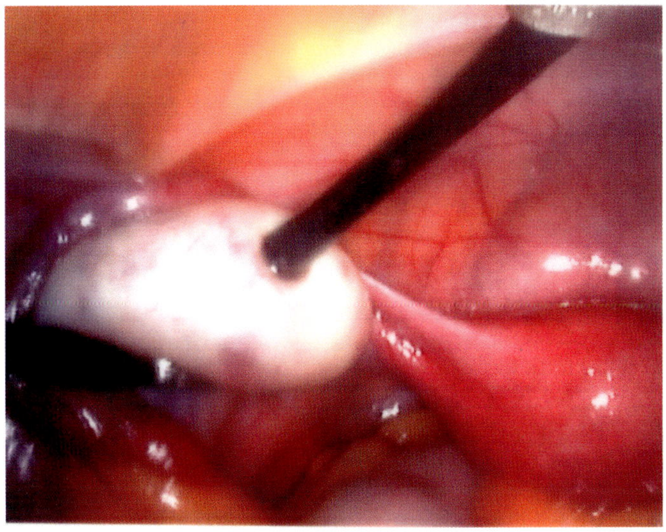

Figure 6 Needle penetration. The full length of the needle is pushed into the ovarian capsule and electricity is activated for five seconds

needle measuring 8 mm in length and 2 mm in diameter and projecting from an insulated solid cone of 6 mm maximum diameter. When the needle penetrates the capsule of the ovary, the insulated cone prevents deep penetration and minimizes thermal damage to the ovarian surface. The needle is applied to the antimesenteric surface of the ovary at right angle to avoid slippage and minimize surface damage (Fig. 5). The site of application should be away from the ovarian hilum and the fallopian tube. This is necessary to avoid damage of the hilum (which can lead to ovarian atrophy) and the fallopian tube (which can cause mechanical infertility). After insertion of the needle through the ovarian capsule (Fig. 6), monopolar coagulation electricity current is activated for five seconds with a power setting of 30 W. Electricity should not be activated before penetrating the surface of the ovary to avoid arcing and minimize the damage to the ovarian surface due to the charring effect, which may later cause adhesion formation. However, it may be necessary to facilitate the needle insertion by a short burst of diathermy. The ovary is then irrigated using Hartmann's solution before releasing it to its normal position (Fig. 7). The techniques are summarized in Table 5.

How Much Energy Should Be Used for LOD?

The amount of thermal energy used and number of punctures made in each ovary varied considerably in different studies. Between 3 and 25 punctures have been reported with power settings between 30 and 400 W (17,43–45). It is important to bear in mind that the number of punctures should be kept to a minimum, in order to avoid excessive ovarian destruction. Studies have shown three to six punctures per ovary to be sufficient to produce the desired effect of LOD (45,46). In a recent

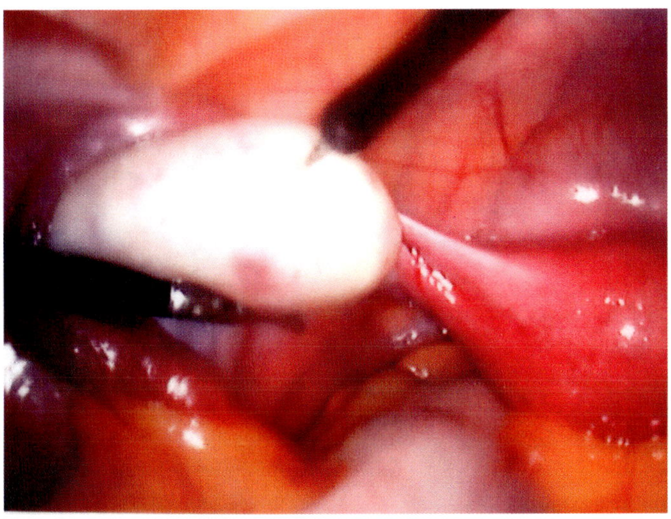

Figure 5 Needle application. With the ovary stabilized in position, the needle is applied to the antimesenteric surface at right angle.

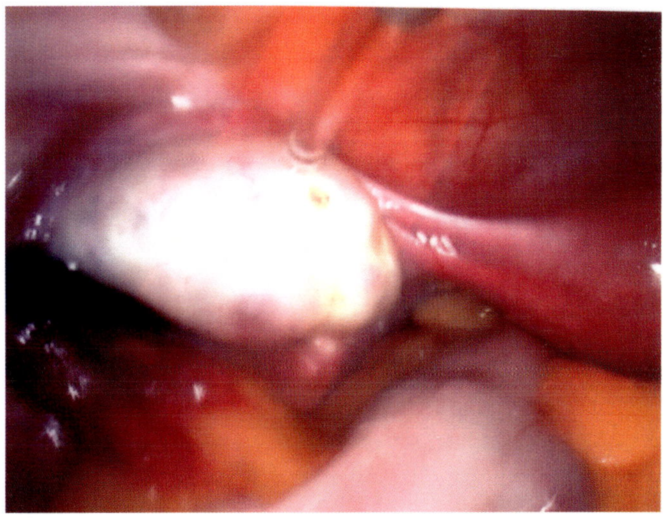

Figure 7 Irrigation after LOD. The ovary is cooled down by irrigation using Hartmann's solution before releasing the ligament.

Table 5 Techniques of LOD Using Electrocautery

1. Three-puncture technique
2. Utero-ovarian ligament is grasped with a pair of atraumatic forceps
3. The ovary is lifted up away from the bowel and stabilized
4. A specially designed monopolar electrosurgery needle probe is used
5. The probe is applied at right angle to the antimesenteric surface of the ovary
6. The probe should be away from ovarian hilum and the fallopian tube
7. Power is set at 30 W (coagulating)
8. The full length of the needle is pushed into the capsule to a depth of 6–8 mm
9. Electricity is activated for 5 sec
10. Four punctures are made in each ovary
11. The ovary is irrigated with saline before releasing the ovarian ligament
12. A crystalloid solution is instilled at the end of the procedure

dose-finding study, using an "up-and-down design," we have found four punctures per ovary at 30 W for five seconds (150 J) per puncture to be the optimum number required to achieve the best result (47).

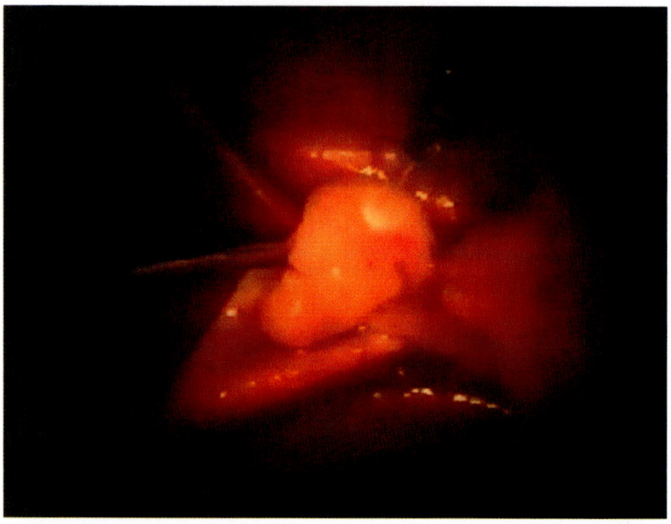

Figure 8 Laparoscopic ovarian drilling with argon laser. The argon laser fiber is introduced through a suction irrigation probe and is applied to the antimesenteric surface of the ovary. The fiber is pushed into the ovarian capsule, and laser is activated for one second with power setting at 6 to 16 W. Twenty to forty punctures are usually made.

Laser Ovarian Surgery

Four lasers, including Nd:YAG, CO_2, argon, and potassium-titanyl-phosphate (KTP) have been used to perform ovarian drilling in women with PCOS. Nd:YAG laser is delivered via a fine quartz fiber and can be used in the contact and noncontact mode. In the noncontact mode, the laser fiber is applied at a distance of 5 to 10 mm of the antimesenteric surface of the ovary, with a power setting of 30 to 100 W. It has been used to make incisions (18) or punctures (48) or to coagulate a wedge-like area (49). In the contact mode, with a sapphire tip screwed on the flexible laser fiber, the probe can be introduced into the ovarian capsule to create punctures (50) or to cut out a wedge-shaped portion (0.5 cm) of the ovary (51). CO_2 laser has been used to drill 10 to 40 craters in the ovarian tissue and to vaporize the visible subcapsular follicles. With power setting of 10 to 30 W in a continuous mode, the laser beam is focused to a spot size of 0.2 mm for 5 to 10 seconds per puncture. Argon and KTP lasers are delivered by flexible fiber, which are used in the contact mode without special tips. With a power setting of 6 to 16 W, all the visible subcapsular cysts can be vaporized and 20 to 40 punctures can be made in each ovary (Fig. 8).

Laser Versus Electrosurgery

It appears that electrocautery is superior to laser for LOD for a number of reasons. First, electrosurgery is more effective than laser in achieving ovulation and pregnancy (48,52,53). Second, laser, especially CO_2 laser, may be associated with a higher risk of adhesion formation because it produces more surface injury than electrosurgery. Third, electrosurgery is less costly and easier to set up. In addition, the effect of diathermy may last longer than the laser effect (52).

The Clinical Outcome of LOD

Immediate Outcome

A very rapid response has been reported following LOD, with ovulation occurring within two to four weeks and menstruation within four to six weeks in the responders. Restoration of regular ovulatory cycles occurs in 70% to 80% of cases. Recently, in a large randomized controlled trial involving 168 CC-resistant PCOS women, Bayram and coworkers reported ovulation rate of 70% per cycle and cumulative conception and live birth rates of 76% and 64%, respectively, following LOD (Table 3) (5).

The main hormonal changes consistently observed after LOD include a rapid and persistent fall of serum concentrations of androgens (testosterone and androstenedione) with a transient increase of gonadotrophins (LH and FSH) during the first 24 to 48 hours, followed later by a gradual fall (45,54–56).

Long-Term Outcome

The favorable clinical and endocrine effects of LOD seem to last for many years (up to 20 years) in a significant proportion of women with PCOS (52,57). In a recent long-term follow-up study involving 116 anovulatory women with PCOS who underwent LOD, we found that the improvements in endocrine parameters, menstrual pattern, and reproductive performance seemed to last for many years in about a third of cases (58,59).

Mechanism of Action of LOD

The mechanism of action of LOD remains largely unexplained. It is likely that LOD exerts its effects via the destruction of androgen-producing tissue in the ovary. The resulting decrease in circulating androgen concentrations may result in a fall in estrone (E1) due to decreased peripheral aromatization of androgens. This fall in E1 then results in decreased positive feedback on LH and decreased negative feedback on FSH at the level of the pituitary. The resulting rise in serum FSH concentrations occurring in the postoperative period results in increased aromatase activity within the follicles. This effect, coupled with a decrease in local androgen concentrations, would convert the intrafollicular environment from being androgen dominant to one that is estrogenic. This may remove an intraovarian block to follicular maturation, allowing follicular development to proceed to subsequent ovulation.

It has also been suggested that ovarian injury leads to the production of nonsteroidal factors, which affect the ovarian–pituitary feedback (60). More recently, it has been hypothesized that the ovary produces a number of growth factors

Table 6 Adhesion Formation after LOD using Monpolar Diathermy

Author	Year	No of patients		Adhesions	
		Total	SLL/CS*	n	Rate**
Greenblatt and Casper[62]	1993	8	8	8	100%
Naether[63]	1995	215	66	12	18%
Saravelos co-workers[64]	1996	21	21	12	57%
Total		244	95	32	34%

*SLL/CS = Second look laparoscopy/Caesarean section.
**Rate per patients who underwent SLL/CS.

(such as IGF-I) in response to tissue injury, which sensitize the ovary to circulating FSH resulting in stimulation of follicular growth.

Predictors of the Outcome of LOD

In a recent study, we investigated various clinical and biochemical factors that may predict the clinical outcome of LOD in 200 PCOS women. We found that marked obesity (BMI $\geq$ 35 kg/m^2), marked hyperandrogenism (testosterone $\geq$4.5 nmol/L or FAI $\geq$15), and/or long duration of infertility (>3 years) seemed to predict resistance to LOD. We also reported that that high preoperative LH concentration ($\geq$10 IU/L) in women who ovulated after LOD appeared to predict higher probability of pregnancy. Age, the presence or absence of acne, the menstrual pattern, LH:FSH ratio, and ovarian volume did not seem to predict the outcome of LOD (61).

Complications of LOD

Intraoperative complications of LOD are rare and include damage to the utero-ovarian ligament, bleeding from the ovary at the diathermy points, and thermal injury to the bowel. Postoperatively, the main drawback of LOD is iatrogenic adhesion formation. An incidence of 30% to 40% has been reported in various studies (Table 6) (62–64). Most studies reported only mild and moderate adhesions, which do not seem to affect the pregnancy rate after LOD. Nevertheless, all precautions should be taken to minimize adhesion formation. This can be achieved by minimizing thermal injury to the ovarian surface (as described above), ample irrigation, and instillation of crystalloid solution at the end of the procedure (64). Another theoretical risk associated with LOD is premature ovarian failure possibly due to excessive destruction of the normal ovarian follicles or the inadvertent damage of the ovarian blood supply. In our cohort of 116 patients with PCOS who were followed up for up to nine years after LOD, no case of premature ovarian failure was observed (59). This risk can largely be avoided by minimizing the number of punctures made and by delivering the energy away from the ovarian hilum.

Failure of Laparoscopic Ovarian Surgery

Women are considered to have failed after LOD if they do not ovulate within six to eight weeks, if they experience recurrence of the anovulatory status after an initial response, or if they fail to conceive despite regular ovulation for 12 months. For anovulatory patients, CC may be restarted. Many studies have demonstrated that LOD renders the ovaries more sensitive to CC (17). If the patient is still anovulatory on CC, the treatment options are (*i*) gonadotrophin ovarian stimulation, (*ii*) metformin, (*iii*) IVF, or (*iv*) repeat LOD. We have recently reported encouraging success rates after repeat LOD in women who previously responded to their first LOD. On the other hand, repeat LOD was not effective in the previous nonresponders (65).

CONCLUSION

Women with PCOS often present with anovulatory infertility, menstrual irregularities, hyperandrogenic skin manifestations, and/or overweight/obesity. The short-term management of this syndrome is symptom oriented. Anovulatory PCOS women who are obese or overweight should first undergo a weight reduction program before embarking on medical treatment. CC remains the standard first-line treatment for ovulation induction in patients with PCOS. LOD has been recommended by many authors as the second line of choice for induction of ovulation in CC-resistant PCOS women, although others have advocated FSH as the preferred treatment. LOD is as effective as FSH ovarian stimulation and has the advantage of avoiding complications such as multiple pregnancies and OHSS. The most widely used technique for laparoscopic ovarian surgery is ovarian drilling using monopolar diathermy needle. Four punctures per ovary at 30 W applied for five seconds per puncture seem to be the optimum amount of energy required for LOD. About two-thirds of women ovulate in response to LOD. Fifty percent of the responders, i.e., about one-third of the total number of patients undergoing LOD, will continue to benefit for several years. The main drawback of LOD is the need for a general anesthetic, an adhesion formation, and a theoretical risk of premature ovarian failure.

REFERENCES

1. Asuncion M, Calvo RM, San Millan JL, et al. A prospective study of the prevalence of the polycystic ovary syndrome in unselected Caucasian women from Spain. J Clin Endocrinol Metab 2000; 85:2434–2438.
2. Hull MG. Epidemiology of infertility and polycystic ovarian disease: Endocrinological and demographic studies. Gynecol Endocrinol 1987; 1:235–245.
3. Rotterdam ESHRE/ASRM-Sponsored PCOS Consensus Workshop Group. Revised 2003 consensus on diagnostic criteria and long-term health risks related to polycystic ovary syndrome. Fertil Steril 2004; 81:19–25.
4. Nestler JE. Role of hyperinsulinemia in the pathogenesis of the polycystic ovary syndrome, and its clinical implications. Semin Reprod Endocrinol 1997; 15:111–122.
5. Bayram N, van Wely M, Kaaijk EM, et al. Using an electrocautery strategy or recombinant follicle stimulating hormone to induce ovulation in polycystic ovary syndrome: Randomised controlled trial. BMJ 2004; 328:192–195.
6. Farquhar C, Lilford RJ, Marjoribanks J, et al. Laparoscopic "drilling" by diathermy or laser for ovulation induction in anovulatory polycystic ovary syndrome. Cochrane Database Syst Rev 2005; 20:CD001122.
7. Moll E, Bossuyt PM, Korevaar JC, et al. Effect of clomifene citrate plus metformin and clomifene citrate plus placebo on induction of ovulation in women with newly diagnosed polycystic ovary syndrome: Randomised double blind clinical trial. BMJ 2006; 24:1485–1488.
8. Legro RS, Barnhart HX, Schlaff WD, et al. Clomiphene, metformin, or both for infertility in the polycystic ovary syndrome. N Engl J Med 2007; 356:551–566.
9. Stein IF, Leventhal ML. Amenorrhoea associated with bilateral polycystic ovaries. Am J Obstet Gynaecol 1935; 29:181–191.
10. Goldzieher JW, Axelrod LR. Clinical and biochemical features of polycystic ovarian disease. Fertil Steril 1963; 14:631–653.
11. Rebar R, Judd HL, Yen SS, et al. Characterization of the inappropriate gonadotropin secretion in polycystic ovary syndrome. J Clin Invest 1976; 57:1320–1329.
12. Raj SG, Thompson IE, Berger MJ, et al. Diagnostic value of androgen measurements in polycystic ovary syndrome. Obstet Gynecol 1978; 52:169–171.

13. Swanson M, Sauerbrie EE, Cooperberg PL. Medical implications of ultrasonically detected polycystic ovaries. J Clin Ultrasound 1981; 9:219–222.
14. Buttram VC, Vaquero C. Post-ovarian wedge resection adhesive disease. Fertil Steril 1975; 26:874–876.
15. Greenblatt RB. Chemical induction of ovulation. Fertil Steril 1961; 12:402–404.
16. Palmer R, de Brux J. Résulats histologiques, biochemiques et therapeutiques obtenus ches les femmes don't les ovaries avaient été diagnostiqués Stein-Leventhal à la coelioscpie. Bulletin Federation Societes de Gynecologie et Obstetrique de Langue Française 1967; 19:405–412.
17. Gjonnaess H. Polycystic ovarian syndrome treated by ovarian electrocautery through the laparoscope. Fertil Steril 1984; 4:20–25.
18. Huber J, Hosmann J, Spona J. Polycystic ovarian syndrome treated by laser through the laparoscope [letter]. Lancet 1988; 2:215.
19. Barbieri RL. The role of adipose tissue and hyperinsulinemia in the development of hyperandrogenism. In: L'Hermite ML, ed. Progress in Reproductive Biology and Medicine, Vol. 14. Basel: Karger, 1990.
20. Dunaif A. Insulin resistance and the polycystic ovary syndrome: Mechanism and implications for pathogenesis. Endocr Rev 1997; 18:774–800.
21. Jensen MD, Haymond MW, Rizza RA, et al. Influence of body fat distribution on free fatty acid metabolism in obesity. J Clin Invest 1989; 83:1168–1173.
22. Yen SS. The polycystic ovary syndrome. Clin Endocrinol (Oxf) 1980; 12:177–207.
23. Franks S. Morphology of the polycystic ovary in polycystic ovary syndrome. In: Dunaif A, Given JR, Haseltine FP, Merriam GR, eds. Polycystic Ovary Syndrome. Boston: Blackwell, 1992:19–28.
24. Balen AH, Conway GS, Kaltsas G, et al. Polycystic ovary syndrome: The spectrum of the disorder in 1741 patients. Hum Reprod 1995; 10:2107–2111.
25. Taylor AE. Polycystic ovary syndrome. Endocrinol Metab Clin North Am 1998; 27:877–902.
26. Dunaif A, Segal KR, Shelley DR, et al. Evidence for distinctive and intrinsic defects in insulin action in polycystic ovary syndrome. Diabetes 1992; 41:1257–1266.
27. Pasquali R, Casimirri F, Venturoli S, et al. Body fat distribution has weight-independent effects on clinical, hormonal, and metabolic features of women with polycystic ovary syndrome. Metabolism 1994; 43:706–713.
28. Barbieri R. Hyperandrogenism. In: Wallach EE, Zacur HA, eds. Reproductive Medicine and Surgery. St Louis, MO: Mosby, 1995:209.
29. Jonard S, Robert Y, Cortet-Rudelli C, et al. Ultrasound examination of polycystic ovaries: Is it worth counting the follicles? Hum Reprod 2003; 18:598–603.
30. Christensen JT, Boldsoen J, Westergaard JG. Ovarian volume in gynecologically healthy women using contraception or using IUD. Acta Obstet Gynecol Scand 1997; 76:784–789.
31. Taylor AE, McCourt B, Martin KA, et al. Determinants of abnormal gonadotropin secretion in clinically defined women with polycystic ovary syndrome. J Clin Endocrinol Metab 1997; 82:2248–2256.
32. Waldstreicher J, Santoro NF, Hall HJE, et al. Hyperfunction of the hypothalamic ± pituitary axis in women with polycystic ovarian disease: Indirect evidence of partial gonadotroph desensitization. J Clin Endocrinol Metab 1988; 66:165–172.
33. Robinson S, Rodin DA, Deacon A, et al. Which hormone tests for the diagnosis of polycystic ovary syndrome? Br J Obstet Gynaecol 1992; 99:232–238.
34. Eden JA, Place J, Carter GD, et al. The diagnosis of polycystic ovaries in subfertile women. Br J Obstet Gynaecol 1989; 96:809–815.
35. Adams J, Polson DW, Franks S. Prevalence of polycystic ovaries in women with anovulation and idiopathic hirsutism. Br Med J 1986; 293:355–359.
36. Legro RS, Kunselman AR, Dodson WC, et al. Prevalence and predictors of risk for type 2 diabetes mellitus and impaired glucose tolerance in polycystic ovary syndrome: A prospective, controlled study in 254 affected women. J Clin Endocrinol Metab 1999; 84:165–169.
37. Lobo RA. A disorder without identity: "HCA," "PCO," "PCOD," "PCOS," "SLS". What are we to call it? Fertil Steril 1995; 63:1158–1160.
38. Carmina E, Wong L, Chang L, et al. Endocrine abnormalities in ovulatory women with polycystic ovaries on ultrasound. Hum Reprod 1997; 12:905–909.
39. Clayton RN, Ogden V, Hodgkinson J, et al. How common are the polycystic ovaries in normal women and what is their significance for the fertility of the population? Clin Endocrinol 1992; 37:127–134.
40. Lord JM, Flight IH, Norman RJ. Metformin in polycystic ovary syndrome: Systematic review and meta-analysis. BMJ 2003; 327:951–953.
41. Palomba S, Orio F Jr, Nardo LG, et al. Metformin administration versus laparoscopic ovarian diathermy in clomiphene citrate-resistant women with polycystic ovary syndrome: A prospective parallel randomized double-blind placebo-controlled trial. J Clin Endocrinol Metab 2004; 89:4801–4809.
42. Farquhar CM. An economic evaluation of laparoscopic ovarian diathermy versus gonadotrophin therapy for women with clomiphene citrate-resistant polycystic ovarian syndrome. Curr Opin Obstet Gynecol 2005; 17:347–353.
43. Naether OGJ, Fischer R, Weise HC, et al. Laparoscopic electrocoagulation of the ovarian surface in infertile patients with polycystic ovarian disease. Fertil Steril 1993; 60:88–94.
44. Felemban A, Tan SL, Tulandi T. Laparoscopic treatment of polycystic ovaries with insulated needle cautery: A reappraisal. Fertil Steril 2000; 73(2):266–269.
45. Armar NA, McGarrigle HHG, Honour J, et al. Laparoscopic ovarian diathermy in the management of anovulatory infertility in women with polycystic ovaries: Endocrine changes and clinical outcome. Fertil Steril 1990; 53:45–49.
46. Amer SA, Li TC, Cooke ID. Laparoscopic ovarian diathermy in women with polycystic ovarian syndrome: A retrospective study on the influence of the amount of energy used on the outcome. Hum Reprod 2002; 17:1046–1051.
47. Amer S, Li TC, Cooke ID. A prospective dose finding study of the amount of energy required for laparoscopic ovarian diathermy in women with polycystic ovarian syndrome. Hum Reprod 2003; 18:1693–1698.
48. Gurgan T, Kisnisci H, Yarali H, et al. Evaluation of adhesion formation after laparoscopic treatment of polycystic ovarian disease. Fertil Steril 1991; 56:1176–1178.
49. Keckstein G, Rossmanith W, Spatzier K, et al. The effect of laparoscopic treatment of polycystic ovarian disease by CO2-laser or Nd:YAG laser. Surg Endosc 1990; 4:103–107.
50. Keckstein J. Laparoscopic treatment of polycystic ovarian syndrome. Baillieres Clin Obstet Gynaecol 1989; 3:563–581.
51. Kojima E, Yanagibori A, Otaka K, et al. Ovarian wedge resection with contact Nd:YAG laser irradiation used laparoscopically. J Reprod Med 1989; 34:444–446.
52. Naether OGJ, Baukloh V, Fischer R, et al. Long-term follow-up in 206 infertility patients with polycystic ovarian syndrome after laparoscopic electrocautery of the ovarian surface. Hum Reprod 1994; 9:2342–2349.
53. Li TC, Saravelos H, Chow MS, et al. Factors affecting the outcome of laparoscopic ovarian drilling for polycystic ovarian syndrome in women with anovulatory infertility. Br J Obstet Gynaecol 1998; 105:338–344.
54. Aakvaag A, Gjonnaess H. Hormonal response to electrocautery of the ovary in patients with polycystic ovarian disease. Br J Obstet Gynaecol 1985; 92:1258–1264.
55. Gjonnaess H, Norman N. Endocrine effects of the ovarian electrocautery in patients with polycystic ovarian disease. Br J Obstet Gynaecol 1987; 94:779–783.

56. Tiitinen A, Tenhunen A, Seppālā M. Ovarian electrocauterization causes LH-regulated but not insulin-regulated endocrine changes. Clin Endocrinol 1993; 39:181–184.
57. Gjonnaess H. Late endocrine effects of Ovarian electrocautery in of women with polycystic ovary syndrome. Fertil Steril 1998; 69:697–701.
58. Amer S, Li TC, Banu Z, et al. Long term follow up of patients with polycystic ovarian syndrome after laparoscopic ovarian drilling: Endocrine and ultrasonographic outcomes. Hum Reprod 2002; 17:2851–2857.
59. Amer S, Li TC, Gopalan V, et al. Long term follow up of patients with polycystic ovarian syndrome after laparoscopic ovarian drilling: Clinical outcome. Hum Reprod 2002; 17:2035–2042.
60. Rossmanith WG, Keckstein J, Spatzier K, et al. The impact of ovarian laser surgery on the gonadotrophin secretion in women with polycystic ovarian disease. Clin Endocrinol (Oxf) 1991; 34:223–230.
61. Amer S, Li TC, Ledger WL. Ovulation induction using laparoscopic ovarian drilling in women with polycystic ovarian syndrome: Predictors of success. Hum Reprod 2004; 19:1719–1724.
62. Greenblatt EM, Casper RF. Adhesion formation after laparoscopic ovarian cautery for polycystic ovarian syndrome: Lack of correlation with pregnancy rate. Fertil Steril 1993; 60:766–770.
63. Naether OGJ. Significant reduction of adnexal adhesions following laparoscopic electrocautery of the ovarian surface (LEOS) by lavage and artificial ascites. Gynaecol Endosc 1995; 4:17–19.
64. Saravelos H, Li TC. Post-operative adhesions after laparoscopic electrosurgical treatment for polycystic ovarian syndrome with the application of Interceed to one ovary: A prospective randomized controlled study. Hum Reprod 1996; 11:992–997.
65. Amer S, Li TC, Cooke ID. Repeated laparoscopic ovarian diathermy is effective in women with anovulatory infertility due to polycystic ovarian syndrome. Fertil Steril 2003; 79:1211–1215.

21

Fallopian tube: physiology, pathophysiology, and occlusive conditions

Peter F. McComb and Victor Gomel

The fallopian tube is a very important organ for the survival of our species. It is the usual meeting place of oocyte and sperm. It is the site of conception. The fallopian tube has several important functions: (*i*) pro-ovarian sperm transport, (*ii*) sperm maintenance and capacitation, (*iii*) ovum capture and transport in prouterine direction, (*iv*) ampullary retention of the ovum, (*v*) provision of a milieu to sustain the ovum and allow fertilization to occur, and finally (*vi*) transport of the zygote from the ampulla to the uterine cavity.

ANATOMY AND PHYSIOLOGY OF THE FALLOPIAN TUBE

Ovum retrieval by the fallopian tube in the human differs from other species. In the rat, the ovary is contained within a bursa, which also includes the fimbriae. In the rabbit and pig, suspensory ligaments link the tube and ovary and thus direct the oocyte within the cumulus oophorus toward the fimbriae. No such ligaments exist in the human. Once ovulation occurs in the human, the cumulus oophorus may adhere to the edge of the ruptured follicle. There appears to be little innate muscular movement of the human fallopian tube (in contrast to lower species). Rather, the small bowel that invests the pelvic organs, may jostle the fallopian tube and ovary to ensure at least random apposition of fimbriae to ovarian surface.

Although direct observation of oocyte and sperm transport in women is not feasible, corresponding data observed directly within the rabbit oviduct may be relevant. After retrieval of the cumulus oophorus and oocyte by the fimbriae, transport by the ciliated mucosa through the ampulla occurs at 0.1 mm/sec until the ampullary–isthmic junction is reached (1). The diminutive diameter of the isthmic lumen and thick isthmic musculature cause the cumulus oophorus to lodge at the junction (Fig. 1). Here, fertilization occurs and the granulosa cells disperse (18 hours postovulation). Once the embryo enters the isthmus, myosalpingeal contractions confer a to-and-fro motion upon the embryo, an individual contraction causing an excursion of up to 10 mm (Fig. 2). After a further 48 hours, the isthmic contractions appear to propel the embryo into the endometrial cavity (2).

In women, oocyte transport across the fimbriae and through the ampulla is a function of cilia-induced fluid currents. Those who have ciliary immotility (Kartagener's syndrome) are infertile (3). Of all portions of the oviduct, the ampullary segment is considered essential. Fertility may be preserved to a variable degree with resection or absence of the cornu, isthmus, and even infundibulum. The fallopian tube is one part of the apparatus that preserves the basic aquatic nature of reproduction in higher forms of life. To put it another way, life began in the sea. With evolution to become higher mammals, we have wrapped the fertilization process within the oviduct, while maintaining the essential fluid basis. An awareness of this original function allows some insight as to why the oviduct is constructed the way it is and also as to how it functions.

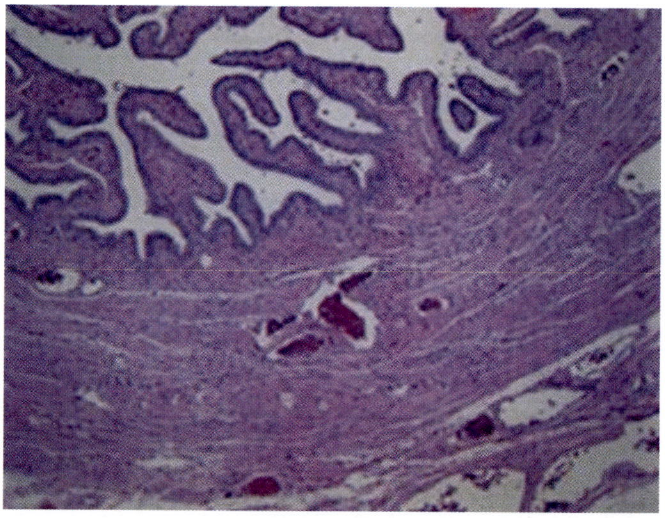

Figure 1 Light microscopy: cross-section of the region of the human ampullary–isthmic junction. Note the thick myosalpinx. (Hematoxylin and eosin stain.)

Anatomy of the Fallopian Tube

In women the fallopian tube is a tubular structure of approximately 9 to 11 cm length; there is wide interindividual

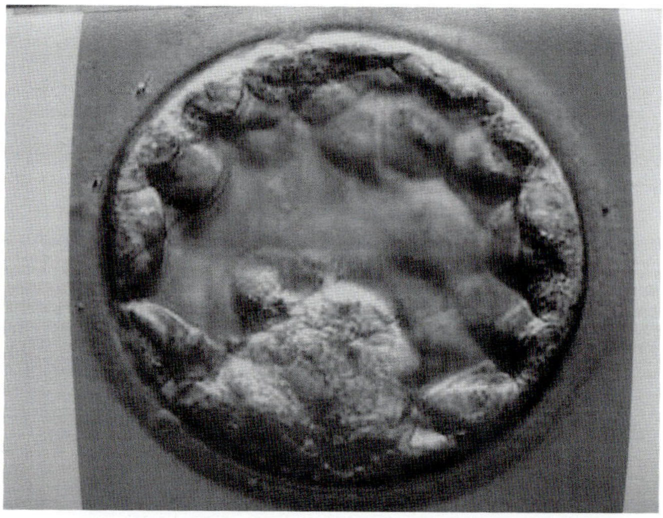

Figure 2 Light microscopy: human embryo at blastocyst stage.

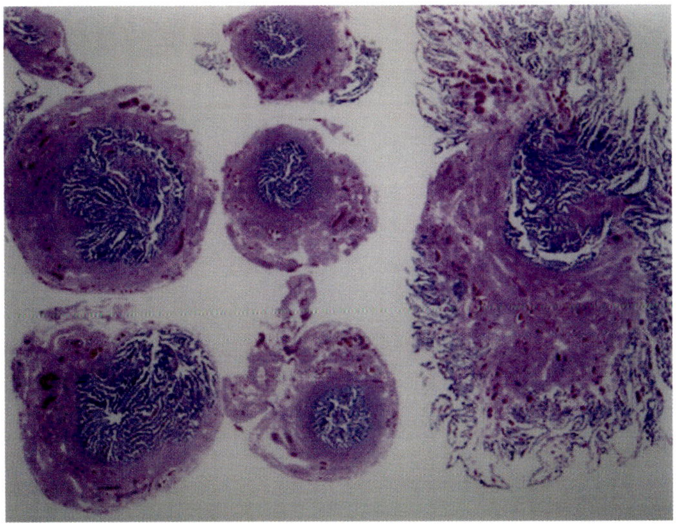

Figure 3 Light microscopy: cross-sections of fimbria (right), ampulla (left), and isthmus (center). (Hematoxylin and eosin stain.)

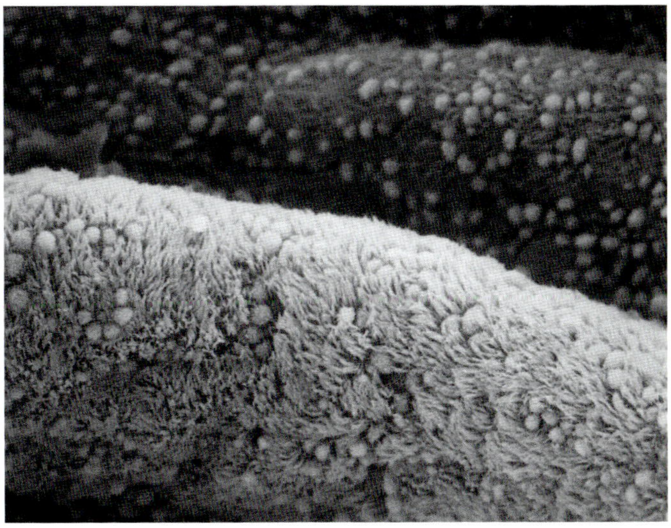

Figure 5 Scanning electron microscopy: ampulla of rabbit oviduct. Rugal fold of endosalpinx showing populations of ciliated and secretory cells. Magnification ×1700.

variation (Fig. 3). It is the site of ovum retrieval, ovum and sperm transport, sperm capacitation, fertilization, and later embryo transport (1). The tubal environment also provides vital nutrient support for the dividing embryo. These mechanisms occur in various anatomic sections of the normal tube.

Cyclical changes in anatomic (ciliation and epithelial height), endocrinological, and mechanical patterns (4–7) have been postulated or proven (8). Although studies have elucidated certain aspects of tubo-ovarian interaction, not all have been verified in humans (8–11).

The oviduct is made up of the fimbriae, infundibulum, ampulla, isthmus, and intramural (interstitial) tube. The fimbriae, the most distal portion of the oviduct, are relatively free and motile. The only attachment to the ovary is via the fimbria ovarica, one of about 25 fimbrial folds. Even this attachment is inconstant. The fimbriae attach to the infundibulum, a trumpet-shaped portion of the fallopian tube of 1 cm length. Like the fimbriae it is thin walled, is densely ciliated (60–80%) (12,13), and has a complex pattern of mucosal folds. Ovum retrieval and initial transport (14) are effected by the close spatial relationship of the fimbriae to the site of ovulation.

The ampulla comprises approximately two-thirds of the total tubal length. Its luminal diameter decreases from 1 cm at the ampullary–infundibular junction to 1 to 2 mm at the ampullary–isthmic junction. The seromuscular layer is thin and comprises an incomplete internal longitudinal, a middle circular, and an external longitudinal layer. The mucosal folds within the ampulla are complex. The lumen is packed with these folds. Approximately 40% to 50% of ampullary cells are ciliated (13) (Figs. 4–8). The inner longitudinal spiral

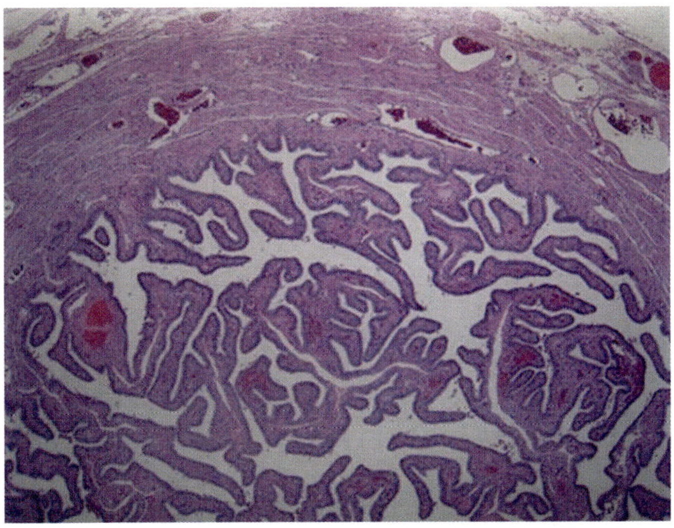

Figure 4 Light microscopy: cross-section of human ampulla demonstrating complex folds of ciliated endosalpinx that fill the lumen. (Hematoxylin and eosin stain.)

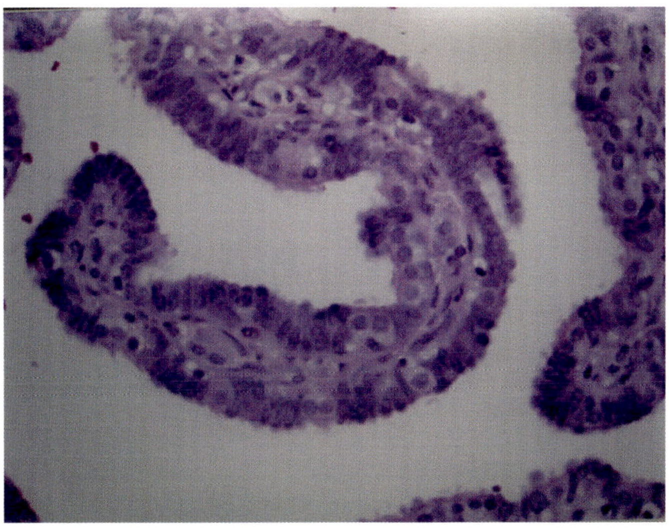

Figure 6 Light microscopy: cross-section of ampullary fold of human endosalpinx.

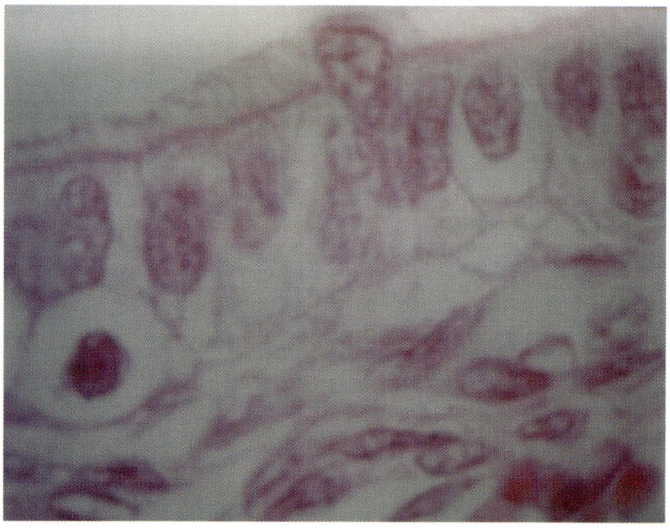

Figure 7 Light microscopy: detail of human ampullary endosalpinx showing ciliated cells. (Hematoxylin and eosin stain.)

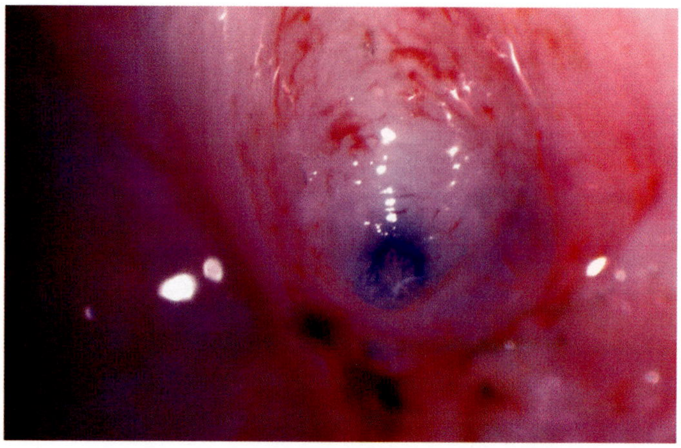

Figure 9 Microphotograph: cut surface of human isthmus.

myosalpingeal layer found in the ampulla is lost at the ampullary–isthmic junction.

The isthmus represents approximately one-third of tubal length (3–3.5 cm) and is considerably narrower than the ampulla (0.1–0.5 mm). The muscular layers are well developed. Isthmic ciliation is less profuse (25–30%) (3) compared to the ampulla. The isthmus has four primary mucosal folds (Figs. 9 and 10).

The intramural or interstitial segment of the tube is short (10 mm) and narrow with either a straight, arched, or convoluted course through the myometrium (14). It has been described as the junction between tube and uterus or, erroneously, as a sphincter although no anatomic correlate to a sphincter has been documented. At the site of junction of the endometrial funnel with the intramural portion of the tube, an abrupt change from endometrial to tubal mucosa occurs (15). A well-developed inner longitudinal muscle layer surrounded by a circular layer is present in the intramural segment. Because of this circular musculature, the uterine cornu can be incised tangentially at the level of the junction of the intramural tube and endometrial cavity without the loss of integrity of the uterus (16).

The vascular supply to the oviduct is derived from the uterine and ovarian arteries. There is a capillary bed within the lateral mesosalpinx and oviduct where the two supplies meet, culminating in a rich vascularity (9) (Fig. 11).

This vascular bed responds to vasoconstrictor solutions (required, e.g., for removal of an ectopic pregnancy). The uterine artery ascends to supply the cornu and then to course laterally beneath the isthmus to dissipate in the lateral mesosalpinx. At tubal surgery, the most prominent and easily injured vessels are those underlying the isthmus.

The function of the autonomic nerve supply to the oviduct is uncertain. It is notable that oviductal transplantation procedures with attendant denervation of the tube have yielded successful pregnancies (17–19).

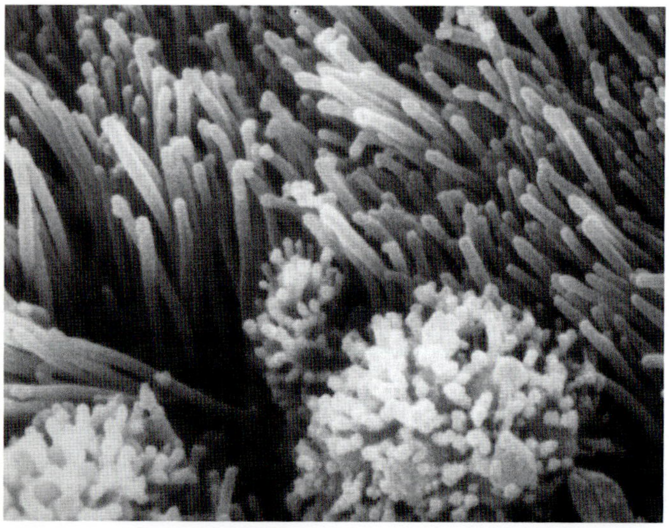

Figure 8 Scanning electron microscopy: ampulla of rabbit oviduct. Detail of ciliated and secretory cells. Magnification ×3400.

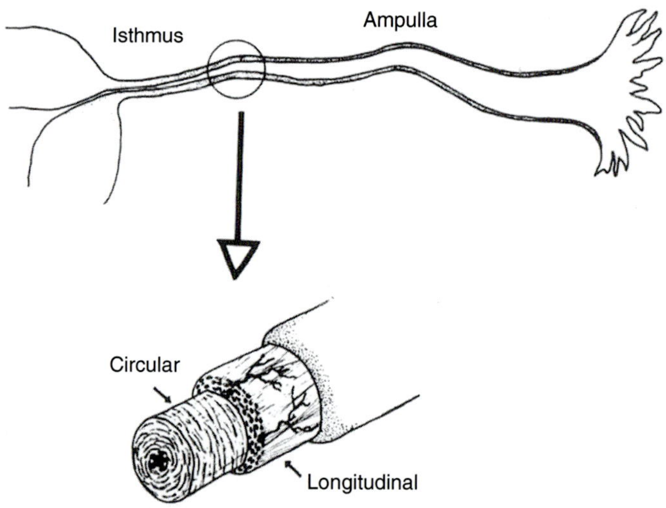

Figure 10 Sketch demonstrating the isthmic musculature.

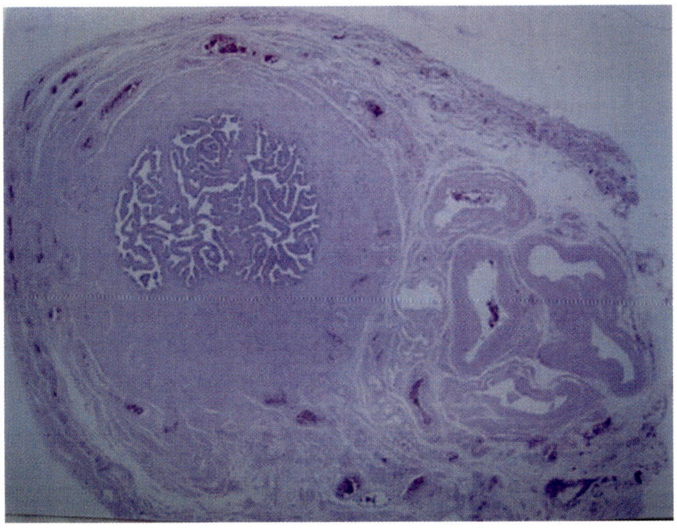

Figure 11 Light microscopy: vessels in the mesosalpinx of the human fallopian tube derived from the ovarian and uterine arteries. (Hematoxylin and eosin stain.)

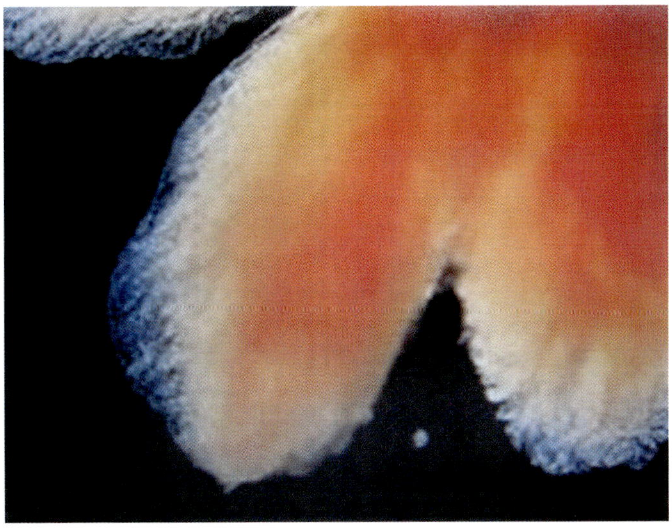

Figure 13 Microphotograph: in vivo observation of lappets of human fimbriae.

Physiology of the Fallopian Tube

A "working model" of the fallopian tube may be described as follows. Much of the detail has been inferred from animal studies, especially the rabbit. At about the time of ovulation, the fimbria is close to the ipsilateral ovary, with some access to the opposite ovary. Bowel invests the adnexa so that there is only a potential space within the pelvis. Peritoneal fluid lubricates the single-cell mesothelial layer of the ovary, serosal surfaces, and peritoneum. Motion is conferred to the pelvis by body movement, bowel peristalsis, and some contraction of the ovarian and tubal mesenteries. With ovulation, the sticky cumulus oophorus unfolds from the follicular cavity and adheres to the follicular stigma assisted by blood clot formation and fibrin deposition.

As the fimbria brushes the ovary, the granulosa cells of the cumulus oophorus are exposed to the fluid currents generated by the rapidly beating cilia that surface the anemone-like folds of the fimbria (Figs. 12 and 13). These currents draw the cloud of granulosa cells toward the ostium of the fallopian tube. As the cumulus is surrounded by more ciliary surface area, it is more tenaciously held. The ovum is carried within the cumulus toward the infundibulum, where the granulosa cells become completely contained within the ampulla (Fig. 14). This process may take minutes to hours. The transport rate across the fimbrial mucosa is about 0.1 mm/sec (20). The ampullary lumen is only a potential space in that the endosalpinx is complex and folded in intricate fronds. Thus, during transport through the ampulla, the cumulus is completely surrounded by ampullary endosalpinx.

Once in the ampulla, the cumulus vehicle has reached a stable environment conducive to fertilization. The complex tertiary mucosal folds are displaced laterally as the cumulus travels through. Ciliary-induced fluid currents serve as

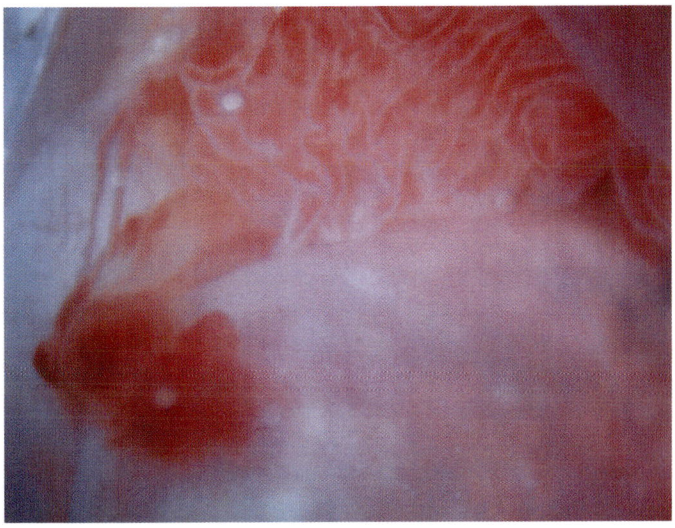

Figure 12 Microphotograph: in vivo observation of rabbit fimbriae and ovulated oocyte and coagulum on ovarian surface.

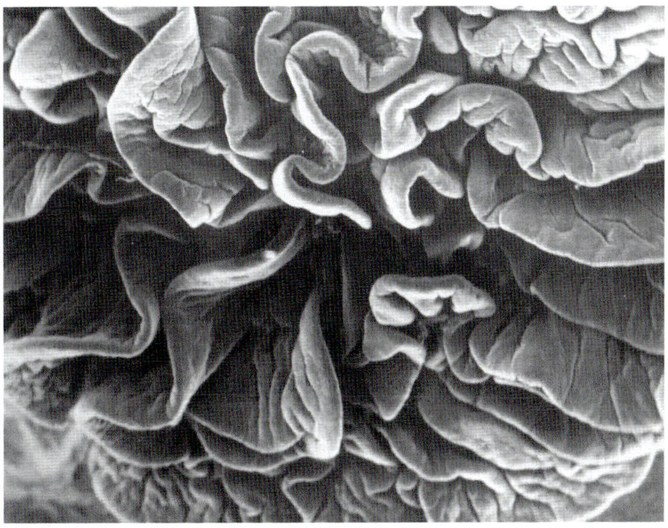

Figure 14 Scanning electron microscopy: fimbria of rabbit oviduct showing complexity of mucosal folds. Magnification $\times 150$.

the major transport mechanism to carry the cumulus to the ampullary–isthmic junction (20), that is, fully two-thirds of the distance from fimbria to uterus. The time elapsed is minutes from the fimbria and hours from first follicular release. The cumulus complex lodges at the ampullary–isthmic junction due predominantly to the volume of the cloud of granulosa cells, the diminutive diameter of the isthmic lumen (1 mm), and the reduced numbers of cilia within the isthmus. The rapid ciliary transport from fimbria and infundibulum delivers the cumulus oocyte complex to the constant nurturing milieu of the proximal ampulla. It is considered that fertilization most often occurs within the ampulla and particularly near the ampullary–isthmic junction.

Once ejaculation of sperm has occurred, spermatozoa are deposited in the vagina as a coagulum. At about the time detumescence of the elastic vaginal tissues has restored a degree of occlusion to the vagina, liquefaction of the seminal coagulum releases the spermatozoa. The periovulatory mucus is cascading from the cervical os. The spinnbarkeit of the mucus causes the previously entangled mucopolysaccharide molecules to align longitudinally; this allows the sperm to form phalanges as they self-propel by axonemal flagellation into the clear copious mucus of the cervical canal. This mucus thereafter acts as a reservoir for the sperm.

Through the uterine cavity, the intramural oviduct, and the isthmus, the spermatozoa appear to move by a combination of self-propulsion and retrograde myometrial and myosalpingeal contraction. Selection of the quickest and most robust sperm cell takes place.

Sperm transport is thought to be a result of a combination of mechanisms, including its innate motility, cilial propulsion, fluid flow, and tubal contractility (21). The number of sperm successfully reaching the fallopian tube is much smaller than that in the ejaculate, a fact partially explained through selection via motility mechanisms. Others postulate the uterotubal junction as a barrier.

Following capacitation of mature spermatozoa in the female oviduct, sperm acquire a hyperactivated motility, which allows them to reach and penetrate the zona pellucida. Capacitation appears to require a minimum oviductal stay of several hours. The acrosome reaction—which is triggered by binding to the zona pellucida and is necessary for penetration of the zona pellucida—occurs only in capacitated spermatozoa. Once the spermatozoa reach the cumulus mass within the ampulla, fertilization may occur. The granulosa cells that surround the oocyte do not interfere with the ability of sperm to fertilize the oocyte.

After 24 hours within the proximal ampulla, the cumulus cells dissipate to facilitate entry of the fertilized ovum/embryo into the isthmus. There is no consensus as to how embryo transport through the human isthmus to the uterine cavity occurs. The embryo stays within the isthmus for two days. Direct observation of the transilluminated rabbit isthmus documents brisk to-and-fro motion of the embryo due to myosalpingeal contraction. This is accompanied by gradual descent of the morula to the uterine cavity (18), where at four days after ovulation the embryo hatches from the zona pellucida to become an expanded blastocyst. Still another three days elapse before implantation.

There is evidence, once more in the rabbit, that a function of the isthmic myosalpinx adjacent to the uterus is to thrust the embryo from the isthmus into the uterine cavity. Of interest, fertility in women is little reduced even when a substantial loss of isthmic length has occurred (compared with the ampulla), suggesting that if this mechanism occurs in the human, then only a short isthmic segment may be needed to perform this function (22).

Before considering the disease states of the oviduct, it is appropriate to review the effects of deletion of segments and deletion of transport function (22,23).

EFFECTS OF DELETIONS OF STRUCTURE AND FUNCTION ON TUBAL PHYSIOLOGY

Structural Deletions

The most frequent structural deletion is that caused by sterilization of women. We can determine the role of each tubal segment, especially with respect to any essential function that it may perform. With a sterilization procedure, the remaining tubal segments are usually healthy with normal muscular, ciliary, and nutritive function. One must also consider the effect of the anastomosis upon the tubal function.

At the outset, one may observe that the process of fertilization is literally essential to the survival of the species. This is reflected in backup mechanisms that may be required if failure or loss of a primary oviductal function occurs. The fimbria has proven to be dispensable (13,24,25). This became evident with the failure rate associated with the fimbriectomy sterilization procedure. In cases of failed sterilization by fimbriectomy, a tongue of fimbrial tissue (usually in the region of the fimbria ovarica) protrudes from a crack in the tubal wall. The function of the fimbria is dependent primarily upon the ciliary mucosa, and the surface area of the mucosa (25) that is available. The ampulla is also richly endowed with ciliated cells. For example, at the surgical reversal of a fimbriectomy, the ampullary mucosa can be fashioned to create a neofimbria albeit with decreased functional surface area.

The ampulla appears to be essential for successful pregnancy. When sterilization reversal is attempted in the absence of the ampulla, for example, by anastomosing infundibulum directly to isthmus, intrauterine pregnancy is rare. The essential function of the ampulla may be as a nutritive site for fertilization (as a containment location for the cumulus oophorus). At least 50% of the ampulla should be present if one is to anticipate successful pregnancies after both ampullary anastomosis and fimbriectomy reversals.

The isthmus and intramural oviduct seem to be the most functionally redundant parts of the human oviduct (26). Ampullary-myometrial anastomosis can lead to successful intrauterine pregnancy. Loss of isthmic length decreases fertility, but not as much as does loss of ampullary length.

Functional Deletion

There are two forms of functional deletion. The first is ciliary and the second muscular. Muscular deletion is seen with a failed sterilization. Usually, the sterilization has been attempted by electrical coagulation of the tubal segment. At reoperation, the surgeon is often able to identify only mucosal tissue between the interrupted tubal segments. Histological section of this intervening tissue demonstrates typically a tunnel of oviductal mucosa linking the two tubal segments. The muscularis of the affected portion of tube had been destroyed at the time of the sterilization and has contracted and retracted. This points to the ability of the layer of ciliary tubal mucosa alone to affect transport of the spermatozoa toward the ovary and that of the embryo toward the uterus. Thus, it can be concluded that the myosalpinx is not essential for oviductal transport of either the gametes or the embryo.

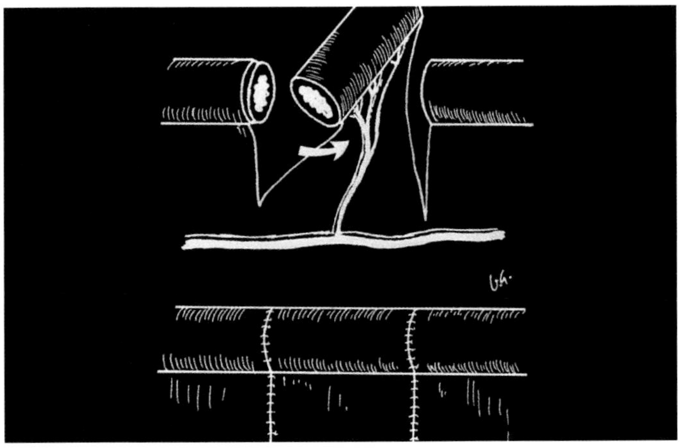

Figure 15 Sketch of reversal of an ampullary segment.

Ciliary deletion has been induced in the rabbit by reversing a segment of ampulla and thereby reversing the direction of ciliary beat (Fig. 15). Infertility was induced in virtually all animals despite the preservation of normal myosalpingeal contractility (20). In women, ciliary deletion is typified by the "immotile cilia" syndrome. Only a small number of those women described as having Kartagener's syndrome (situs inversus and bronchiectasis) or "ciliary dyskinesia" will have absolutely immotile cilia (Figs. 16 and 17) (27).

Various intraciliary ultrastructural defects may be related to varied forms and degrees of ciliary dyskinesis. These defects may involve the mechanochemical coupling between the ATPase containing outer dynein arms of the A microtubule with the B microtubule and other skeletal derangements. In women who have ciliary immotility documented by phase contrast microscopy, there is associated infertility (3). This points to the essential nature of ciliary transport through the oviduct.

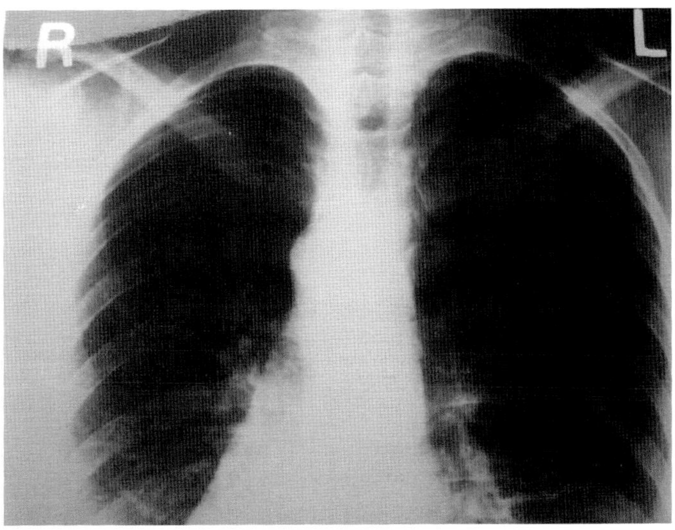

Figure 16 Radiograph: chest film demonstrating dextrocardia in an infertile woman with Kartagener's syndrome.

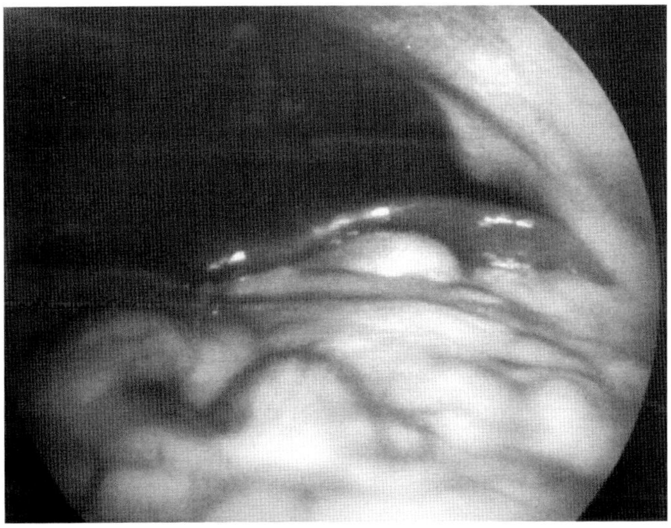

Figure 17 Laparoscopy: view of liver and gall bladder in an infertile woman with situs inversus and Kartagener's syndrome.

PATHOPHYSIOLOGY OF TUBAL DISEASE AND CAUSES OF TUBAL OCCLUSION

Most tubal lesions interfere with fertility by distortion of normal anatomy and occlusion of the tube. Interference through alteration of normal function is less well understood. The primary pathogenesis of tuboperitoneal disease is due to ascending infection from the lower genital tract through the uterus and the fallopian tubes to ovary and peritoneum. The other causes include tubal disease of other etiology, congenital abnormalities, inflammatory diseases of the bowel and pelvis, and previous surgical interventions. It is important to differentiate between those oviductal lesions that are caused by disease as opposed to those that are iatrogenically caused.

Lesions in Otherwise Normal Tubes

The segmental deletion due to sterilization of normal fallopian tubes usually leaves the tubal tissue that is intrinsically normal. One exception to this is the endometriosis that may damage the proximal segment of oviduct after sterilization (28,29). It is postulated that the menstrual fluid that would ordinarily traverse the oviduct to reach the peritoneal cavity instead becomes loculated in the proximal tubal stump. The endometrial tissue so entrapped initiates endometrial gland formation within the isthmic myosalpinx. The subsequent reactive fibrosis further damages the proximal tubal stump to render it useless for reconstruction. Development of these poststerilization lesions does appear to accord with the time elapsed since the sterilization (30).

Ascending Genital Tract Infection

Background, Symptoms, and Signs

From the perspective of infertility history taking, researchers have long documented the fact that tubal damage can be sustained without the apparent overt knowledge of the woman (31,32). Of all symptoms and signs associated with salpingitis, pus in the cervical mucus is the most constant predictive sign and constitutes an indication for treatment (32–34). Others perform a laparoscopy to confirm or refute the diagnosis, so as to treat aggressively when indicated. Unarguably, there is a direct increase in the likelihood of infertility due to tubal disease with each episode of laparoscopically verified acute salpingitis (35). *Chlamydia* is often considered the primary infective agent—largely inferred because of correlation between evidence of chronic tubal damage and presence of antibodies to heat shock proteins detectable in the serum (36,37) and DNA in tubal tissue (38). Much less defined is the point at which *Chlamydia* becomes a clinically relevant infection—as opposed to a localized colonization of the cervical glands. Of interest, the prevalence of positive cervical chlamydial cultures is 3% to 22% in asymptomatic heterosexual women (39). This far exceeds the purported prevalence of salpingitis due to *Chlamydia* in the same populations.

Although most women do not experience symptoms or signs of overt salpingitis, there are certain details from the history from infertile women due to known tubal disease that can predict the outcome of therapy (40). We have shown that the occurrence of intrauterine pregnancy after laparoscopic salpingostomy for distal tubal occlusion is predicted by a history of previous pregnancy and gonococcal infection (40). Occurrence of ectopic pregnancy subsequent to salpingostomy is predicted by a lack of previous ectopic pregnancy, negative history of use of an intrauterine device (IUD), and positive history of pelvic inflammatory disease (PID). Clearly then, what a woman tells us (although she may not specifically know whether she has incurred tubal disease) is clinically useful. Such historical events may, to a large extent, be predictive by virtue of the fact that they can be clearly defined and recalled.

One may also observe that sexually transmitted diseases (STDs) are not static in a given population. If we cast our minds back to the time of earliest recognition of STD, it has been defined by occurrence of disease subsequent to sexual activity (33). The communal baths of 1100 AD, the "hot stews" in United Kingdom, and prostitution in Europe fomented transmission. Through these medieval times to the late 19th century, "therapy" consisted of attempts to change sexual behavior—motivated mostly by the need for disease-free armed forces.

Even with the advent of antibiotic treatment in the 1940s and 1950s, any population benefit was soon overwhelmed by the permissive sexual behavior of the 1960s. In this decade, the bulge of the baby boomer cohort became pubertal coincident with the liberal availability of nonbarrier contraceptives—both oral contraceptives and IUDs. In this era of "sex, drugs, and rock and roll," the resultant increase in salpingitis (34,41) formed the basis for the career opportunities of many reproductive surgeons through the next several decades. In parallel, over the same millennium, the character of STD has transformed from the clinically flamboyant to the occult. Syphilis, a parasitic spirochete, is the great masquerader that mimics a variety of illnesses from tumor to psychosis. Gonorrhea, due to intracellular diplococci, is more clinically subtle but often manifests as membranous mucopurulent discharge or even arthritis. *Chlamydia* is an obligate intracellular organism with virus-like properties associated with subclinical, "silent" salpingitis. HIV, the latest known behaviorally defined infection, is a virus with a prolonged latent phase that defies clinical detection.

Only change in sexual behavior has proven to be effective for control of STD. In contemporary societies, age of onset of intercourse and number of lifetime sexual partners predict likelihood of diagnosis of STD (42,43). STD is not static in a community. This is clearly reflected in the rise in incidence of salpingitis in the 1960s (that preceded increased rates of tubal infertility/ectopic pregnancy) up to the 1990s (41). Even within this period, the causative bacteria known to be associated with tubal disease altered—a dramatic example is the emergence of penicillin-resistant *Gonococcus* that emanated from Vietnam. Presently, in British Columbia, there is an increase in the incidence of case reports of *Chlamydia*. This has increased from 120 cases per 100,000 women in 1993 to 225 in 2004. This rise predicts that in subsequent years, cases of tubal infertility and ectopic pregnancy will burgeon. In summary, to some extent we can determine the risk of tubal disease from history taking and, in some cases, predict from that history who will benefit from therapy. A vaccine for Chlamydia is developmental.

Pathophysiology

PID and its sequelae appear to be on the rise in industrialized countries. The majority represent sexually transmitted cases, although postoperative, postinstrumentation, puerperal, or secondary (associated with appendicitis, diverticulitis, or *Mycobacterium tuberculosis*) infections do occur. Only about 40% of women with tuboperitoneal infertility and evidence of previous intraperitoneal inflammation give a history of PID. Pathological changes such as deciliation, flattened mucosal folds, and degeneration of secretory cells are observed in cases of both overt and silent PIDs (44).

The classical concept is that of an ascending, monoorganism (*Neisseria gonorrhoeae*) infection. Evidence has accumulated that the majority of cases of PID represent a multiorganism infection commonly involving *Chlamydia trachomatis* and anaerobic organisms. Significant regional differences in the prevalence of pathogens appear to exist. A hematogenous (i.e., tuberculosis) or lymphatic (streptococci, staphylococci, and coliform bacilli) spread is postulated for certain organisms, but the more common pathway of bacterial infection appears to involve an ascent of pathogens from the endocervix via the endometrium to the endosalpinx. In particular, gonococci tend to invade and spread along mucosal surfaces.

Tubal Occlusion and Lesions

Proximal Tubal Occlusion

In a series of 360 infertile women, an initial hysterosalpingographic study (HSG) suggested an incidence of unilateral proximal tubal obstruction in 18 and a bilateral obstruction in 22 women. When the HSG was repeated one month later, the unilateral obstruction persisted in 12 (3.3%) and the bilateral obstruction in 9 (1.1%) women (45). In one series, obliterative fibrosis was the most common cause (38%) and chronic tubal inflammation was the next most commonly identified lesion (21%) (46). Other causes of proximal obstruction include salpingitis isthmica nodosa (SIN), tubal endometriosis (this includes endometrial colonization), chronic ectopic pregnancy, and congenital disease. Tubal polyps rarely lead to complete obstruction. One study reported that 11 of 18 cases of purported proximal tubal obstruction failed to have histological evidence of occlusion. Amorphous tubal casts or plugs were found in six, no pathology in three, and some pathology but no obstruction in eight patients (47). This finding highlights the need to investigate extensively with repeated evaluations of tubal patency before surgery is undertaken, so as to minimize the false-positive findings. Ancillary measures such as selective HSG or tubal cannulation can assist. Tubal cornual obstruction usually affects the intramural tube and the contiguous isthmus. More extensive disease tends to encroach laterally into the isthmus.

Following unilateral tubocornual anastomosis (TCA) and contralateral salpingostomy, pregnancy rates are (48) more consistent with rates found following pure TCAs than after salpingostomies. Taking into consideration the poor success after repair of bipolar disease (disease located at both ends of the oviduct), it is postulated that proximal tubal occlusion represents one extreme of a disease spectrum. An ascending infective process is thought to first involve the tubocornual junction. This may lead to obstruction at the tubocornual junction and thereby impede further ascent of the infectious agent. When the inflammation does not cause obstruction, the infection may spread transmucosally to involve the distal tube to culminate in distal occlusion. Bipolar damage reflects progression of the proximal disease in the presence of distal occlusion and therefore represents involvement of the entire length of the oviduct. This explains the poor outcome associated with tubal reconstruction in this situation (49,50).

Obliterative Fibrosis

In tubal occlusion caused by obliterative fibrosis, the tubal lumen is completely obliterated by dense collagenous connective tissue. No other preceding or predisposing condition can be identified. The tubal epithelium is completely destroyed. Obliterative fibrosis has been viewed as a nonspecific response of the tubal epithelium to a variety of stimuli, including inflammation or infection (Fig. 18) (46). On inspection or palpation, the tube may appear completely normal.

Salpingitis Isthmica Nodosa

SIN was first described by Chiari (51) in 1887 as epithelial inclusions within the tubal wall. In its more advanced stage, the fibrosis induced by SIN may occlude the tube. It is considerably less common than distal tubal disease but is thought to be responsible for up to 5% of female infertility. At elective sterilization, less than 1% of tubes show evidence of SIN (52). SIN is identified as the causative histological abnormality in 23% to 60% (48,53–55) of cases of proximal tubal occlusion. Of 37 cases of women with isthmic ectopic pregnancy and no other predisposing factors, 46% were found to have SIN in the involved tube (56). Others have found SIN in 57% of fallopian tubes in a series of 100 ectopic pregnancies (57). Despite this prevalence, SIN has been acknowledged and thus sought after as a potential cause of ectopic pregnancy only recently. Both clinician and pathologist must operate with a high index of suspicion to identify SIN. The documentation of SIN within a woman's fallopian tubes has implications for future management and follow-up both for infertility and for ectopic pregnancy.

Age distribution

SIN is a disease of woman in the reproductive age, with a range of 26 to 30 years (57). It has rarely been described in premenarchal or postmenopausal women. A higher incidence has been noted in the black population in North America and in Jamaicans in retrospective, uncontrolled series (58,59).

Site

In one study that established the radiological appearance of SIN, the lesion was identified in 45 patients (in 70 tubes) from 1194 HSGs. Of these lesions, 35.7% were bilateral and 50% were located only in the proximal tube, 28% only in the midtubal region, and 3% only in the distal tube. In 7% the entire tube and in 11% both proximal and midportion were involved. Other authors have reported up to 85% bilaterality and >65% isthmic involvement (60). A histological review of 100 ectopic pregnancies found the lesions of SIN to be located predominantly in the isthmus (63%) rather than in the ampulla (37%) (57).

Histology

Histologically, SIN is characterized by nodular hyperplasia and hypertrophy of the muscularis surrounding pseudo-gland-like structures that are lined by tubal epithelium. The lining epithelium consists of columnar to cuboidal cells with occasional ciliated cells (Fig. 19). An attempt to grade the severity of SIN has proposed that the depth of glandular invasion into the myosalpinx should be taken into consideration. No clinical correlation with the outcome is available (57).

In a large number of cases, endometrial-like stromal cells may be seen clustered around the diverticula. By contrast, if tubal epithelium is not present and if both endometrial stroma and endometrial glands are seen, a diagnosis of endometriosis must be made, as distinct from SIN. There is no documented correlation of SIN with endometriosis clinically. Few have been able to identify histologically the direct connection

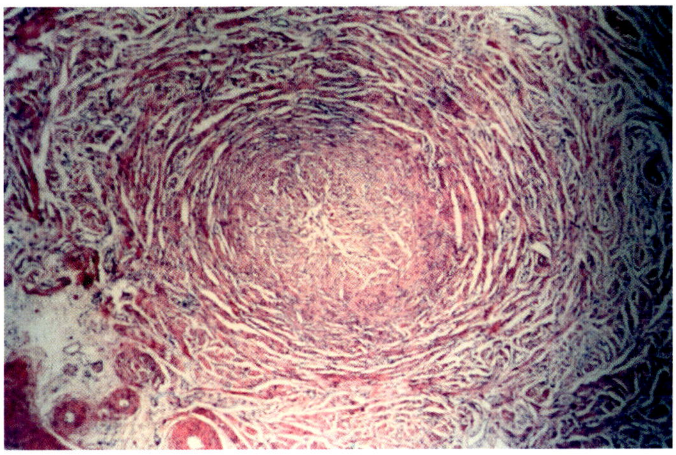

Figure 18 Light microscopy: obliterative fibrosis. The tubal lumen is completely obliterated by dense collagenous connective tissue. (Hematoxylin and eosin stain.)

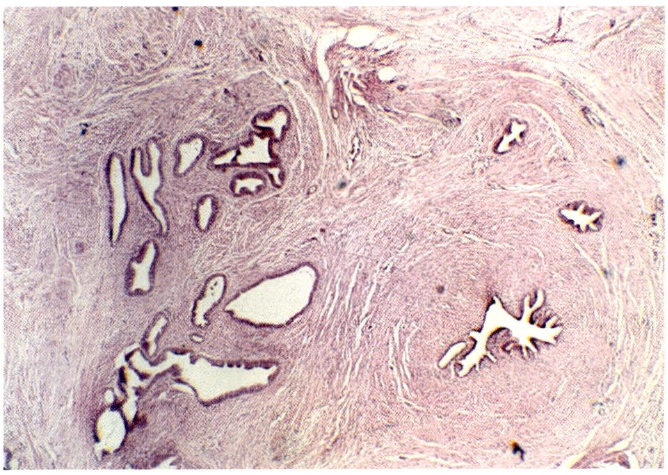

Figure 19 Light microscopy: cross-section of nodule of salpingitis isthmica nodosa showing diverticula composed of tubal epithelium adjacent to lumen of isthmus. (Hematoxylin and eosin stain.)

from the tubal lumen to the pseudogland that is seen at HSG and thereby show direct extension of tubal epithelium from the oviductal lumen to the diverticular pouch (57). In one case of ectopic pregnancy, implantation was observed within an SIN diverticulum. This prompted the assumption that the mechanical arrest of ovum transport may lead to nidation within a pseudogland. Apart from isthmic and ampullary pregnancies, SIN has also been reported as the underlying etiology in a case of interstitial pregnancy (61).

Many authors have found histological evidence of chronic inflammation manifest as lymphocytic infiltration coexisting with SIN as well as evidence of previous infection elsewhere in the pelvis (55). Others have not been able to demonstrate a difference in the presence of chronic salpingitis in tubes that contain an ectopic pregnancy as well as an SIN compared with tubes that contain an ectopic without an SIN (57). Various synonyms have been used for SIN: tubal diverticulosis, adenomyosalpingitis, epitheliomyosis, adenosalpingitis, adenomyohyperplasia, and adenomyosis. Some have used the term endosalpingiosis interchangeably (60) with SIN, although these are considered two distinct entities by most. Others have described SIN and adenomyosis-like features within the tubal wall following tubal electrocautery (62). This is in contrast to the usual histological diagnosis of endometriosis after tubal sterilization. These postcauterization lesions lack the feature of (reactive) muscular hypertrophy and have been coined endosalpingoblastosis as opposed to endosalpingiosis. Since both uterine and tubal features may be found in the same specimen, their origin is postulated to be from pluripotent coelomic stem cells (63). We suggest that the terminology remain as SIN.

Diagnosis

The mainstays of diagnosis are the distinctive radiological and laparoscopic appearances. SIN is radiologically characterized by single or multiple diverticula or tracts in close proximity to the tube. The incidence reported varies from 3.9% to 8.7% (62) of HSGs, likely because of differences in the populations studied or differing indications for the HSGs. The differential diagnosis includes contrast extravasation (this disappears on late films), tubal endometriosis, and tuberculosis (these are usually associated with other radiological features). In one study, a hysteroscopic finding of endosalpingeal hyperplasia of the tubal ostium correlated with SIN on histology in six cases (64). At laparoscopy, one characteristically notes a nodular, fusiform enlargement with thickening and induration of the isthmus. With transcervical injection of a dye solution, characteristic diverticula may become visible. The serosa is usually smooth and intact (see further chapters 23 and 24).

Etiology

Divergent theories as to the etiology of SIN have been advanced: congenital, inflammatory, hormonal, and mechanical. SIN has rarely been reported in prepubertal females, although a case report of this occurrence exists in a diethylstilbestrol (DES)-exposed teenager (65). Infertility and ectopic pregnancies are common sequelae in DES-exposed woman, but SIN has not frequently been described in association with DES exposure. Neonatal mice injected with DES manifest SIN-like tubal lesions. Continuing hormonal stimulation produces a steady progression of the tubal lesion as well as ovarian cyst formation. This is an indirect evidence of a possible hormonal mechanism in the genesis of SIN in women. The absence of muscular hypertrophy in the animal model could implicate a cofactor, possibly inflammation in humans (66). Others support this theory with the observation that the SIN disease process is similar to adenomyosis. That is, a hormonally sensitive mullerian tissue derivative responds to unknown stimuli by slow proliferation (65). Others postulate that chronic tubal spasm of the thick isthmic muscle results in pulsion diverticula akin to diverticulosis coli (51).

The etiology of SIN is thus still unclear, although it is likely to be an acquired condition. An inflammatory/infectious etiology is favored by most investigators. The evidence supporting this view is circumstantial, based predominantly on historical, histological, serological, and radiological evidence of associated inflammation or infection (52,55,57,65). In retrospective series, an association has been found between SIN and primary infertility and ectopic pregnancy. This casual linkage (51,56) has prompted some to advocate TCA whenever SIN is detected, despite patency in the diseased tubes. The decision to advise a TCA in these circumstances is based on the severity of the SIN lesion, the length of time of preceding infertility, and other intercurrent factors such as history of ectopic pregnancy.

SIN appears to be a progressive disease, with an initial increase in size of lesions eventually leading to complete obliteration of the tubal lumen despite lack of evidence of a continuing stimulus (67). This observation suggests that a recent HSG should be available for evaluation before reconstructive surgery is undertaken. It is also recommended that an HSG be performed after an ectopic pregnancy so as to search for SIN.

SIN is a distinct disease of the proximal tube that has only recently been associated with a high incidence of infertility and ectopic pregnancy. The progressive nature of SIN poses unique diagnostic and therapeutic challenges to both pathologist and clinician. Of all the current pathophysiological conditions of the oviduct, this disease warrants most research.

DISTAL TUBAL DISEASE

The degree of damage to the pelvis may range from a few filmy peritubal adhesions with tubal patency to a "frozen pelvis" and an occluded distal oviduct. The anatomical distortion may be categorized as peritubal, occlusive tubal, and ciliary.

The peritubal adhesions are best considered for their potential for repair: (*i*) if the fallopian tube is freely mobile with space between the tube, ovary, and pelvic sidewall, and the adhesions are easily transected, then the prospects for restoration of tubal function are reasonable; (*ii*) if the adhesive process has fused the tube to the ovary—usually with dense adhesions—then the probability of successful correction is diminished; and (*iii*) if the ovary and/or oviduct have fused additionally to the pelvic sidewall, often with loss of ovarian volume, then the prospects for effective repair are guarded.

Occlusive-tubal damage may be represented by fimbria encased completely or in part by adhesions, fimbrial phimosis, or total distal tubal occlusion (hydrosalpinx). Each is attended by a different extent of mucosal damage. Intratubal adhesions may further reduce potential transport function. The ciliated cells are also ablated by inflammation to a varied extent (42,68). A direct ciliostatic effect of *Mycoplasma hominis* has been reported (69).

In terms of tubal function, the physical quality of the oviduct is the best predictor. Prospective scoring systems have been proposed for prediction of fertility based on the distal ampullary diameter, tubal wall thickness, appearance of the mucosal folds at the neostomy site, and the extent and character of adhesions. One of these was approved by the American Fertility Society, currently the American Reproductive Society (70,71). Surgery is capable of restoring patency in more than 75% of hydrosalpinges (72); however, the subsequent overall intrauterine pregnancy rate is around 30% to 35%. This rate is much lower when the tubal epithelium is greatly affected and higher when mildly affected (73). This discrepancy in reproductive outcome has also been demonstrated by salpingoscopy; the pregnancy outcome was inversely proportional to the degree of damage exhibited by the ampullary epithelium (74).

Distal tubal disease induces poor retrieval and ampullary containment of the cumulus oophorus. Scarring, limited tubo-ovarian mobility, reduced ovarian surface, and compromised ovulatory function may compound the abnormal transport. Delay in retrieval or transport of the cumulus complex may result in blastocyst formation within the oviduct, and an ectopic implantation (6).

Sterilization Reversal

Female sterilization by surgical occlusion of the fallopian tubes is the most widely used contraceptive method worldwide, accounting for 10% to 40% of contraceptive methods (75). Globally, some 60 million women undergo tubal sterilization annually. In the United States, 20% of sterilized women seek a reversal, but less than half of these will actually undergo reversal of sterilization (76).

The most common reason for reversal of sterilization is change in marital status, especially in women younger than 30 years of age at the time of sterilization (77,78). Much less often, the reason involves the death of a child, either from sudden infant death syndrome or from accident (78). Other women regret being sterilized per se—citing insufficient time to consider fully the implications of sterilization, feeling pressured to have the sterilization, or wishing to restore childbearing potential (79). In addition to fertility, some studies suggest that reversal of sterilization (ROS) helps restore body-image and self-esteem (80).

Inflammatory Disorders of the Bowel

Appendicitis

Appendicitis is a cause of adnexal inflammation. However, in our experience it is an unusual cause, unless it is complicated by rupture and its sequelae. As one of the common differential diagnoses to acute salpingitis, an early diagnostic laparoscopy is indicated. Often the diagnosis of appendicitis has been delayed. This occurs more frequently when appendicitis complicates pregnancy.

Crohn's disease

Crohn's disease is a chronic transmural inflammatory disease of the bowel. The peak incidence of the disease is between ages 14 and 24 years and so affects the female during reproductive life. There have been conflicting reports in the literature regarding the prevalence of infertility in the patients; furthermore, most studies pertain to heterogenous groups of women who may or may not have active disease, or medical therapy or bowel surgery. However, the majority of the studies report compromised fertility in patients with Crohn's disease (81–83). Pelvic adhesions are often encountered in this group of patients either as a result of the surgery such as bowel resection or as complications of the disease that include fistula and abscess formation.

Congenital Abnormalities

Congenital abnormalities of the female reproductive tract (abnormalities of the mullerian ducts) occur in 1 in 500 women in a general gynecological practice (84). Congenital fallopian tube anomalies include accessory ostia, multiple lumina, accessory tubes (85), duplication (86), and complete (87) or segmental deletions (88–100). Complete absence of the oviduct may occur with or without absence of the ipsilateral ovary. Autoamputation may explain some of these occurrences (101).

Parafimbrial Cysts

These may distort the apposition of fimbria and ovary.

Hydatid of Morgagni

A hydatid of Morgagni is composed of cyst attached by a peritoneal strand to the ampulla. The blood supply to the cyst may be compromised with consequent inflammatory adhesion of the ischemic cyst to adjacent pelvic structures.

Accessory Tubal Ostia

An ampullary ostium on a tissue stalk may/may not communicate with the tubal lumen. The fimbria may have supernumery ostia. Coelomic invagination has been postulated as the causative mechanism for accessory ostia and multiple lumina. An association with infertility and ectopic pregnancy has been suggested (85).

Rudimentary Horn

A uterine horn that does not communicate with the cervical canal may or may not have an endometrial cavity. A cavity with functional endometrial lining may manifest clinically with episodic dysmenorrheal. If there is no cavity, a diminutive horn constitutes a cornual occlusion. The presence of a rudimentary or noncommunicating uterine horn may be misdiagnosed as an occluded proximal tube.

Segmental Atresia

Congenital segmental deletions occur in the proximal (93–95,99), mid (88–92,98,99), and distal (96) portions of the oviduct. These abnormalities are often discovered during investigation for infertility (90). Usually, the diagnosis is of hydrosalpinx of infectious etiology. Rarely is ampullary atresia suspected. In this case, there is total absence of the distal ampulla. Only a web of mesosalpingeal tissue links the terminus of the occluded ampulla with the isolated fimbrial tissue (see further chapter 24).

Prefimbrial Phimosis

Prefimbrial phimosis may be a partial expression of the process that leads to ampullary atresia. This appears to be an intermediate degree of stenosis between a normal distal ampulla and an ampullary atresia. There is ballooning of the ampulla proximal to the stenotic ampullary region.

Abdominal Ovaries

In this rare condition, the infundibulopelvic ligaments are short and the ovarian ligaments are commensurately longer. The ovaries nestle at the pelvic brim at some distance from the fimbriae.

Elongated Fallopian Tubes

We have seen an unusual case of elongated fallopian tubes. In this woman, the ovaries were located at the pelvic brim, superior to the normal location.

Tuberculosis

Tuberculosis as tuberculous salpingitis has been estimated to account for 1% of infertility in the United States, as compared with 10% in India (102). The damage associated with tubal tuberculosis is diffuse. Although the initial oviductal infection is mucosal, thereafter the muscularis and serosa are involved. Tuberculosis has a proclivity to infect tubal mucosal epithelium (as it does the endometrium) by hematogenous spread. At first, the disease is a microscopic infection secondary to a primary focus (usually respiratory). It then may progress to become nodular, albeit with preservation of fimbria, or adhesive with distortion of the adnexa. In the exudative form of tuberculous salpingitis, caseated granulomata can coalesce to simulate a pyosalpinx.

The consequence of this infection is to obstruct the tube (most often at the proximal ampulla) and to further interfere with ovum retrieval and transport by the adhesion formation. The rigidity of the oviduct reflects the transmural damage. The extensive tubal damage caused by this disease is such that tubal repair cannot yield functional fallopian tubes. Hysterosalpingography provides pathognomonic images resulting from these changes (see chapter 23).

Tubal Polyps

Tubal polyps are usually located within the intramural segment and less often in the isthmus. They consist of polypoid functional endometrial tissue anchored on a stalk that extends from the cornual endometrium. They are often bilateral with a single polyp at each site and range from a few millimeters to over a centimeter in size. Microscopically, they are composed of endometrial-type mucosa (103). Tubal polyps have been described in association with tubal infertility, although their exact correlation with infertility is still unclear. Polyps have been identified in up to 10% of HSGs performed for the investigation of infertility (104) and 11% of hysterectomy specimens (105). Obstruction of the tubal lumen is possible but rare. We note an association with endometriosis and/or anovulation.

REFERENCES

1. Gomel V, McComb P. Microsurgery in reproductive physiology. In: Gomel V, ed. Microsurgery in Female Infertility. Boston: Little Brown and Co., 1983:29–50.
2. McComb P, Halbert SA, Gomel V. Pregnancy, ciliary transport and the reversed ampullary segment of the fallopian tube. Fertil Steril 1980; 34:386–390.
3. McComb P, Verdugo P, Langley L. The oviductal cilia and Kartagener's syndrome. Fertil Steril 1986; 46:412–416.
4. Bonilla-Musoles F, Ferrer-Barriendos J, Pelliger A. Cyclical changes in the epithelium of the fallopian tube. Clin Exp Obstet Gynecol 1983; 10:79–86.
5. Donnez J, Casanas-Roux F, Caprasse J, et al. Cyclic changes in ciliation, cell height, and mitotic activity in human tubal epithelium during reproductive life. Fertil Steril 1985; 43:554–559.
6. Helm G, Owman C, Sjoeberg NO, et al. Motor activity of the human fallopian tube in vitro in relation to plasma concentration of oestradiol and progesterone, and the influence of noradrenaline. J Reprod Fertil 1982; 64:233–242.
7. Jansen RPS. Endocrine response in the fallopian tube. Endocr Rev 1984; 5:525–551.
8. McComb PF, Moon Y. Prostaglandin E and F concentration in the fimbria of the rabbit fallopian tube increases at the time of ovulation. Acta Eur Fertil 1985; 16:423–426.
9. Gomel V. Microsurgery in Female Infertility. Boston: Little Brown and Co, 1983.
10. McComb P, Bourdage RJ, Halbert SA. Suppressed ovulatory function and oviductal microsurgery in the rabbit. Fertil Steril 1981; 35:481–482.
11. McComb P, Delbeke L. Decreasing the number of ovulations in the rabbit with surgical division of the blood vessels between the fallopian tube and ovary. J Reprod Med 1984; 29:827–829.
12. Critoph FN, Dennis KJ. Ciliary activity in the human oviduct. Br J Obstet Gynaecol 1977; 84:216–218.
13. Halbert SA, McComb P, Patton DL. Function and structure of the rabbit oviduct following fimbriectomy: Part I: Distal ampullary salpingostomy. Fertil Steril 1981; 35:349–354.
14. Gaddum-Rosse P, Blandau RJ. In vitro studies on ciliary activity within the oviduct of the rabbit and pig. Am J Anat 1973; 136:91–104.
15. Merchant RN, Prabhu SR, Chougale A. Uterotubal junction-morphology and clinical aspects. Int J Fertil 1983; 28:199–205.
16. McComb P. Microsurgical tubocornual anastomosis for occlusive cornual disease: Reproducible results without the need for tubouterine implantation. Fertil Steril 1986; 46:571–574.
17. McComb P, Filmar S, Pabuccu R. Successful transplantation of a free fimbrial graft to the peritoneum. J Reprod Med 1989; 34:55–58.
18. McComb PF. Free autologous graft of fimbria to ampulla with subsequent oviductal function. J Reprod Med 1992; 37:223–226.
19. Winston RML, McClure-Browne JC. Pregnancy following autograft transplantation of fallopian tube and ovary in the rabbit. Lancet 1974; 2:494–495.
20. McComb P, Gomel V. The effect of segmental ampullary reversal on the subsequent fertility of the rabbit. Fertil Steril 1979; 31:83–85.
21. Harper MJK. Gamete and zygote transport. In: Knobil E, Neill J, et al., eds. The Physiology of Reproduction. New York, NY: Raven Press, 1988:103–134.
22. McComb P, Gomel V. The influence of fallopian tube length on fertility in the rabbit. Fertil Steril 1979; 31:3–6.
23. McComb P, Halbert SA. Reproduction in rabbits after excision of the oviductal isthmus, ampullary-isthmic junction and utero-isthmic junction. Fertil Steril 1981; 35:669–677.
24. Halbert SA, McComb P, Patton DL. Function and structure of the rabbit oviduct following fimbriectomy: Part II: Proximal ampullary salpingostomy. Fertil Steril 1981; 35:355–358.
25. Coppo M, McComb P, Halbert S. The functional potential of the fimbria in the rabbit. J Reprod Med 1984; 29:731–735.
26. Halbert SA, McComb PF, Bourdage RJ. The structural and functional impact of microsurgical anastomosis on the rabbit oviductal isthmus. Fertil Steril 1981; 36:653–658.
27. Lurie M, Tur-Kaspa I, Weill S, et al. Ciliary ultrastructure of respiratory and fallopian tube epithelium in a sterile woman with Kartagener's syndrome. Chest 1989; 95:578–581.
28. Donnez J, Casanas-Roux F, Ferin J, et al. Tubal polyps, epithelial inclusions, and endometriosis after tubal sterilization. Fertil Steril 1984; 41:564–568.
29. Rock JA, Parmley TH, King TM, et al. Endometriosis and the development of tuboperitoneal fistulas after tubal ligation. Fertil Steril 1981; 35:16–20.
30. Vasquez G, Winston RML, Boeckx W, et al. Tubal lesions subsequent to sterilization and their relation to fertility after attempts at reversal. Am J Obstet Gynecol 1980; 138:86–92.
31. Gomel V. Surgical correction of sequelae of pelvic inflammatory disease. J Reprod Med 1983; 2:718–726.
32. Hubacher D, Grimes D, Lara-Ricalde R, et al. The limited clinical usefulness of taking a history in the evaluation of women with tubal infertility. Fertil Steril 2004; 81:6–10.
33. Westrom L, Mardh P-A. Pelvic inflammatory disease. I: Epidemiology, diagnosis, clinical manifestations, and sequelae. In: Holmes KK, Mardh P-A, eds. International Perspectives on Sexually Transmitted Diseases: Impact on Venereology, Fertility, and Maternal and Infant Mortality. New York, NY: McGraw-Hill, 1982.

34. Wiesenfeld HC, Hillier SL, Krohn MA, et al. Lower genital tract infection and endometritis: Insight into subclinical pelvic inflammatory disease. Obstet Gynecol 2002; 100:456–463.
35. Westrom L, Joesoef R, Reynolds G, et al. Pelvic inflammatory disease and fertility. A cohort study of 1,844 women with laparoscopically verified disease and 657 control women with normal laparoscopic results. Sex Transm Dis 1992; 19:185–192.
36. Nelson DB, Ness RB, Peipert JF, et al. Factors predicting upper genital tract inflammation among women with lower genital tract infection. J Womens Health 1998; 7:1033–1040.
37. Mol BWJ, Dijkman B, Wertheim P, et al. The accuracy of serum chlamydial antibodies in the diagnosis of tubal pathology: A meta-analysis. Fertil Steril 1997; 67:1031–1037.
38. Johnson NP, Taylor K, Nadgir AA, et al. Can diagnostic laparoscopy be avoided in routine investigation for infertility? BJOG 2000; 107:174–178.
39. Hinton EL, Bobo LD, Wu TC, et al. Detection of *Chlamydia trachomatis* DNA in archival paraffinized specimens from chronic salpingitis cases using the polymerase chain reaction. Fertil Steril 2000; 74:152–157.
40. Taylor RC, Berkowitz J, McComb PF. Role of laparoscopic salpingostomy in the treatment of hydrosalpinx. Fertil Steril 2001; 75:594–600.
41. Selvin M. Changing medical and societal attitudes toward sexually transmitted diseases: A historical overview. In: Holmes KK, Mardh P-A, Sparling PF, Wiesner PJ, eds. Sexually Transmitted Diseases. New York, NY: McGraw-Hill, 1984:3–19.
42. Kamwendo F, Forslin L, Bodin L, et al. Epidemiology of ectopic pregnancy during a 28 year period and the role of pelvic inflammatory disease. Sex Transm Infect 2000; 76:28–32.
43. Shrikhande SN, Zodpey SP, Kulkarni HR. Risk factors and protective factors of pelvic inflammatory disease: A case control study. Indian J Public Health 1998; 42:42–47.
44. Patton DL, Moore DE, Spadoni LR, et al. A comparison of the fallopian tube's response to overt and silent salpingitis. Obstet Gynecol 1989; 73:622–630.
45. Dessole S, Meloni GB, Capobianco G, et al. Canalis GCA second hysterosalpingography reduces the use of selective technique for treatment of a proximal tubal obstruction. Fertil Steril 2000; 73:1037–1039.
46. Fortier J, Haney AF. The pathologic spectrum of uterotubal junction obstruction. Obstet Gynecol 1985; 65:93–98.
47. Sulak PJ, Letterie GS, Coddington CC, et al. Histology of proximal tubal obstruction. Fertil Steril 1987; 48:437–440.
48. McComb PF, Lee NH, Stephenson MD. Reproductive outcome after unilateral tubocornual anastomosis and contralateral salpingostomy by microsurgery. Fertil Steril 1991; 55:1011–1013.
49. McComb PF, Lee NH, Stephenson MD. Reproductive outcome after microsurgery for proximal and distal occlusions in the same fallopian tube. Fertil Steril 1991; 56:134–135.
50. Patton PE, Williams TJ, Coulam CB. Results of microsurgical reconstruction in patients with combined proximal and distal tubal occlusion: Double obstruction. Fertil Steril 1987; 48: 0–4.
51. Chiari H. Zur pathologischen Anatomie des Eileitercatarrhs. Z Heilkunde 1887; 8:457–473.
52. Honore LH. Salpingitis isthmica nodosa in female infertility and ectopic pregnancy. Fertil Steril 1978; 29:164–168.
53. Donnez J, Casanas-Roux F. Histology: A prognostic factor in proximal tubal occlusion. Eur J Obstet Gynecol Reprod Biol 1988; 29:33–38.
54. Jansen RPS. Tubal resection and anastomosis. II. Isthmic salpingitis. Aust N Z J Obstet Gynaecol 1986; 26:300–304.
55. Punnonen R, Soederstroem KO, Alanen A. Isthmic tubal occlusion: Etiology and histology. Acta Eur Fertil 1984; 15:39–42.
56. Homm RJ, Holtz G, Garvin AJ. Isthmic ectopic pregnancy and salpingitis isthmica nodosa. Fertil Steril 1987; 48:756–760.
57. Majmudar B, Henderson PH, Semple E. Salpingitis isthmica nodosa: A high-risk factor for tubal pregnancy. Obstet Gynecol 1983; 62:73–78.
58. Creasy JF, Clark RL, Cuttino JT, et al. Salpingitis isthmica nodosa: Radiologic and clinical correlates. Radiology 1985; 154:597–600.
59. Persaud V. Etiology of tubal ectopic pregnancy. Radiologic and pathologic studies. Obstet Gynecol 1970; 36:257–263.
60. Donnez J, Casanas-Roux F. Prognostic factors influencing the pregnancy rate after microsurgical cornual anastomosis. Fertil Steril 1986; 46:1089–1092.
61. Petersen LK, Clausen I. Repeated contralateral ectopic pregnancy. Int J Gynecol Obstet 1989; 29:185–187.
62. Karasick S, Karasick D, Schilling J. Salpingitis isthmica nodosa in female infertility. J Can Assoc Radiol 1985; 36:118–121.
63. McCausland A. Endosalpingiosis ("endosalpingoblastosis") following laparoscopic tubal coagulation as an etiologic factor of ectopic pregnancy. Am J Obstet Gynecol 1982; 143:12–22.
64. Vancaillie T, Schmidt EH. The uterotubal junction. J Reprod Med 1988; 33:624–629.
65. Benjamin CL, Beaver DC. Pathogenesis of salpingitis isthmica nodosa. Am J Clin Pathol 1951; 21:212–222.
66. Newbold RR, Bullock BC, McLachlan JA. Diverticulosis and salpingitis isthmica nodosa (SIN) of the fallopian tube. Am J Pathol 1984; 117:333–335.
67. McComb PF, Rowe TC. Salpingitis isthmica nodosa: Evidence it is a progressive disease. Fertil Steril 1989; 51:542–545.
68. Vasquez G, Winston RML, Boeckx W, et al. The epithelium of human hydrosalpinges: A light optical and scanning microscopic study. Br J Obstet Gynaecol 1983; 90:764–770.
69. Baldetorp B, Mardh P-A, Weström L. Studies on ciliated epithelia of the human genital tract. Sex Transm Dis 1983; 11(Suppl):363–365.
70. Boer-Meisel ME, te Velde ER, Habbema JDF, et al. Predicting the pregnancy outcome in patients treated for hydrosalpinx: A prospective study. Fertil Steril 1986; 45:23–29.
71. American Fertility Society. The American Fertility Society classification of adnexal adhesions, distal tubal occlusion, tubal occlusion secondary to tubal ligation, tubal pregnancies, mullerian anomalies and intrauterine adhesions. Fertil Steril 1988; 49:944–955.
72. McComb PF, Paleologou A. The intussusception technique for the therapy of distal oviductal occlusion at laparoscopy. Obstet Gynecol 1991; 78:443–447.
73. Gomel V, Frenus M. Salpingostomy by Microsurgery. The American Fertility Society, 46th Annual Meeting. Program Supplement (Abstracts); 1990: P-097, S-106.
74. Marana R, Catalano GF, Muzii L, et al. The prognostic role of salpingoscopy in laparoscopic tubal surgery. Hum Reprod 1999; 14:2991–2995.
75. Ryder RM, Vaughan MC. Laparoscopic tubal sterilization. Methods, effectiveness, and sequelae. Obstet Gynecol Clin North Am 1999; 26:83–97.
76. Baill IC, Cullins VE, Pati S. Counseling issues in tubal sterilization. Am Fam Physician 2003; 67:1287–1294.
77. Gomel V. Profile of women requesting reversal of sterilization. Fertil Steril 1978; 30:39–41.
78. Hillis SD, Marchbanks PA, Tylor LR, et al. Poststerilization regret: Findings from the United States Collaborative Review of Sterilization. Obstet Gynecol 1999; 93:889–895.
79. Abraham S, Jansen R, Fraser IS, et al. The characteristics, perceptions and personalities of women seeking a reversal of their tubal sterilization. Med J Aust 1986; 145:4–7.
80. Langer M, Hick P, Nemeskeri N, et al. Psychological sequelae of surgical reversal or of IVF after tubal ligation. Int J Fertil Menopausal Stud 1993; 38:44–49.
81. Hudson M, Flett G, Sinclair TS, et al. Fertility and pregnancy in inflammatory bowel disease. Int J Gynaecol Obstet 1997; 58:229–237.
82. Lindhagen T, Bohe M, Ekelund G, et al. Fertility and outcome of pregnancy in patients operated for Crohn's disease. Int J Colorectal Dis 1986; 1:25–27.
83. Wikland M, Jansson I, Asztely M, et al. Gynaecological problems related to anatomical changes after conventional

procto-colectomy and ileostomy. Int J Colorectal Dis 1990; 5: 49–52.
84. Woolf RB, Allen WM. Concomitant malformations: The frequent simultaneous occurrence of congenital malformations of the reproductive and urinary tracts. Obstet Gynecol 1953; 2:236–265.
85. Beyth Y, Kopolovic J. Accessory tubes: A possible contributing factor in infertility. Fertil Steril 1982; 38:382–383.
86. Daw E. Duplication of the uterine tube. Obstet Gynecol 1973; 43:137–138.
87. Eustace DL. Congenital absence of fallopian tube and ovary. Eur J Obstet Gynecol Reprod Biol 1992; 46:157–159.
88. Kistner RW, Patton GW. Atlas of Infertility Surgery. Boston: Brown, 1975:146.
89. Szlachter N, Weiss G. Distal tubal pregnancy in a patient with a bicornuate uterus and segmental absence of the fallopian tube. Fertil Steril 1979; 32:602–603.
90. Farber M, Mitchell GW. Bicornuate uterus and partial atresia of the fallopian tube. Am J Obstet Gynecol 1979; 134:881–884.
91. Richardson DA, Evans MI, Talerman A, et al. Segmental absence of the mid-portion of the fallopian tube. Fertil Steril 1982; 37:577–579.
92. Kanter E. Segmental absence of the mid-portion of the fallopian tube. Fertil Steril 1983; 40:551–552.
93. Silverman AY, Greenberg EI. Absence of a segment of the proximal portion of a fallopian tube. Obstet Gynecol 1983; 62:90s–91s.
94. Paterson PJ, Chan CL. Congenital absence of fallopian tube segments. Aust N Z J Obstet Gynaecol 1985; 25:130–131.
95. Wanerman J, Wulwick R, Brenner S. Segmental absence of the fallopian tube. Fertil Steril 1986; 46:525–527.
96. McBean JH, Brumsted JR. Pregnancy after laparoscopic neosalpingostomy in a patient with atresia of the distal fallopian tubes. Fertil Steril 1994; 61:1163–1164.
97. Goldberg JM, Freidman CI. Noncanalization of the fallopian tube. A case report. J Reprod Med 1995; 40:317–318.
98. Polasek PM, Erickson LD, Stanhope CR. Transverse vaginal septum associated with the tubal atresia. Mayo Clin Proc 1995; 70:965–968.
99. Kozlowski D, Luciano AA. Bilateral atresia of the proximal ampullary segment of the fallopian tubes. J Am Assoc Gynecol Laparosc 1995; 3:99–101.
100. Johnston AC, McComb PF. Fertility potential of women with congenital ampullary atresia of the fallopian tube. Fertil Steril 2003; 79:431–433.
101. Bates GW, Abide JK. Bilateral autoamputation of the fallopian tubes. Fertil Steril 1982; 38:253–254.
102. Schaefer G. Tuberculosis of the female genital tract. Clin Obstet Gynecol 1970; 13:965–998.
103. Gordts S, Boeckx W, Vasquez G, et al. Microsurgical resection of intramural polyps. Fertil Steril 1983; 40:258–259.
104. Reasbeck J, Wynn-Williams G, Gillett W. Tubal intramural polyps: Incidence and radiographic demonstration. Australas Radiol 1988; 32:117–121.
105. Lisa JR, Gioia J, Rubin IC. Observations of the interstitial portion of the fallopian tube. Surg Gynecol Obstet 1954; 99:159–169.

22

Investigation of tubal and peritoneal causes of infertility

Victor Gomel and Peter F. McComb

The investigation of the infertile couple should be concluded rapidly, accurately, and inexpensively, with as little invasion as possible. In addition, the emotional needs of the couple must be recognized and addressed (1). This chapter will primarily discuss investigations specific to tubal and peritoneal factors of infertility.

The investigation of the infertile couple can now be simplified, thanks to the scientific and technical progress realized in the past two decades. These include progress in imaging technology (ultrasonography, computer-assisted tomography, and magnetic resonance imaging), significant improvement in the outcomes of IVF, and the introduction of intracytoplasmic sperm injection (ICSI), which proved to be a panacea in the treatment of male infertility. Indeed, the outcomes of IVF with ICSI produce similar outcomes in couples with and without male factor (2).

Investigation must commence with a thorough clinical assessment of the couple. A detailed history followed by a physical examination permits the physician to establish the initial investigatory tests to undertake. A positive history for ruptured appendicitis has a predictive value of tubal pathology of OR 4.4 (2.5–7.6) and that of having had sexually transmitted infection or the finding of *Chlamydia* antibodies of OR 3.7 (1.7–8.4) (3).

Most gynecologists include pelvic ultrasonography as part of the physical examination, since their offices are equipped and since they have had the necessary training to perform it themselves. This examination will confirm a clinical impression (fibroids, for example) or reveal a significant finding (an intrauterine lesion, for example).

Clinical assessment will determine the need for requesting specific endocrine and other blood tests and any further investigation. Evidence of ovulation should be sought in the female partner and a semen analysis performed in the male. These are simple inexpensive tests that must be done before undertaking more complex or invasive investigations. We have all been referred couples, the female partner of whom had been submitted to extensive investigation while the male partner had not been clinically assessed and not even a semen analysis performed.

INVESTIGATION OF TUBAL AND PERITONEAL CAUSES OF INFERTILITY

Hysterosalpingography (HSG), to which selective salpingography and tubal cannulation may be added as indicated, and laparoscopy are the principal investigations of tuboperitoneal causes of infertility. Other currently employed techniques include salpingosonography and hydroculdoscopy. Falloposcopy (transcervical microendoscopic evaluation of the inner tubal architecture) and radionuclide HSG (a scintigraphic procedure designed to evaluate the spontaneous pro-ovarian transport of microspheres in the genital tract (a test designed to assess primarily the sperm transport function of the uterus and tubes) are experimental procedures not used clinically.

Hysterosalpingography

HSG is a radiologic contrast study of the cervical canal, uterine cavity, and fallopian tubes. It is a simple, rapid, safe, and relatively inexpensive diagnostic procedure. When performed properly, HSG provides valuable information about the uterine cavity and fallopian tubes, including their inner architecture.

Contraindications to HSG are possible pregnancy, acute pelvic inflammatory disease (PID), uterine bleeding, lower genital tract infection, and allergy to the contrast material that contains iodine. When proper technique is adhered to, complications are rare. Complications include bleeding from the tenaculum site, uterine perforation, and PID.

In women with a history of recurrent PID, or any suggestion of a recent exacerbation, there is a significant risk of reactivation of quiescent PID. This occurs in about 3% of such patients. To combat this risk, many centers prophylactically administer antibiotics. During the preliminary history and physical examination, the physician must search for possible contraindications to HSG, and lower genital tract infection must be ruled out (4).

We will not review the technique of HSG in detail, for which the reader is referred to prior publications (4,5). Briefly stated, (*i*) the procedure is timed to occur between the complete cessation of menstruation and ovulation; (*ii*) administration of one of a nonsteroidal anti-inflammatory before the procedure is very helpful, as it reduces the patient's discomfort due to uterine cramping and thus diminishes diagnostic errors; (*iii*) the procedure is performed under fluoroscopic control with image intensification; (*iv*) contrast material is injected very slowly to avoid discomfort, uterine contractions, and tubal spasm (Fig. 1A and 1B); (*v*) the uterus is manipulated with the cannula, as necessary, to better display uterine lesions and specific tubal segments; (*vi*) films are taken at appropriate phases of the procedure and when abnormal findings are encountered; in certain cases, a true lateral film may be necessary to determine such features as the position of the uterus, the location of intrauterine lesions, and the course and configuration of the tubes; and (*vii*) when water-soluble medium is used, the patient is re-examined fluoroscopically and an additional film is taken, 10 to 20 minutes after removal of the cannula. This examination and film may yield information about the external contour of the internal genitalia, the shape of the ovarian fossa, and the presence of periadnexal adhesions (4).

Both oil- and water-soluble contrast media are available for HSG. Although the use of oil-soluble media results in subsequent greater pregnancy rates when compared to

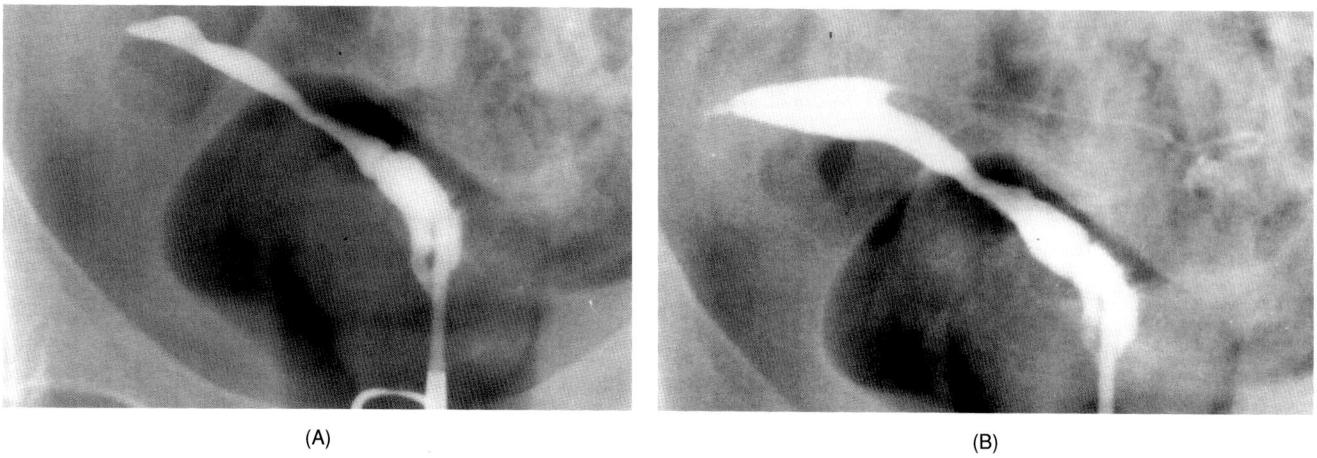

Figure 1 Hysterosalpingography: (A) Uterus exhibiting marked contractions in response to the injection of contrast material, likely under excessive pressure. (B) After a period of rest, the uterus relaxes and contrast commences to enter into the left oviduct; the right cornu demonstrates a degree of spasm.

water-soluble media (OR 1.92; 95% CI: 1.60–2.29) (6), water-soluble media are most widely used. Water-soluble media is much better tolerated by the patients; it coats the epithelial surfaces without sticking to them, producing sharp and finely shaded images and greater visual detail of the lesions, characteristics that enable better assessment of the intraluminal architecture (Fig. 2A to 2C). This contrast material is eliminated within 30 minutes and does not cause pelvic granuloma formation, which has been reported after use of oil-soluble media.

HSG provides valuable information about the uterus and oviducts. Abnormal uterine findings include fusion anomalies of the uterus: septate uterus (Fig. 3); bicornuate uterus (Fig. 4); uterus didelphus (Fig. 5); unicornuate uterus (Fig. 6); arcuate uterus (Fig. 7), T-shaped uterus, usually caused by intrauterine exposure to diethylstilbestrol (DES) (Fig. 8); intrauterine synechiae (Figs. 9, 10A and 10B); fibroids, submucous (Figs. 11 and 12) intramural, intramural distorting the cavity (Figs. 13 and 14), and calcified; polyps (Fig. 15); endometrial hyperplasia; and intra-adenomyosis (Fig. 16).

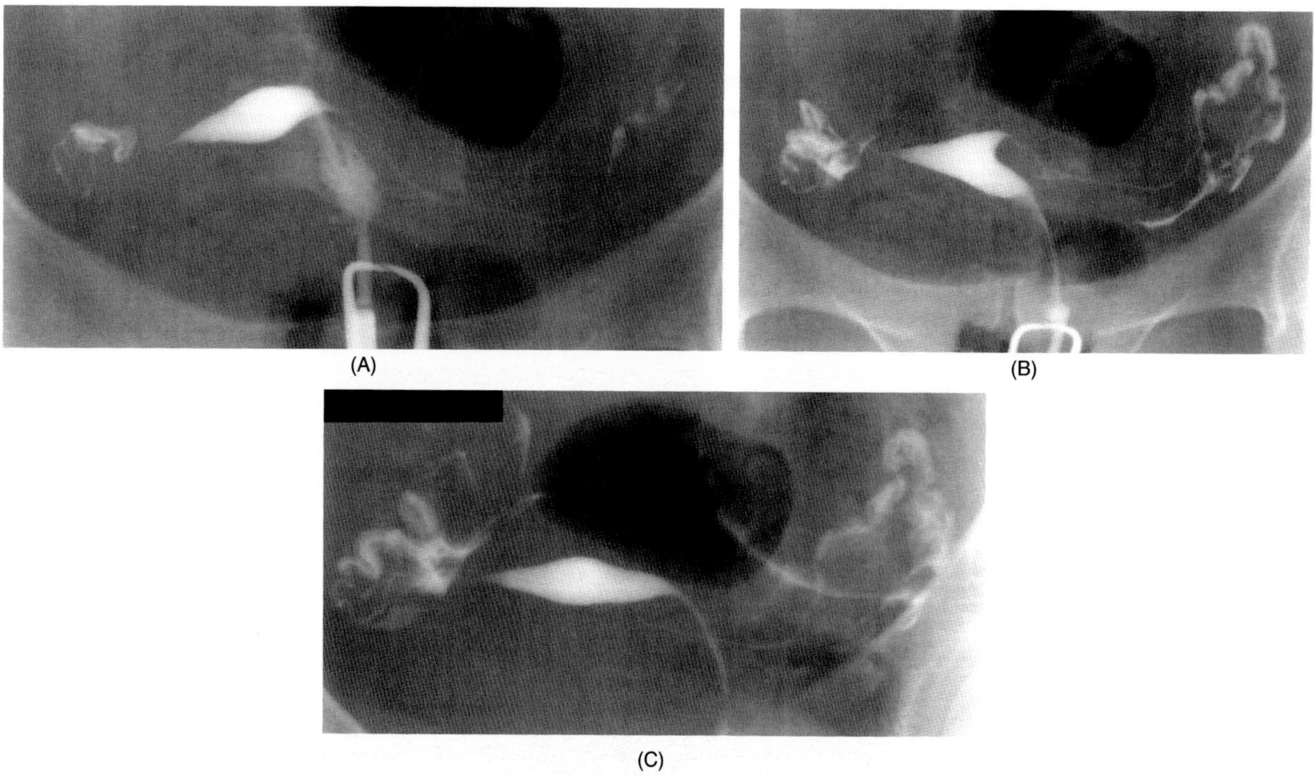

Figure 2 Hysterosalpingography: (A). Early phase: the contrast outlines a normal cervical canal and uterine cavity and has started to enter the tubes, up to the proximal ampulla. (B) Both tubes are patent and demonstrate normal ampullary mucosal folds. (C) Late film showing dispersion of the contrast material in the peritoneal cavity.

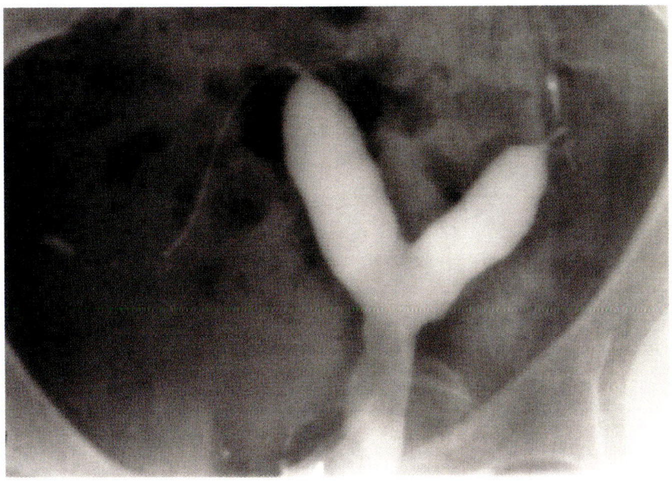

Figure 3 Hysterosalpingography: septate uterus in a patient with prior tubal sterilization.

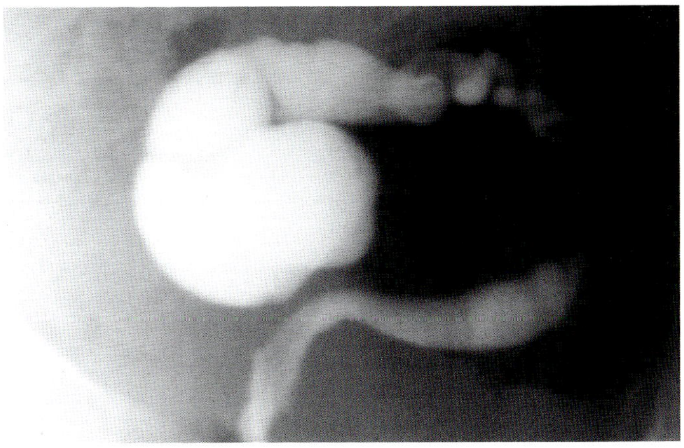

Figure 6 Hysterosalpingography: unicornuate uterus with a large hydrosalpinx.

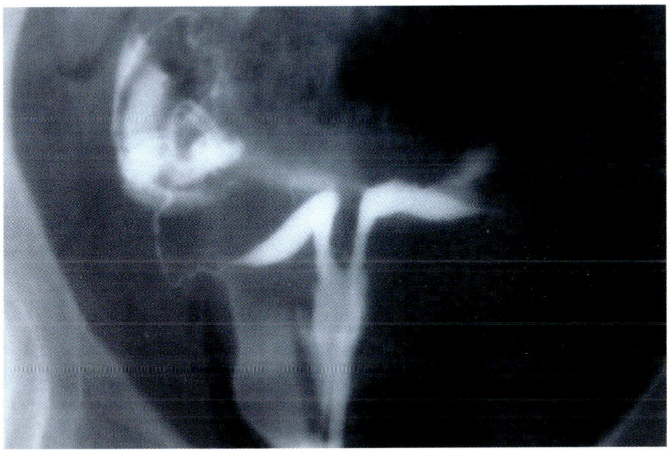

Figure 4 Hysterosalpingography: bicornuate uterus with patent fallopian tubes.

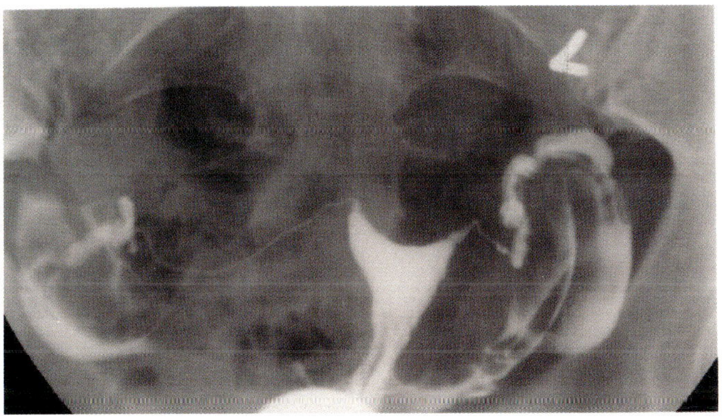

Figure 7 Hysterosalpingography: arcuate uterus with normal fallopian tubes.

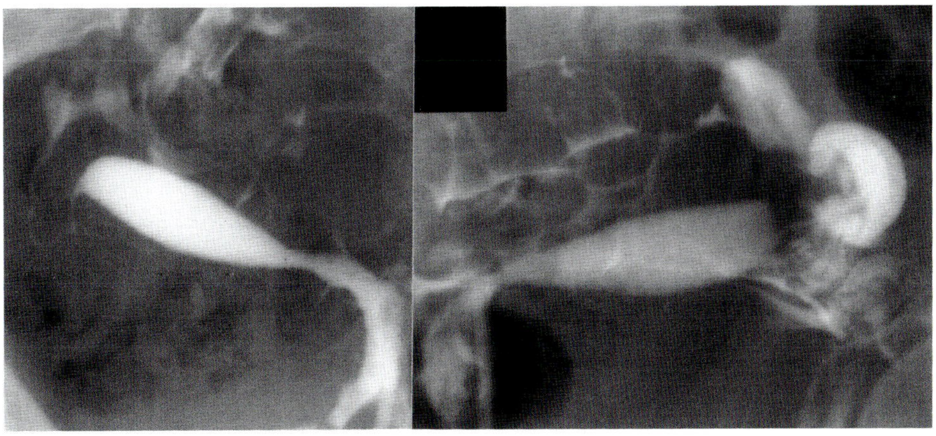

Figure 5 Hysterosalpingography: didelphus, complete duplication with two cervices and uteri.

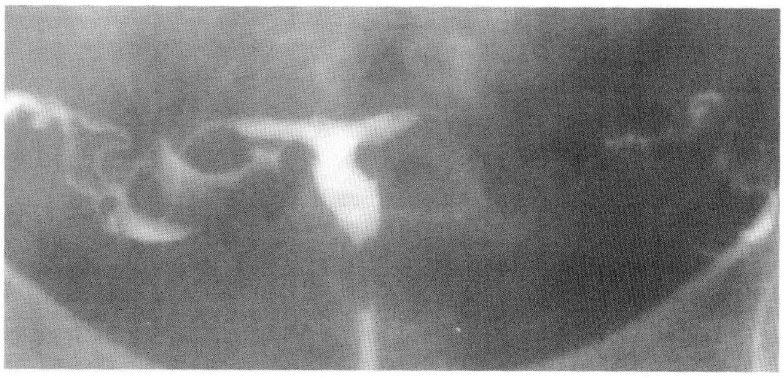

Figure 8 Hysterosalpingography: T-shaped uterus. Note the dilated intramural tubal segments.

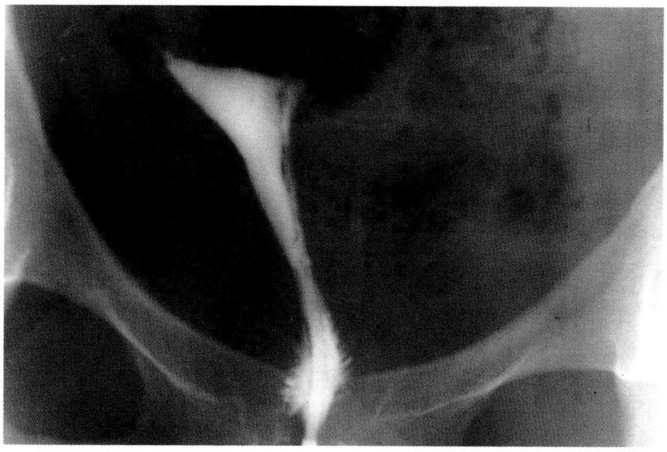

Figure 9 Hysterosalpingography: intrauterine synechiae on the left lateral aspect of the uterine cavity.

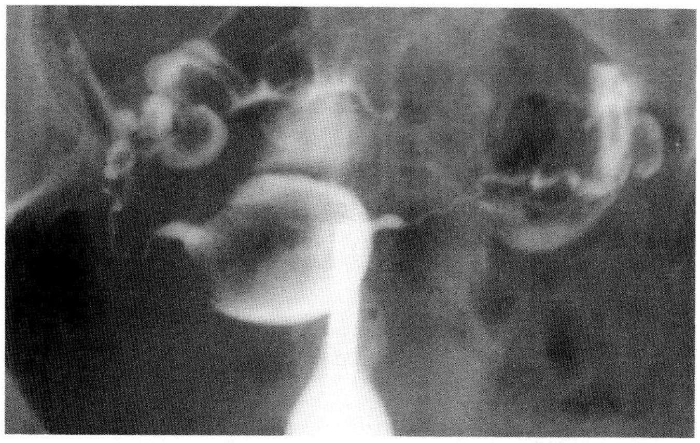

Figure 11 Hysterosalpingography: large intrauterine fibroid, with normal patent fallopian tubes.

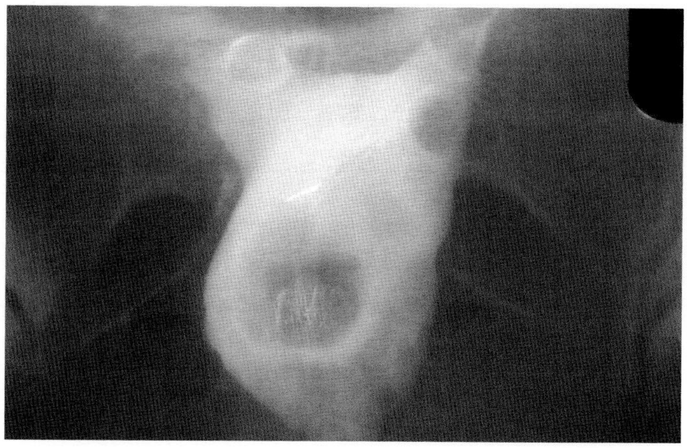

Figure 12 Hysterosalpingography: numerous intrauterine fibroids.

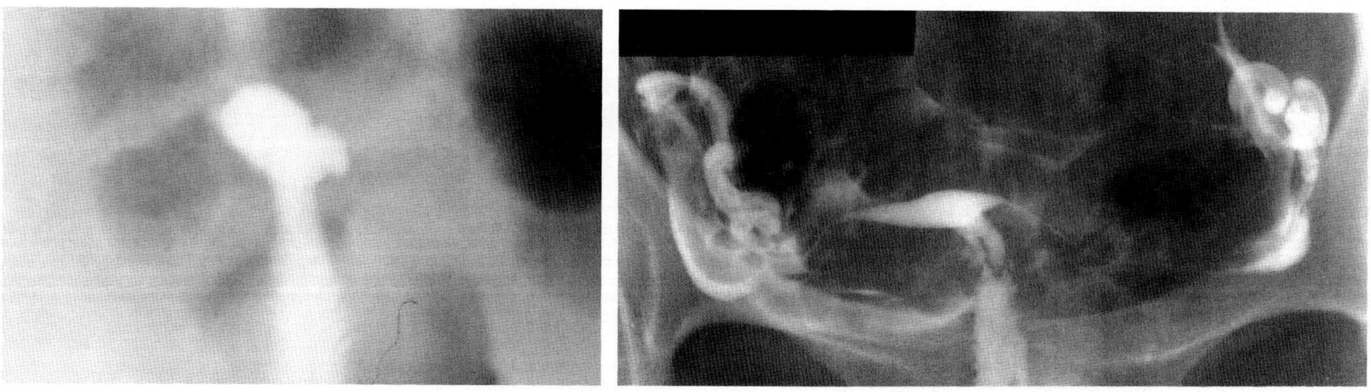

(A) (B)

Figure 10 Hysterosalpingography: (A) Severe synechiae; the contrast material outlines only the cervical canal. (B) HSG of the same patient after hysteroscopic adhesiolysis.

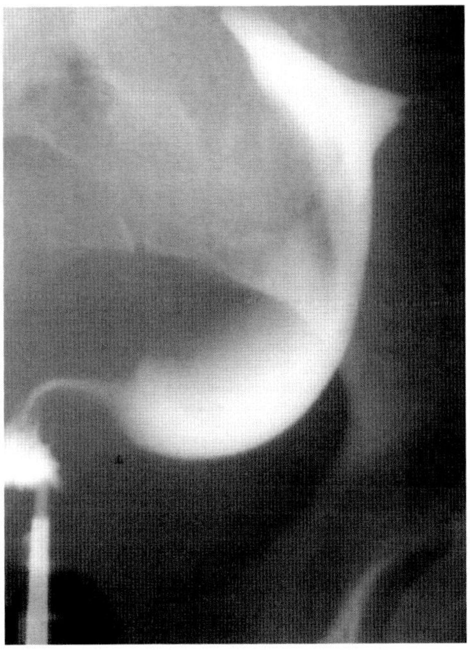

Figure 13 Hysterosalpingography: large intramural fibroid, significantly deforming the uterine cavity.

Tubal findings include normal findings, tubal occlusion (proximal, midtubal, and distal), lesions (salpingitis isthmica nodosa (SIN), endometriosis, and trophoblast), and specifics of intratubal architecture (dilatation, rugae, intratubal adhesions, and pathognomonic findings of prior tuberculous salpingitis) (Table 1) (7,8).

Failure of contrast to enter the tube may be unilateral or bilateral. It may simply be due to tubal spasm, which can be prevented by premedication and use of a gentle technique. Other causes include a mucous plug, synechiae, or more important lesions (obliterative fibrosis, SIN, endometriosis, prior surgery, etc.) as outlined in chapter 21.

SIN is a relatively frequent cause of proximal tubal disease and/or occlusion (see chap. 21 for details about this condition). The characteristic image of SIN is that of periluminal diverticula within the myosalpinx of the proximal oviduct. Radiographically, it appears as speckles of contrast radiating from the tubal lumen (Figs. 17–19). Endometriosis is encountered less frequently, usually when the tube is distally occluded, including postfimbriectomy. The radiographic image resembles SIN, but the speckles are much more pronounced (Fig. 20). Cornual polyps only rarely cause a proximal tubal occlusion. Radiographically, they appear as small globular or elongated vacuoles surrounded by contrast medium (Fig. 21).

One of the frequent challenges with HSG is the lack of passage of the contrast material into the fallopian tubes, suggesting cornual or proximal tubal obstruction (Fig. 22). The association of HSG with false-positive results in this regard is largely due to the lack of preparation of the patient for the procedure and use of a poor technique. This was clearly demonstrated by Lang and Dunaway (9). Out of 400 cases diagnosed as having cornual occlusion with a prior HSG elsewhere, simple premedication with aspirin before repeat HSG demonstrated tubal patency in one or both tubes in 82 cases. The use of selective salpingography in the others revealed

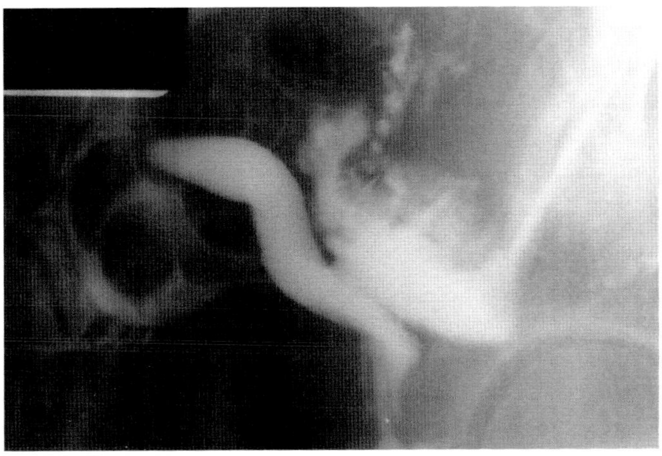

Figure 14 Hysterosalpingography: lateral view of the uterus demonstrating a large intramural fibroid with a necrotic cavity that is communicating with the uterine cavity. Note the intravasation of the contrast material through the fibroid.

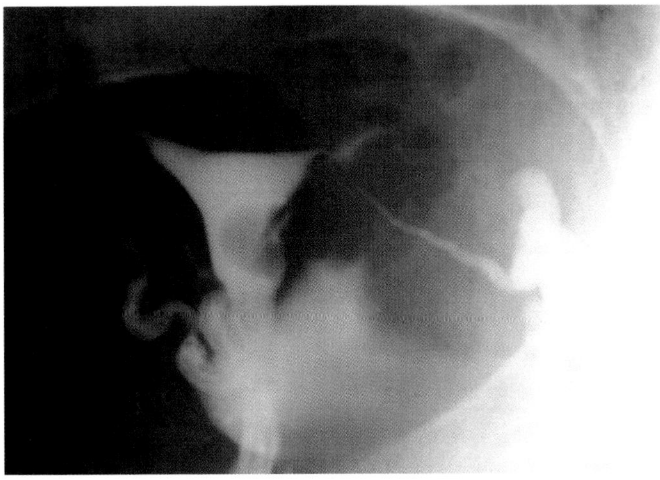

Figure 15 Hysterosalpingography: uterus demonstrating large filling defect due to an endometrial polyp.

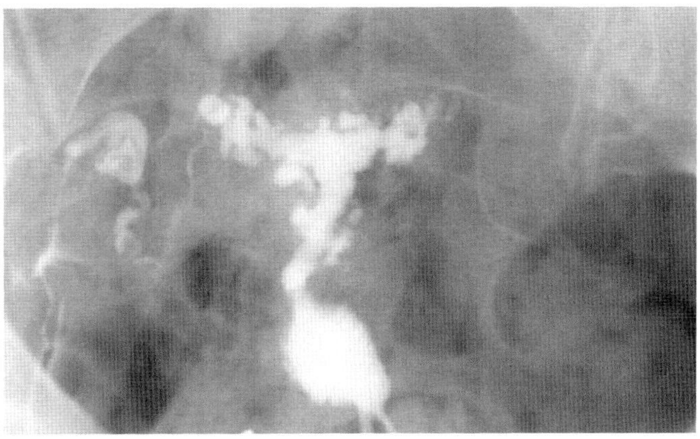

Figure 16 Hysterosalpingography: severe adenomyosis; the contrast material enters the endometrial glands infiltrating the myometrium.

Table 1 Hysterosalpingography: Abnormalities of the Fallopian Tube

Abnormality	Appearance	Comments
Tubocornual region		
Failure of contrast to enter tube	Simple obstruction	May be due to tubal spasm, presence of mucous plug, synechia, or lesions. May be unilateral or bilateral
Salpingitis isthmica nodosa (SIN)	Appears as speckles of contrast radiating from the tubal lumen. The tube may be patent or occluded	May be unilateral or bilateral
Endometriosis	Similar to SIN, usually with more pronounced punctate pattern	May be unilateral or bilateral
Polyps	Small globular or elongated vacuole surrounded by contrast medium	May be unilateral or bilateral
Isthmus		
Occlusion	Contrast outlines portion of the isthmic segment only	Commonly due to prior sterilization or tubal pregnancy, less commonly due to SIN, and uncommonly due to endometriosis and tuberculosis
Ampulla		
Midampullary occlusion	The contrast material outlines only varying lengths of the proximal portion of the ampulla. The intratubal architecture is usually normal	Most likely prior excision of distal ampulla for tubal sterilization or ectopic pregnancy. May also be congenital. Rarely signs specific to tuberculosis may be observed
Intraluminal adhesions	Patchy filling defects. Leopard skin appearance	Caused by endosalpingeal infection
Tubal pregnancy	Obstruction, stenosis, round defect, and occasionally calcification	Usually unilateral
Infundibulum		
Hydrosalpinx	Obstruction usually bilateral	Most common type of occlusion
Phimosis of distal tubal ostium	Intraluminal retention of contrast medium and slow intraperitoneal spill from stenosed tube	Both conditions are usually sequelae of pelvic inflammatory disease
Intraperitoneal spread		
Adhesions	Localized pooling and loculation of contrast medium around distal end of oviducts	

Source: Modified from Ref. 1.

tubal patency in one or both tubes in 131 of 318 cases. The remaining 187 women were submitted to tubal cannulation; this procedure was successful, in one or both tubes, in 145 and failed in 42 women (9). This study also demonstrates that selective salpingography, followed by tubal cannulation, when the former fails, should be performed when HSG suggests cornual occlusion; this should ideally be done in the same setting (see below).

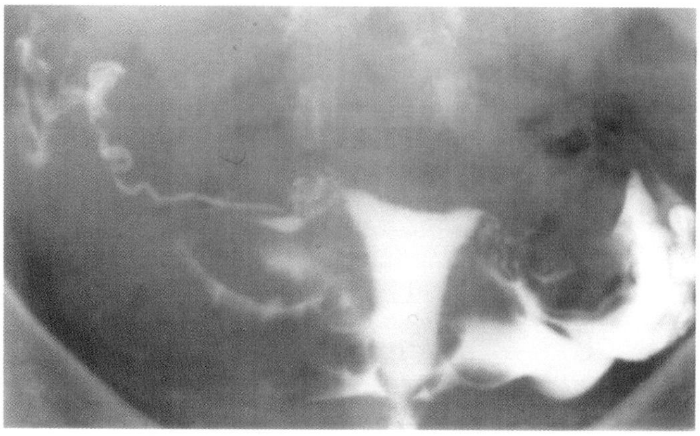

Figure 17 Hysterosalpingography: bilateral salpingitis isthmica nodosa. Large lesions, with typical appearance, are present on both cornual regions. The tubes are patent.

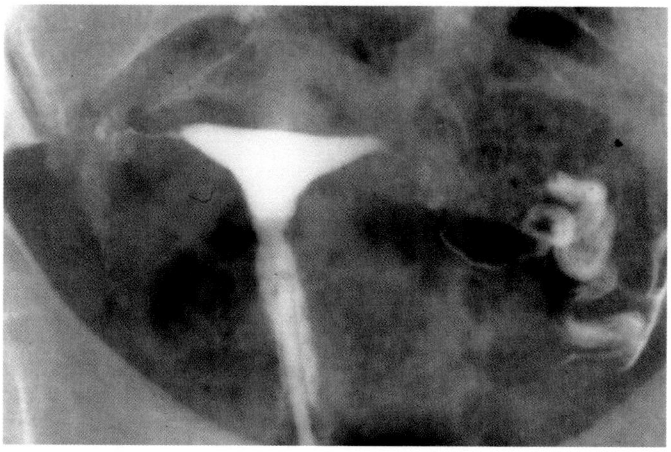

Figure 18 Hysterosalpingography: bilateral salpingitis isthmica nodosa. The left tube is patent. The right tube is occluded immediately adjacent to the lesion, which demonstrates the progressive nature of the lesion.

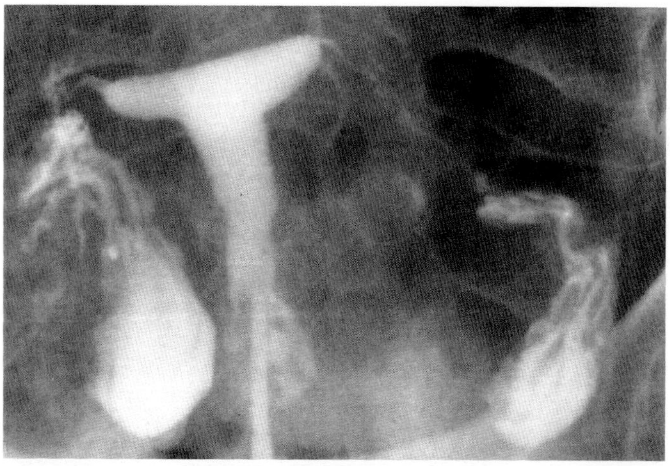

Figure 19 Hysterosalpingography: bilateral salpingitis isthmica nodosa. Both tubes are dilated and occluded distally (hydrosalpinx). In view of the finding of bipolar, distal and proximal, disease reconstructive surgery is not recommended.

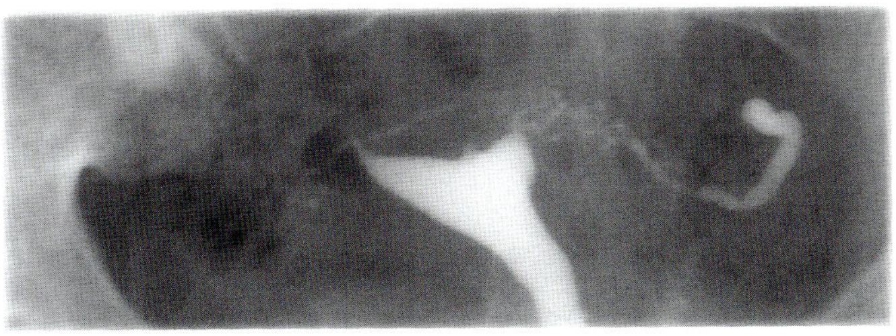

Figure 20 Hysterosalpingography: extensive endometriosis of the left tube, in a patient with prior excision of the distal tubal segments for permanent contraception. The speckles within the lesion are more pronounced than those in SIN.

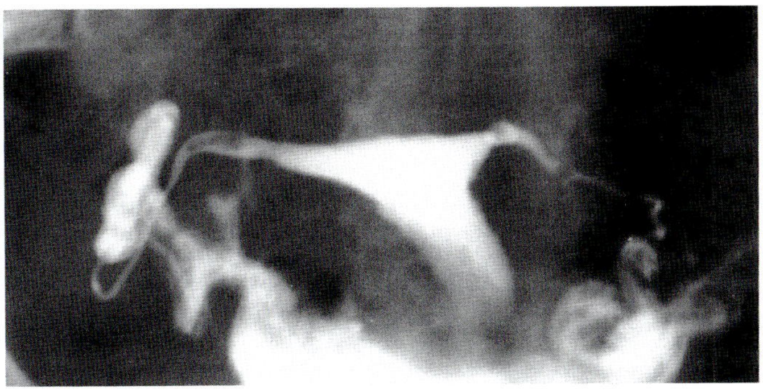

Figure 21 Hysterosalpingography: bilateral tubal polyps, in the presence of patent fallopian tubes.

Occlusion within the isthmic segment of the tube is commonly due to prior sterilization or tubal pregnancy, less commonly SIN, and uncommonly to endometriosis and tuberculosis. Contrast outlines portion of the isthmic segment only. The finding of a midampullary occlusion may also pose a diagnostic challenge. This, not infrequently, is interpreted as a "hydrosalpinx." In the absence of previous surgery (e.g., tubal sterilization, tubal pregnancy, etc.), it may be an ampullary atresia or may be caused by chorionic tissue from an expired tubal pregnancy that has not been totally resolved or calcified

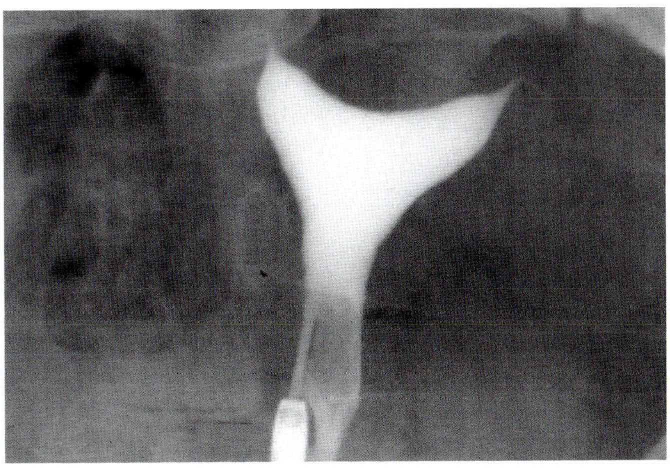

Figure 22 Hysterosalpingography: bilateral cornual occlusion. The intramural segments have been opacified and appear normal as does the uterus.

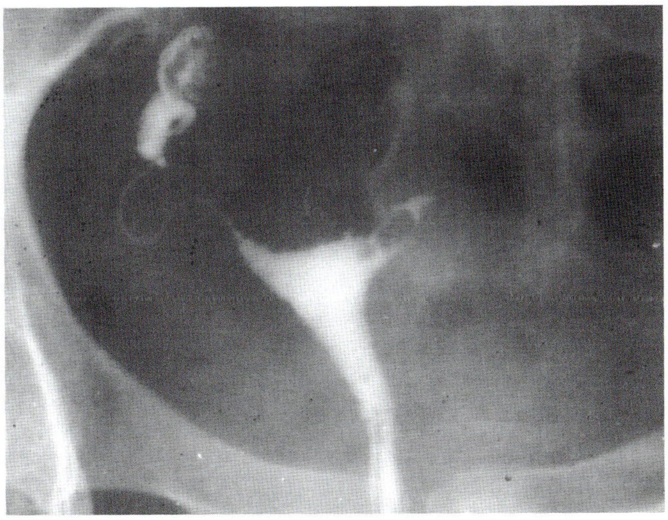

Figure 23 Hysterosalpingography: a calcified ectopic pregnancy occludes the ampullary segment of the right fallopian tube. The patient's left tube had been removed because of a tubal pregnancy.

(Fig. 23). Rarely, signs specific to tuberculosis may be observed in what appears as a tube with a shortened ampullary segment.

Complete distal occlusion of the tube is termed hydrosalpinx, the most common cause of which is salpingitis (see chap. 21); at HSG, there is no spill of contrast material from the distal end of the tube into the peritoneal cavity (Fig. 24). In some instances, the occlusion is incomplete and a small opening remains; this is termed phimosis of the distal tubal ostium. At HSG, there is retention of contrast medium within the tube with dilatation of the ampulla and eventual slow spill into the peritoneal cavity (Fig. 25).

Salpingography provides information in regard to the intratubal architecture, which is predictive of the prognosis of conception. Filling defects may be noted within an otherwise patent tube; these may be due to a prior spontaneously arrested tubal pregnancy or one treated with methotrexate, a finding that is usually unilateral (Figs. 23 and 26). In the event of a hydrosalpinx, the appearance of the tubal epithelium and the degree of tubal dilatation are important prognostic factors (Figs. 24 and 27). Presence of intratubal adhesions, even if there

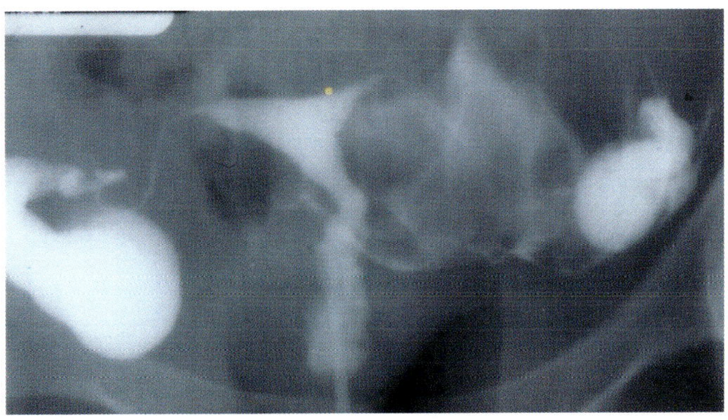

Figure 24 Hysterosalpingography: bilateral hydrosalpinx. With further injection of contrast material, increased tubal distention, and pressure, some contrast escaped through a crack on the distal end of the left tube.

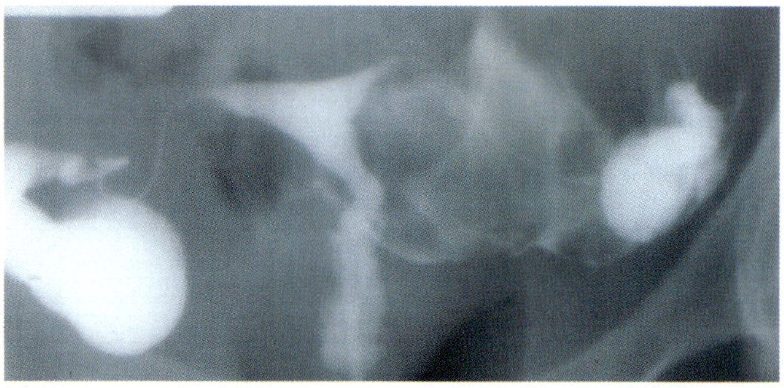

Figure 25 Hysterosalpingography: left tubal phimosis. After distention of the left ampullary segment, contrast slowly escapes into the peritoneal space. Right hydrosalpinx.

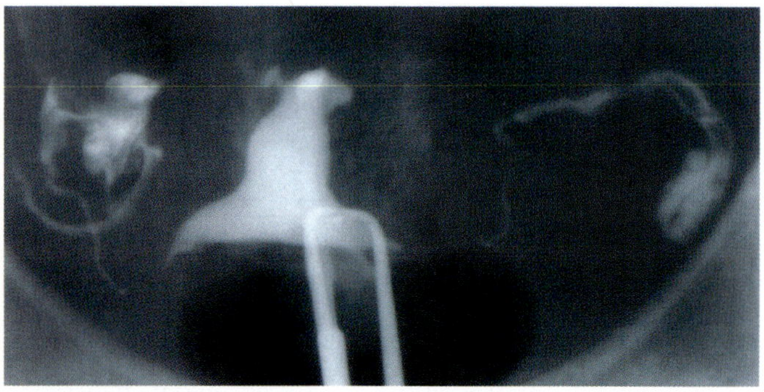

Figure 26 Hysterosalpingography: this film taken when the initial spill occurred from the right fallopian tube outlines a round defect in the ampulla of the same tube, at the site of a prior ectopic pregnancy treated with methotrexate. The left tube appears distally occluded.

is evidence of contrast spill, represents a very poor prognosis for successful conception (Figs. 28 and 29). Salpingography is a poor predictor of periadnexal adhesions, although not infrequently they prevent the dissemination of the contrast material that remains confined. This radiographic appearance is suggestive of adhesions (Fig. 30). Occasionally one encounters surprises, as we had in a 29-year-old woman with a very large pelvic mass in whom we carried out an HSG, which demonstrated the mass to be a giant hydrosalpinx, weighing 3145 g (10) (Fig. 31).

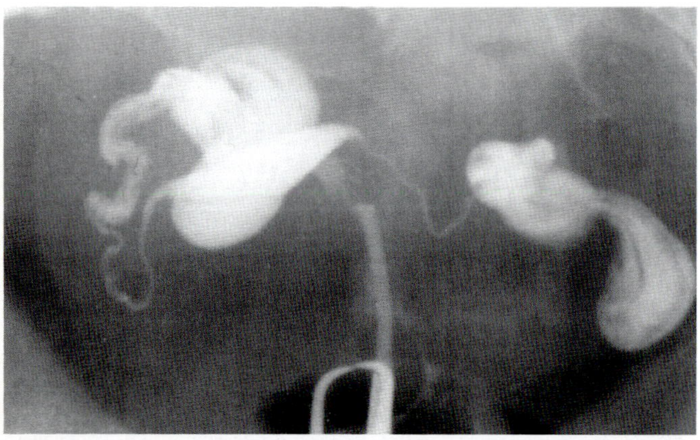

Figure 27 Hysterosalpingography: bilateral hydrosalpinx. Both tubes exhibit prominent ampullary folds, a good prognostic sign.

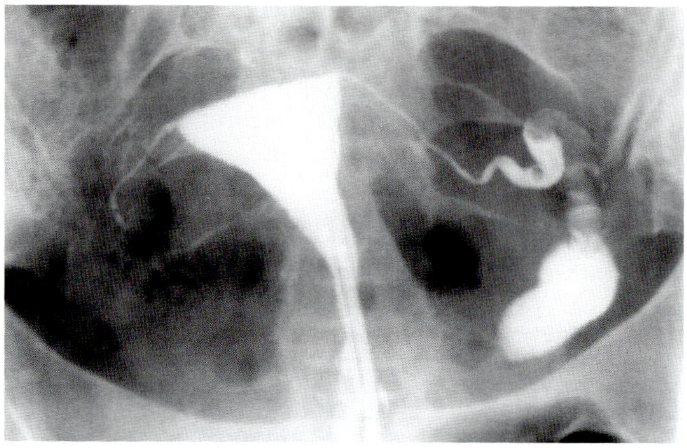

Figure 28 Hysterosalpingography: there are significant intratubal adhesions in the ampullary region of the left tube, which is a hydrosalpinx: a poor prognostic sign. The major part of the right tube had been previously removed.

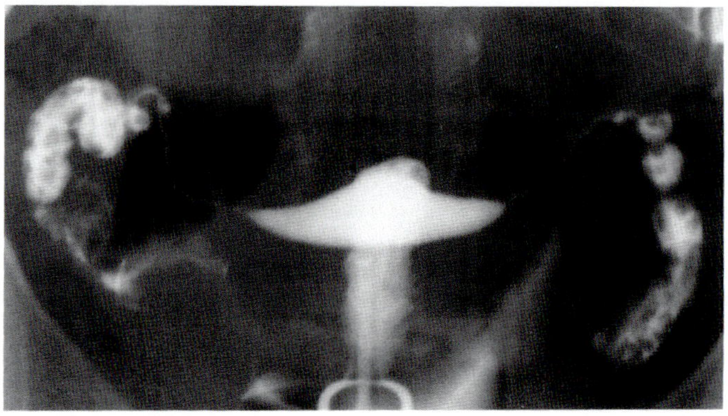

Figure 29 Hysterosalpingography: severe bilateral intratubal adhesions producing a honeycomb appearance.

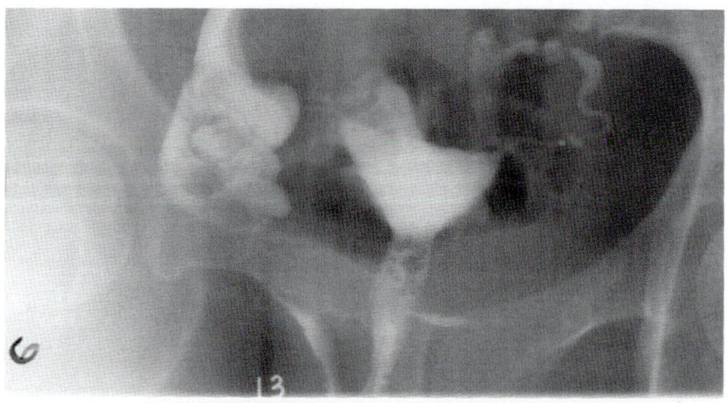

Figure 30 Hysterosalpingography: right periadnexal adhesions. The contrast material remains confined around the opacified fallopian tube.

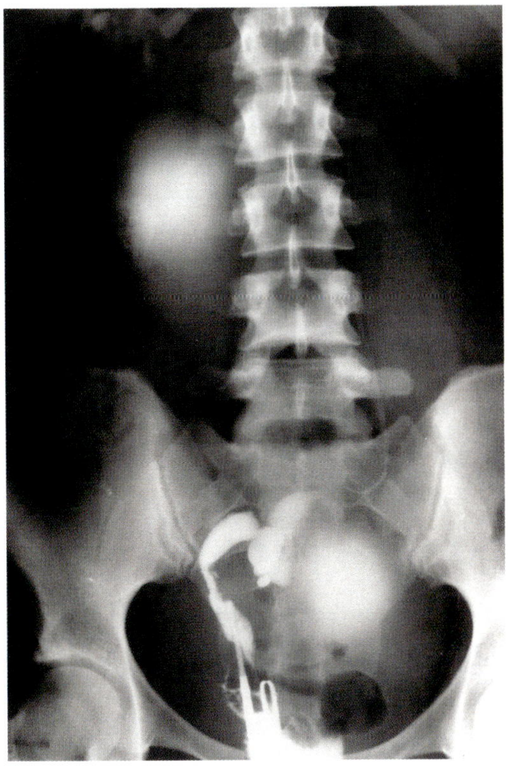

Figure 31 Hysterosalpingography: giant hydrosalpinx. The uterus is of normal size; the left hydrosalpinx is quite large and is confined to the pelvis. The right tube forms a very large mass that extends high into the abdominal cavity.

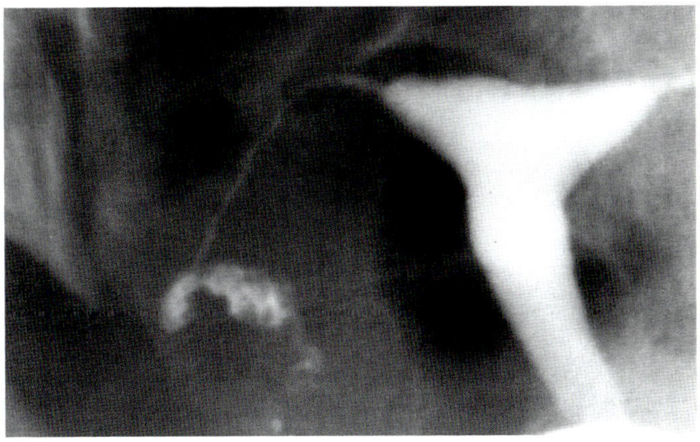

Figure 33 Hysterosalpingography: tuberculosis. The right tube is occluded in the proximal ampullary region, which demonstrates significant intratubal adhesions.

Prior genital tuberculosis frequently yields pathognomonic HSG images. One may encounter one or more of the following: intravasation of the contrast material into the uterine vessels and lymphatics, frequently with uterine synechiae (Fig. 32); a rigid shortened tube occluded usually at the level of the proximal ampulla, usually with a cotton wool appearance distal to it (Figs. 33 and 34); a beaded appearance of the lumen of the distally occluded tube, with dilatation alternating with stenosis; intratubal adhesions with or without diverticula; and a "rosette" or "Maltese cross" image of the distal oviduct (Fig. 35). Calcified pelvic lymph nodes may also be present.

There is a pronounced association between SIN and ectopic pregnancy. Florid SIN may be apparent at surgery, performed to remove the ectopic pregnancy. However, edema, hemorrhage, and anatomic distortion may not permit adequate evaluation. For this reason, an HSG is recommended in a woman who wishes to have another pregnancy, once the hCG assay is negative and normal menses has re-established (Fig. 36).

Selective salpingography is the injection of contrast medium directly into the uterine tubal ostium. This is achieved with the use of a special radiopaque cannula inserted through the cervix and guided toward the uterine tubal ostium. The contrast material is injected into the ostium. The increased pressure generated by the direct injection helps to overcome obstructions associated with mucus plugs or minor synechiae, in which case it may help outline either a normal tube or a pathologic tube, which may be patent or occluded (Fig. 37A and 37B).

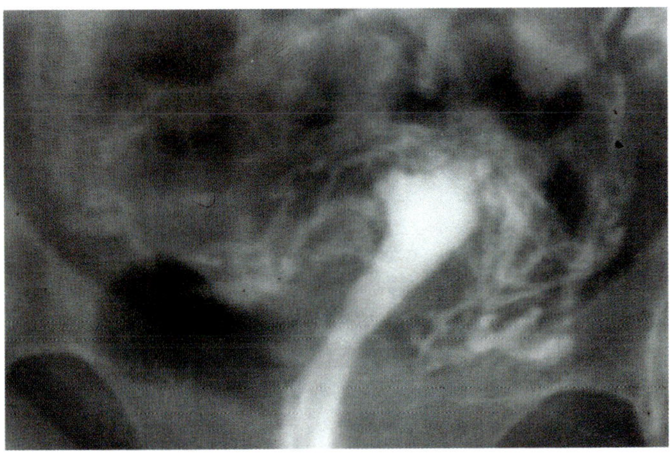

Figure 32 Hysterosalpingography: tuberculosis. In addition to extensive fundal synechiae, there is massive intravasation of the contrast material. The tubes are not outlined, likely due to the synechiae.

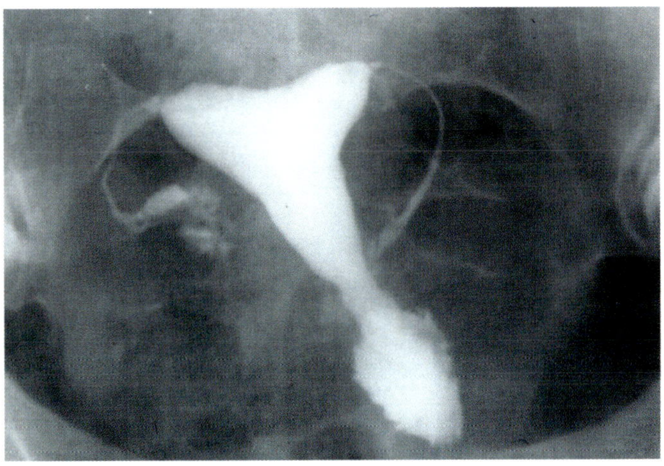

Figure 34 Hysterosalpingography: tuberculosis. The uterus appears normal. Both tubes appear rigid; only the proximal portions of the tubes are opacified until the proximal ampulla, distal to which the contrast material produces the so-called "cotton wool" image.

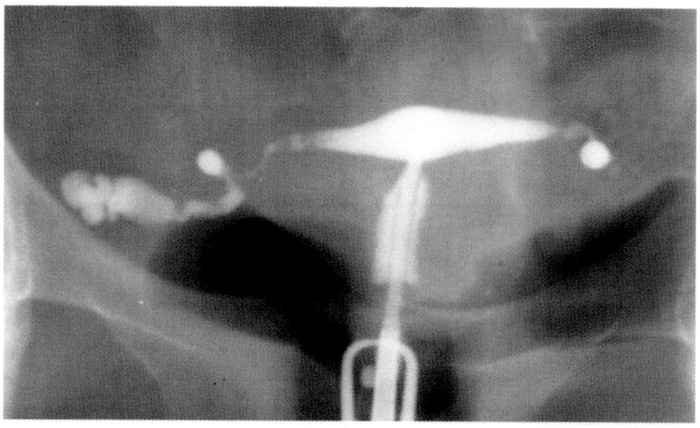

Figure 35 Hysterosalpingography: tuberculosis. The uterus appears normal. Only a very short portion of the left tube is opacified. The right tube, which is almost completely opacified, has dilated and constricted sections and terminates in the shape of a Maltese cross.

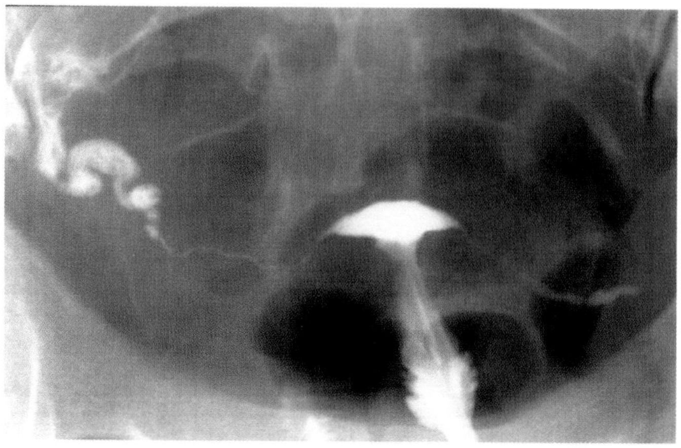

Figure 36 Hysterosalpingography performed some six weeks after the excision of a cornual pregnancy demonstrates a normal uterine cavity and right fallopian tube. The left tube had previously been removed.

Tubal cannulation requires the use of a special flexible guide wire and narrow-gauge cannula. This cannulation system is introduced through the larger cannula used for selective salpingography. These techniques are useful in differentiating true from false cornual occlusion. The therapeutic benefits of this approach have been shown for apparent cornual spasm, obstructions caused by amorphous material (tubal plugs), and tubal synechiae in the region of the uterine tubal ostium. It is doubtful that these techniques have a real therapeutic effect on occlusions owing to obliterative fibrosis, chronic follicular salpingitis, SIN, or endometriosis. Selective salpingography and tubal cannulation have diagnostic role as well, by outlining a normal-appearing tube or adversely a tubal occlusion, distal or elsewhere, or a diseased tube that appears inoperable (Figs. 38 and 39) (4,8). By demonstrating tubal pathology that is inoperable, both selective salpingography and tubal cannulation avoid further invasive investigation, including a laparoscopy, and permits the physician to recommend recourse to assisted reproduction (ART).

There are those who argue in favor of an immediate laparoscopy bypassing HSG. An analysis of 18 published series demonstrates good congruence between laparoscopic and HSG findings. These collected data indicate that the sensitivity and specificity of HSG are around 76% and 83%, respectively (11). These studies represent a selected population of patients in whom the prevalence of tubal occlusion was 38%. This prevalence figure falls to 10% in studies of large numbers of unselected patients, which reflects more accurately the general population (12,13). If the sensitivity and specificity figures reported above are applied to a hypothetical group of patients with a 10% rate of tubal occlusion, 3% of those with a normal HSG will have an abnormal laparoscopy. Thus, the laparoscopy will be normal in about 97% of patients.

The preceding clearly demonstrates the advantages of an initial HSG for the investigation of uterine and tubal causes of infertility. The information yielded by a well-performed HSG significantly helps in directing further investigation or treatment. In the event endoscopy is to be undertaken next, the

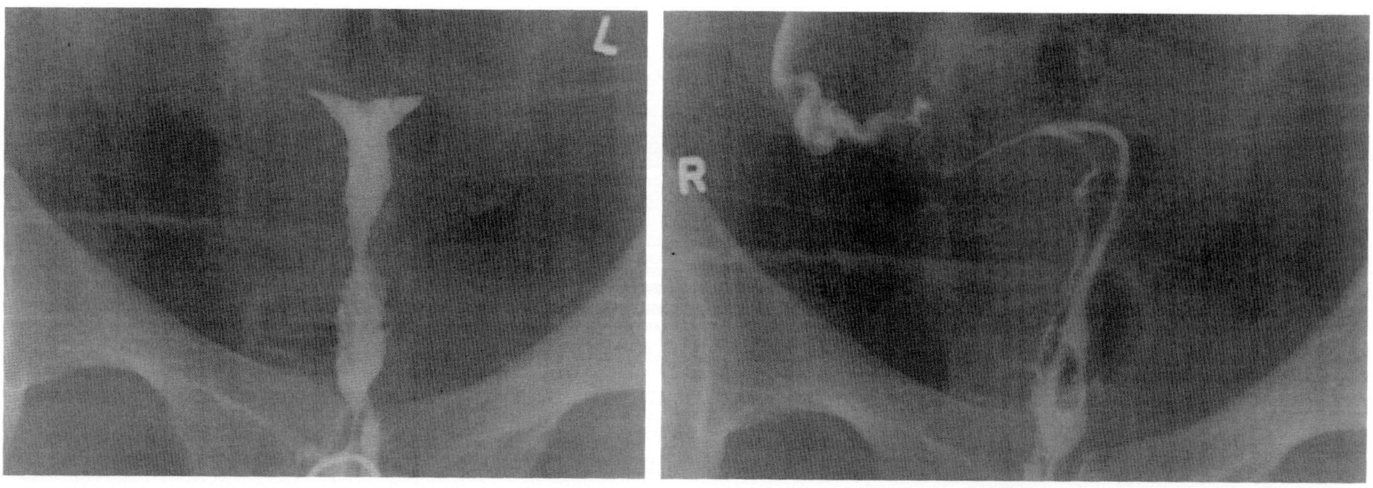

(A) (B)

Figure 37 Hysterosalpingography: (A) bilateral cornual occlusion, followed by (B) selective salpingography with opacification of the right tube.

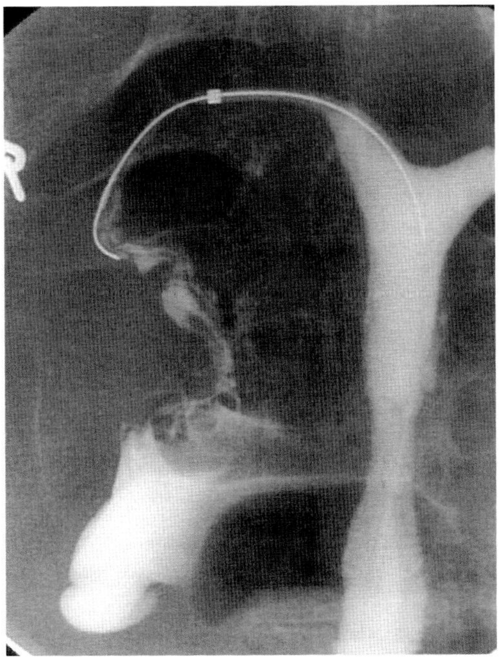

Figure 38 Tubal cannulation: cannulation and opacification of the right tube that is patent.

surgeon will be prepared to use the endoscopic procedure for both confirmation and treatment of the lesion(s). In many instances, HSG demonstrates the presence of severe tubal damage or conditions that are considered as contraindications of reconstructive surgery: severe intratubal adhesions and distal tubal occlusion in association with proximal tubal disease (e.g., SIN). In such instances, the couple may be advised of the significance of the findings, and ART may be recommended as primary treatment, without recourse to laparoscopy.

Evident limitations of HSG include a low positive predictive value in the diagnosis of periadnexal adhesions and endometriosis. According to the guidelines of the National Institute of Clinical Excellence (NICE-NHS) in the United Kingdom, "laparoscopy may be indicated in the initial evaluation of infertile women who have significant symptoms of endometriosis or who have a history of appendicitis, previous pelvic surgery, pelvic inflammatory disease, or other conditions that suggest pelvic pathology" (14). We question the wisdom of this recommendation, in patients presenting with infertility, since knowledge about the uterus and tubes would be of great value when undertaking the laparoscopy (with or without hysteroscopy), permitting the surgeon to better counsel the patient (couple) before the intervention, better plan the surgery, and treat the disease during the same laparoscopy. "The temptation to proceed to immediate laparoscopy should be resisted . . . A useful rule of thumb is to perform laparoscopy to confirm diagnosis formulated clinically, particularly if the condition will be amenable to laparoscopic treatment" (15). Laparoscopy ideally should be undertaken in a center able to perform the necessary procedures to treat the disease, during the same setting (16).

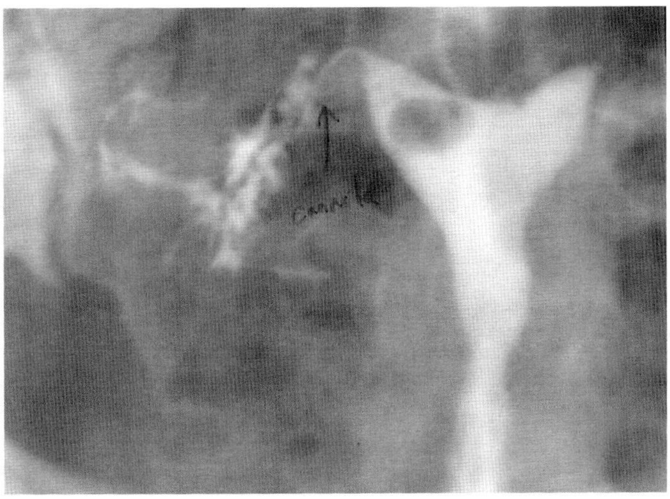

Figure 39 Tubal cannulation: cannulation of the right tube outlines a severely diseased isthmic portion.

Hysterocontrast Sonography (Salpingosonography)

Hysterocontrast sonography (HyCoSy) or salpingosonography is a sonographic technique designed to asses the uterus and the patency of the fallopian tubes. The technique includes the following steps: a Foley catheter is inserted into the cervix and transvaginal sonography is carried out to assess the pelvis. A 20-mL syringe is filled with 10 mL of saline solution followed by 10 mL of air. Air is injected first, slowly, and the passage is followed through the tube; saline is then injected to cause the air bubbles to flow more visibly through the tube (17). Air-filled albumin microspheres have also been used for this purpose (18).

With this method, with regard to tubal patency, a concordance with laparoscopy of more than 80% has been reported. The reported concordance with HSG is 72% to 90% (17–21). While the reported concordance with HSG with regard to passage of contrast into the peritoneal cavity appears high, it is important to note that, in contrast to HSG, HyCoSy does not provide any information with regard to the intratubal architecture. Yet, the pain scores associated with both of these techniques were comparable, as demonstrated in a prospective study (18).

Laparoscopy

Laparoscopy permits direct visualization of the entire peritoneal cavity, the pelvis, and internal reproductive organs. Intraoperative chromopertubation tests tubal patency. It is the most accurate way to identify periadnexal adhesive disease and endometriosis. Laparoscopy is an invasive procedure that usually requires a general anesthetic. It must be noted that most of major vascular and bowel injuries occur with the initiation of laparoscopy (introduction of the Veress needle, principal trocar, and ancillary trocars) (22,23). Laparoscopy also provides the necessary surgical access to perform surgical procedures. Hysteroscopy and salpingoscopy, when indicated, may be performed during the same setting. Abdominal, pelvic, and periadnexal adhesions may impede laparoscopic access to the pelvis and the adnexa, necessitating preliminary adhesiolysis.

A thorough laparoscopic survey will identify abdominal and pelvic lesions and permit assessment of the uterus, ovaries, and tubes. The information yielded by the prior HSG, together with this survey, enables the surgeon to undertake reconstructive laparoscopic surgery or surgery by open access when this form of access is indicated or recommend ART.

It is not the purpose of this chapter to describe in detail the laparoscopy technique. After the introduction of the laparoscope, it is imperative to thoroughly inspect the whole abdominal cavity commencing with the upper abdomen and including the liver and the undersurface of the diaphragm, while the operating table is in the horizontal position. Perihepatic "violin string" adhesions suggest prior salpingitis. Rarely, the undersurface of the diaphragm may reveal presence of endometriotic lesions; other lesions may be noted in the liver or other organs.

Attention is then focused on the lower abdomen and pelvis. To improve visibility, the patient is placed in the Trendelenburg position and the bowel is displaced upward. A general panoramic inspection of the pelvis, with the laparoscope at a distance, may suggest the cause of the infertility. Adhesions and peritoneal scarring are evidence of a previous inflammatory process, infectious or postsurgical. Evidence of endometriosis may be noted.

The laparoscope is then advanced; appropriate manipulation of the uterus, with the cervical cannula placed before the initiation of laparoscopy, and manipulation of the organs, with an appropriate instrument introduced through an ancillary port, enhance the visibility of specific pelvic organs that are inspected in turn. With the uterus moved backward, its anterior surface, the vesicouterine pouch, and the dome of the bladder are assessed (Fig. 40). The uterus is then moved into anteversion; the uterine fundus and its posterior surface, the uterosacral ligaments, and the pouch of Douglas are thoroughly inspected (Fig. 41). If fluid is present in the pouch, its nature is noted. It may be necessary to aspirate the fluid, with a suction cannula that can also be used as a manipulating probe, to properly inspect the underlying peritoneal surfaces. The aspirated fluid can be sent for microbiologic, histologic, or biochemical studies as necessary. The cul-de-sac and the lateral peritoneal surfaces are inspected for any scarring or evidence of endometriosis.

The extent and type of pelvic and periadnexal adhesions are noted. Each tube and ovary and the respective pelvic sidewalls are thoroughly scrutinized. Once the anterior surface of the ovary is inspected, the ovary is elevated and flipped upward, with a manipulating probe or other appropriate instrument, to expose its posterior surface, the fossa ovarica, and the pelvic sidewall down to the level of the uterosacral ligament (Fig. 42). If the ovary is adherent within the fossa ovarica, gentle release of the ovary will permit visualization of its posterior surface and the pelvic sidewall; this will reveal the cause, which is frequently endometriosis (Fig. 43). The tube is inspected from the proximal to the distal end. Attention is paid to any evidence of fusiform swelling at the uterotubal junction, usually caused by SIN (Fig. 44) or less frequently by endometriosis; presence of fimbrial phimosis or frank distal tubal occlusion (hydrosalpinx); or other abnormalities. The ovarian fimbrial relation is assessed, and the fimbriae are examined by close observation (Figs. 45 and 46). Once the other adnexum is similarly assessed, chromopertubation is carried out by injection of dilute indigo carmine or methylene blue solution through the uterine cannula. The passage of the dye solution is followed through the tube, and the nature of the spill is examined by viewing the fimbriae to search for evidence of prefimbrial phimosis or fine fimbrial adhesions that may impede ovum pickup (Figs. 47 and 48) (8).

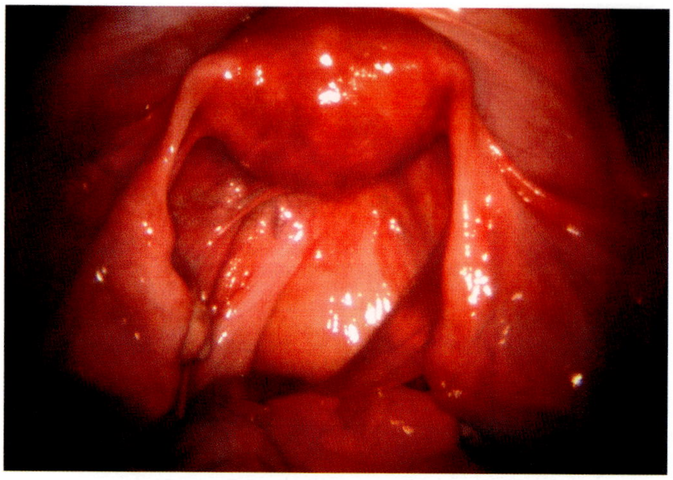

Figure 41 Laparoscopy: panoramic view of the pelvis.

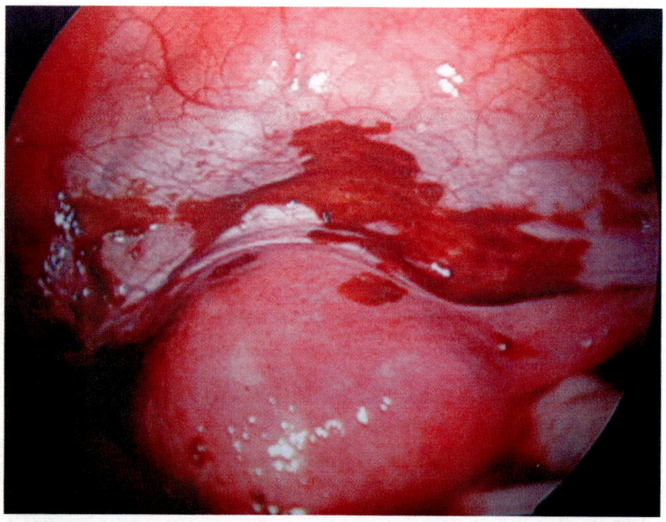

Figure 40 Laparoscopy: large patch of endometriosis over the bladder peritoneum and anterior surface of the uterus.

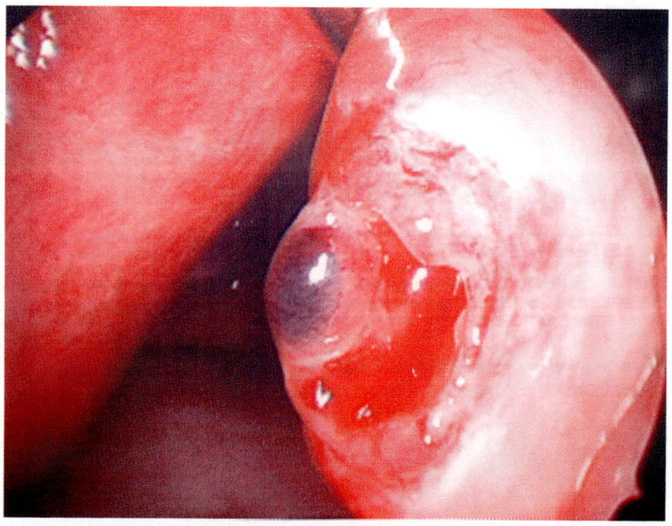

Figure 42 Laparoscopy: recent ovulation in a normal ovary.

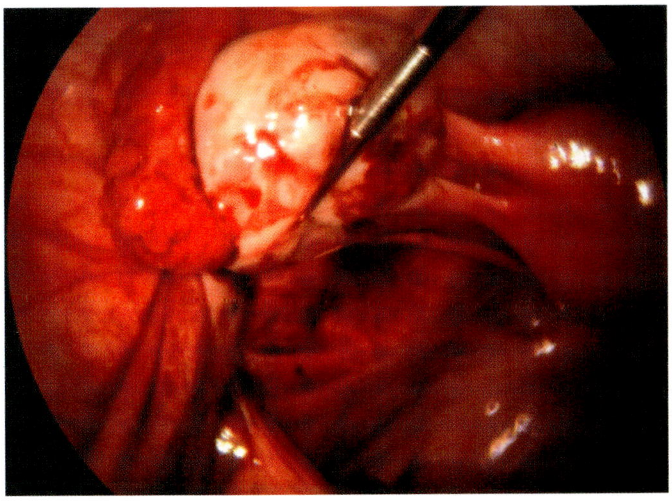

Figure 43 Laparoscopy: endometriosis on the posterior surface of the left ovary and in the fossa ovarica, to which the ovary had been adherent.

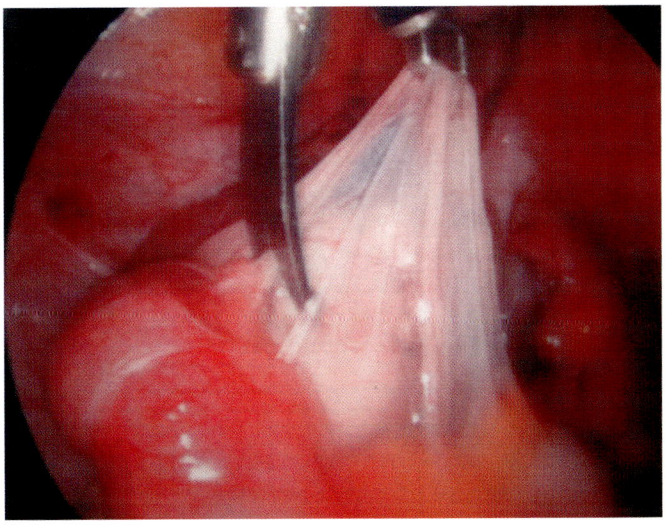

Figure 45 Laparoscopy: peritubal adhesions encasing the ovary.

Laparoscopy may be complemented with hysteroscopy, as necessary, to confirm a diagnosis and/or treat a lesion noted at HSG. Laparoscopic surgical access is used extensively in reproductive surgery as well as in many other reconstructive and ablative gynecologic procedures; these are discussed in many chapters of this book.

Hysteroscopy

Hysteroscopy permits direct visualization of the cervical canal and the uterine cavity. It also provides surgical access to permit therapeutic surgical procedures, previously performed blindly by vaginal route or via abdominal access and a hysterotomy to access the uterine cavity.

Initially described as "a technique looking for an indication," the impact of hysteroscopy in our specialty has been radical. This came about when hysteroscopy started to be used as a new mode of surgical access into the uterus. This revolutionized and greatly simplified many procedures that previously required a laparotomy and a hysterotomy to access the uterine cavity: lysis of severe uterine synechiae, metroplasty for septate uterus, excision of symptomatic intrauterine fibroids, and endometrial polyps. These, after all, are common conditions; hysteroscopy has simplified these procedures and significantly reduced their morbidity (24). These conditions, their relationship to subfertility and other symptoms, and the procedures themselves have been discussed in other chapters of this book. Tubal cannulation may also be performed by hysteroscopy; this is usually done under laparoscopic control, when the latter procedure is also indicated (Fig. 49).

Technical progresses in instrumentation, the production of mini hysteroscopes that provide excellent vision, now permit out patient "office hysteroscopy." The procedure is usually performed with mild analgesia using the "vaginoscopic technique." As opposed to the traditional approach, a vaginal speculum and a cervical tenaculum are not used. The

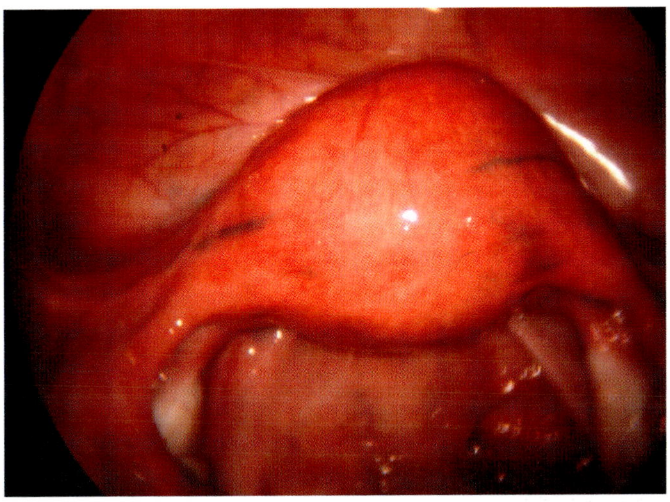

Figure 44 Laparoscopy: bilateral cornual occlusion. Note the fusiform shape of the cornua and the intravasation of the blue dye solution in the superficial vessels of the fundus.

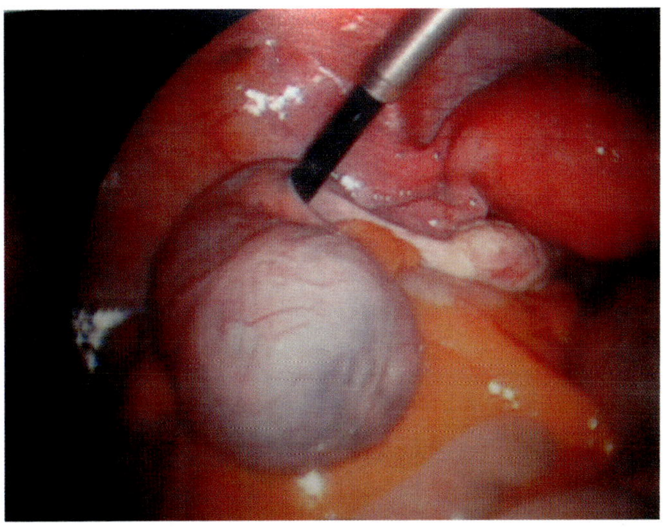

Figure 46 Laparoscopy: left hydrosalpinx.

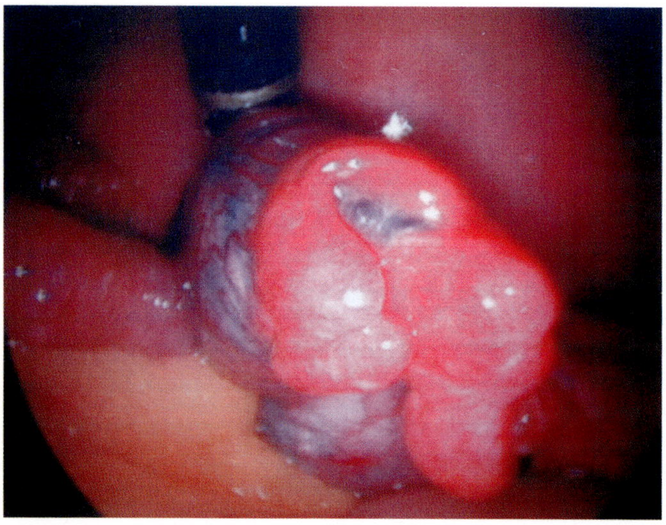

Figure 47 Laparoscopy: prefimbrial distal occlusion of the left tube. The blue dye solution has distended the whole ampulla until the infundibulum, without any spill. The fimbriae are visible distal to the site of occlusion.

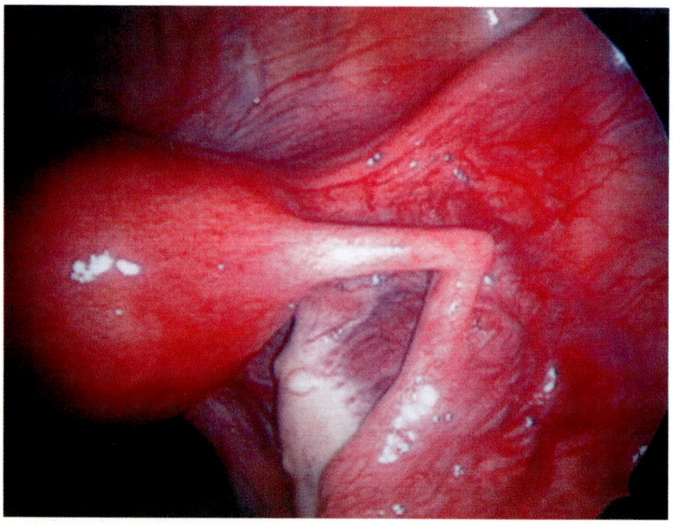

Figure 49 Laparoscopy: laparoscopic view of hysteroscopic tubal cannulation.

hysteroscope is introduced into the vagina, which is distended with saline solution. This permits inspection of the vagina and cervix. The cervical canal is entered under direct vision while continuing to distend the canal and uterine cavity with the saline solution. In addition to its diagnostic potential, this approach also permits minor interventions to be performed using special instruments that are introduced though the shaft of the hysteroscope (25). Hysteroscopy and hysteroscopic procedures are discussed in chapter 6.

Salpingoscopy

Salpingoscopy is the endoscopic examination of the ampullary portion of the tubal lumen. Visualization of the ampullary lumen may be accomplished at laparoscopy with a small-gauge rigid or flexible endoscope introduced through an

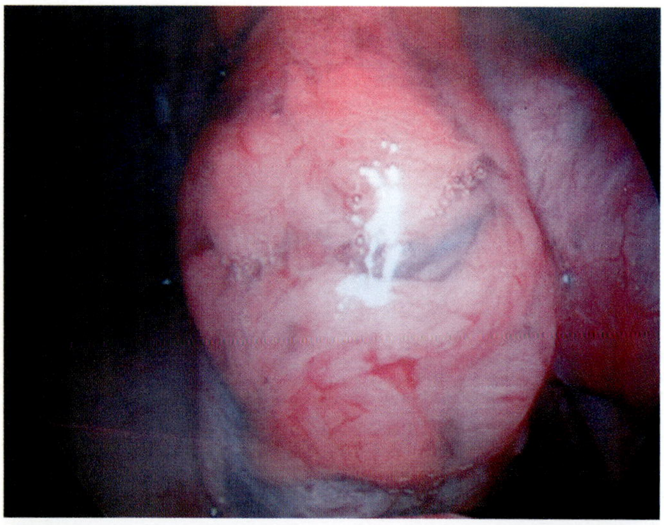

Figure 48 Laparoscopy: distal tubal occlusion due the entrapment of the fimbriae by a fibrous adhesion that covers the terminal end of the tube. The tube is distended with blue dye solution, which is visible through the adhesion.

ancillary portal. The endoscope is introduced through fimbrial ostium. The tube is distended with physiologic solution injected through the outer sheath of the rigid endoscope or the channel of the flexible endoscope, for proper visualization. The endoscope is advanced gradually within the distended ampulla; thus, it is possible to assess most of the ampulla. To perform a salpingoscopy in a hydrosalpinx, a small opening is made in its distal portion, as is done to start a salpingostomy, to permit the introduction of the endoscope. The findings have been classified into five grades (26):

Grade 1—normal mucosal architecture
Grade 2—tubal mucosa with variable degrees of flattening of both major and minor mucosal folds that are largely preserved
Grade 3—focal adhesions between mucosal folds
Grade 4—extensive intraluminal adhesions or disseminated flattened epithelial areas
Grade 5—tubes that are rigid and hollow, with a complete loss of epithelial folds

Salpingoscopic evaluation appears to have a good prognostic predictive value in regard to future pregnancy, as demonstrated by numerous workers in this field (26–28).

Hydroculdoscopy

Hydroculdoscopy has been introduced as a means to visualize the cul-de-sac of Douglas, the ovaries, and the fallopian tubes. The technique is an elegant modification of the traditional culdoscopy. It was introduced under the name of "fertiloscopy" as a diagnostic technique to replace a laparoscopy in the investigation of infertile women (29).

The technique includes exposure of the posterior fornix of the vagina, the initial introduction of some 200 to 250 mL of saline solution into the pouch of Douglas with a Veress type needle, and the subsequent insertion of a trocar/cannula that permits the introduction of a small-caliber endoscope. The procedure permits the visualization of the pouch of Douglas, the posterior surface of the uterus, the fallopian tubes, and ovaries. Tubal patency can be ascertained by introduction of a dilute methylene blue solution into uterine cavity, through an appropriate cannula. If tubal damage is suspected, a salpingoscopy may be performed during the same procedure.

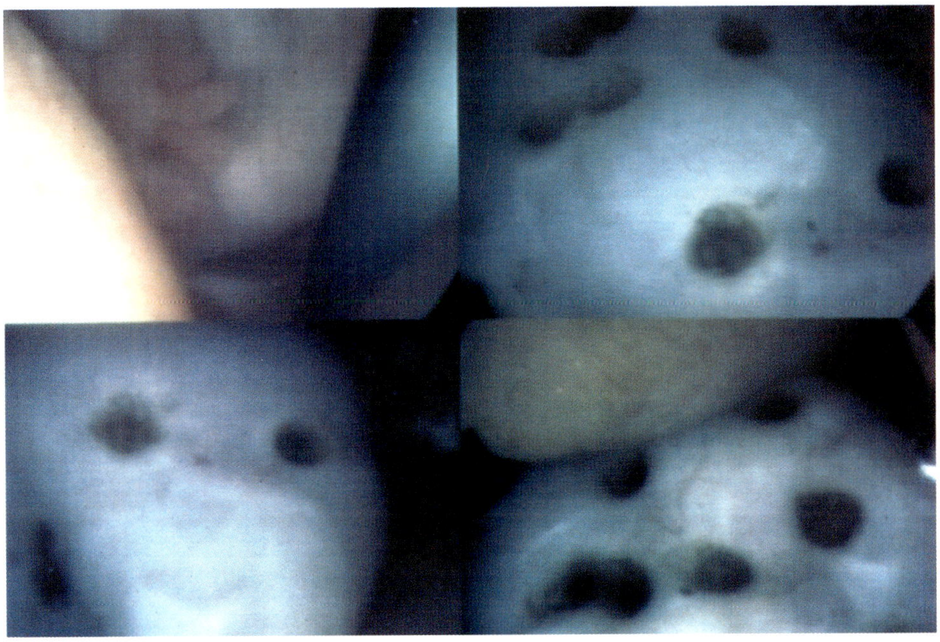

Figure 50 Hydroculdoscopy: four views of ovarian drilling via hydroculdoscopy, using a bipolar electrode.

Initially introduced as a diagnostic tool, the technique has also provided surgical access for certain therapeutic procedures, including minor adhesiolysis and ablation of minor endometriotic lesions. The first ovarian drilling with this approach was performed, in France in 1999, at the Antoine Beclère Hospital by Hervé Fernandez on my suggestion and assistance, introducing a bipolar Versapoint® probe into the pouch of Douglas through a site lateral to that of the endoscope. The patient was markedly obese and was found to have polycystic ovaries (30) (Fig. 50). Ovarian drilling using this access has since been performed in many centers; the reported results appear similar to those performed by laparoscopy (31).

It is evident that the procedure cannot be undertaken if the cul-de-sac of Douglas is occluded. The view with hydroculdoscopy is localized and very different from the panoramic view obtained by laparoscopy and does not offer the wide surgical applications that laparoscopic surgical access offers. However, it does have a role, in replacing a laparoscopy, in appropriately selected patients.

SUMMARY

- The investigation of the infertile couple should be concluded rapidly, accurately, and inexpensively, with as little invasion as possible.
- The many important technological advances realized in imaging and ART during the last 30 years have led to the simplification the investigation of infertility.
- The investigation should be individualized, based on the findings of the clinical assessment of the couple. Evidence of ovulation should be sought in the female partner and a semen analysis performed in the male early on.
- HSG remains the initial test in the investigation of uterine and tubal causes of infertility. When performed properly, HSG provides valuable information about the uterine cavity and the tubes including their inner architecture.
- Advances in imaging and laboratory medicine have significantly decreased the diagnostic role of endoscopy in infertility. A useful rule of thumb is to perform endoscopy to confirm a diagnosis formulated clinically, particularly if the condition will be amenable to endoscopic treatment. Furthermore, endoscopy should preferably be undertaken in a center able to treat the anomaly and/or condition, affecting the patient, during the same setting.

REFERENCES

1. Gomel V, Taylor PJ. Diagnostic and Operative Gynecologic Laparoscopy. St Louis: Mosby, 1995:105.
2. Centers for Disease Control and Prevention. 2003 Assisted Reproductive Technology (ART) Report. Web site: www.cdc.gov/ART/ART2003.
3. Luttjeboer FY, et al. 23rd Annual Meeting ESHRE, 2007:O-061.
4. Gomel V, Taylor E. Reconstructive tubal surgery. In: Rock JA, Jones HW III, eds. Te Linde's Operative Gynecology, 10th ed, Philadelphia: Wolters Kluwer, 2008:404.
5. Musset R. An Atlas of Hysterosalpingography. Quebec: Les Presses de l'Université Laval, 1979.
6. Watson A, Vandekerckhove P, Lilford R, et al. A meta-analysis of the therapeutic role of oil soluble contrast media at hysterosalpingography: A surprising result? Fertil Steril 1994; 61:470–477.
7. Gomel V. Recent advances in surgical correction of tubal disease producing infertility. Curr Probl Obstet Gynecol 1978; 10:1–60.
8. Gomel V, Taylor PJ. Diagnostic and Operative Gynecologic Laparoscopy. St Louis: Mosby, 1995:99–113.
9. Lang EK, Dunaway HH. Recanalization of obstructed fallopian tube by selective salpingography and transvaginal bougie dilatation: Outcome and cost analysis. Fertil Steril 1996; 66:210.
10. Gomel V, Munro MG. Giant hydrosalpinx. J Reprod Med 1980; 25:129–131.
11. Taylor PJ, Collins JA. Unexplained Infertility. Oxford: Oxford University Press, 1992.
12. Collins JA, Wrixon W, Jans LB, et al. Treatment-independent pregnancy among infertile couples. N Engl J Med 1983, 309:1201–1206.
13. Hull MGR, Glazener CMA, Kelly NJ. Population study of causes, treatment and outcome of infertility. Br Med J 1985; 291:1693–1697.

14. NICE, NHS. Fertility: Assessment and Treatment for People with fertility Problems—Full Guideline. London: RCOG Press, 2004.
15. Taylor PJ, Gomel V. Pelvic pain. Curr Prob Obstet Gynecol Fertil 1987; 9:395–437.
16. Gomel V. Chronic pelvic pain: A challenge. J Minim Invasive Gynecol 2007; 14:521–526.
17. Heikkinen H, Tekay A, Volpi E, et al. Transvaginal salpingosonography for the assessment of tubal patency in infertile women: Methodological and clinical experiences. Fertil Steril 1995; 64:293–298.
18. Cheong YC, Li TC. Evidence based management of tubal disease and infertility. Curr Obstet Gynaecol 2005; 15:306–313.
19. Chenia F, Hofmeyr GJ, Moolla S, et al. The assessment of endometrial pathology and tubal patency: A comparison between the use of ultrasonography and X-ray hysterosalpingography for the investigation of infertility patients. Br J Radiol 1997; 70: 833–836.
20. Inki P, Palo P, Anttila L. Vaginal sonosalpingography in the evaluation of tubal patency. Acta Obstet Gynecol Scand 1998; 77:978–982.
21. Strandell A, Bourne T, Bergh C, et al. Sonographic hydrotubation using agitated saline: A new technique for improving fallopian tube visualization. Ultrasound Obstet Gynecol 1999; 14:200–204.
22. Chapron C, Querleu D, Bruhat MA, et al. Surgical complications of diagnostic and operative gynaecological laparoscopy: A series of 29,966 cases. Hum Reprod 1998; 13:867–872.
23. Marret H, Harchaoui Y, Chapron C, et al. Trocar injuries during laparoscopic gynaecological surgery. Report from the French Society of Gynaecological Laparoscopy. Gynaecol Endosc 1998; 7:235–241.
24. Gomel V. Foreword. In: Donnez J, ed. Atlas of Operative Laparoscopy and Hysteroscopy. 3rd ed. London: Informa, 2007.
25. Bettocchi S, Ceci O, Di Venere R, et al. Advanced operative office hysteroscopy without anaesthesia: Analysis of 501 cases treated with a 5 Fr bipolar electrode. Hum Reprod 2002; 17:2435–2438.
26. Henry-Suchet J, Loffredo V, Tesquier L, et al. Endoscopy of the tube (= tuboscopy): Its prognostic value for tuboplasties. Acta Eur Fertil 1985; 16:139–145.
27. Brosens I, Boeckx W, Delattin P, et al. Salpingoscopy: A new preoperative diagnostic tool in tubal infertility. Br J Obstet Gynaecol 1987; 94:768–773.
28. Marana R, Catalano GF, Muzii L, et al. The prognostic role of salpingoscopy in laparoscopic tubal surgery. Hum Reprod 1999; 14:2991–2995.
29. Watrelot A, Nisolle M, Chelli H, et al. International Group for Fertiloscopy Evaluation. Is laparoscopy still the gold standard in infertility assessment? A comparison of fertiloscopy versus laparoscopy in infertility. Results of an international multicentre prospective trial: The 'FLY' (fertiloscopy-laparoscopy) study. Hum Reprod 2003; 18:834–839.
30. Fernandez H, Alby JD, Gervaise A, et al. Operative transvaginal hydrolaparoscopy for treatment of polycystic ovary syndrome: A new minimally invasive surgery. Fertil Steril 2001; 75:607–611.
31. Fernandez H, Watrelot A, Alby JD, et al. Fertility after ovarian drilling by transvaginal fertiloscopy for treatment of polycystic ovary syndrome. J Am Assoc Gynecol Laparosc 2004; 11:374–378.

23

Reproductive surgery

Victor Gomel

Reproductive surgery encompasses much more than simply procedures designed to improve fertility, as understood by some. In fact, in addition to fertility-promoting procedures, such us tubal reconstruction, it includes all surgical procedures performed on the pelvic organs of female children, adolescents, and childbearing-aged women, and not only when performed in those who present with infertility. It must be stressed that "female infertility is frequently caused by misdiagnosis or delayed diagnosis and treatment of acute conditions in young and/or reproductive age women, such as pelvic inflammatory disease, ectopic pregnancy, appendicitis, etc. It is also caused by surgical procedures that are unnecessary, unnecessarily extensive and/or traumatic, resulting in damage to or loss of normal reproductive organs and development of post-operative adhesions" (1). These observations clearly demonstrate the need to stress the importance of reproductive surgery and to avail surgeons and especially gynecologists with training opportunities in this field.

Most of the reconstructive gynecologic procedures have been discussed in other chapters of this book and will not be reiterated here. This chapter will primarily review procedures designed to treat tubal factor infertility.

DEVELOPMENTS AND TRENDS

Until the mid-1980s, reconstructive surgery was the only therapeutic option for infertility caused by tubal and peritoneal factors. Traditional techniques yielded poor outcomes, often as a result of extensive postoperative adhesions. In my textbook *Microsurgery in Female Infertility*, I wrote "I have vivid recollections of the frustration and disappointment I felt, when assisting as a resident at second-look laparotomies for removal of prosthetic devices such as Mulligan hoods, at finding extensive adhesions in the peritoneal cavity; with bowel, omentum, and the internal genitalia adherent to one another. Extensive adhesiolysis and separation of these structures were often necessary in order to visualize the oviducts and remove the prosthetic devices left in situ during the prior reconstructive operation." Many important developments followed. Gynecologic microsurgery was introduced in the early 1970s (2–4); simultaneously, laparoscopic access was being explored for tubal reconstruction (5,6), especially in distal tubal disease. Initially used by laparotomy, microsurgical tenets were also being applied by laparoscopic access (7,8). The use of magnification and especially microsurgical principles yielded significantly improved outcomes, especially in tubal anastomosis (9). Laparoscopic access provided the advantages that are now well recognized: less postoperative discomfort and analgesic requirement, shorter hospital stay and period of convalescence, frequently reduced costs, and cosmetically preferable (10). Many of these laparoscopic interventions became ambulatory procedures. It also did not take long to realize that this mode of surgical access yielded results that were not dissimilar to those obtained via laparotomy, provided of course the technique used was the same (11). Experience with laparoscopy permitted modification of open interventions for more complex cases, such as tubocornual anastomosis, where a small minilaparotomy incision replaced a formal laparotomy, permitting such procedures also to be performed on ambulatory basis (12).

The assimilation of these techniques and microsurgical principles into our specialty made the gynecologist much more conscious of avoiding peritoneal trauma and more careful in tissue handling and tissue care. It made the gynecologist more conscious of conservation and overall a better surgeon (11), skills that may well be lost with lack of teaching of reconstructive microsurgery.

The scene for reconstructive tubal surgery started to change once success rates of in vitro fertilization (IVF) reached more credible levels, as it offered an alternative treatment modality, especially in those in whom surgery offered a poor prognosis. The first survey of outcomes carried out by Seppälä (13) was an international survey; it included 10,028 cycles that resulted in 523 births (5.2%). The U.S. results for the years 1985 and 1986, as reported by the National Registry of IVF and ET, were as follows: the total number of cycles for these two years were only 3921 and 4867, respectively, resulting in total annual births of 257 (6.6% of births per initiated cycle) and 311 (6.4%) (14). It is of interest to note the high prevalence of spontaneous abortions (more than one-third of clinical pregnancies) in both reports: 324 in Seppälä's survey, and 140 and 151 in the United States for the respective years of 1985 and 1986.

The 1990s witnessed improvements in IVF outcomes that were truly significant. In the United States, these rates progressed from 12.3% of births per initiated cycle, in 1990 (15), to 25.4% in 1999 (16). This rate seems to have reached a plateau around 28% since 2002 (17,18). The 1990s also witnessed the introduction and acceptance of intracytoplasmic sperm injection (ICSI) (19), which proved to be a panacea in the treatment of male infertility.

The significant improvement in the outcomes of assisted reproduction techniques (ART) was largely due to the simplification of techniques, both clinical and laboratory; progress made in cryopreservation; and the replacement of multiple embryos. Another important factor was the industrialization of these services, which proved lucrative. The number of IVF programs in the United States increased from 267 in 1994 to 461 in 2004, and the number of cycles performed quadrupled during the intervening 20 years from about 32,000 to 128,000, which represents a 1.25 billion dollar business. During the same period, there has been a significant decline in the use and teaching of reconstructive infertility surgery. IVF started increasingly to be offered, as primary treatment option, in most cases of tubal factor infertility. These changes have occurred despite the acceptance of laparoscopic access to perform many of the reconstructive tubal operations and the use of minilaparotomy incision for more complex anastomotic procedures, both of which have become day care procedures (20). Concerned with this trend, as early as 1992, we emphasized that both therapeutic options had a place that treatment should be individualized based on the clinical findings and circumstances of the couple and that these two options were not competitive but rather complementary (21). We are of the same opinion today.

IVF VERSUS RECONSTRUCTIVE TUBAL SURGERY

Assisted reproduction has dramatically changed the treatment of infertility for the good. As discussed in an earlier chapter, it has permitted to streamline the investigation of the couple presenting with infertility. It has offered couples the opportunity to attempt conception with a new therapeutic modality, and by the development of ICSI with an effective way to overcome most types of male infertility. Indeed, the outcomes for IVF with ICSI are similar, in couples with and without male infertility, within the same age groups (17). Furthermore, IVF has permitted the development of preimplantation genetic diagnosis.

This discussion must also include other important aspects of ART. Based on the current U.S. outcomes of a birth rate of 28% per initiated cycle, the cumulative probability of live birth after three cycles of treatment would be around 52%. However, several studies have shown conclusively that a large percentage of couples do not wish to complete three cycles of IVF, even when these are subsidized (22,23). There are others who refuse to have IVF for religious or ethical reasons, and many would find the cost of IVF prohibitive, since the procedure is not covered in many states or countries while other treatment modalities are, as is the case in British Columbia in Canada.

A recent study has demonstrated this in two groups of infertile women: one with tubal factor and the other with endometriosis. The cumulative birthrate after fresh and frozen embryo transfer cycles was 43.7% for those with tubal infertility, and 55.8% and 40.3%, respectively, for those with stages I and II, and III and IV endometriosis (24).

ART is associated with a tremendous increase in preterm births and its important sequelae of perinatal mortality and morbidity, including cerebral palsy (25). The rates of preterm births for singletons, singletons from multiple fetuses, twins, triplets, and greater order of multiples are 12.5%, 18.3%, 63.3%, and 95.3%, respectively. The perinatal mortality was 1.9% in the IVF group, almost double that of the controls (25). In the United States, in 2006, of the 34,719 pregnancies resulting from ART, 28% were twins and 3.8% were triplets and greater order of multiples; of the resulting 28,404 births, 28.8% were twins, and the rate of the triplets and greater order of multiples decreased to 1.9% either by fetal reduction and/or spontaneously (18). The large proportion of multiple births with the associated increased obstetrical complications, and neonatal complications and deaths, causes great societal costs and significant financial burden and emotional costs for parents. This is the reason for which single embryo transfer is being actively investigated, especially in younger women (26). The number of embryos to be transferred has even been legislated in certain jurisdictions.

For the infertile woman with tubal damage, there are only two realistic options to achieve a pregnancy: reconstructive surgery or IVF. The presence of a credible alternative, in IVF, permits the reproductive surgeon to operate on cases with a better prognosis, which was not the case before the end of the 1980s (8). We have known for a long time that one of the important factors influencing surgical outcome was the degree of tubal damage, which led to the development of various classifications (8,27–31). Operating on patients with better prognosis will translate in superior outcomes as has been well demonstrated.

There are those who consider reproductive surgery obsolete (32). This lacks thoughtfulness and eliminates a credible alternative for patients with tubal infertility, recognizing the limitations and other factors regarding IVF discussed earlier. The choice of the primary treatment and any subsequent treatment should be dependent on a careful consideration of both nontechnical and technical factors. These must be individualized for each patient (21).

Nontechnical considerations include age, cost, and wishes of the couple. The age of the female partner is a very important factor in the outcome, irrespective of the treatment selected. For those in late reproductive age, it is prudent to attempt IVF since the result is immediate. Health insurance coverage and the cost of the procedure, depending on the jurisdiction, and the resources of the couple play important roles in the decision-making process. Another, often underestimated, potential factor is the economic impact of a multiple pregnancy, which occurs much more frequently with IVF.

Technical considerations result from proper investigation of the couple. For example, ICSI within the IVF setting is the only option in the presence of severe male factor infertility. IVF clearly represents the only therapeutic option for those with inoperable fallopian tubes due to severe tubal damage and tubal disease coincident with another important infertility factor. For others whose sole cause of infertility is tubal factor that is operable, surgery, if successful, will offer multiple cycles to achieve conception and the opportunity to have more than one pregnancy (1).

The choice of the primary and any subsequent treatments depends on careful consideration of both nontechnical and technical factors. These must be individualized to the circumstances of each couple. Information about success and complication rates of the available treatment options must accurately reflect local experience. Active involvement of the couple in the decision-making process is more likely to result in resolution of the conflict of infertility should treatment proves unsuccessful (21).

FERTILITY-PROMOTING PROCEDURES

The goal of fertility-promoting surgery is to restore the anatomic and functional integrity of the reproductive organs. Restoration of the anatomic integrity does not equate with the restoration of functional integrity, since the latter is dependent on of the extent to which it was damaged prior to surgery. This is why proper selection of cases is an important factor in the outcome. As mentioned earlier, because of ART, the reproductive surgeon today has the luxury of operating on cases with a more favorable prognosis and, thus, improves the success rate of a given procedure.

Fertility-promoting procedures require the use of a special delicate technique frequently referred to as "microsurgical technique." Some equate microsurgery with surgery under magnification. In fact, magnification is only a single facet of the technique that embraces a broad concept of tissue care, designed to minimize tissue trauma. In the abdominal cavity, the peritoneal surfaces are kept moistened with a physiologic solution to avoid drying. The introduction of foreign substances is avoided; hemostasis is achieved with fine instruments and appropriate level of energy to minimize adjacent tissue damage; abnormal tissues are excised completely; and tissues such as segments of oviduct, requiring approximation, are aligned precisely and tissue planes apposed with fine and least reactive suture materials. Magnification, used when necessary, permits better appreciation of normal and pathologic morphologic details and facilitates the application of the preceding principles; it also enables the use of microsurgical instruments and very fine sutures. It is useful to conclude the procedure with a thorough "pelvic lavage" to remove from the peritoneal cavity any blood clots, foreign bodies, or debris that may be present (4,33). These principles can be applied irrespective of the access route: laparotomy, minilaparotomy, laparoscopy, etc.

With all of these procedures, it is useful to have pertinent information of the case and the hysterosalpingography images in view in the operating theatre. In most cases, it is important to place a pediatric Foley catheter or an appropriate cannula into the uterine cavity to permit intraoperative chromopertubation. Preoperative prophylactic antibiotics are used as necessary.

RECONSTRUCTIVE SURGERY FOR DISTAL TUBAL DISEASE

These procedures are salpingo-ovariolysis, fimbrioplasty, and salpingostomy. These are some of the first procedures performed by laparoscopic access at the start of operative laparoscopy; they were performed with monocular view, and with essentially blind assistance (5–7,10). They are indeed all very amenable to be performed by this access, which has been our approach from the beginning. They should be undertaken as part of any diagnostic laparoscopy performed as part of an infertility investigation.

Salpingo-ovariolysis

Pelvic and periadnexal adhesions, in reproductive-age women, frequently are the sequelae of PID. These adhesions may be broad or shallow; they are usually not too vascular and extend from one structure to another, from tube to ovary, uterus to adnexa, pelvic side wall to adnexa, etc. In doing so, they tend to leave a space or potential space between the involved structures, a characteristic that facilitates adhesiolysis (Fig. 1A and B). Dense cohesive adhesions, where adjacent structures are intimately conglutinated, often result from prior surgery. The adherent area is devoid of the superficial, mesothelial layer of peritoneum. In other words, the underlying stromal layers of the two structures coalesce. The lysis of such an adhesive process is technically difficult and is associated with a very high percentage of recurrence, unless the two denuded surfaces are separated with an antiadhesive barrier.

Periadnexal adhesions may be the sole abnormality causing infertility; they encapsulate an otherwise patent tube and/or the ovary and prevent the oocyte to be captured by the fimbriae. Periovarian adhesions may also affect follicular development, as has been demonstrated in both animal and human studies. In rare cases, adhesions can fix the fimbriated end of the patent tube at a distance from the ovary, distorting the spatial and hence the functional relationship that exists between these two organs, and prevent ovum pickup. In most such cases, salpingo-ovariolysis will restore fertility. Periadnexal adhesions often coexist with various types of tubal occlusion, and, by necessity, the procedure becomes an integral part of other reconstructive procedures.

Technique

The pelvic organs are thoroughly inspected and the location, extent, and nature of adhesions assessed. We use mechanical division of adhesions with sharp scissors and obtain hemostasis, as necessary, by desiccation of the individual bleeders, preferably using a microbipolar electrode. Dissection should commence in a well-exposed area (Fig. 2A).

Safety requires clear identification and exposure of each adhesive layer and its attachments and recognition of what lies behind before starting the dissection. Each layer of adhesion is grasped and retracted, and divided along the organ of interest (Fig. 2B). On the tubal extremity of the adhesion, division is effected 1 mm from the surface to preclude denudation of the serosa. It is important to note that these adhesions are frequently composed of two layers, even when they appear to be single, and affix at different sites of the particular organ. Identification and transection of each of the separate layers avoids damaging the surface of the organ to which they are attached, which is a frequent occurrence if the two layers are transected together.

The usual sequence of steps is as follows: the adhesion is grasped with a suitable forceps, gentle traction exposes one of its attachments, and a small incision is made over a clear area to determine what lies behind the adhesion and whether it is composed of a single or two layers. The adhesion is divided parallel to the target organ, remaining at a 1-mm distance and pausing to secure any obvious blood vessels prior to division. Broad adhesions are dissected free from all their attachments

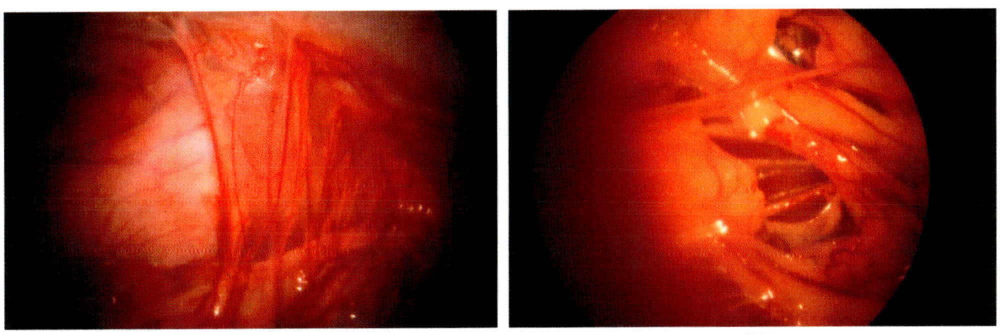

(A) (B)

Figure 1 Pelvic adhesions. (A) Vascular adhesions. (B) Omental adhesions.

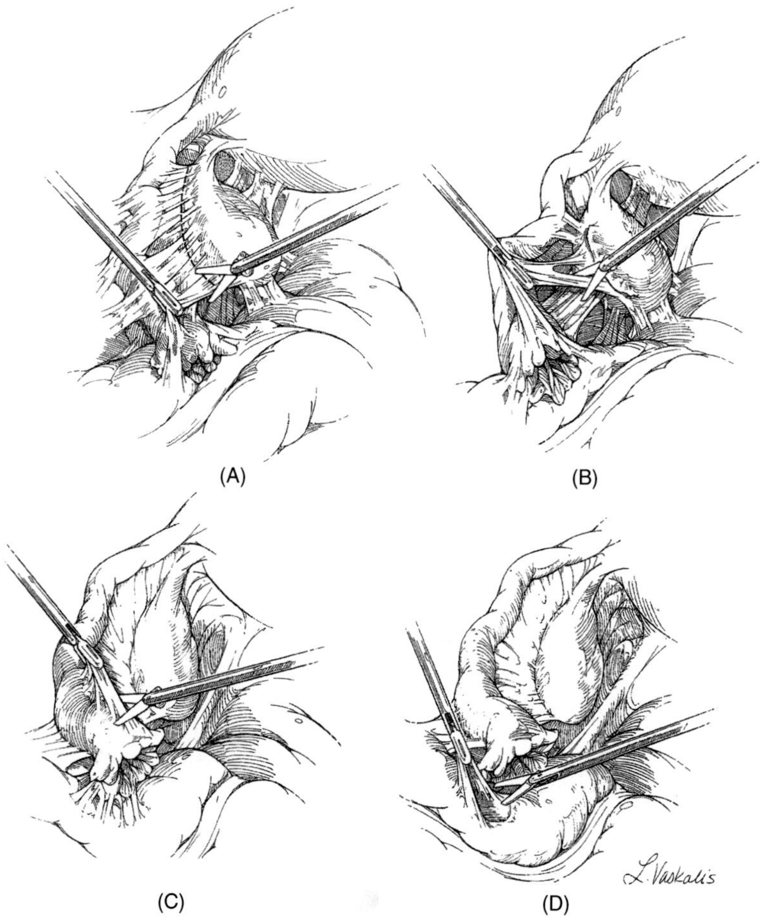

Figure 2 Salpingo-ovariolysis. **(A)** Dissection commences in a well-exposed area. **(B)** Each layer of adhesion is grasped and retracted and divided along the organ of interest. **(C)** Broad adhesions are dissected free from all their attachments and removed from the peritoneal cavity. **(D)** The procedure is being completed. *Source*: From Ref. 34.

and removed from the peritoneal cavity (Fig. 2C and 2D). Shallow adhesions are simply divided. The procedure is concluded with a pelvic lavage.

Cohesive adhesions between two structures requires the identification of the dissection plane, by making a small incision and developing a tissue plane either by spreading the jaws of the scissors, by blunt dissection, or by hydrodissection. Thermal energy should not be used in such cases (34).

Occasionally salpingo-ovariolysis reveals unexpected findings, even malignancy, as shown in Figures 3A to 3C. Thin periovarian adhesions enveloped the ovary; when these were lysed, an exophytic tumor was exposed, which proved to be a borderline carcinoma of the ovary.

Results

In the early stages of development of operative laparoscopy, we demonstrated that, for salpingo-ovariolysis, laparoscopic access yields results that are similar to those obtained by open access. We also stressed the importance of adhering to microsurgical principles in the performance of such procedures by laparoscopic access. We reported later a series of 92 patients who underwent salpingo-ovariolysis by laparoscopy. The duration of involuntary infertility was longer than 20 months for all. Periadnexal adhesions were severe in 79 and moderate in 13; furthermore, the series included only those patients in whom ovum pickup by the tube on the side with lesser disease was deemed impossible or greatly hampered. At the time of the survey, the patients had been monitored postoperatively for a period of nine months or longer. Of the 92 patients, 57 (62%) achieved at least one intrauterine pregnancy, 54 (59%) had one or more live births, and 5 (5.4%) had ectopic pregnancies. After the publication of this study, among the patients who could not be contacted and reported as failures, we became aware of four additional women who had live births (35).

Similar results were corroborated by other centers in Europe and North America; the reported intrauterine pregnancy rates range from 51% to 62%, and ectopic pregnancy rates range from 5% to 7.5% of operated cases (36–39). The outcome is certainly affected by the extent and type of adhesions. The rate of ectopic pregnancy clearly demonstrates that periadnexal disease is not an entity confined to periadnexal structures alone and that the infection would have caused concomitant damage to the tubal endothelium, despite its normal appearance and evident patency.

Fimbrioplasty

Fimbrioplasty refers to the reconstruction of existing fimbria of a partially or totally occluded fallopian tube (fimbrial phimosis). The agglutinated fimbriae often leave a small opening at the distal end of the tube; chromopertubation will distend the ampulla before the escape of dye solution from the tube. The agglutinated fimbrial end may also be covered by an adhesion, which may cause complete occlusion of the terminal end of the tube. Less frequently, the tube is stenosed at the level of the abdominal tubal ostium, located at the apex of the infundibular portion; this is termed prefimbrial phimosis. In

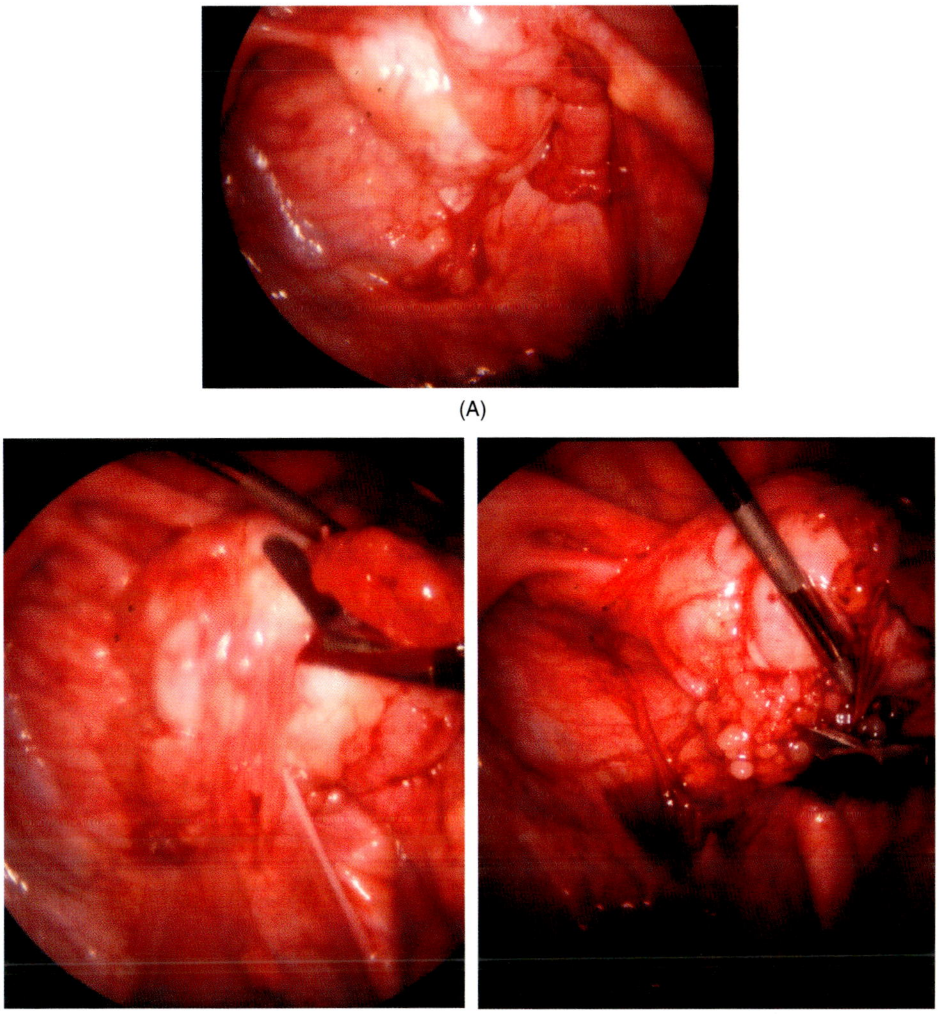

Figure 3 Salpingo-ovariolysis. **(A)** Filmy adhesions extending from the fallopian tube have enveloped the ovary. **(B)** Division of adhesions begins along the tube. **(C)** Adhesiolysis reveals an exophytic tumor of the ovary.

such cases, the fimbriae may have a normal appearance. Frequently, periadnexal adhesions will be present. The condition represents the sequel of a more advanced inflammatory process. In our series of salpingo-ovariolysis discussed earlier, 12 of the 92 subjects had unilateral fimbrial phimosis in their adnexa with greater pathology (35).

Technique

In the presence of periadnexal adhesions, it will be necessary first to perform a salpingo-ovariolysis. This will permit better assessment of the tube and ovary. Chromopertubation at this point will distend the tube and permit better assessment of the distal end. A small opening is usually present at the distal end of the tube unless this opening is covered by fibrous tissue, in which case it will be necessary to incise or excise it using small sharp scissors, to expose the agglutinated fimbriae. The tube is stabilized with an atraumatic grasping forceps for this purpose. Once the agglutinated fimbriated end is exposed, a 2 to 3 mm grasping or alligator-jawed forceps, with jaws closed, is introduced through the phimotic fimbrial opening, while the tube is distended by chromopertubation (Fig. 4A). Once within the tube, the jaws of the forceps are opened, and the forceps are gently withdrawn keeping the jaws open to break down some of the adhesive process (Fig. 4B). It will be necessary to repeat these steps several times, altering the axis of in which the jaws are opened, until satisfactory disagglutination is obtained (Fig. 4C). When sufficient gentleness is used during this manipulation, bleeding is usually negligible.

In prefimbrial phimosis, the fimbriae may have a normal appearance. However, when chromopertubation is performed, the ampullary portion of the tube distends before any exit of dye solution. Correction requires placement of an incision on the antimesosalpingeal border of the tube, which commences at the infundibulum and continues past the stenotic area into the distal ampulla, to relieve the stenosis. The tube is stabilized with an atraumatic grasping forceps and held against the uterine fundus. A thin Teflon probe is inserted through the stenotic ostium, into the distal ampulla. An incision is placed along the antimesosalpingeal border of the tube, electrosurgically using a needle electrode. This incision is started at the fimbriated and continued into the ampulla past the divided stenotic abdominal tubal ostium (Fig. 5A and 5B). Alternatively, the area can be injected with 1 mL of dilute vasopressin solution (1 IU in

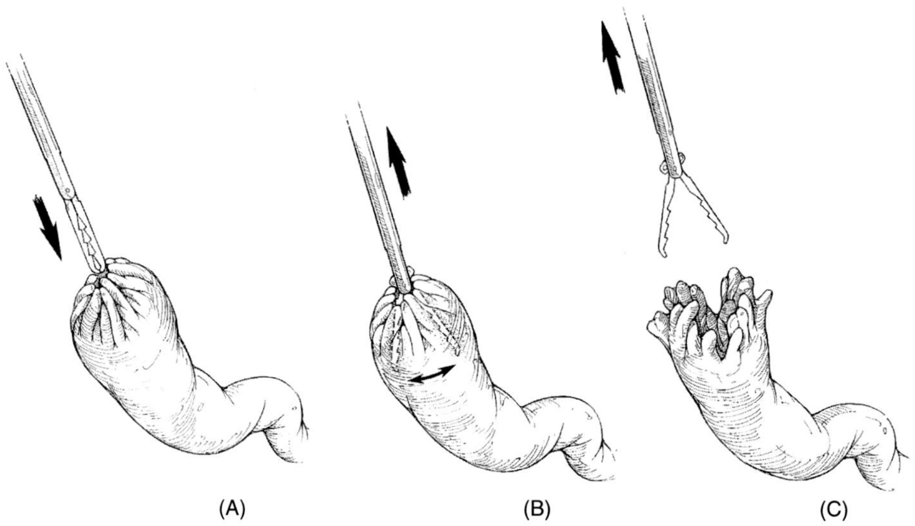

Figure 4 Fimbrioplasty: disagglutination of fimbriae. **(A)** A 2- to 3-mm alligator-jawed forceps, with jaws closed, is introduced through the phimotic fimbrial opening. **(B and C)** The jaws of the forceps are opened within the tube, and the forceps are gently withdrawn, keeping the jaws open, to break down some of the adhesive process. It will be necessary to repeat these steps several times, altering the axis. *Source*: From Ref. 34.

20 mL of normal saline) and the incision made mechanically with microsurgical scissors. Any bleeding points are desiccated electrosurgically with the needle electrode. To maintain tubal patency, it may be necessary to place interrupted sutures, of 7-0 or 6-0 size, at the apices of each of the flaps created by the incision; this is our preferred approach (Fig. 5C). Alternatively the serosal aspect of the flaps can be lightly desiccated, causing them fold backward.

Results

Very few investigators have classified fimbrioplasty as an independent procedure. Most include such patients in their salpingostomy series. French and Belgian centers include fimbrioplasty (correction of partial distal tubal occlusion) as stage 1 in their salpingostomy series. We reported a study on 40 such patients, all treated by laparoscopic access. Live births occurred in 19 patients (48%), and 2 patients (5%) had tubal gestations (33).

Patton, in a series of 40 patients submitted to open fimbrioplasty procedures, reported total intrauterine and ectopic pregnancy rates of 63% (25 patients) and 5% (2 patients), respectively, after 24 months' follow-up. The outcome of the intrauterine pregnancies and the live birthrates were not provided (40). Donnez and Casanas-Roux, in an open series of 100 patients, reported a total pregnancy rate of 61%. The location and outcome of these pregnancies were not provided (41). Canis et al. included 32 such patients with their salpingostomy series of patients performed by laparoscopy; 16 (50%) of these achieved intrauterine pregnancies, but the outcome was not reported. Surprisingly, there were no tubal pregnancies (42).

While these studies suffer from having been uncontrolled, laparoscopic and open fimbrioplasty procedures

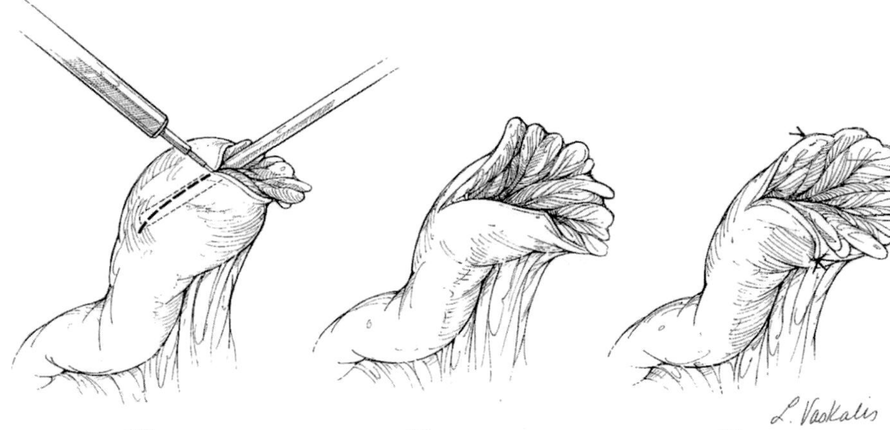

Figure 5 Fimbrioplasty: correction of prefimbrial phimosis. **(A and B)** An incision is placed along the antimesosalpingeal border of the tube and extended into the ampulla, past the divided stenotic abdominal tubal ostium. **(C)** Completed procedure with flaps everted. *Source*: From Ref. 34.

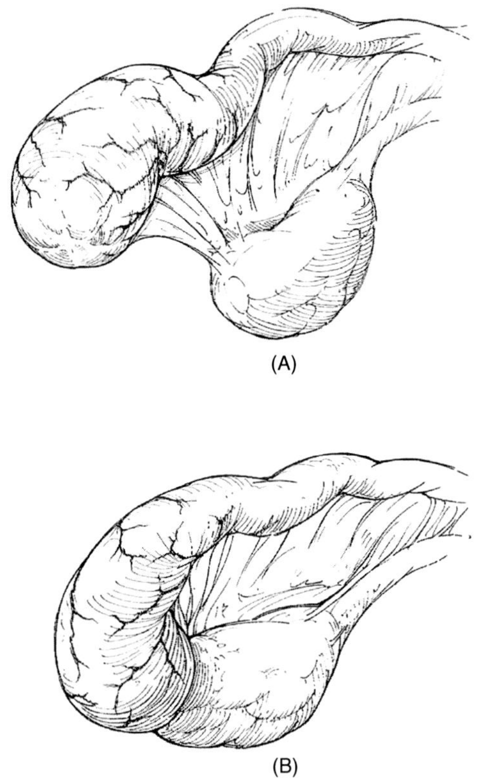

Figure 6 Hydrosalpinx. (A) The occluded distal tube is free. (B) The occluded distal tube is adherent to the ovary. *Source*: From Ref. 34.

appear to yield comparable outcomes. Undoubtedly, laparoscopic access and the opportunity to perform these procedures as part of a diagnostic laparoscopy provide the patient with considerable advantages.

Salpingostomy

Salpingostomy, or salpingoneostomy, is the creation of a new stoma in a fallopian tube that has a completely occluded distal end, commonly called hydrosalpinx. This represents the sequel of an even more advanced inflammatory process. Periadnexal and pelvic adhesions are frequently part of the picture. Depending on the anatomic location at which the new stoma is fashioned, salpingostomy may be terminal, ampullary, or isthmic. Isthmic and ampullary salpingostomy are of historic interest, except for the reversal of prior fimbriectomy (Kroener's sterilization), where ampullary salpingostomy may have a place, if more than one-half of the ampulla is conserved.

Technique

It is necessary to first complete the salpingo-ovariolysis. It is then important to closely examine the distal end of the tube, to ensure that it is not adherent to the ovary or any other structures. If the distal tube is adherent, it must be dissected free until the tubo-ovarian ligament is exposed (Fig. 6A and 6B). Only by freeing the tube can the surgeon be certain that the neostomy is being performed at the appropriate site. At this point, the tube is distended by transcervical chromopertubation. The occluded terminal end of the tube is examined under magnification; this permits recognition of the relatively avascular zones that radiate from a central punctum in a cartwheel manner. The tube is entered at this central point with use of fine scissors (Fig. 7A and 7B), and the incision is extended toward the ovary over an avascular line. This incision fashions a new fimbria ovarica that maintains the tubo-ovarian relation. At this point in the procedure, the tube is visualized from within to place additional incisions along its circumference, to complete the creation of a new stoma (Fig. 7C). These additional incisions are made between endothelial folds, over avascular areas. In doing so, one avoids cutting through vascular mucosal folds, which will be shaped as fimbriae, and bleeding is minimized as a result (Fig. 7D). Any bleeders that occur are

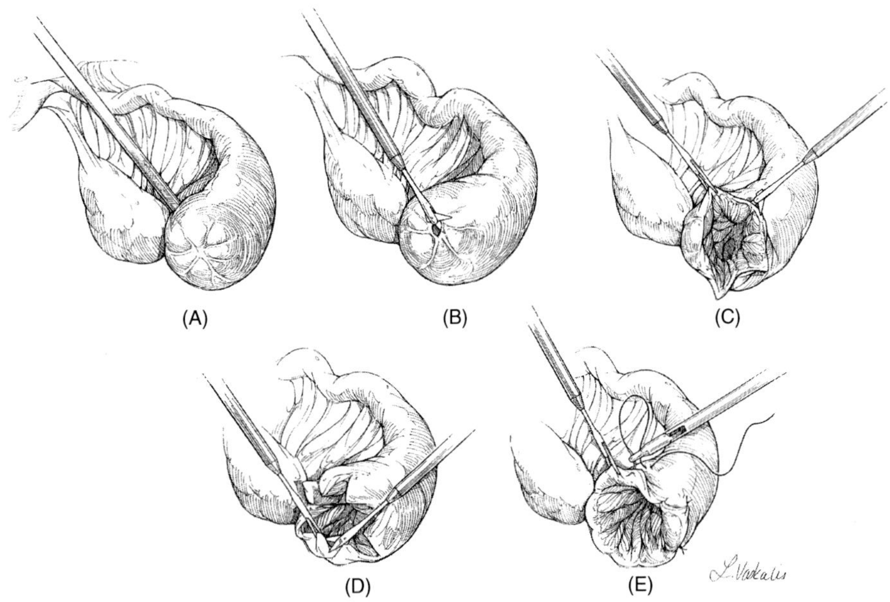

Figure 7 Salpingostomy. (A) The occluded terminal end of the tube exhibits relatively avascular zones that radiate from a central punctum in a cartwheel manner. (B) The tube is entered at this central point with use of fine scissors, and the incision is extended toward the ovary over an avascular line. (C) Viewing the tube from within, additional incisions are placed. (D) This is continued along the circumference of the tube until a satisfactory stoma is fashioned. (E) The main flaps, created in the process, are everted using 7-0 sutures. *Source*: From Ref. 34.

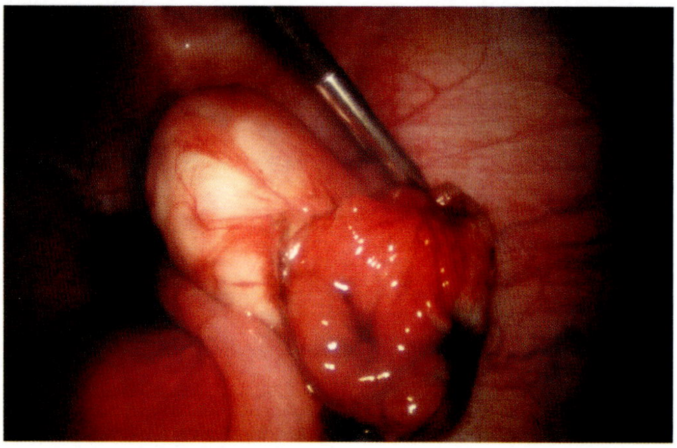

Figure 8 Salpingostomy by laparoscopy. Completed salpingostomy.

exposed under a jet of irrigation fluid and desiccated individually with a needle electrode or microbipolar forceps. Once a satisfactory stoma is achieved, the flaps created in the process are everted, by securing them without tension to the ampullary seromuscularis with interrupted 7-0- or 8-0-size Vicryl sutures (Figs. 7E and 8) (6,8,10,34,43,44). Desiccation of the serosal surface of the flaps will also cause them to fold backward.

If the surgeon wishes to carry out a salpingoscopy to assess the ampullary mucosa, the most appropriate time to do this is after the initial opening into the tube is made; the opening is slightly enlarged to permit introduction of a small-caliber scope, which is passed down through one of the ancillary portals (see chap. 22).

The technique of salpingostomy is identical irrespective of the access route. However, there is scant indication today to submit the patient to an open procedure.

Results

As indicated earlier, it has become evident that the major determinants of the outcome of salpingostomy are the degree of preexisting tubal damage and the extent and nature of periadnexal adhesions. It is essentially these two factors that explain the difference in outcomes reported from well-trained and equipped centers. The reported live birthrates from microsurgical series performed by laparotomy (3,8,29,41,43,45–50) or by minilaparotomy (30) range from 17% to 37%. Most of these series predate the early 1990s. Thereafter, the number of salpingostomies performed decreased in step with improvements in the outcomes of IVF, and those performed were largely done by laparoscopic access. The major laparoscopic series report similar results (7,39,42,51–54). Unfortunately, not all series, both open and laparoscopic, reported live birth rates.

We were the first to describe laparoscopic salpingostomy, in a small series of nine patients, published in 1997. Eight of these women had previously undergone a failed salpingostomy by laparotomy, elsewhere. Four women conceived and later delivered live infants. The one patient in whom the laparoscopic approach was the primary surgery was among the successes (7).

We have also reported a series of 90 patients who underwent microsurgical salpingostomy using a minilaparotomy incision (30). Nineteen (21.1%) were lost to follow-up and were considered failures. Twenty-seven (30%) patients achieved one or more intrauterine pregnancies, and eight (8.9%) had tubal pregnancies. Ectopic gestations occurred in two patients who also had intrauterine pregnancies. Twenty-three (25.6%) women were successful in having one or more live births. These 90 patients were assessed using the American Fertility Society (AFS) classification. On the basis of this classification, 73 patients had extensive (severe) damage, and 17 had limited (mild) damage. In the group of 73 patients, 15 (20.5%) had one or more intrauterine pregnancies and 13 (17.8%) had one or more live births. In the "mild" group of 17 patients, 12 (70.6%) had one or more intrauterine pregnancies and 10 (58.8%) had one or more live births. We have learned much about the factors that adversely affect the outcome of salpingostomy, and many classifications have been proposed. Having a credible alternative treatment with IVF, we now have the opportunity to select cases with a good prognosis, and the luxury to perform the procedure by laparoscopy as part of a diagnostic laparoscopy and obtain better results. This emphasizes the need for proper investigation of the couple and individualization of treatment.

Since the early 1990s, some researchers considered salpingostomy an obsolete procedure (55) and others argued against this opinion. The preceding observations and previous discussion about IVF versus surgery make it evident that salpingostomy is not obsolete, provided it is performed in appropriate cases.

We have been made aware of the deleterious effect of hydrosalpinx on the outcome of IVF treatment (56–58). This deleterious effect is more evident with large hydrosalpinges, visible at sonography. It has been demonstrated that in such cases, salpingectomy before IVF clearly improves the outcome of this treatment (59,60). It has also become evident that the detrimental effect is due to a "wash-out effect" owing to the passage of the collected tubal fluid to the uterine cavity at the time, or soon after the transfer of the embryos to the uterine cavity. This wash-out effect may also occur some time after transfer; as evidence suggests, many embryos ascend to the tube after transfer and eventually return to the uterus when the tube assumes a prouterine transport. It is at this time that the fluid contained in the hydrosalpinx, by passing to the uterus, may wash the embryos out. There were other hypotheses such as toxic factors adversely affecting the embryo or endometrial receptivity; these have largely been disproved (61).

The assumption that the deleterious effect of large hydrosalpinges may be owing to a washout of the transferred embryos is supported by a study of Van Voorhis et al. (62). They compared women with hydrosalpinges ($n = 34$) with women who had tubal disease but no hydrosalpinges ($n = 124$), undergoing IVF treatment. Women with hydrosalpinges were found to have a reduced clinical pregnancy rate (18% vs. 37%, $p = 0.053$), a reduced ongoing pregnancy rate (15% vs. 34%, $p = 0.051$), and reduced implantation rate (7% vs. 18%, $p = 0.003$) after IVF procedures. Among women who had hydrosalpinges, 16 had their hydrosalpinges aspirated at the time of oocyte retrieval and 18 did not. Aspiration of hydrosalpinges was associated with a higher clinical pregnancy rate (31% vs. 5%, $p = 0.07$), a higher ongoing pregnancy rate (31% vs. 0%, $p = 0.015$), and a higher implantation rate (14 vs. 1%, $p = 0.015$) (60). Others have suggested that aspiration of hydrosalpinx fluid, prior to oocyte retrieval or embryo transfer, is of little value.

A study from our department demonstrated that performing a salpingostomy in the terminally occluded fallopian tube of women with a unilateral hydrosalpinx and a contralateral patent tube significantly improved embryo implantation (63). Twenty-three such patients, with a duration of infertility of 19 to 146 months (mean 53.6 months), were submitted to laparoscopic salpingostomy. The subsequent intrauterine and ectopic pregnancy rates were 43.5% and 4%, respectively. The average time to conception was 13.4 months (range 0–71 months). Exclusion of a single patient whose surgery–pregnancy interval was 71 months reduces the average time frame of the others to seven months. Both the high intrauterine pregnancy and low ectopic pregnancy rates and the short surgery–pregnancy time frame strongly suggest that these conception occurred through the previously patent (lesser damaged) oviduct. It also suggests that the salpingostomy alleviates the deleterious effect of the unilateral hydrosalpinx on embryo implantation. The beneficial effect of salpingostomy in IVF was demonstrated earlier in a small number of cases (58). Obviously salpingostomy, in addition, offers the woman the potential of achieving a pregnancy naturally. This and other evidence suggest that there may well be a place for laparoscopic salpingostomy, instead of salpingectomy, in selected cases who will undergo IVF.

Salpingostomy for Reversal of Fimbriectomy

This subject is more of historic interest, since this type of sterilization is much less frequently being performed today. We have reported a small series of 14 patients submitted to ampullary salpingostomy for reversal of sterilization. They all met the requirement of having more than one-half of ampulla preserved, at least on one side (Fig. 9). Six of these women had one or more intrauterine pregnancies (42.9%), of whom five had live births (35.7%) and the other had midtrimester abortion. There were no ectopic pregnancies (64). Subsequently performed experiments on rabbits corroborated the necessity of having one-half of more of the ampulla preserved (65,66). This recommendation has been corroborated further in a much more recent study, by Tourgeman et al., reporting on 41 women who had fimbriectomy reversal (67).

TUBAL ANASTOMOSIS

Tubal anastomosis may be undertaken to overcome an occlusion of the fallopian tube located anywhere between the two tubal ostia, from the uterine to the abdominal, occlusion that is caused by a disease process, congenital or iatrogenic, or to excise a nonoccluding tubal lesion. There has been a significant decline in the procedures undertaken for pathologic tubal occlusions. Most occlusions caused by a disease process are located in the intramural and proximal isthmic portions of the tube; a tubal anastomosis at this location (tubocornual anastomosis) is one of the more challenging fertility-promoting procedures. Such patients now are frequently referred for IVF, as discussed earlier in this chapter. Congenital occlusions are rare and are usually due to segmental atresia. The iatrogenic occlusions are by and large prior tubal sterilization cases. Although performed less frequently than before, reversal procedures have as yet not suffered the abandonment other anastomotic tubal procedures have experienced. Yet, microsurgery finds its ultimate application in tubotubal anastomosis. The precision afforded by the microsurgical technique allows total excision of occluded or diseased portions, proper alignment, and excellent apposition of each layer of the proximal and distal tubal segments.

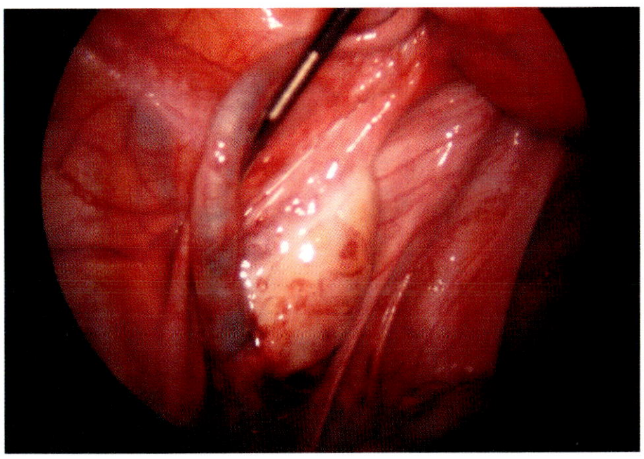

Figure 9 Prior fimbriectomy. More than half of the ampulla has been preserved.

Principles of Microsurgical Tubal Anastomosis

The principles of tubotubal anastomosis are the same, irrespective of the mode of access used: laparoscopy, minilaparotomy, or laparotomy. The procedure is performed under magnification with an operating microscope, a minilaparotomy, or the laparoscope when laparoscopic access is used. After proper inspection and preparation of the site, including salpingo-ovariolysis for periadnexal adhesions, the steps of the procedure are as follows. The tube is appropriately exposed; its proximal segment is distended with transcervical chromopertubation to identify the site of occlusion (Figs. 10A and 11A). The tube is then transected at right angle, with straight sharp scissors or a sharp microblade, adjacent to the site of occlusion. The incision is carried to the mesosalpinx, but not further, to avoid damaging the adjacent vascular arcade (Figs. 10B and 11B). Dye solution will escape from the transected tubal lumen. The cut surface of the tube is examined under magnification, to ensure that it is normal; otherwise the tube is transected again 1 to 2 mm further, until normal tissue is reached. The cut surface of a normal tube is devoid of scarring and exhibits normal muscular and vascular architecture, together with intact mucosal folds. The tube is then transected immediately distal to the diseased segment in a similar manner (Figs. 10C and 11C). Distending the distal segment by introducing of a few milliliters of fluid through the fimbriated helps identify the distal limit of the occluded portion. The diseased portion of tube is excised from the mesosalpinx with scissors or electrosurgically with an insulated microelectrode, keeping the line of incision close to the tube, to avoid damaging the vascular arcade mentioned earlier (Fig. 10D). Hemostasis is obtained by precise electrodesiccation of the more significant bleeders; on the cut surface of the tube, these are located between the serosa and muscularis. Each is exposed by irrigation and desiccated with an insulated microelectrode. If open access is used, a gentle compression of the tube between thumb and forefinger facilitates this process. Desiccation of minor bleeders is unnecessary, since they stop spontaneously. In the process, it is important to avoid damaging the tubal epithelium in order not to adversely affect future tubal function. Major tubal vessels (such as those composing the vascular arcade) may be divided inadvertently or by necessity. These can be desiccated with mono- or bipolar current. It is imperative to avoid overzealous desiccation to prevent devitalization of the anastomosis site. Anastomosis of the tubal segments is performed in two layers, the first of these apposes the muscularis and epithelium and the second the serosa. To properly align the two segments, it is important to place the first musculoepithelial suture at the point the mesosalpinx joins the tube (6-o'clock position); this suture is tied (Figs. 10E, 10F, and 11D and 11E). This and

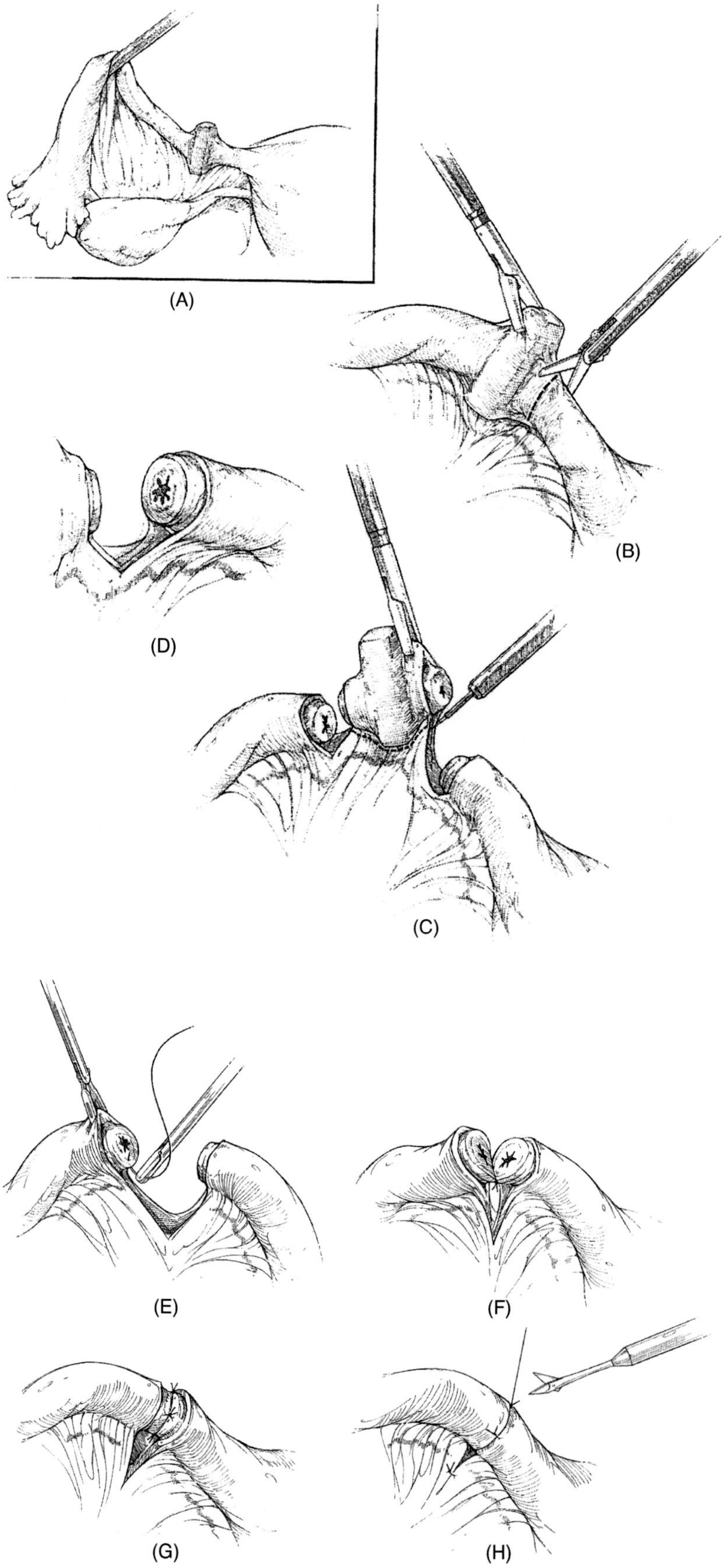

Figure 10 Isthmic–isthmic anastomosis. (**A**) Prior clip sterilization. (**B**) The tube is elevated and transected at right angles, with straight sharp scissors, proximal and distal to the clip. (**C**) The portion of tube enclosed in the clip, including the clip, is excised from the mesosalpinx, electrosurgically using a microelectrode. (**D**) The cut surface of the tube is examined under magnification, to ensure that it is normal, (**E**) The fist suture is placed at 6-o'clock position, in a way that positions the knots peripherally, and (**F**) tied. (**G**) Apposition of the inner musculoepithelial layer is completed with the placement of additional sutures. (**H**) Approximation of the serosa and mesosalpinx completes the anastomosis. *Source*: From Ref. 34.

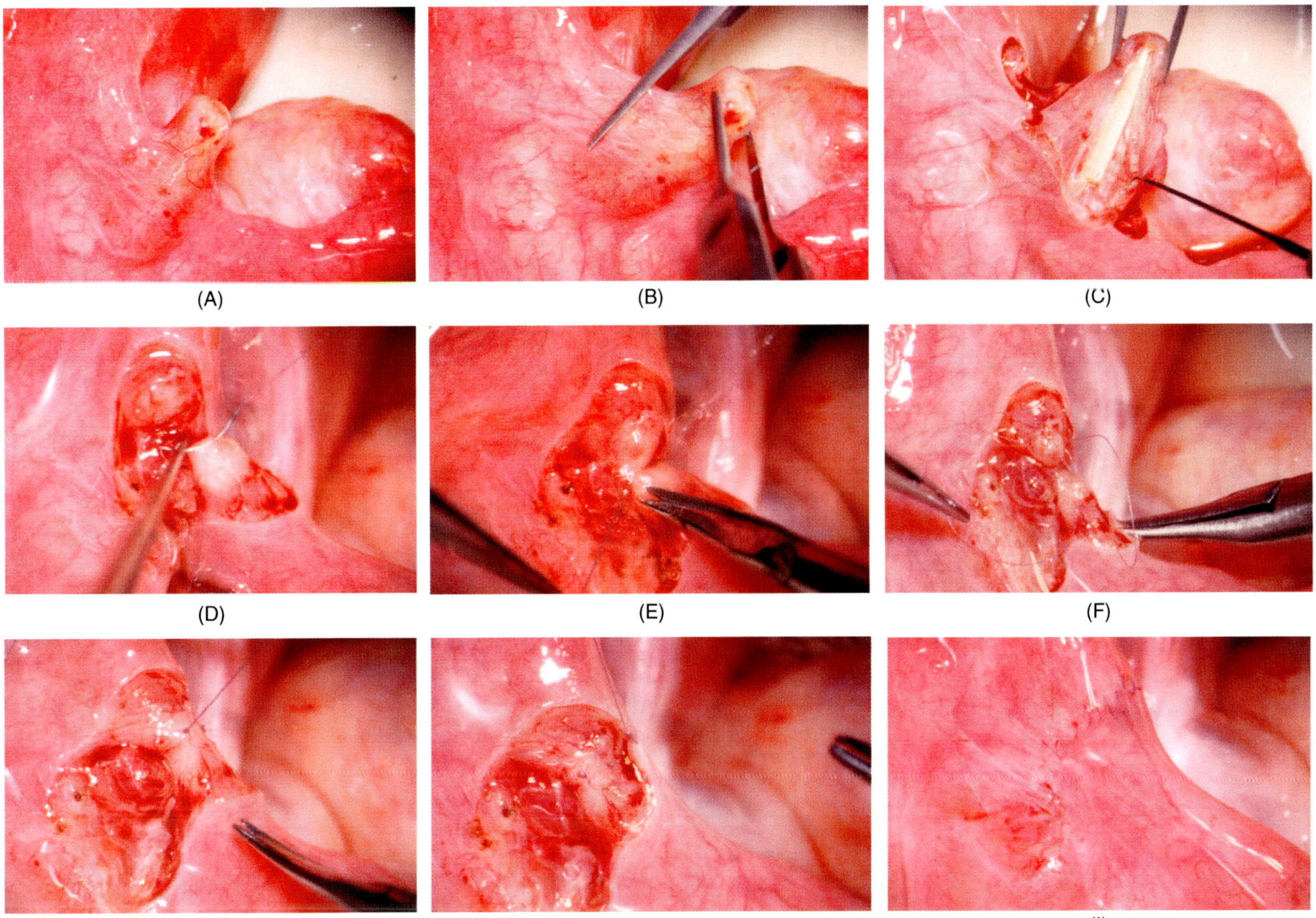

Figure 11 Isthmic–isthmic anastomosis. **(A)** Prior clip sterilization. **(B)** The tube is elevated and transected at right angles, with straight sharp scissors, proximal and distal to the clip. **(C)** The portion of tube enclosed in the clip, including the clip, is excised from the mesosalpinx, electrosurgically using a microelectrode. **(D)** The fist suture is placed at 6-o'clock position, in a way that positions the knots peripherally, and **(E)** tied. **(F)** Subsequent sutures may be placed using a single strand of suture as a continuous series of loops. **(G)** The sutures are still tied individually, after the division of the loop between each successive suture. **(H)** Apposition of the inner musculoepithelial layer is completed; the serosa will be approximated with a continuous 8-0 suture. **(I)** Approximation of the serosa and mesosalpinx completes the anastomosis.

subsequent sutures incorporate the muscularis and the lower part of the epithelium and are placed in a way that positions the knots peripherally. We generally use no. 8-0 Vicryl suture swaged on a 130-micron-shaft, 4- or 5-mm-long, taper-cut needle. Depending on the site of the anastomosis, three or more additional sutures placed equidistantly will be necessary to join this layer. These additional sutures can be placed one at a time and tied; they can also be placed using a single strand of suture as a continuous series of loops, in which case the sutures are still tied individually, after the division of the loop between each successive suture (Fig. 11F). This approach facilitates and speeds up suture placement. We recommend against the use of a luminal splint, as it complicates the procedure and may traumatize the endothelium. After the apposition of the first layer (Figs. 10G and 11G), the serosa is joined next either with interrupted sutures or with two continuous sutures, one that runs anteriorly and the other posteriorly (Fig. 11H); finally, the defect in the mesosalpinx is repaired (Figs. 10H and 11I). In exceptional circumstances when the distance between the two segments is great, the mesosalpinx may be approximated with one or two interrupted no. 6-0 or 7-0 sutures first, to bring the tubal segments into close proximity, in order to facilitate suture placement and reduce the tension while tying the sutures (4,9,10,12,27,34,68,69).

Technical Variations

Minor technical variations are required depending on the type of tubal anastomosis, which can be intramural–isthmic, intramural–ampullary, isthmic–isthmic, isthmic–ampullary, or ampullary–infundibular.

Intramural-Isthmic Anastomosis

This is the type of anastomosis most often performed to treat cornual disease; it is also termed tubocornual anastomosis. When performed for cornual disease, it is one of the most challenging of anastomotic procedures, the details of which will be treated separately.

In cases of reversal of sterilization, even if the site of tubal resection is adjacent to the cornu, the intramural segment is usually intact; there may also be a very short isthmic segment, which is frequently adherent to the side of the uterus as a result of retraction of the adjacent mesosalpinx, thus giving the

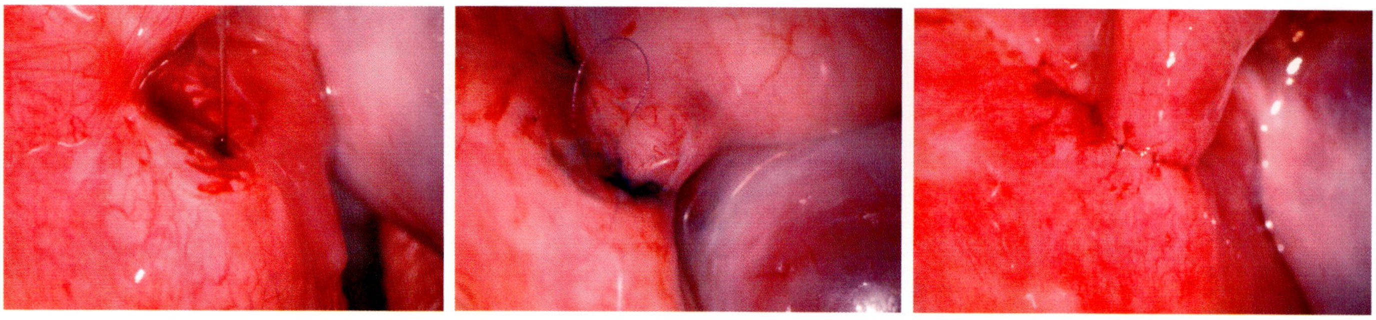

(A) (B) (C)

Figure 12 Intramural–isthmic anastomosis. **(A)** Dye solution streams out of the prepared intramural segment. **(B)** Suturing of the inner layer of the two segments. **(C)** Completed anastomosis.

appearance of total absence of the proximal tube. The presence of a portion of isthmus would have been evident from HSG. Transcervical chromopertubation distends this small segment of isthmus, facilitating identification of its distal margin and its dissection from the uterus. The conservation and appropriate preparation of this segment, even when very small, convert the anastomosis to an isthmic–isthmic type.

In the absence of any isthmus (as may be the case subsequent to either a tubal sterilization or an excision of an isthmic pregnancy), distention of the uterus by chromopertubation will indicate the site of the intramural segment, between the uterine insertion points of the round and ovarian ligaments. Excision of the serosa and underlying scar tissue over the distended area will result in the dye solution to stream out of the intramural segment. In some instances, it will be necessary to excise 1 or 2 mm more of the intramural segment (Fig. 12A). Prior dissection of the tubal muscularis of this segment from the surrounding uterine muscle will facilitate this step. The distal segment is prepared, and a two-layer anastomosis is done as previously described (Fig. 12B). The only variation here is as follows: the serosa and the superficial muscle of the cornual region are approximated to the serosa of the isthmus, and the defect under the tube is repaired by suturing the mesosalpinx to the serosa of the lateral edge of the uterus (Fig. 12C) (9,68–70).

Intramural–Ampullary Anastomosis

This type of anastomosis is now very rarely performed. The salient issue here is the considerable luminal disparity that exists between the intramural and ampullary segments. The technique to overcome this problem will be described under isthmic–ampullary anastomosis, which is frequently performed.

Isthmic–Isthmic Anastomosis

This is the simplest type of anastomosis to perform. The lumina are comparable in size. The technique is the same as that described earlier under basic principles of tubotubal anastomosis.

Isthmic–Ampullary Anastomosis

This type of anastomosis is most frequently performed for sterilization reversal and rarely after excision of midtubal disease. The latter include endometriosis and tubal pregnancy, usually undiagnosed or treated by observation. Tubal stenosis or occlusion may also occur at the site of a tubal pregnancy treated medically with methotrexate or surgically by linear salpingotomy. Treatment of tubal pregnancy by segmental excision will leave the tube in two segments, as with tubal sterilization. Rare causes include tuberculosis in which case reconstruction is contraindicated and segmental agenesis.

In the case of an occlusive lesion as referred above, the proximal and distal segments of tube are prepared as described under basic principles of tubotubal anastomosis. As a result, if the there is no great disparity between the caliber of the lumina, the anastomosis can be realized as described. However, if the disparity is great, it will be necessary to enlarge the isthmic lumen or narrow the ampullary lumen, at the anastomotic site. To enlarge the isthmic lumen, a 2- to 3-mm slit is made, with sharp microscissors, at its antimesosalpingeal border. Excision of a tiny portion of tissue of each of the corners created will result in an enlarged oval opening (Fig. 13A). In this particular situation, to approximate the inner musculoepithelial layer, the 6-o'clock suture is placed first and tied. Five additional sutures are usually required, and these are placed as described earlier. The 12-o'clock suture must incorporate the muscularis and epithelium of the ampulla and the same tissues at the apex of the isthmic slit (Fig. 13B). Approximation of the serosa and closure of the defect in the mesosalpinx complete the anastomosis. The alternative approach is to reduce the size of the large ampullary opening. This is achieved by plicating the muscular layer surrounding the ampullary lumen with interrupted sutures, following which the epithelial fronds that prolapse out of the lumen must be replaced. The anastomosis is performed as described, being very careful about incorporating only the thin ampullary muscularis within the sutures of the inner layer, avoiding the copious epithelial fronds (9,68,69).

As stated earlier, the great majority of this type of anastomosis is performed for sterilization reversal. With the majority of these cases, it is possible to gage the size of the ampullary opening, since the occluded end of the ampullary stump is usually free. The technical details are as follows. The isthmic segment is prepared as described. To better identify the occluded proximal end of the ampullary segment, which may be buried between the leaves of the mesosalpinx, the tube is distended with a few milliliters of fluid introduced through the fimbriated end. If adherent to, or buried within the mesosalpinx, the occluded end is dissected free. The serosa over the tip of the ampullary stump is exposed; this and successive steps may be facilitated by inserting a blunt probe into the tube, through the fimbriated end. The serosa is incised in a

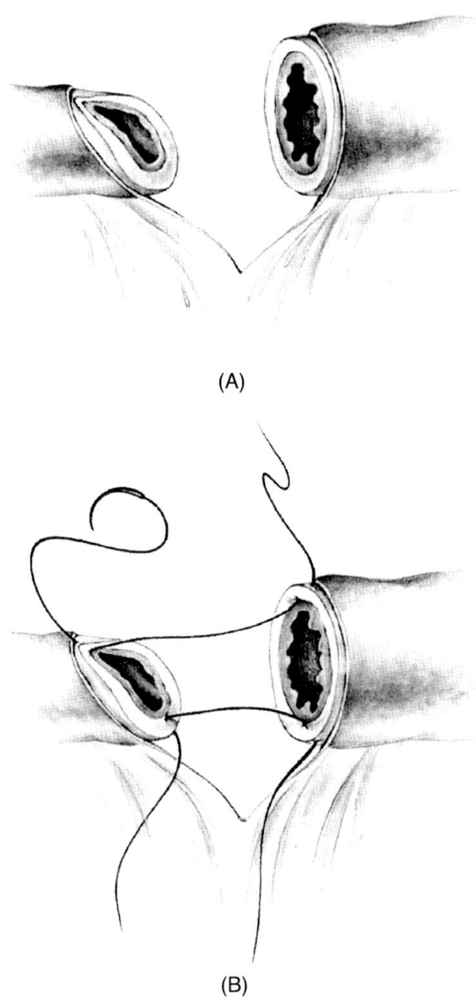

Figure 13 Isthmic-ampullary anastomosis in the presence of significant luminal disparity. (A) Enlargement of the isthmic lumen. (B) Placement of the 6- and 12-o'clock sutures. *Source*: From Ref. 71.

circular manner, using microscissors (Figs. 14A and 15A and 15B). This tiny portion of serosa and any scar tissue under it are then excised to expose the muscularis of the occluded end. The center point of the exposed muscularis is grasped with toothed microforceps, and a small incision is made into the ampullary lumen with the microscissors. This opening is enlarged, to correspond in size to the lumen of the proximal tubal segment, by excising a tiny circular portion of muscularis and epithelium (Figs. 14B and 15C). The resulting opening is slightly larger than the intramural lumen, but because of the absence of significant disparity, a two-layer anastomosis of the two segments can be performed as described earlier (Fig. 15D) (9,68,69).

Ampullary–Ampullary Anastomosis

The majority of ampullary–ampullary anastomoses are performed for sterilization reversal. Occasionally, excision of lesions described under isthmic–ampullary anastomosis may require an ampullary–ampullary anastomosis. The proximal ampullary segment is transected near the occluded end, which is then excised from the mesosalpinx as previously described. An opening that corresponds in size to the lumen of the proximal segment is made in the occluded end of the distal ampullary segment, as described under isthmic–ampullary anastomosis.

In this type of anastomosis, the major irritant is the propensity of the ampullary epithelium to prolapse through the lumen (Fig. 16A). Although investigators such as Winston have advocated excision of these epithelial fronds, we recommend against this approach, as it creates a potential for intratubal adhesions at the anastomosis site. The epithelial fronds should be replaced with pressure from the irrigating solution or with the tip of the plain microforceps, while the successive sutures of the inner layer are tied. One must be careful not to include these epithelial fronds within a suture or knot or between the segments that are being approximated (Fig. 16B). The larger circumference of the ampulla will require a greater number of interrupted sutures to complete the anastomosis (9,68,69).

Ampullary–Infundibular Anastomosis

These are rarely performed. It may be required to reconstruct a tube with distal segmental atresia when the infundibulum is present and occasionally for sterilization reversal where the most distal ampullary portion of the tube was ablated or excised. The occluded ampulla is prepared as described previously. To permit anastomosis of the two segments, it will be necessary to fashion an opening on the apex of the infundibular portion. To do so, a Teflon probe with a conical tip is introduced into the infundibulum from the fimbriated end, and a circular opening is fashioned with microscissors, from the medial side, corresponding in size to the lumen of the ampullary segment. A two-layer anastomosis is then performed (9,68,69).

Results of Tubotubal Anastomosis for Reversal of Sterilization

Microsurgery finds its ultimate application in tubotubal anastomosis. The precision afforded by this technique and the use of magnification allows precise dissection of the occluded ends, proper alignment of the two segments, and excellent apposition of each layer with very fine nonreactive sutures. Furthermore, since in the vast majority of cases of reversal of tubal sterilization the available tubal segments are normal, the outcome is an anatomically and physiologically normal, albeit shortened, fallopian tube (9,70–72).

The major published, open microsurgical series report live birth rates between 54% and 81%; the ectopic gestation rates are usually low (9,73–89). In the absence of a male factor, and presuming a good surgical technique, the most important two factors that affect the outcome are the age of the woman, which plays a paramount role on fertility, irrespective of treatment, and the length of the reconstructed tube(s), which is obviously dependent on the prior sterilization. In regard to its length, it is important for the tube to have a sufficiently long ampullary infundibular segment to permit oocyte pickup and retention. Therefore, the outcome depends on the degree of rigor in selection criteria and the quality of the surgical technique. This is also corroborated by relatively recent reports on sterilization reversal, which include two large series from Korea (86,87). In our experience, in the absence of a male factor, the two most important parameters that predict outcome are the age of the female partner and the length of the reconstructed tube. It is interesting to note the significant difference in the outcomes of the two studies from Korea: one included 387 patients (86); the birth rate was reported as 76.2% as opposed to the other, which was 32.7% among 1118 patients included (87).

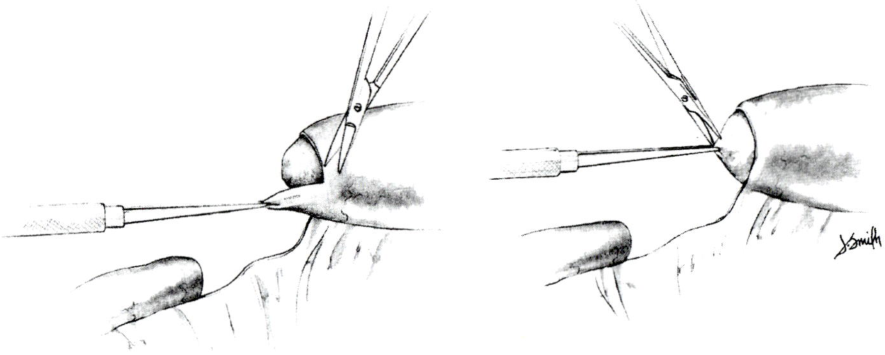

(A) (B)

Figure 14 Isthmic-ampullary anastomosis. Preparation of the ampulla to avoid luminal disparity. (**A**) The serosa over the tip of the ampullary stump is exposed, incised in a circular manner using microscissors, and excised. (**B**) The center point of the exposed muscularis is grasped with toothed microforceps, and a small opening is made into the ampullary lumen. *Source*: From Ref. 71.

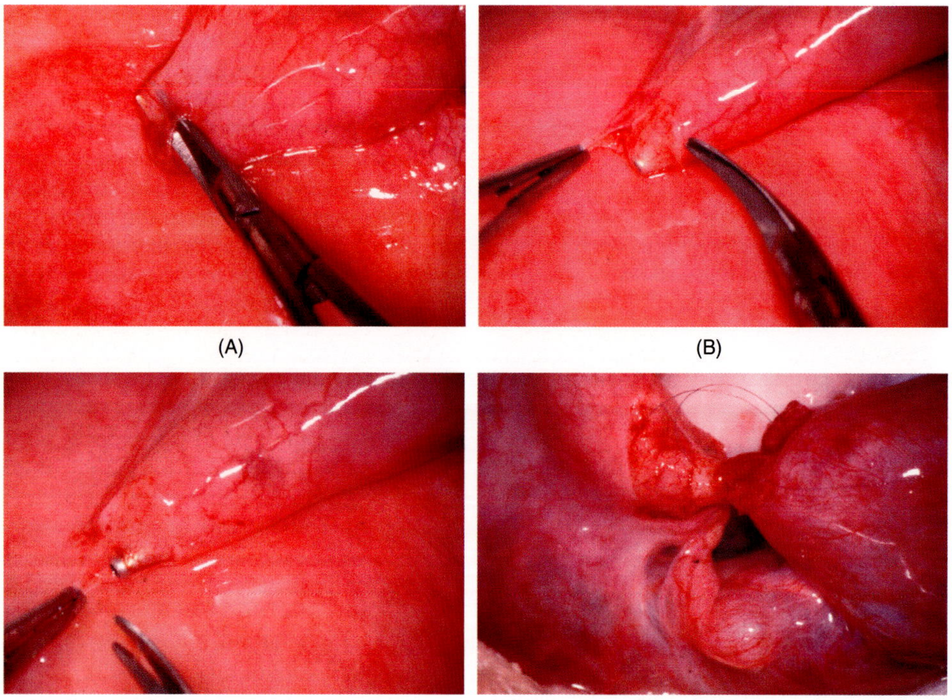

(A) (B) (C) (D)

Figure 15 Isthmic-ampullary anastomosis. Preparation of the ampulla to avoid luminal disparity. (**A**) The serosa over the tip of the ampullary stump is exposed, dissected, and (**B**) incised in a circular manner. (**C**) A small opening is made into the ampullary lumen. (**D**) Anastomosis of the two segments becomes possible without difficulty.

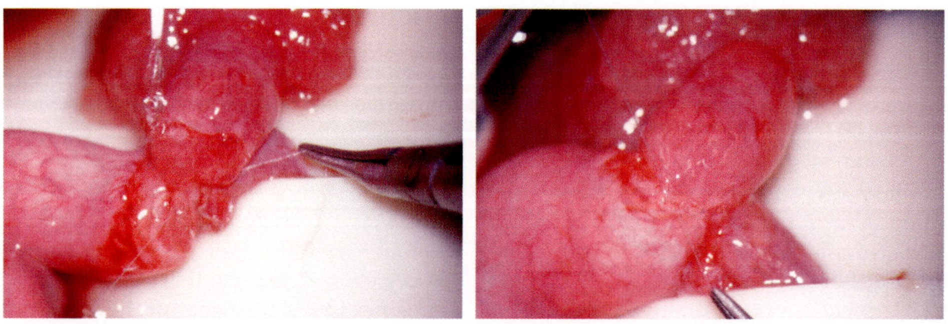

(A) (B)

Figure 16 Ampullary-ampullary anastomosis. (**A**) In this type of anastomosis, the ampullary epithelium prolapses through the lumen. (**B**) The epithelial fronds should be replaced while the successive sutures of the inner layer are tied.

The highest birthrate, 81.2%, was reported from Shanghai, China (83); the majority of these patients had a reversal because of loss of a child and were in the same marital relationship, with previous proven fertility.

Tubotubal anastomosis, by laparoscopic access, for reversal of sterilization is being performed in several centers. The reported outcomes with this approach are inferior in comparison to open access (88–95). This is largely due to modification of the proven microsurgical technique, in order to make the laparoscopic procedure easier to perform. Most surgeons, who attempted tubotubal anastomosis by laparoscopic access, using the technique described earlier in this text, found that the operating time is too long. Many attempted to simplify the technique, by using tissue glue or clips instead of sutures, or using only two sutures for the apposition of the prepared tubal segments, as first reported by Dubuisson and Swolin (90). In this technique, the first suture (4/0 Vicryl) approximates the mesosalpinx immediately beneath the two segments of tube, and the second (6/0 Vicryl) approximates the tube at 12-o'clock position. The second suture incorporates the serosa and muscularis of the two segments of tube. There are several reports in the literature with the use of this modified technique. There are also publications reporting on the laparoscopic use of a truly microsurgical, two-layer anastomosis technique. One of these is a series by Yoon et al., from Korea (93), which includes 202 cases. Fifteen of these were lost to follow-up, and one had no partner. Among the 186 who had follow-ups, 154 achieved intrauterine pregnancies; this represents an intrauterine pregnancy rate of 76.6% if we consider, as most series do, the 15 cases lost to follow-up as failures. Ninety-eight delivered healthy infants, 25 pregnancies ended in abortion, and 31 patients had ongoing pregnancies at the time of the survey. If all 31 ongoing pregnancies would have resulted in live births, the total number of patients having a live birth would have been 129 and represent a live birthrate of 64.5%. There were five cases of ectopic pregnancy. These results are not too dissimilar to those reported by open access, which confirms the importance of good surgical technique, irrespective of the mode of access. Cha et al., also from Korea, further support this assumption (88). In their study, they compare the fertility outcome in 81 women who had microsurgical reversal of sterilization, 37 by laparoscopic and 44 by open access. Both intrauterine and tubal pregnancy rates were similar in both groups. Attempts to develop simpler techniques for laparoscopic access continue to be explored, including the use of robotics (96). Use of robot is associated with increased operating time and costs (97).

Tubocornual Resection and Anastomosis for Proximal Tubal Disease

The proximal tubal region can be affected and occluded by various disease processes. An early study from France evaluated histologically tissues excised from 131 cases of cornual occlusion (98). The following lesions were identified: salpingitis isthmica nodosa (34%), inflammatory and obliterative fibrosis (31.9%), endometriosis (19%), ectopic gestation (4.5%), and tuberculosis (3.5%), and in 6.1% no lesions were found. The latter is a constant finding in a small proportion of cases of every reported series. We have since come to recognize that occlusion may be caused by a mucous plug, synechiae, and may even be an effect caused by spasm during the investigative procedure, hence the reason for meticulous investigation, including cannulation before contemplating reconstructive surgery, as discussed in the investigation chapter of this book. Ascending infections that affect the oviduct may be impeded, by the very occlusion it produces in the proximal tube, and may spare the remainder of the tube, ovary, and periadnexal areas from the inflammatory process. The outcomes reported with tubocornual resection and anastomosis (TCA) reflect the preservation of relatively healthy distal tube.

The management strategy in proximal tubal occlusion must take into account other variables, including the condition of the distal tube, the extent and nature of pelvic adhesions, the presence of associated pelvic disease, and the status of other fertility parameters, especially male factor infertility. This strategy must also respect the following principles: simplicity, reproducibility, and cost effectiveness. The selection of treatment must be individualized according to the investigative findings, the wishes of the couple, the expertise of the surgeon, and the results achieved by the center in which the couple will be managed (21,69).

Technique

The introduction of the microsurgical techniques into fertility surgery has enabled the performance of a tubocornual anastomosis and supplanted tubal implantations performed earlier. We were the first to report on microsurgical tubocornual anastomosis (2,99). Central to this approach is the complete excision of the affected portion of tube, intramural and/or isthmic. In many cases of pathologic occlusion, a portion of the intramural tube is spared, permitting often the conservation of part of this segment. In other instances, the whole intramural segment is involved in the disease process and must be excised; this will require an anastomosis to be performed between the uterine tubal ostium and the healthy portion of isthmus. Depending on the extent of intramural tube that is excised and thus the site at which the anastomosis is performed, tubocornual anastomosis may be juxtamural, intramural, or juxtauterine (Fig. 17).

Surgical Access

These are complex cases; for TCA and other complex cases, we prefer a minilaparotomy as surgical access, an approach we have used since 1985 (12,69). We place a suprapubic transverse incision, unless a midline or paramedian scar is present,

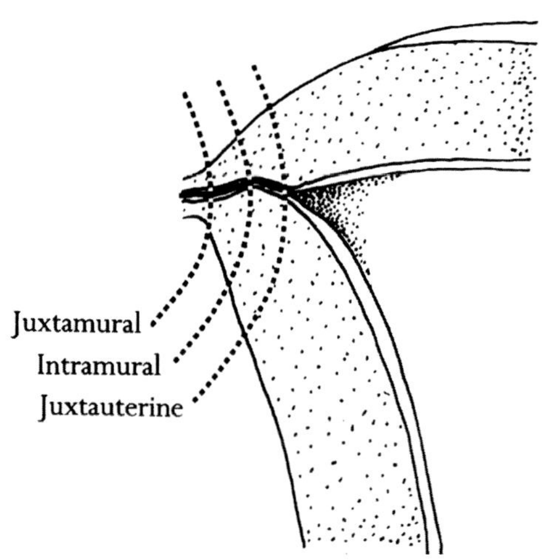

Figure 17 Tubocornual anastomosis. Depending on the extent of intramural tube that is excised, a tubocornual anastomosis becomes juxtamural, intramural, or juxtauterine. *Source*: From Ref. 100.

of 4.5 to 6 cm in length, depending on the depth of the patient's subcutaneous adipose layer. The site of the proposed incision is first infiltrated with a long-acting anesthetic agent such as 0.25% bupivacaine (Marcaine) solution. The incision is made and extended down to the fascia. The subcutaneous fat is dissected over the fascia, in the midline upward and downward. The fascia is then incised vertically in the midline, and recti muscles separated. The peritoneum is incised vertically, with the incision curbed laterally at the lower end to avoid the bladder. Once the abdomen is entered we introduce a Protractor®, a disposable device that combines the functions of wound protector and retractor, providing circumferential retraction with maximal exposure for the incision size. Before closure of the skin incision, the subcutaneous tissues are reinfiltrated with the same local anesthetic solution. Thereafter, a bilateral ilioinguinal nerve block is established. The small size of the incision and the precautions taken; the lack of bowel manipulation, along with gentle handling of tissues during the procedure; and the use of local anesthesia reduce postoperative discomfort and analgesia requirements. This approach permits prompt mobilization of the patient and discharge from the hospital or surgical center within 4 to 24 hours. Most of our patients are discharged on the same day. These patients return to normal activity almost as rapidly as those who have had less complex procedures performed by laparoscopic access.

Surgical Technique

Once the patient is anesthetized, prepped, and draped, the bladder is drained with a Foley catheter and connected to a drainage bag. A pediatric Foley catheter is introduced into the uterine cavity and connected to a syringe filled with dilute methylene blue solution to permit intraoperative chromopertubation. The vagina may be packed, as necessary, to elevate the uterus. Surgical access is obtained as described above. A pad soaked in heparinized (5000 U/L) lactated Ringer solution may be introduced into the pouch of Douglas to further elevate the uterus and isolate the bowel already displaced by a mild (10–15°) Trendelenburg tilt. With the surgical site well exposed, the operating microscope is positioned. Although the operating microscope may be draped, we have not found this to be necessary, particularly if foot pedals control the microscope. For intraoperative irrigation, heparinized, lactated Ringer solution, in an intravenous bag that is elevated and connected with intravenous tubing to a Gomel microsurgical irrigator, is used. This enables periodic irrigation of the exposed peritoneal surfaces and ovaries to prevent desiccation and clear the surgical site, instead of sponging, and to visualize individual bleeders to permit precise desiccation with a microelectrode.

The cornual region being very vascular, it is infiltrated with 2 mL dilute vasopressin solution, administered in a circular fashion, under the serosa 1 cm medial to the uterotubal junction (UTJ), using a 30-gauge needle on a 3-mL syringe (Fig. 18A). Vasoconstriction is recognized by serosal blanching. In most such cases, the proximal isthmus is indurated and demonstrates a fusiform enlargement. Even all of the intramural segment may be similarly affected. The cornu, at the UTJ, is incised down to the level of the periphery of the tubal musculature. If the tube at this level is indurated and enlarged, it may be dissected from the surrounding uterine musculature for a few millimeters (Fig. 18B). The tube is transected being careful not to divide the arteriovenous arcade at its mesosalpingeal margin. Patency of the intramural segment is assessed by transcervical chromopertubation, and the cut surface is evaluated under high magnification (Figs. 18C and 19A). If the tube is occluded or abnormal, its muscularis is dissected from the surrounding uterine muscle, 1 to 2 mm at a time, and transected again until normal patent tube is reached (Figs. 18D and 18E and 19B). The small portion of tube thus dissected is transected, and the cut surface is reassessed. The preoperative HSG usually provides information about the length of the normal intramural segment and the extent of excision required. Successive portions of the intramural tube can be transected using sharp, curved microscissors or an especially designed cornual blade (Gomel cornual blade, Spingler-Tritt, Jestetten, Germany). By limiting the excised tissue to the intramural tube, there is little risk of creating a large defect at the cornu.

After the preparation of the cornual end, the occluded or abnormal isthmic segment is prepared by making serial cuts 1 to 2 mm apart, as described earlier under principles of microsurgical tubal anastomosis. Patency of the distal segment is confirmed by descending hydropertubation, injecting of a few milliliters of dye or irrigation solution through the fimbriated end. The intervening abnormal tubal segments are excised from the mesosalpinx and hemostasis obtained (Figs. 18F and 19C). Anastomosis is achieved by placing the first suture, as always, at the 6-o'clock position (Fig. 19D). If the anastomosis is superficial (juxtamural type), the suture is tied. However, for an anastomosis deep in the cornu, as in intramural or juxtauterine types, the 6-o'clock suture is held with a clip until the remaining sutures have been placed. Tying the initial 6-o'clock suture would make placement of the subsequent sutures difficult if not impossible. Once this initial suture is placed and held, the subsequent sutures are placed with a continuous strand of suture, as described earlier (Figs. 18G and 20A and 20B). This approach facilitates suture placement and prevents the individual sutures from becoming tangled. Three additional sutures, placed at cardinal points, are usually sufficient to join the inner layer (Figs. 18H and 19E). If the cornual crater is deep and the placement of sutures is difficult, this task can be facilitated by making a coronal incision on the uterus, above the cornual crater. The edges of this incision must be properly approximated after all the sutures of the inner layer are tied. After approximation of the first layer, the seromuscularis of the uterus is joined to the serosa of the tube with no. 7-0 or 8-0 sutures. The defect under the tube is closed by approximating the mesosalpinx to the lateral edge of the uterus (Figs. 18I and 19F) (69,72,99,100).

Results

Compared with tubouterine implantation, microsurgical tubocornual anastomosis offers several advantages: it largely maintains the integrity of the uterine cornu; preserves a longer tube; obviates the need for a Caesarean section, except for obstetric reasons; and yields better results. The published series report a live birth rate from 33% to 54% (4,11,64,99–106). Most of these studies were published before 1990; there is a paucity of recent publications, which also demonstrates decreased utilization of this procedure. A study published in 1996 is interesting and clearly demonstrates that reconstructive surgery and ART are complementary rather than competitive procedures (105). In this study, 59 women with occlusive proximal disease were submitted to TCA; 27 (45.8%) of these had live births and 3 ectopic pregnancies. Of the 32 women who had no births within two years following surgery, 21 agreed to undergo IVF; 66 cycles of IVF resulted in live births for 12 of them, increasing the total live birth rate of the 59 women to 66.1% ($n = 39/59$) (105).

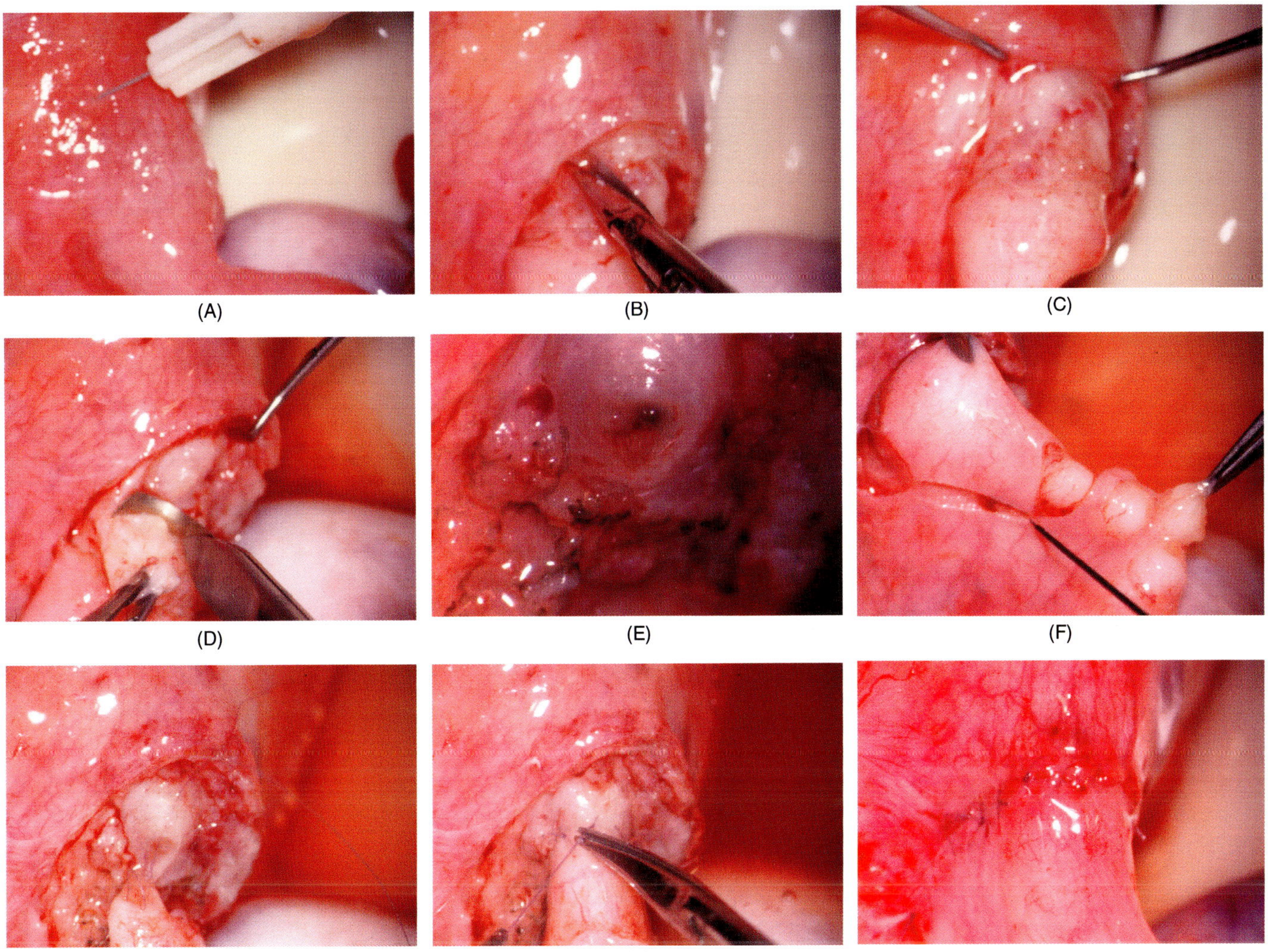

Figure 18 Tubocornual anastomosis. (**A**) 2 mL of dilute vasopressin solution is injected under the serosa of the cornual region, 1 cm medial to the uterotubal junction, using a 30-gauge needle on a 3-mL syringe. (**B**) The indurated portion of the intramural tube may be dissected from the surrounding uterine musculature. (**C**) The tube is transected and the cut surface is evaluated under high magnification (still occluded and abnormal). (**D**) The tube is dissected further and transected again. (**E**) The normal intramural tube is reached; in this case, it is almost at the level of the uterine ostium. (**F**) The isthmic segment is prepared by making serial cuts 1 to 2 mm apart, commencing at the UTJ, until normal isthmus is reached; the abnormal tubal segments are excised. (**G**) After placement of the 6-o'clock suture, subsequent sutures are being placed with a continuous strand of suture. (**H**) Tying of cardinal sutures completes apposition of the inner layer. (**I**) The seromuscularis of the uterus is joined to the serosa of the tube, and the defect under the tube is closed by approximating the mesosalpinx to the lateral edge of the uterus.

RARE AND COMPLEX PROCEDURES

Before the 1980s, when IVF got initiated, many unusual and rare procedures, including tubal transplantation, were performed with scant evident success. Introduction of microsurgical techniques, in the early 1970s, provided relative success with many rare procedures such as double anastomosis on the same tube; anastomosis of the proximal portion of on tube to the distal portion of the contralateral tube; approximation of the fimbriated end of the tube to the ovary located on the opposite side, when on one side there is a tube but no ovary and on the opposite side the contrary, and ovarian transposition for the same condition, etc. Significant improvement in IVF outcomes by the mid-1980s made many of these interventions unnecessary. I was privileged to perform a number of these procedures during the first two decades of gynecologic microsurgery (107). I also had the opportunity to do a case of microsurgical transposition of the fallopian tube and ovary in a woman with a left unicornuate uterus (108) (see below). Many of these are complex procedures. The technical difficulty of a procedure must be differentiated from the prognosis it offers. Difficulty is a relative term, since what is commonplace work for some may be difficult or even impossible for others. From the patient's standpoint, what is important is the prognosis, the yield associated with the procedure. Furthermore, prognosis is not necessarily inversely proportional to the technical difficulty of the procedure.

Tubo-ovarian Transposition

We performed a tubo-ovarian transposition in a woman who was refused both IVF and surgery in several institutions. She had a single left unicornuate uterus whose ipsilateral tube and ovary were removed subsequent to a left tubal pregnancy. Laparoscopy confirmed presence of a left unicornuate uterus with total absence of the left adnexa; on the right side it

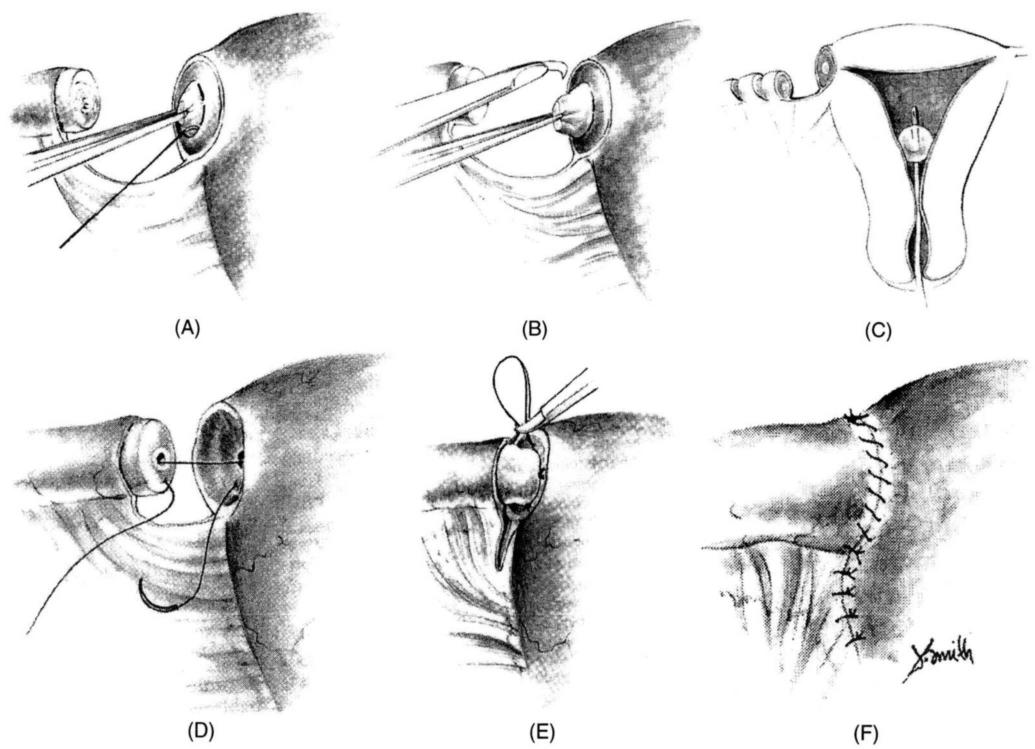

Figure 19 Tubocornual anastomosis for proximal tubal disease. **(A)** The tube is transected at the tubocornual junction, and the cut surface is assessed under high magnification. **(B)** The intramural portion of tube is dissected from the surrounding uterine musculature, 1 to 2 mm at a time, and transected, until normal tube is reached. **(C)** The isthmic segment is prepared by making serial cuts 1 to 2 mm apart, commencing at the UTJ, until normal isthmus is reached; the abnormal tubal segments are excised. **(D)** The first anastomotic suture is placed at the 6-o'clock position. **(E)** Placement of cardinal sutures completes apposition of the inner layer. **(F)** The seromuscularis of the uterus is joined to the serosa of the tube and the defect under the tube is closed by approximating the mesosalpinx to the lateral edge of the uterus. *Source*: From Ref. 71.

revealed, placed high on the pelvic sidewall, a normal appearing ovary and a short oviduct, composed of infundibulum and ampulla (Figs. 21A and 22A). Hysterosalpingography, in addition to unicornuate uterus with a moderate-size uterine cavity, demonstrated the presence of a short segment of intramural tube.

Technique

To mobilize the uterus toward the center of the pelvis, the left round ligament was divided near its inguinal insertion and dissected from the broad ligament with its vascular supply intact (Fig. 21A). The divided end of the round ligament was affixed to the right inguinal region (Fig. 21B). With transuterine

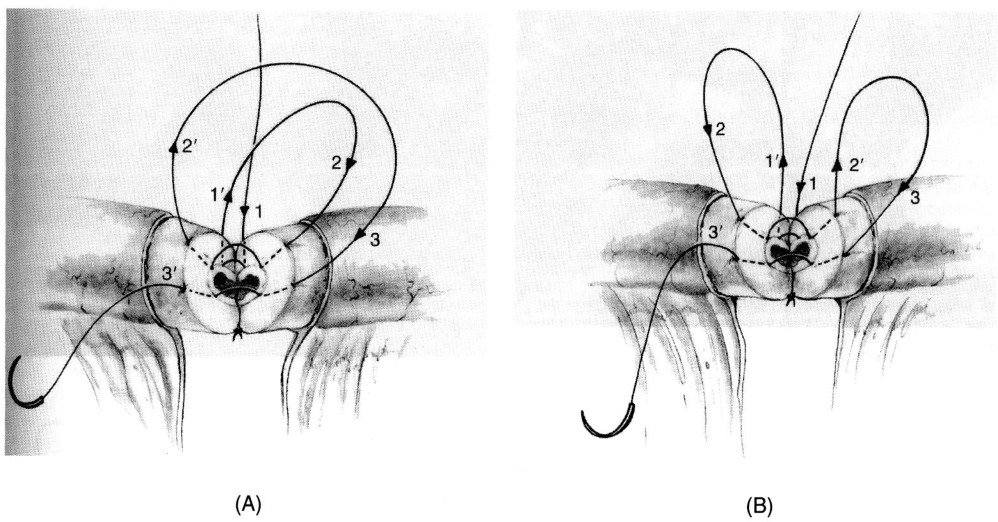

Figure 20 Tubotubal anastomosis. Placement of sutures, using a single strand of suture, as a continuous series of loops. *Source*: From Ref. 71.

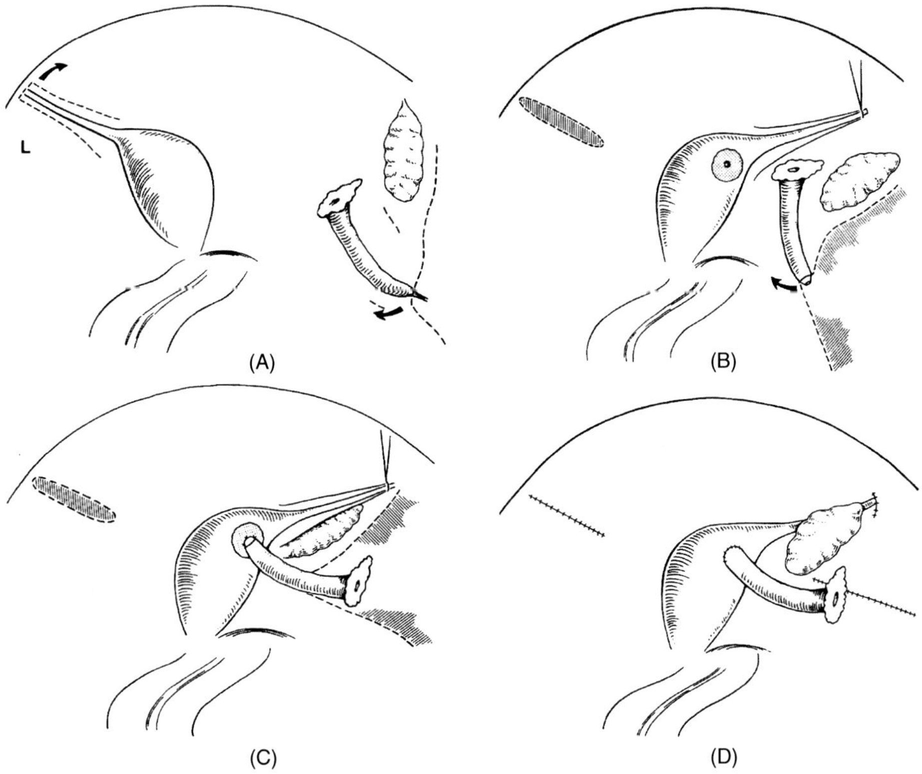

Figure 21 Tuboovarian transposition. **(A)** Schematic drawing of the findings. The dotted lines indicate the peritoneal incisions made during the procedure (l = left side). **(B)** The uterus was centered by moving the left round ligament and attaching it to right inguinal fossa. The intramural segment of the left tube is identified. **(C)** The right adnexa is mobilized, with its vascular pedicle intact. The right tube is rotated clockwise to bring its ampullary stump in proximity of the left intramural segment and permit a two-layer anastomosis to be performed. **(D)** The anastomosis is completed by apposition of the cornual seromuscularis to the serosa of the tube. All peritoneal incisions are closed. *Source*: From Ref. 108.

chromopertubation and with successive excision of thin sections of the cornu, the intramural tube was identified (Figs. 21B and 22B). The right ovary and tube were transposed while preserving intact their vascular supply (Figs. 21C and 22C). This permitted a two-layer anastomosis between the left intramural and right ampullary–infundibular tubal segments (Figs. 21C and 21D and 22D, 22E, and 22F). The ovary was mobilized further to achieve a normal spatial relationship with the fimbrial extremity of the tube (Fig. 22H). The reconstructed oviduct measured 5.5 cm from cornu to the fimbrial extremity. In the third postoperative cycle, the patient was successful in achieving an intrauterine pregnancy, which resulted in a normal live birth (108). After this birth she had two more children. Since the publication of this report in May 1985, there have been at least five case reports of successful transposition of the fallopian tube without the ovary. These reports clearly illustrate the potential of surgery, even though technically difficult, in restoring fertility in the face of unusual pelvic anatomy.

SUMMARY

Reproductive surgery encompasses a large surgical field, of which fertility-promoting procedures are only a part. It includes all surgical procedures performed on the pelvic organs of female children, adolescents, and childbearing-aged women. Reproductive surgery enjoyed significant developments since the early 1970s. These include the introduction of microsurgery, which markedly improved outcomes; introduction of laparoscopic and hysteroscopic access for many reproductive procedures; and greater utilization of minilaparotomy, instead of laparotomy.

Assisted reproduction has dramatically changed treatment of infertility for good. It has permitted streamlining investigation of the infertile couple. It has also offered couples the opportunity to attempt conception with a new therapeutic modality and by the development of ICSI with an effective way to overcome most types of male infertility.

In step with improvements in IVF results, there has been a decrease in the practice and teaching of reproductive surgery, although presence of this credible alternative permits the reproductive surgeon of today to operate on cases with a better prognosis and obtain better overall results. This is a retrogressive step, as it denies the couple with tubal infertility an effective option of treatment. Even if a couple is willing to undergo three successive cycles of IVF, based on the current U.S. outcomes, around 50% of the couples would not have a take-home baby. Furthermore, several studies have shown conclusively that a large percentage of couples do not wish to complete three cycles of IVF-ET, even when these are subsidized. There are others who refuse to have IVF for religious or ethical reasons, and many would find the cost of IVF prohibitive, since the procedure is not covered in many states or countries while other treatment modalities are, as is the case in my province, British Columbia in Canada.

It is worth stressing that successful surgery offers the couple multiple cycles in which to achieve conception naturally, and the opportunity to have more than one pregnancy

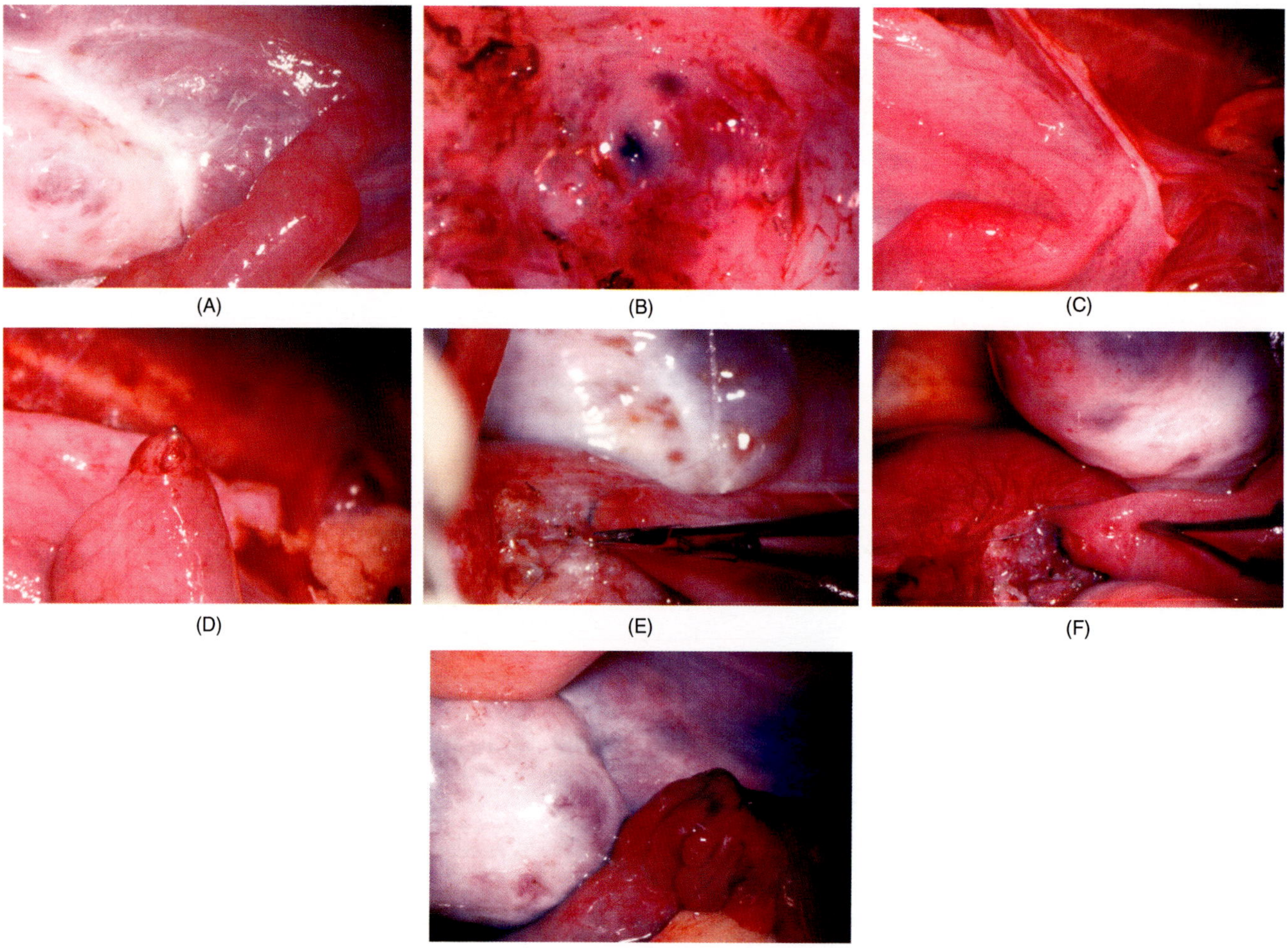

Figure 22 Tubo-ovarian transposition. (**A**) The ampullary stump and ovary on the right side. (**B**) The intramural segment of the left tube is identified. (**C**) The right adnexa is mobilized, with its vascular pedicle intact. (**D**) The right tube has been rotated clockwise to bring its ampullary stump in proximity of the left intramural segment. A small opening is made into the ampullary lumen. (**E**) The inner layer of the intramural–ampullary anastomosis has been completed. (**F**) The seromuscular layer of the cornu is being approximated to serosa of the tube to complete the anastomosis. (**G**) The ovary has been mobilized to achieve a normal spatial relationship with the fimbrial extremity of the tube. Chromopertubation demonstrates patency of the reanastomosed tube.

after a single surgical intervention. For a couple with tubal infertility, the choice of the primary treatment and any subsequent treatment should be dependent on careful consideration of both nontechnical and technical factors, discussed in detail in this text. These must be individualized to the circumstances of each couple. Information about success and complication rates of the available treatment options must accurately reflect local experience. Active involvement of the couple in the decision-making process is more likely to result in resolution of the conflict of infertility should treatment proves unsuccessful.

REFERENCES

1. Gomel V. Reproductive surgery. Minerva Ginecol 2005; 57: 21–28.
2. Gomel V. Tubal reconstruction by microsurgery. Presented at the Eighth World Congress on Fertility and Sterility (IFFS) Buenos Aires; Argentina; 1974; Abstract No. 391.
3. Swolin K. Electro microsurgery and salpingostomy: Long-term results. Am J Obstet Gynecol 1975; 121:418.
4. Gomel V. Tubal anastomosis by microsurgery. Fertil Steril 1977; 28:59–65.
5. Gomel V. Laparoscopic tubal surgery in infertility. Obstet Gynecol 1975; 46:47–49.
6. Gomel V. Reconstructive surgery of the oviduct. J Reprod Med 1977; 18:181–190.
7. Gomel V. Salpingostomy by laparoscopy. J Reprod Med 1977; 18:26–28.
8. Gomel V. Salpingostomy by microsurgery. Fertil Steril 1978; 29:380–387.
9. Gomel V. Microsurgical reversal of sterilization: A reappraisal. Fertil Steril 1980; 33:587–597.
10. Gomel V. Recent advances in surgical correction of tubal disease producing infertility. Curr Probl Obstet Gynecol 1978; 1(10): 1–60.
11. Gomel V. An odyssey through the oviduct. Fertil Steril 1983; 39:144–156.
12. James C, Gomel V. Surgical management of tubal factor infertility. Curr Opin Obstet Gynecol 1990; 2:200–206.
13. Seppälä M. The world collaborative report on in vitro fertilization and embryo replacement: Current state of the art in January 1984. Ann N Y Acad Sci 1985; 442:558.
14. National IVF/ET Registry. Medical Research International. The American Fertility Society Special Interest Group. In vitro

fertilization/embryo transfer in the United States: 1985 and 1986 results. Fertil Steril 1988; 49:212–215.
15. Medical Research International, Society for Assisted Reproductive Technology (SART), The American Fertility Society. In vitro fertilization-embryo transfer (IVF-ET) in the United States: 1990 results from the IVF-ET Registry. Fertil Steril 1992; 57:15–24.
16. Society for Assisted Reproductive Technology, American Society for Reproductive Medicine. Assisted reproductive technology in the United States: 2000 results generated from the American Society for Reproductive Medicine/Society for Assisted Reproductive Technology Registry. Fertil Steril 2004; 1:207–220.
17. CDC. Reproductive health. Available at: www.cdc.gov/ART/ART2003.
18. CDC. Reproductive health. Available at: www.cdc.gov/ART/ART2006.
19. Palermo G, Joris H, Devroey P, et al. Pregnancies after intracytoplasmic injection of single spermatozoon into an oocyte. Lancet 1992; 340:17–18.
20. Gomel V. Operative laparoscopy: Time for acceptance. Fertil Steril 1989; 52:1–11.
21. Gomel V, Taylor PJ. In vitro fertilization versus reconstructive tubal surgery. J Assist Reprod Genet 1992; 9:306–312.
22. Land JA, Courtar DA, Evers JL. Patient dropout in an assisted reproductive technology program: Implications for pregnancy rates. Fertil Steril 1997; 68:278–281.
23. Olivius C, Friden B, Borg G, et al. Why do couples discontinue in vitro fertilization treatment? A cohort study. Fertil Steril 2004; 81:258–261.
24. Kuivasaari P, Hippeläinen M, Anttila M, et al. Effect of endometriosis on IVF/ICSI outcome: Stage III/IV endometriosis worsens cumulative pregnancy and live-born rates. Hum Reprod 2005; 20:3130–3135.
25. Bergh T, Ericson A, Hillensjo T, et al. Deliveries and children born after in-vitro fertilization in Sweden 1982–95: A retrospective cohort study. Lancet 1999; 354:1579–1585.
26. Karlström PO, Bergh C. Reducing the number of embryos transferred in Sweden-impact on delivery and multiple birth rates. Hum Reprod 2007; 22:2202–2207.
27. Gomel V. Causes of failure of reconstructive infertility microsurgery. J Reprod Med 1980; 24:239–243.
28. Gomel V, ed. Microsurgery in Female Infertility. Boston: Little, Brown & Company, 1983:247–248.
29. Boer-Meisel ME, te Velde ER, Habbema JD, et al. Predicting the pregnancy outcome in patients treated for hydrosalpinx: A prospective study. Fertil Steril 1986; 45:23–29.
30. Gomel V, Erenus M. Salpingostomy by microsurgery. The American Fertility Society, 46th Annual Meeting. Program Supplement; 1990; P-097, S-106 (Abstract).
31. The American Fertility Society. The American Fertility Society classifications of adnexal adhesions, distal tubal occlusion, tubal occlusion secondary to tubal ligation. Fertil Steril 1988; 49:944–954.
32. Feinberg EC, Levens ED, DeCherney AH. Infertility surgery is dead: Only the obituary remains? Fertil Steril 2008; 89:232–236.
33. Gomel V. Microsurgery in Female Infertility. Boston: Little, Brown & Company, 1983:147–149.
34. Gomel V, Taylor PJ. Fertility promoting procedures and assisted reproductive technology. In: Gomel V, Taylor PJ, eds. Diagnostic and Operative Gynecologic Laparoscopy. St. Louis: Mosby, 1995:169–180.
35. Gomel V. Salpingo-ovariolysis by laparoscopy in infertility. Fertil Steril 1983; 34:607–611.
36. Bruhat MA, Mage G, Manhes H, et al. Laparoscopy procedures to promote fertility ovariolysis and salpingolysis: Results of 93 selected cases. Acta Eur Fertil 1983; 14:113.
37. Fayez JA. An assessment of the role of operative laparoscopy in tuboplasty. Fertil Steril 1983; 39:476.
38. Donnez J, Nisolle M, Casanas-Roux F. CO2 laser laparoscopy in infertile women with adnexal adhesions and women with tubal occlusion. J Gynecol Surg 1989; 5:47.
39. Milingos S, Kallipolitis G, Loutradis D, et al. Adhesions: Laparoscopic surgery versus laparotomy. Ann N Y Acad Sci 2000; 900:272–285.
40. Patton GW Jr. Pregnancy outcome following microsurgical fimbrioplasty. Fertil Steril 1982; 37:150–155.
41. Donnez J, Casanas-Roux F. Prognostic factors of fimbrial microsurgery. Fertil Steril 1986; 46:200–204.
42. Canis M, Mage G, Pouly JL, et al. Laparoscopic distal tuboplasty: Report of 87 cases and a 4-year experience. Fertil Steril 1991; 56:616–621.
43. Gomel V, Swolin K. Salpingostomy: Microsurgical technique and results. Clin Obstet Gynecol 1980; 23:1243–1258.
44. Gomel V. Microsurgery in Female Infertility. Boston: Little, Brown & Company, 1983:159–169.
45. Larsson B. Late results of salpingostomy combined with salpingolysis and ovariolysis by electromicrosurgery in 54 women. Fertil Steril 1982; 37:156–160.
46. Verhoeven HC, Berry H, Frantzen C, et al. Surgical treatment for distal tubal occlusion: A review of 167 cases. J Reprod Med 1983; 28:293.
47. Tulandi T, Vilos GA. A comparison between laser surgery and electrosurgery for bilateral hydrosalpinx: A two year followup. Fertil Steril 1985; 44:846.
48. Kosasa TS, Hale RW. Treatment of hydrosalpinx using a single incision eversion procedure. Int J Fertil 1988; 33:319.
49. Schlaff WD, Hassiakos DK, Damewood MD, et al. Neosalpingostomy and distal tubal obstruction: Prognostic factors and impact of surgical technique. Fertil Steril 1990; 54:984.
50. Winston RML, Margara RA. Microsurgical salpingoscopy is not an obsolete procedure. Br J Obstet Gynaecol 1991; 98:637–642.
51. Daniell JF, Herbert CM. Laparoscopic salpingostomy using the CO_2 laser. Fertil Steril 1984; 41:558.
52. Dubuisson JB, Chapron C, Morice P, et al. Laparoscopic salpingostomy: Fertility results according to the tubal mucosal appearance. Hum Reprod 1994; 9:334.
53. Oh ST. Tubal patency and conception rates with three methods of laparoscopic terminal salpingostomy. J Am Assoc Gynecol Laparosc 1996; 3:519.
54. Taylor RC, Berkowitz J, McComb PF. Role of laparoscopic salpingostomy in the treatment of hydrosalpinx. Fertil Steril 2001; 75:594–600.
55. Lilford RJ, Watson AJ. Has in vitro fertilization made salpingostomy obsolete? Br J Obstet Gynaecol 1990; 97:557–560.
56. Zouves C, Erenus M, Gomel V. Tubal ectopic pregnancy after in vitro fertilization and embryo transfer: A role for proximal occlusion or salpingectomy after failed distal tubal surgery? Fertil Steril 1991; 56:691–695.
57. Strandell A, Waldenstrom U, Nilsson L, et al. Hydrosalpinx reduces in-vitro fertilization/embryo transfer pregnancy rates. Hum Reprod 1994; 9:861–863.
58. Murray DL, Sagoskin AW, Widra EA, et al. The adverse effect of hydrosalpinges on in vitro fertilization pregnancy rates and the benefit of surgical correction. Fertil Steril 1998; 69:41–45.
59. Strandell A, Lindhard A, Waldenstrom U, et al. Hydrosalpinx and IVF outcome: A prospective, randomized, multicentre trial in Scandinavia on salpingectomy before IVF. Hum Reprod 1999; 14:2762.
60. Strandell A, Lindhard A, Waldenstrom U, et al. Hydrosalpinx and IVF outcome: Cumulative results after salpingectomy in a randomized, controlled trial. Hum Reprod 2001; 16:2403.
61. Strandell A, Sjögren A, Bentin-Ley U, et al. Hydrosalpinx fluid does not adversely affect the normal development of human embryos and implantation in vitro. Hum Reprod 1998; 13:2921–2925.
62. Van Voorhis BJ, Sparks AE, Syrop CH, et al. Ultrasound guided aspiration of hydrosalpinges is associated with improved pregnancy and implantation rates after in-vitro fertilization cycles. Hum Reprod 1998; 13:736.
63. McComb PF, Taylor RC. Pregnancy outcome after unilateral salpingostomy with a contralateral patent oviduct. Fertil Steril 2001; 76:1278–1279.

64. Gomel V. Clinical results of infertility microsurgery. In: Crosignani PG, Rubin BL, eds. Microsurgery in Female Infertility. London: Academic Press, 1980:77.
65. Halbert S, McComb PF, Patton DL. Function and structure of the rabbit oviduct following fimbriectomy. I. Distal ampullary salpingostomy. Fertil Steril 1981; 35:349.
66. Halbert S, McComb PF. Function and structure of the rabbit oviduct following fimbriectomy. II. Proximal ampullary salpingostomy. Fertil Steril 1981; 35:355.
67. Tourgeman DE, Bhaumik M, Cooke GC, et al. Pregnancy rates following fimbriectomy reversal via neosalpingostomy: A 10 years retrospective analysis. Fertil Steril 2001; 76:1041.
68. Gomel V. Microsurgery in Female Infertility. Boston: Little, Brown & Company, 1983:183–200.
69. Gomel V. Reconstructive tubal surgery. In: Rock HA, Jones HW III, eds. Te Linde's Operative Gynecology, 9th ed. Philadelphia: Lippincott Williams & Wilkins, 2003:557–593.
70. Gomel V, McComb PF. Microsurgery for tubal infertility. J Reprod Med 2006; 51:177–184.
71. Gomel V, Taylor E. Reconstructive tubal surgery. In: Rock HA, Jones HW III, eds. Te Linde's Operative Gynecology, 10th ed. Philadelphia: Lippincott Williams & Wilkins, 2008:403–437.
72. Gomel V. Reversal of tubal sterilization versus IVF in the era of assisted reproductive technology: A clinical dilemma. Reprod Biomed Online 2007; 15:403–407.
73. Winston RML. Reversal of sterilization. Clin Obstet Gynecol 1980; 23:1261.
74. Gomel V. Microsurgery in Female Infertility. Boston: Little, Brown & Company, 1983:225–244.
75. DeCherney AH, Mezer HC, Naftolin F. Analysis of failure of microsurgical anastomosis after mid-segment, non-coagulation tubal ligation. Fertil Steril 1983; 39:618–622.
76. Schlösser HW, Frantzen C, Mansour N, et al. Sterilisation Refertilisierung. Erfahrungen und Ergebnisse bei 119 microchirurgisch refertilisierten Frauen. Geburtshilfe Frauenheilkd 1983; 43:213.
77. Silber SJ, Cohen R. Microsurgical reversal of tubal sterilization: Factors affecting pregnancy rate, with long-term follow-up. Obstet Gynecol 1984; 64:67–82.
78. Henderson SR. The reversibility of female sterilization with the use of microsurgery: A report on 102 patients with more than one year of follow-up. Am J Obstet Gynecol 1984; 149:57–61.
79. Paterson PJ. Factors influencing success of microsurgical tuboplasty for sterilization reversal. Clin Reprod Fertil 1985; 3:57–64.
80. Spivak MM, Librach CL, Rosenthal DM. Microsurgical reversal of sterilization: A six-year study. Am J Obstet Gynecol 1986; 154:355–361.
81. Boeckx W, Gordts S, Buysse K, et al. Reversibility after female sterilization. Br J Obstet Gynaecol 1986; 93:839–842.
82. Rock JA, Guzick DS, Katz E, et al. Tubal anastomosis: Pregnancy success following the reversal of Falope ring or monopolar cautery sterilization. Fertil Steril 1987; 48:13–17.
83. Xue P, Fa Y-Y. Microsurgical reversal of female sterilization. J Reprod Med 1989; 34:451–455.
84. Putman JM, Holden AEC, Olive DL. Pregnancy rates following tubal anastomosis: Pomeroy partial salpingectomy versus electrocautery. J Gynecol Surg.1990; 6:173–178.
85. teVelde ER, Boer ME, Looman CWN, et al. Factors influencing success or failure after reversal of sterilization: A multivariate approach. Fertil Steril 1990; 54:270–277.
86. Kim JD, Kim KS, Doo JK, et al. A report on 387 cases of microsurgical tubal reversals. Fertil Steril 1997; 68:875.
87. Kim SH, Shin CJ, Kim JG, et al. Microsurgical reversal of tubal sterilization: A report on 1118 cases. Fertil Steril 1997; 68: 865.
88. Cha SH, Lee MH, Kim JH, et al. Fertility outcome after tubal anastomosis by laparoscopy and laparotomy. J Am Assoc Gynecol Laparosc 2001; 8:348–352.
89. Wiegerinck MA, Roukema M, van Kessel PH, et al. Sutureless re-anastomosis by laparoscopy versus microsurgical reanastomosis by laparotomy for sterilization reversal: A matched cohort study. Human Reprod 2005; 20:2358–2005.
90. Dubuisson JB, Swolin K. Laparoscopic tubal anastomosis (the one stitch technique) preliminary results. Hum Reprod 1995; 10:2044–2046.
91. Dubuisson JB, Chapron C. Single suture laparoscopic tubal reanastomosis. Curr Opin Obstet Gynecol 1998; 10:307–313.
92. Bisonette F, Lapensee L, Bouzayen R. Outpatient laparoscopic tubal anastomosis and subsequent fertility. Fertil Steril 1999; 72:549.
93. Yoon TK, Sung HR, Kang HG, et al. Laparoscopic tubal anastomosis: Fertility outcome in 202 cases. Fertil Steril 1999; 72:1121–1126.
94. Mettler L, Ibrahim M, Lehmann-Willenbrock E, et al. Pelviscopic reversal of tubal sterilization with the one- to two-stitch technique. J Am Assoc Gynecol Laparosc 2001; 8:353–358.
95. Ribeiro SC, Tormena RA, Giribela CG, et al. Laparoscopic tubal anastomosis. Int J Gynaecol Obstet 2004; 84:142–146.
96. Degueldre M, Vandromme J, Huong PT, et al. Robotically assisted laparoscopic microsurgical tubal reanastomosis: A feasibility study. Fertil Steril 2000; 74:1020–1023.
97. Rodgers AK, Goldberg JM, Hammel JP, et al. Tubal anastomosis by robotic compared with outpatient minilaparotomy. Obstet Gynecol 2007; 109:1375–1380.
98. Madlenat P, DeBrux J, Palmer R. L'etiologie des obstructions tubaires proximales et son róle dans le prognostic des implantations. Gynecologie 1977; 28:47–53.
99. McComb P, Gomel V. Cornual occlusion and its microsurgical reconstruction. Clin Obstet Gynecol 1980; 23:1229–1241.
100. Gomel V. Microsurgery in Female Infertility. Boston: Little, Brown & Company, 1983:171–181.
101. Winston RM. Microsurgery of the fallopian tube: From fantasy to reality. Fertil Steril 1980; 34:521–530.
102. Donnez J, Casanas-Roux F. Prognostic factors influencing the pregnancy rate after microsurgical cornual anastomosis. Fertil Steril 1986; 46:1089–1092.
103. McComb P. Microsurgical tubocornual anastomosis for occlusive cornual disease: Reproducible results without the need for tubouterine implantation. Fertil Steril 1986; 46:571–577.
104. Gillett WR, Herbison GP. Tubocornual anastomosis: Surgical considerations and coexistent infertility factors in determining the prognosis. Fertil Steril 1989; 51:241.
105. Tomazevic T, Ribic-Pucelj M, Omahen A, et al. Microsurgery and in-vitro fertilization and embryo transfer for infertility resulting from pathological proximal tubal blockage. Hum Reprod 1996; 11:2613.
106. Awartani K, McComb PF. Microsurgical resection of nonocclusive salpingitis isthmica nodosa is beneficial. Fertil Steril 2003; 79:1199–1203.
107. Gomel V. Microsurgery in Female Infertility. Boston: Little, Brown & Company, 1983:209–219.
108. Gomel V, McComb PF. Microsurgical transposition of the human fallopian tube and ovary with subsequent intrauterine pregnancy. Fertil Steril 1985; 43:804–808.

24

General principles in preservation of fertility in gynecologic surgery

Recai Pabuccu and Victor Gomel

Infertility, in young and/or reproductive age women, is frequently caused by misdiagnosis or delayed diagnosis and treatment of acute conditions, such as pelvic inflammatory disease, appendicitis, ectopic pregnancy, etc. It is also caused by surgical procedures that are unnecessary, unnecessarily extensive, and/or traumatic, resulting in damage to or loss of normal reproductive organs and the development of postoperative adhesions (1). Our purpose in this chapter is to increase awareness about these issues.

Surgical procedures in the peritoneal cavity are associated with postoperative adhesions, irrespective of the access mode. We have come to better understand the importance of postoperative adhesions. They can cause pelvic pain including dyspareunia, bowel obstruction, and infertility. It has clearly been shown that one-third of the patients who have had abdominal surgery subsequently have adhesion-related hospital admissions. These individuals are re-admitted an average of two times in the 10 years following the surgery. The re-admission rate is similar whether the procedure is performed on the female reproductive tract or other intraperitoneal organs (2–4).

POSTOPERATIVE ADHESIONS

Postoperative adhesions have been the *bête noire* of surgeons for time immemorial. We have come to recognize that they are an important clinical problem. Pelvic adhesions have been found in 56% to 100% of patients undergoing early second-look laparoscopy after primary gynecological surgery (5–7). The ovary appears to be the most adhesion-prone organ in the pelvis (8). These data make clearly evident the importance of preventing adhesions in female children, adolescents, and reproductive age women.

While our knowledge of the pathophysiology of adhesion formation has greatly increased and many preventive agents have been produced and marketed, reduction of trauma during surgery remains the most important initial step in the cascade of postoperative adhesion formation (7,9). This led to the introduction of microsurgical techniques (10–13) (discussed in detail in chap. 23).

The subject of postoperative adhesions has been reviewed in several chapters of this book including chapters 2 and 12 and will not be further addressed here, except for stressing its importance as has been done above.

INFECTION AND INFERTILITY

Many microorganisms affect the female reproductive tract. Some are more important than others in regard to their deleterious effect on fertility. Common vaginal infections caused by *Trichomonas vaginalis*, *Gardnerella vaginalis*, or *Candida albicans* are relatively easy to treat and do not affect fertility in the long term. Endometritis, usually a posttraumatic or postabortal infection, may cause uterine synechiae that may adversely affect future fertility. This topic is discussed further in this chapter. The most important and common organisms that affect fertility are *Chlamydia trachomatis* and *Neisseria gonorrhea*. These sexually transmitted organisms ascend through the genital tract causing endocervicitis and may progress into pelvic inflammatory disease (PID), adnexitis, and even local or diffuse peritonitis, and abscess formation. Pelvic inflammatory disease is the major cause of tubal damage (14–16). In addition to tubal damage involving principally the epithelium, and tubal occlusion, extension of the infection into the peritoneal cavity may cause extensive periadnexal, pelvic, and abdominal adhesions (17,18).

Tubal factor infertility remains an important cause of female infertility. *Chlamydia trachomatis* is the principal pathogen of PID, although frequently other organisms are associated. This is a sexually transmitted disease that remains an important social problem (15). The condition may be associated with only subtle symptoms; hence it is important to examine the cervix for evidence of lower genital tract infection. In addition to obtaining material for culture, endocervical material should be examined microscopically for evidence of infection. Considering the ascending nature of this type of infection, it is prudent to do the same microscopic examination prior to referring a woman for hysterosalpingography or other invasive intrauterine procedure; this will decrease the incidence of PID associated with these interventions.

With PID, subsequent fertility is directly related to delay in diagnosis and treatment. Early diagnosis of this condition is essential to prevent infertility; however, in many instances, this is not possible by clinical means alone. A more liberal use of laparoscopy with or without endometrial biopsy to establish the diagnosis and to institute appropriate therapy is preferable to a wait-and-see attitude. This is especially important in the young and nulliparous patient. Early institution of high-dose, intravenous antibiotic therapy that takes into account the polymicrobial etiology of salpingitis is the only means at our disposal to improve the very bad prognosis associated with this condition (18). After a single episode of PID, the relative risk for tubal factor infertility is approximately 10%. Each repeat episode of PID doubles the risk and so it is approximately 23% after two episodes and almost 54% after three or more episodes. Seroepidemiological studies suggest that chlamydial infection may account for a large proportion of cases of tubal factor infertility and ectopic pregnancy (19). Adolescents and women younger than 24 years of age are at an increased risk of contracting such infections. In addition to lack of significant symptoms, diagnosis and treatment is often hindered by concern for screening and treatment confidentiality and lack of knowledge about community medical resources (20).

ABORTION AND INFERTILITY

The incidence of postoperative infection after first trimester therapeutic abortion is low. But, increasing numbers of women are undergoing repeated pregnancy terminations, which increases their risk of cervical and/or uterine trauma and infection. The incidence of infertility, midtrimester abortion, or prematurity does not seem to be increased significantly after a first trimester pregnancy termination. However, the reported deleterious outcomes after multiple abortions are contradictory (21). Obviously, they pale in comparison to the serious complications and the deleterious outcomes on fertility and health associated with the so called "illegal abortions."

Uterine synechiae and Asherman's syndrome occurs after trauma to the basalis layer of the endometrium generally after endometrial curettage, most frequently of a gravid uterus (13,21). The condition was first described by Heinrich Fritsch in 1894 (22). Asherman's experience was based on a series of postabortal and postpartum cases submitted to uterine curettage. He suggested that the syndrome was the consequence of trauma to the endometrium, producing partial or complete obliteration of the uterine cavity, and/or the cervical canal, resulting in symptoms including menstrual abnormalities, infertility, and recurrent pregnancy loss. It is now recognized that trauma to nongravid uterus may also cause intrauterine adhesions and endometrial fibrosis (23). However, gravidity remains the major factor. In 1856 cases of Asherman's syndrome reviewed by Schenker and Margalioth, gravidity was the dominating predisposing factor in 90.8% of cases submitted to curettage (66.7% postabortal, 21.5% postpartum, 2% after cesarean section, and 0.6% after evacuation of a hydatidiform mole) (24). These findings have been confirmed in other studies (25–27).

One of the possible explanations for the gravid uterus being a major predisposing factor for the development of Asherman's syndrome is the low estrogen status at the time of the operation or immediately afterward, as the endometrium depends on estrogen for regeneration. Another possible explanation could be the physiologic changes that occur in a gravid uterus around the pregnancy period. The uterus could be in a vulnerable state after pregnancy, making the basal layer of endometrium more easily damaged by any trauma, especially curettage (22,23).

PREVENTION OF UTERINE SYNECHIAE AND ASHERMAN'S SYNDROME

Trauma to the nongravid uterus may cause Asherman's syndrome. The reported rates are as follows: 1.6% after diagnostic curettage, 1.3% after abdominal myomectomy, 0.5% after cervical biopsy or polypectomy, 0.2% after insertion of an intrauterine device (24). Intrauterine adhesions can also result from various types of hysteroscopic surgery. In a study comprising 95 women who underwent hysteroscopic surgery, Asherman's syndrome was found to have occurred in 6.7% (1 out of 15) of patients after resection of septa and in 31.3% (10 out of 32) and 45.5% (9 out of 20), respectively, of patients after hysteroscopic resection of solitary fibroids and multiple fibroids (28).

Postabortal or post-postpartum curettage, for retained products, may be replaced by hysteroscopic evacuation. Goldenberg et al. (29) used operative hysteroscopy with a cutting loop, used as a curette, for selective removal of the adherent residual tissue while avoiding interference with the rest of the endometrial surface. They found that selective curettage of residual trophoblastic tissue directed by hysteroscopy is an easy, short procedure that may be preferable to conventional, nonselective, blind curettage. If surgical evacuation is indeed required in the puerperium or after miscarriage, suction evacuation of the uterus should be undertaken by a senior obstetrician. It should be performed gently, with the use of either suction or a blunt (not sharp) curette to avoid unnecessary trauma to the basal layer of the endometrium (23,29–31).

General measures to reduce postoperative intrauterine adhesions resulting from hysteroscopic surgery include avoiding trauma to healthy endometrium and myometrium surrounding the lesions to be removed, reducing the usage of electrosurgery whenever possible especially during the removal of myomas with extensive intramural involvement, treating opposing myomas at a subsequent procedure, and avoiding forced cervical manipulation.

Some researchers suggest early second-look hysteroscopy as an effective preventive and therapeutic strategy (32). The use of prophylactic antibiotics in hysteroscopic surgery, to avoid infection and to prevent postoperative IUA, has not been uniformly recommended (7,32). GnRH analogues and Danazol are commonly administered before certain hysteroscopic procedures such as metroplasty and myomectomy to suppress ovarian function in order to reduce endometrial vascularity and edema during the procedure and reduce perioperative complications. The role of endometrial suppression before resectoscopic surgery on the frequency of postoperative IUA has been questioned (7). It has also been demonstrated that the frequency of postoperative IUA was dependent on the pathology initially treated with no difference between placebo and Danazol-treated (200 mg twice/day) groups (28). Data pertaining to the role of preoperative GnRH analogues on the development and/or re-development of IUA after hysteroscopic surgery were not found in the English language literature.

The postoperative administration of conjugated estrogens (doses of 1.25–5 mg daily) and progestins, in a cyclic regimen for 30 to 60 days, has been recommended to stimulate the re-epithelialization of the scarred surfaces (33). However, the efficacy of this approach requires validation by appropriately designed studies.

Separation of traumatized endometrial surfaces is considered essential in the prevention and in the reformation of synechiae after intrauterine surgery. For many years, the placement of an IUD in the uterine cavity, for three months, was considered the standard method to separate the apposing surfaces. However, the specific type of IUD for this purpose remains controversial. The copper-bearing IUDs and the levonorgestrel intrauterine system (IUS) have too small a surface area to achieve this purpose; furthermore, IUDs containing copper might induce an excessive inflammatory reaction. In theory, the Lippes-IUD may be the most efficacious by keeping the raw dissected surfaces separated during the initial healing phase, reducing the chance of re-adherence (34–36). An alternative approach has been to place a pediatric Foley catheter into the uterine cavity, inflate its balloon, and leave it in place for several days. Vaginal discomfort and uterine pain limits the duration of residence of the catheter. For this purpose, a triangular-shaped flat balloon with a short tail, through which it is inflated after placement, is commercially available. In a recent study, Pabuccu et al. (37) reported that insertion of a Lippes IUD during the initial hysteroscopic assessment of the uterine cavity, after lysis of some of the adhesions, greatly facilitated complete adhesiolysis during a subsequent hysteroscopy undertaken one week later. The

IUD "indicated the right pathway within the uterine cavity to the fundus and tubal orifices." The IUD was left in place for two months during which cyclical estrogen and progesterone was administered (37).

Preliminary studies have demonstrated that the intrauterine application of autocross linked hyaluronic acid gels (ACP) following hysteroscopic adhesiolysis significantly reduces the reformation of postoperative IUA. In a randomized controlled study, Guida et al. demonstrated that ACP also significantly reduces the incidence and severity of de novo formation of IUA after resectoscopic removal of myomas, polyps, and septa (38). Seprafilm (Genzyme Corporation, Cambridge, Massachusetts) is a bioresorbable membrane of chemically modified HA and carboxymethylcellulose; it has been shown to be effective in reducing adhesion formation after suction curettage for incomplete and missed abortion (39). These findings should be confirmed in prospective cohort studies.

OVARIAN SURGERY

Surgery for endometriosis, endometriomas, and other conditions of the ovary has been discussed in other chapters of this book (chaps. 9 and 10). Therefore, our remarks here will be limited to concerns of fertility preservation with such procedures. These include prevention of adhesions and reduction of ovarian reserve. The ovary is the most adhesiogenic organ in the pelvis (8); hence conservative surgery requires the use of microsurgical principles and technique to minimize tissue trauma.

Ovaries affected with endometriosis frequently are adherent to the ipsilateral fossa ovarica or to other organs. When the ovary is released from the pelvic wall, the incidence of re-adherence is extremely high unless an effective barrier is placed between the apposing damaged surfaces or the ovary elevated with an absorbable suture that will keep the ovary temporarily away from the fossa ovarica (temporary ovarian suspension).

During excision, endometriomas frequently rupture causing spillage of contents into the peritoneal cavity. Spillage also occurs when the technique comprises intentional cyst rupture. Do the endometrioma contents stimulate adhesions to form? The answer is not clear; however, it would be preferable to evacuate the contents of the endometrioma, at the outset by careful suction, to prevent large amounts of its contents to contaminate the peritoneal cavity. It would also be prudent to carry out a thorough lavage at the close of the surgery, which will also remove blood and surgical debris from the peritoneal cavity (40).

The other issue is preservation of the ovarian reserve. While striving to remove completely the diseased tissues, it is necessary to preserve as much of the surrounding ovarian cortical tissues as possible, and avoid damaging the cortex and the ovarian vascular supply by careless use of energy and/or sutures.

Another issue is whether or not to reconstruct the ovary after removal of a cyst. Our practice have been to approximate the edges of the cortex either with a subepithelial continuous fine suture such as 6–0 Vicryl® or with interrupted sutures of the same material, taking care to place the knots internally (40). It is important to avoid deep sutures in order to prevent occlusion of the blood vessels that supply the ovary through its hilum (40). A recent study has reported that reconstructing ovaries treated for endometriomas results in a lower rate of postoperative adhesions (41).

Dermoid cysts represent 10% to 15% of all ovarian tumors. Having a proper capsule, they are more easily amenable to intact removal. Avoidance of rupture is important because of the irritant and fatty nature of the contents of the teratomas. With laparoscopic access, removal of the cyst from the abdominal cavity should be done within an appropriate laparoscopic bag to avoid rupture and intraperitoneal spillage of its contents (40). Spillage may be associated with peritonitis, adhesions, and subsequent impaired fertility. In the event of spillage, copious peritoneal lavage is used (40,42). The perception is that suction of released teratoma contents, followed by copious irrigation and suction until the affluent is clear of fat globules and other debris, reduces postoperative adhesions (40,42).

MYOMECTOMY

Uterine leiomyomas (their relationship with infertility), myomectomy (by hysteroscopic and laparoscopic access), and use of laparoscopic access versus laparotomy have been discussed in three other chapters (chaps. 6, 7, and 19) and will not be recapitulated here.

The primary issue regarding myomectomy in a patient who wishes to retain her fertility or an infertile patient is indication for the procedure. This is important because not all myomas adversely affect fertility and also because myomectomy is a procedure that results in significant postoperative adhesions that involve not only the site of primary surgery but frequently also the adnexae. Periovarian and peritubal adhesions may hinder normal ovulation, prevent ovum pick-up by the fimbriae and thus impair fertility.

The goals of myomectomy, in the group of patients in question, are to remove all of the tumors, without damaging the uterine cavity; restore the uterine anatomy to normal with proper apposition of the uterine incisions; and the use of a gentle and careful technique to reduce postoperative adhesions. Such an approach will prevent reduction of the fertility potential of the patient as a result of the surgery and significantly reduce the rate of uterine rupture in the event of pregnancy.

TUBAL PREGNANCY

Early diagnosis of ectopic pregnancy and prompt treatment prevents the various, including serious, complications that may result from delayed diagnosis. Progress in laboratory medicine and imaging has greatly simplified early diagnosis of tubal pregnancy. Provided the condition is suspected, measurement of β-hCG level and use of transvaginal ultrasonography, both of which are readily available, permits a diagnosis to be made in the majority of cases. These diagnostic measures have greatly decreased the diagnostic role of laparoscopy, which was frequently used in the past. Laparoscopy is now used largely to gain access to the peritoneal cavity, when surgical treatment is required (43).

There has also been significant progress in the treatment of ectopic pregnancy partly because of our ability to diagnose the condition early. The role and place of medical treatment has been clarified. The available tools of measurement of β-hCG levels, use of transvaginal ultrasonography, and other ancillary blood tests as necessary as well as the clinical status of the patient permit the condition to be treated expectantly, medically, or surgically (43–45).

The advantages of using laparoscopic access in surgical treatment of tubal pregnancy became evident in the seventies (46–48). In addition to recognized advantages of less postoperative discomfort and reduced analgesic requirement, a shorter hospital stay and period of convalescence, and frequently reduced costs, laparoscopy also permits a more thorough assessment of the pelvic and abdominal cavities and results in less postoperative adhesions (49,50). Therapeutic details have been discussed in chapter 13 and will not be discussed here.

Several factors affect future fertility after a tubal pregnancy, and one of the most important of these is the status of the contralateral tube (51,52). Because of this, future fertility appears to be comparable after salpingotomy and salpingectomy (52). As for all cases of reproductive surgery, a delicate atraumatic technique should be employed to prevent further deterioration of the patient's fertility potential.

REFERENCES

1. Gomel V. Reproductive surgery. Minerva Ginecol 2005; 57: 21–28.
2. Ellis H, Moran BJ, Thompson JN, et al. Ahesion-related hospital readmissions after abdominal and pelvic surgery: A retrospective cohort study. Lancet 1999; 353:1476–1480.
3. Ellis H. The clinical significance of adhesions: Focus on intestinal obstruction. Eur J Surg Suppl 1997; 577:5–9.
4. Lower AM, Hawthorn RJS, Ellis H, et al. The impact of adhesions on hospital readmissions over ten years after 8849 open gynaecological operations (an assessment from the Surgical and Clinical Adhesions Research Study). Br J Obstet Gynaecol 2000; 107:855–862.
5. Schwartz LB, Diamond MP. Formation, reduction and treatment of adhesive disease. Semin Reprod Endocrinol 1991; 9: 89–99.
6. Diamond MP, Daniell JF, Feste J. Adhesion formation and de novo adhesion formation after reproductive pelvic surgery. Fertil Steril 1987; 47:864–866.
7. Nappi C, Di Spiezio Sardo A, Ereco E, et al. Prevention of adhesions in gynaecological endoscopy. Hum Reprod Update 2007; 13:379–394.
8. Diamond MP. Surgical aspects of infertility. In: Sciarra JJ, SimpsonJL, Speroff L, eds. Gynecology and Obstetrics. Vol. 5. Philadelphia, PA: JB Lippincott Co, 1991:1–23.
9. Gomel V, Urman B, Gurgan T. Pathophysiology of adhesion formation and strategies for prevention. J Reprod Med 1996; 41:35–41.
10. Gomel V. Tubal reanastomosis by microsurgery. Fertil Steril 1977; 28:59–65.
11. Gomel V. Reconstructive surgery of the oviduct. J Reprod Med 1977; 18:181–190.
12. Gomel V. From microsurgery to laparoscopic surgery: A progress? Fertil Steril 1995; 63:464–468.
13. Gomel V. Microsurgery in Female Infertility. Boston, USA: Little, Brown and Co., 1983.
14. Tiitinen A, Surcel HM, Halttunen M, et al. *Chlamydia trachomatis* and chlamydial heat shock protein 60-specific antibody and cell-mediated responses predict tubal factor infertility. Hum Reprod 2006; 21:1533–1538.
15. Paavonen J, Eggert-Kruse W. *Chlamydia trachomatis*: Impact on human reproduction. Hum Reprod Update 1999; 5:433–447.
16. den Hartog JE, Ouburg S, Land JA, et al. Do host genetic traits in the bacterial sensing system play a role in the *C. trachomatis*-associated tubal pathology in subfertile women? BMC Infect Dis 2006; 6:122.
17. Pellati D, Mylonakis I, Bertoloni G, et al. Genital tract infections and infertility. Eur J Obstet Gynecol 2008; 140:3–11.
18. Lauper U, Schalter C. Adnexitis and pelvic inflammatory disease. Gynakol Geburtshilfliche Rundsch 2005; 45:14–18.
19. Westrom I. Incidence, prevalence, and trends of acute pelvic inflammatory disease and its consequences in industrialized countries. Am J Obstet Gynecol 1980; 138:880.
20. Tarr ME, Gilliam ML. Sexually transmitted infections in adolescent women. Clin Obstet Gynecol 2008; 51:306–318.
21. Huggins ER, Cullins VE. Fertility after contraception or abortions. Fertil Steril 1999; 54:559–573.
22. Dan Yu MM, Yat-May MRCOG, Cheong Y, et al. Asherman syndrome-one centry later. Fertil Steril 2008; 89:759–779.
23. Valle RF, Sciarra JJ. Intrauterne adhesions: Hysteroscopic diagnosis, classification, treatment, and reproductive outcome. Am J Obstet Gynecol 1988; 158:1459–1470.
24. Schenker JG, Margolioth EJ. Intrauterine adhesions: An updated appraisal. Fertil Steril 1982; 37:593–610.
25. Smid I, Bedo T. Curettage during puerperum and its late consequences. Zentralbl Gynakol 1978; 100:916–920.
26. Westendorp IC, Ankum WM, Mol BW, et al. Prevalance of Asherman's syndrome after secondary removal of placental remnants or a repeat curettage for incomplete abortion. Hum Reprod 1998; 13:3347–3350.
27. Friedler S, Margalioth EJ, Kafka I, et al. Incidence of post-abortion intra-uterine adhesions evaluated by hysteroscopy—a prospective study. Hum Reprod 1993; 8:442–444.
28. Taskin O, Sadik S, Onoglu A, et al. Role of endometrial suppression on the frequency of intrauterine adhesions after resectoscopic surgery. J Am Assoc Gynecol Laparosc 2000; 7:351–354.
29. Goldenberg M, Schiff E, Achiron R, et al. Managing residual trophoblastic tissue. Hysteroscopy for directing curettage. J Reprod Med 1997; 42:26–28.
30. Schenker JG. Etiology of and therapeutic approach to synechia uteri. Eur J Obstet Gynecol Reprod Biol 1996; 65:109–113.
31. Alcazar JL. Transvaginal ultrasonography combined with color velocity imaging and pulsed Doppler to detect residual trophoblastic tissue. Ultrasound Obstet Gynecol 1998; 11: 54–58.
32. Wheeler JM, Taskin O. Second-look office hysteroscopy following resectoscopy: the frequency and management of intrauterine adhesions. Fertil Steril 1993; 60:150–156.
33. Orhue AAE, Aziken ME, Igbefoh JO. A comparison of two adjunctive treatments for intrauterine adhesions following lysis. Int J Gynecol Obstet 2003; 82:49–56.
34. Farhi J, Bar Hava I, Homburg R, et al. Induced degeneration of the endometrium following curettage for abortion: a comparative study. Hum Reprod 1993; 8:1143–1144.
35. March CM. Intrauterine adhesions. Obstet Gynecol Clin North Am 1995; 22:491–505.
36. Al-Inany H. Intrauterine adhesions. Acta Obstet Gynecol Scand 2001; 80:986–993.
37. Pabuccu R, Onalan G, Kaya C, et al. Efficiency and pregnancy outcome of serial intrauterine device-guided hysteroscopic adhseiolysis of intrauterine synechiae. Fertil Steril 2008; 90:1973–1977.
38. Guida M, Acunzo G, Di Spiezio Sardo A, et al. Effectiveness of auto-cross-linked hyaluronic acid gel in the prevention of intrauterine adhesions after hysteroscopic adhesiolysis: a prospective randomized, controlled study. Hum Reprod 2004; 19:1461–1464.
39. Tsapanos VS, Stathopoulou LP, Papathanassopoulou VS, et al. The role of Seprafilm bioresorbable membrane in the prevention and therapy of endometrial synechiae. J Biomed Mater Res 2002; 63:10–14.
40. Gomel V, Taylor PJ. Ovarian surgery. In: Gomel V, Taylor PJ, eds. Diagnositic and Operative Gynecologic Laparoscopy. St. Louis: Mosby, 1995:189–199.
41. Pellicano M, Bramante S, Guida M, et al. Ovarian endometrioma: Postoperative adhesions following bipolar coagulation and suture. Fertil Steril 2008; 89:796–799.

42. Tsikouras P, Liberis V, Galazios G, et al. Laparoscopic treatment of ovarian dermoid cysts. Clin Exp Obstet Gynecol 2008;3 5:124–129.
43. Gomel V, Taylor PJ. Tubal pregnancy. In: Gomel V, Taylor PJ, eds. Diagnositic and Operative Gynecologic Laparoscopy. St. Louis: Mosby, 1995:157–168.
44. Stovall TG, Ling FW. Single-dose methotrexate: An expanded clinical trial. Am J Obstet Gynecol 1993; 168:1759–1762.
45. Lipscomb GH, McCord ML, Stovall TG, et al. Predictors of success of methotrexate treatment in women with tubal ectopic pregnancies. N Engl J Med 1999; 341:1974–1978.
46. Gomel V. Laparoscopy in the diagnosis and treatment of ectopic gestation. Gine Dips. 1978; 2:85–87
47. Stangel J, Gomel V. Techniques in conservative surgery for tubal gestation. Clin Obstet Gynecol 1980; 23:1221–1228.
48. Zouves C, Gomel V. Tubal pregnancy: Management by operative laparoscopy versus laparotomy. Infertility 1989; 12: 23–29.
49. Lundorff P, Thorburn J, Hahlin M, et al. Laparoscopic surgery in ectopic pregnancy. A randomized trial versus laparotomy. Acta Obstet Gynecol Scand 1991; 70:343–348.
50. Vermesh M, Silva PD, Rosen GF, et al. Management of unruptured ectopic gestation by linear salpingostomy: A prospective, randomized clinical trial of laparoscopy versus laparotomy. Obstet Gynecol 1989; 73:400–404.
51. Urman B, Zouves C, Gomel V. Fertility outcome following tubal pregnancy. Acta Eur Fertil 1991; 22:205–208.
52. Hajenius PJ, Mol BWJ, Bossuyt PMM, et al. Interventions for tubal ectopic pregnancy. Cochrane Database Syst Rev 2000; (2):CD000324.

25

Preservation of fertility in gynecologic malignancy

Denis Querleu

Gynecological malignancies may affect women in their reproductive age. As a consequence, loss of fertility is a concern for those women who have not fulfilled their desire for maternity. On the other hand, it has been recognized for years that subsequent pregnancy does not adversely affect the outcome of patients managed for cancer and that the majority of drugs currently used for the treatment of gynecological malignancies do not impair ovarian function. On the contrary, the dose of pelvic radiation therapy required to control pelvic malignant conditions definitively inhibits the reproductive and hormonal function of the ovaries, and impairs the ability of the uterus to maintain a viable pregnancy.

As a consequence, preservation of fertility in the management of gynecologic malignancies requires the maintenance of at least the uterus and one ovary without radiation therapy, if possible without inducing pelvic adhesions impairing fertility, though the latter can be overcome using assisted reproductive technologies. This chapter will provide the available evidence that selected gynecologic malignancies may be safely managed by conservative surgery alone or medical treatment. Conservative surgery is defined as surgery with complete staging and preservation of at least the uterine corpus and at least part of one ovary.

CARCINOMA OF THE UTERINE CERVIX

With the development of the screening policies, more and more women are likely to be diagnosed during early cervical tumor. For the younger patients, the question of fertility potential is raised in addition of the treatment of their malignancy. The concept of radical trachelectomy (1) is designed to answer this question. It consists of the resection of cervix, upper vagina, proximal parametria, and the reanastomosis of the uterine corpus to the vagina.

Initially described in 1956 by Aburel as an open procedure—with no reported pregnancy—the operation was updated in 1987 by Dargent, who designed a combination of a transvaginal radical trachelectomy reproducing the initial steps of a modified Schauta operation and a laparoscopic pelvic lymphadenectomy.

Surgical Technique

The operation starts with a laparoscopic pelvic lymph node dissection. The rationales for lymph node dissection are multiple: comprehensive staging and therapy, selection of node-negative patients, knowing that node-positive patients are usually offered definitive radiation, and chemotherapy without consideration for later pregnancies. The rationale for the use of laparoscopic techniques is the reduction of de novo adhesion formation after laparoscopy as compared to laparotomy (2). As per surgeon's preference, laparoscopic lymph node dissection is performed as a staging operation before definitive pathology of nodes and final decision or as part of the same operation. If the latter option is favored, frozen section of nodes are required, with a 89% sensitivity (3). Sentinel node identification may in the future improve the accuracy of frozen section, as a tool to send a limited number of relevant nodes to the pathologist (4). If the nodes are positive, surgery of the primary tumor is aborted, an aortic node dissection is performed, and the patient is offered radiation and concurrent chemotherapy.

The vaginal step of the operation (5,6) is illustrated in Figures 1 to 7. To summarize, the technique is similar to a Schauta (radical vaginal) hysterectomy up to the point when the cardinal ligaments are divided. As this point, uterine arteries are identified and spared, cervical arteries are divided, the isthmus is identified, and the endocervix is divided at least 5 mm below the isthmus, according to Dargent, or preferably 10 mm, according to the Quebec team (7). After removal, the specimen is optionally sent for frozen section (8). Frozen section is not performed when a diagnostic cone biopsy has removed in toto the disease. When some disease is remaining in the cervix, frozen section evaluates the upper margin of resection and the gross distance between malignant growth and margins. Additional excision of the endocervix may be indicated. When the requirements for clear margins cannot be fulfilled without definitively impairing reproductive function of the uterus, the Schauta operation is completed.

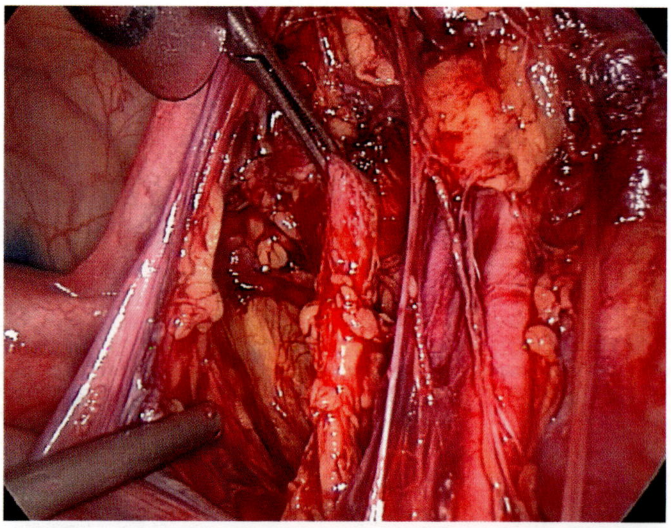

Figure 1 Right pelvic dissection. (Right to left) Psoas muscle, genitofemoral nerve, external iliac artery, external iliac vein, obturator nodes (grasped by the forceps), and paravesical space. The obliterated umbilical artery is moved medially by the suction cannula.

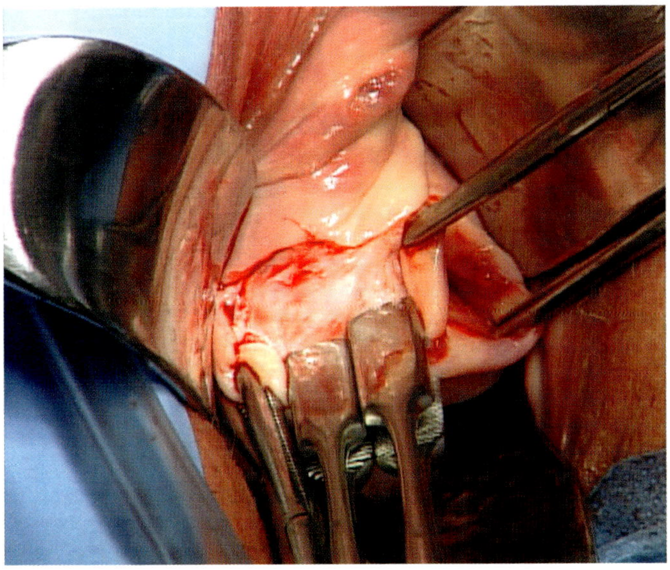

Figure 2 Vaginal incision. The upper vagina is enclosed in a series of forceps.

When the margins are found to be clear, a permanent cerclage is placed around the isthmus. The suture starts, and finally the knot is tied, posteriorly. This avoids later discharge secondary to the exposition of the knot, which occurs more frequently when the knot is tied anteriorly (9). The uterine cervix is then re-anastomosed to the vagina using interrupted sutures or partial Sturmdorf sutures, taking care not to cover the internal os. A Foley catheter is placed in the bladder. In our experience, the bladder catheter is removed on the second postoperative day and bladder function is checked.

Other Techniques

More recently, the historical Aburel abdominal approach has been revisited, with subsequent pregnancies (10,11).

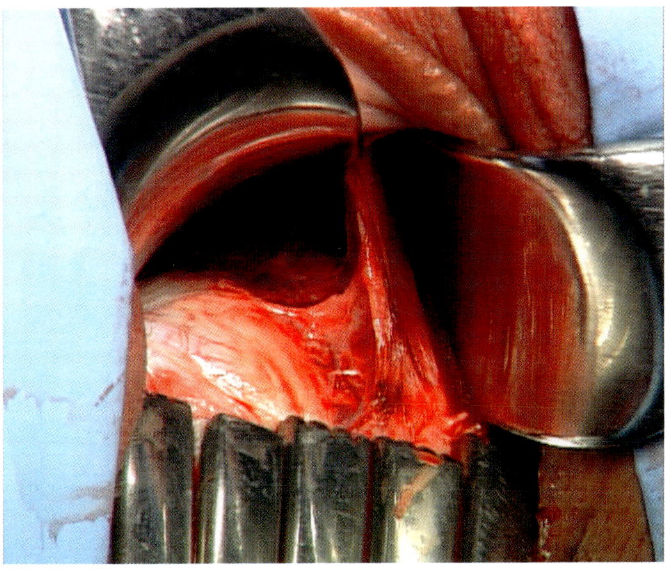

Figure 3 The vesicovaginal space and the left paravesical space are opened. The bladder pillar is visible. It contains the ureter.

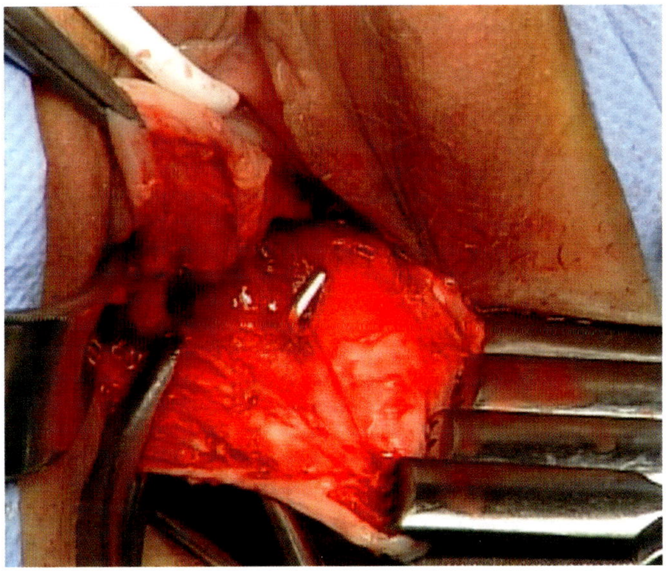

Figure 4 The right paracervix (cardinal ligament) is clamped. The tip of the clamp is placed close to the knee of the ureter. The paraisthmic window separated the cervix, upper vagina, and paracervix, from the uterine corpus and its blood supply by the uterine artery.

The abdominal technique is similar to the original vaginal approach, although uterine arteries may have to be divided during the process, with or without reanastomosis. It may be elected by surgeons who are not at ease with radical vaginal procedures. The laparoscopic variant, which mimics the abdominal operation, has also been described (12,13). In addition, less than radical surgery, involving simple trachelectomy, may be accepted in selected cases of early cervical cancer with negative nodes (14), although this cannot be accepted as a standard.

Oncological Outcome

A case–control study comparing conservative versus radical management has provided evidence of the safety of the

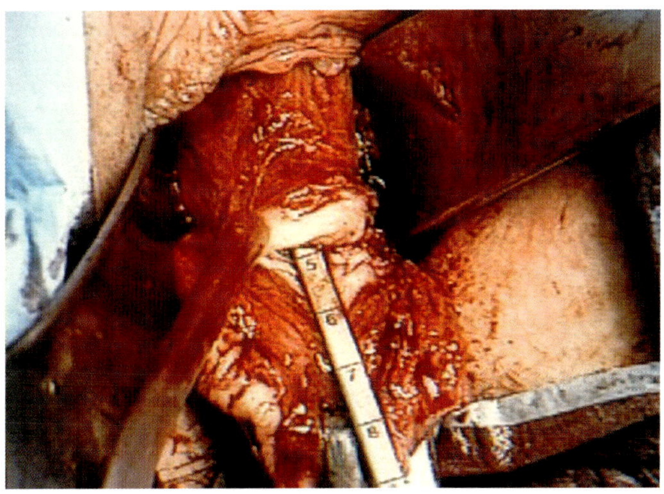

Figure 5 The anterior half of the cervix has been divided, the cervical canal is catheterized, and the size of the remaining uterus is assessed.

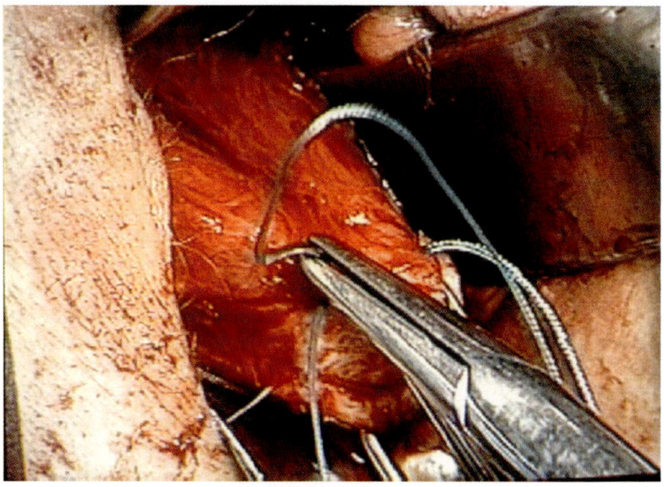

Figure 6 A permanent cerclage is placed around the isthmus.

concept (15). Central as well as lateropelvic or distant metastases have been described (16,17). An ovarian recurrence has been reported (18).

The most recent information about long-term oncological results has been presented in 2006 at the 11th Biennial Meeting of the International Gynecologic Cancer Society (IGCS), Santa Monica, California (19). A combination of databases of seven major centers in Canada, Germany, United States, and France totaled 532 patients. Incidentally, duration of surgery was 232 minutes and hospital stay averaged 4.7 days in this large collaborative series. The intraoperative and postoperative complications secondary to lymph node dissection and trachelectomy, were 1% and 1.4%, and 5.6% and 15.3% respectively. Thirty-two patients had some adjuvant therapy impairing fertility as a result of positive nodes or margins. In the remaining 500 patients, 18 recurrences were observed, 7 of them were central recurrences. Six patients died of disease.

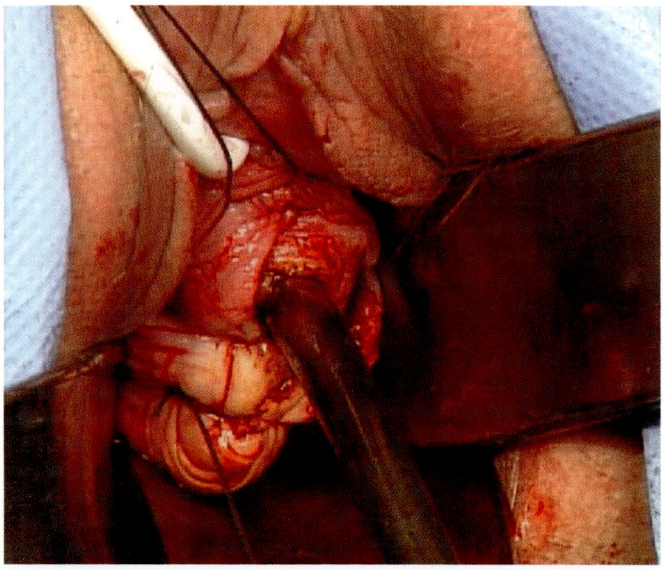

Figure 7 The vagina is re-anastomosed to the uterine isthmus.

No influence of pathologic subtype was found, which means that adenocarcinoma is an acceptable indication. Lymph vascular space invasion (LVSI) and tumor diameter were strongly related to the risk of recurrence. Tumor diameter was available in 189 patients. Two patients out of 22 presenting with tumors larger than 2 cm had recurrence compared to 4 out of 167 patients presenting with tumors less than 2 cm ($P < .001$). Information on peritumoral LVSI was available in 403 patients. A significant proportion (11 out of 99, 11%) of patients with LVSI had recurrence compared to 4 out of 304 patients without LVSI ($P < .001$).

This large series provides a clear information available for a safe selection of patients: only node-negative patients, less than 2 cm squamous cell or adenocarcinoma of the uterine cervix, without LVSI. Other pathologic subtypes are excluded. Patients with polypoid tumors larger than 2 cm with a narrow implantation base on the cervix, far from the endocervical canal may be accepted. The presence of LVSI is a strong argument against the indication.

Obstetrical Outcome

Although Dargent's operation is reserved to young women with a real desire of childbearing, some patients do not really desire pregnancy. Preserving at least the option of future childbearing may be the only goal of the operation. Infertility related to the reduction of cervical function does exist but is becoming less frequent as a result of a trend toward strict selection of patients allowing to preserve a 10 mm endocervix (7). Patients presenting with evidence of impaired fertility may be included as long as the infertility factor is curable. Assisted reproductive techniques including in vitro fertilization, intrauterine insemination, and ovarian stimulation have been used after radical trachelectomy (20).

Pregnancies occur in approximately half of patients. There is a definite risk of premature birth or late abortion, which is only partially prevented by permanent isthmic cerclage and additional cervical closure during pregnancy. Early reports by the Lyon team and others (20) found an average 17% of second trimester loss. This can be overcome only by maintaining 10 mm of endocervix (7,21).

Preoperative Workup and Selection of Patients

Selection of patients is crucial to ensure oncological safety and prevent second trimester abortions and premature deliveries. Specific preoperative workup includes MRI and cone biopsy. MRI allows to precisely assess the maximum diameter of the tumor, selecting with a few exceptions patients with tumors less or equal to 2 cm. Localization of the upper limit of the tumor is another essential information that helps to predict the requirements for endocervical resection and estimate the length of remaining endocervix.

A majority of patients are referred after diagnostic cone biopsy. Careful review of the report and whenever necessary review of slides is mandatory. Special attention is given to the identification of lymph-vascular space invasion. The adverse prognosis attached to the presence of LVSI is important enough to advise preoperative cone biopsy in all cases, although repeat multiple biopsies may help to rule out this prognostic factor, this is considered by many researchers as a contraindication to conservative surgery and an indication for adjuvant external radiation therapy.

Another issue is the required upper margin since much of the endocervix should be retained in order to avoid impairing fertility and to improve the obstetrical outcome. On the other hand, a 8 mm clear pathologic margin is theoretically required for squamous cell cancer, as observed in vulvar cancers (22). There is obviously a trade-off between fertility preservation and oncological safety that also affects patient selection: location of the upper endocervical limit of the tumor must be compatible with the dual requirement of sufficient clear margin and sufficient remaining endocervix.

Finally, aggressive pathologic subtypes such as neuroendocrine carcinomas are absolute contraindication. Overall, after a careful selection process, up to 40% of patients presenting with cervical cancer before the age of 40 might still be candidate to conservative management (23).

Other Fertility Preserving Options

Neoadjuvant chemotherapy followed by simple conization has also been proposed (24-26). Although investigational, this option is the only one available for patients with tumors larger than 2 cm.

EPITHELIAL OVARIAN CANCER

Conservative treatment of at least a part of one ovary and the uterus in order to preserve fertility in young patients can be proposed in selected patients with epithelial ovarian cancer (EOC). However, the results and limits of such treatment remain unclear. Only three studies involving a large number of patients have been published on the results of conservative management of EOC (27–29). The largest and the only one to include a centralized pathologic review of the ovarian tumor by the same pathologist is the French study (29). Thirty-four patients of this study fulfilled all inclusion criteria. Thirty patients had stage IA disease (G1, $n = 13$; G2, $n = 14$; G3, $n = 3$), three patients has stage IC, and one patient had stage IIA. Ten patients received postoperative chemotherapy. Eleven patients recurred: 10 patients had invasive disease and 1 had borderline recurrence. Among the 10 patients with invasive recurrence, initial stage and grade were as follows: stage IA G1, $n = 1$; stage IA G2, $n = 4$; stage IA G3, $n = 1$; stage $\geq$ IC, $n = 4$. Overall, all patients with stage > IA had recurrence. Ten pregnancies were observed in 9 patients. The conclusion is that conservative management is safe in stage IA grade 1 patients, can be discussed in stage IA grade 2 and in selected small volume stage IA grade 3 patients, but patients in stages IC and over must be excluded. Comprehensive staging including peritoneal cytology, peritoneal biopsies, omentectomy, systematic bilateral pelvic and aortic lymph node dissection, and dilatation and curettage is mandatory to correctly stage candidate patients and exclude occult advanced stage disease. Pathological examination by a pathologist experienced in ovarian malignancy is mandatory.

As far as the affected ovary is concerned, unilateral salpingo-oophorectomy is advised as a standard. The technique is straightforward, although the need for an oncologically safe removal, without any rupture or morcellation and consequent contamination of the peritoneal cavity or abdominal wall, must be stressed. In this regard, laparoscopic technique or small transverse incisions may adversely affect the outcome if they lead to faulty technique and contamination of the abdominal wall. On the other hand, laparoscopic surgery is adapted to the reassessment of apparent stage I diagnosed during primary surgery (30). Laparoscopic surgery by an experienced surgeon allows careful examination of the contralateral ovary, is an adapted tool to rule out peritoneal growth, and has been found to be a safe technique to perform advanced staging operation such as omentectomy and pelvic/aortic lymph node dissection (31).

Some reports of pregnancy after chemotherapy for advanced ovarian cancer are available in the literature (32). Anecdotically, pregnancies have been reported in patients previous managed by normothermic or hyperthermic intraperitoneal chemotherapy (33).

GERM CELL TUMORS OF THE OVARY

Germ cell tumors are rare, but prefentially occur in adolescent or young women (34). As the patients are usually curable with fertility preservation at all stages of disease including stage III, fertility preservation is a mainstay of surgical management. This also holds in the setting of residual masses after chemotherapy, which may be benign. Preoperative diagnosis is essential, and involves a routine performance of specific markers in all young women that present with a pelvic mass. Elevated alpha-fetoprotein for the diagnostic of yolk sac tumors and human chorionic gonadotrophin for the diagnosis of choriocarcinoma are diagnostic of an ovarian germ cell tumor. CA-125, lactate dehydrogenase, and placental alkaline phosphatase are less sensitive and less specific. Diagnosis of malignant transformation of mature teratomas is more difficult and depends on the size and squamous cell carcinoma marker of apparently benign dermoid cysts. Diagnosis of nonsecreting dysgerminomas and immature teratomas is obtained only at final pathology. Thus, conservative management is advisable in young patients even in the case of advanced disease with peritoneal implants. Frozen section is not reliable enough to decide a hasty radical surgery. Unilateral salpingo-oophorectomy is safe, but is too radical if the tumor is benign. Cystectomy may thus be acceptable (35).

Most patients, but those with stage I dysgerminomas or low-grade immature teratomas, will receive platinum- and etoposide-based chemotherapy, with or without bleomycin. Fertility is not impaired after chemotherapy for germ cell tumor of the ovary (36).

BORDERLINE OVARIAN TUMORS

As the majority of borderline ovarian tumors (BOT) are observed in patients of reproductive age, fertility is a major issue in young female patients presenting with suspicious adnexal masses. It must be stressed that BOT are not precursors of ovarian cancer, and recurrence as a malignant tumor is observed in only 2% of cases (37,38). BOT are almost invariably controlled by surgical management, and the use of chemotherapy is limited to the infrequent occurrence of invasive peritoneal implants. Recurrence is possible, but can still be controlled by repeat surgery (39,40). Prognosis is excellent, with 97% to 98% long-term survival in early stages and 92% in advanced stage serous BOT. Advanced stage mucinous BOT carry a worse prognosis, but the difficulties of differential diagnosis with invasive adenocarcinoma might account for the apparent difference in prognosis.

In general, definitive pathology by an experienced pathologist is required for the diagnosis of BOT in order to rule out invasive disease and to identify micropapillary serous BOT, which carry a worse prognosis and are classified by some researchers as "low-grade carcinomas" rather than

BOT. When a doubt persists at the time of surgery and frozen section, conservative management and then referral to an oncological team including experienced surgeons and pathologists is advised.

The mainstay of management of BOT in young female patients is conservative surgery. Total hysterectomy and bilateral salpingo-oophorectomy is no longer advocated in young patients, whatever the stage. Unilateral salpingo-oophorectomy is standard. Cystectomy is accepted only when the tumor is bilateral or develops on a remaining ovary. When a BOT is diagnosed after cystectomy of an apparent benign ovarian cyst, complementary salpingo-oophorectomy is indicated only in multifocal or large tumors, and/or when complete removal has not been clearly obtained. Conservative surgical management of advanced stage BOT is acceptable after extensive discussion and informed consent of a patient eagerly desiring children (41).

Surgical staging is based on careful macroscopic examination of the contralateral ovary and peritoneum. Biopsy of the contralateral ovary is not advised as it may induce adhesions without improving the detection of implants compared to visual examination of the ovary. Removal and pathological examination of any extraovarian growth is mandatory to completely manage the disease and detect invasive implants. Node dissection is not standard. Omentectomy, and appendectomy in mucinous tumors, is part of surgical staging and management. However, the low yield of restaging surgery in incompletely staged patients does not justify routine reoperation for the only purpose of random biopsies (42).

Recurrence rate is definitely higher after conservative surgery: 7% of patients experience recurrence, most frequently on the contralateral ovary, after unilateral salpingo-oophorectomy. Recurrences on the affected ovary are observed in patients managed by cystectomy only, accounting for an overall recurrence rate of 23% (40). Repeat fertility-preserving surgery is acceptable (38). Fertility-inducing methods, including ovarian stimulation, have been shown not to impair the outcome (43). However, most researchers advise limitation of the number of stimulation cycles.

SEX CORD STROMAL TUMORS

Sex cord stromal tumors may occasionally carry a malignant evolution. The majority of unilateral sex cord stromal tumors can be managed conservatively in patients of reproductive age, as the survival for patients who undergo unilateral salpingo-oophorectomy is similar to patients who are managed by hysterectomy (44). Standard staging is similar to BOT. The need for lymph node dissection is not clearly established, as the yield of lymph node dissection is quite low at the time of primary management, while late node recurrences account for a significant proportion of long-term recurrences (45). However, radical surgery and chemotherapy are indicated in advanced stage disease.

ENDOMETRIAL ADENOCARCINOMAS

Multiple reports have proposed a conservative management of early clinical stage and low-grade adenocarcinoma of the uterus by using hormonal therapy in patients younger than 40 years. An extensive review of the English literature up to December 2003 is available on the topic (46). The study included 81 patients, from 27 papers, who were given progestin therapy, mainly medroxyprogesterone acetate or megestrol acetate: 19 patients (24%) did not respond; 62 patients (76%) responded after a median time of 12 weeks (range 4–60), but 15 of them later recurred after a median time to recurrence of 19 months (range 6–44); 10 patients ultimately had total hysterectomy; and overall, 20 patients-approximately 1 out of 4-experienced at least one pregnancy. No patient included in this review died of disease.

An additional major paper has been published in 2007, reporting a series of nine patients who were given 400 mg of medroxyprogesterone per day for six months; four out of eight married women conceived; two patients recurred but none died of disease (47). However, publication bias may overestimate the safety of conservative management via underreporting of failures.

The only accepted indication is stage IA grade 1 endometrial cancer. After office diagnostic endometrial biopsy, the final step of diagnosis and first step of treatment is a dilatation and curettage, which ensures an accurate grading performed by an experienced pathologist. Careful workup is mandatory to rule out myometrial invasion and extrauterine disease. In this regard, magnetic resonance imaging (MRI), ideally performed before dilatation and curettage by an experienced radiologist, is essential. However, specificity of MRI in ruling out minimal myometrial invasion is not 100%, and this is one of the limitations of the indications for conservative managements. In addition, diagnostic laparoscopy is advised. Peritoneal cytology sampling, examination of the peritoneal cavity, and careful examination of the ovaries in order to rule out ovarian disease is mandatory (48). Lymph node dissection is not mandatory, knowing the occurrence of positive node is quite uncommon in stage IA grade 1 endometrial cancers, but could be decided as an additional precaution considering that MRI is not totally accurate and that positive lymph nodes have been reported in stage IA grade 1 patients (49).

There is currently no standard regimen for the choice of drug, dosage, and evaluation of response. Intrauterine progesterone delivered via a progesterone-containing intrauterine device has also been used in 12 patients. Results of biopsies were negative in 7 of 11 patients at 6 months and 6 of 8 patients at 12 months (50). Daily administration of a synthetic progestin during 12 weeks is generally accepted as a minimal option before a first evaluation of response by repeat dilatation and curettage. Duration of therapy is not standardized. The median duration of treatment in patients who respond is 24 weeks (46). Optimal time from completion of progesterone therapy to attempting pregnancy is still unknown. Considering that young women who develop endometrial adenocarcinoma are typically affected by polycystic ovarian syndrome and chronic anovulation, fertility is affected in this group of patients and ovarian stimulation or surgical techniques may be required to favor ovulation and pregnancy.

Atypical endometrial hyperplasia, which is a precursor of endometrial cancer, can be managed in a similar way. However, inclusion of endometrial hyperplasia patients in series is not advisable, as it may artificially lead to the conclusion that hormonal therapy is safe only in early endometrial cancer. As a consequence, pathology of the dilatation and curettage must be reviewed in order to rule out noninvasive disease. Gynecologists must be aware that the differential diagnosis between atypical hyperplasia and early endometrial cancer is subtle and that discrepancies between pathologists does exist. As atypical endometrial hyperplasia may not respond to curettage and hormonal therapy, close follow-up of this group of patients with serial endometrial biopsies is mandatory.

As a conclusion of this section, many questions are still unanswered. The safety of conservative management of endometrial cancers in young women is not definitively established. Comprehensive counseling, careful workup, and close follow-up are mandatory.

UTERINE SARCOMAS

It is widely accepted that uterine sarcomas require upfront surgical management including total hysterectomy. In addition, low-grade endometrial stromal sarcomas are hormone dependent, which means that bilateral oophorectomy is an essential feature of surgical management. Even though carcinosarcomas are managed as adenocarcinomas, they are assimilated to grade 3 adenocarcinomas and therefore cannot be managed conservatively.

Exceptions to the rule are few: Low-grade uterine sarcomas found after myomectomy in young patients have been managed conservatively after extensive imaging and counseling (51). Mullerian adenosarcomas presenting as polyps may also be managed conservatively under the same restrictions.

On the other hand, preferential management of vaginal and cervical rhabdomyosarcomas in children is definitely conservative, based on chemotherapy completed by surgery or radiation therapy only in those girls who do not achieve complete remission (52).

TROPHOBLASTIC DISEASE

Although trophoblastic disease is beyond the scope of this book, a few basic principles must be recalled. Malignant trophoblastic disease typically occurs in patients of reproductive age. Cure rates after chemotherapy are high even in the setting of advanced disease. Fertility after single or multiagent chemotherapy for persistent trophoblastic disease is not impaired, and no adverse effects on offspring have been observed (53). Fertility outcome of patients is excellent and can only be impaired by the faulty performance of repeat curettage inducing intrauterine adhesions or expeditive hysterectomy in the context of bleeding or suspicious uterine mass. Uterine masses suspicious at ultrasound in young patients with a recent history of pregnancy require blood tests to detect trophoblastic disease, which may be diagnostic, and avoid faulty radical surgery. Indications for surgery in the setting of persistent uterine choriocarcinomas without extrauterine disease are rare. Local excision has been described and may be therapeutic in selected patients with minimal residual choriocarcinoma or placental site trophoblastic tumor after chemotherapy (54).

CANCER AND CONCURRENT PREGNANCY (55)

Radical surgery and/or termination of pregnancy is not a standard feature of management of gynecologic malignancies in pregnant patients. Fetal outcome is good whenever pregnancy has been preserved (56).

A delay to initiation of therapy is accepted in the majority of third trimester and late second trimester patients. Cesarean section in the presence of a gynecologic oncologist ensures the dual purpose of adequate perinatologic care and standard oncological management. Surgical staging and/or management according to standards can be performed at the time of laparotomy for cesarean section.

Patients in the first or early second trimester must be counseled and managed by an experienced team. Early carcinomas of the cervix can be staged using MRI and/or laparoscopic lymph node dissection and then managed conservatively using cone biopsy only or radical trachelectomy according to the extent of disease. Cone biopsy is indicated only in the case of early invasive (IA1) disease, or, in the case of completely removed IA2 disease without LVSI. Vaginal or abdominal trachelectomy is possible in patients with early IB1 cervical cancers without node metastasis (1,57). More advanced cervical cancers can be staged during pregnancy by using MRI and laparoscopic lymph node dissection. Some of them can be managed after informed consent by neoadjuvant chemotherapy during pregnancy (58). Adnexal malignancies can be managed by unilateral or bilateral salpingo-oophorectomy along with comprehensive staging and cytoreduction. Chemotherapy during pregnancy followed by definitive surgical management at the time of cesarean section has been proposed in advanced ovarian cancer (59). Vulvar cancer is managed in a standard fashion while preserving the pregnancy; but not in the case of node-positive disease found at the time of early pregnancy, a condition that imposes groin radiation therapy.

FERTILITY AFTER RADICAL SURGERY OR DEFINITIVE RADIATION THERAPY OF GYNECOLOGIC MALIGNANCY

Fertility is still a concern in patients who cannot be managed conservatively. The impact of medically assisted reproductive technologies must be taken into account. Preservation of the ovaries along with total hysterectomy may preserve the possibility of oocyte retrieval, in vitro fertilization, and surrogate pregnancy (60–63).

The option is reasonable, after informed consent, when the risk of ovarian metastasis is minimal. An additional advantage is avoiding the need for hormone replacement therapy. The case of early stage carcinoma of the cervix not amenable to radical trachelectomy is definitely acceptable, as the risk of ovarian metastasis in the case of early squamous cell cervical cancer is negligible, which is not true in the case of large tumoral volume, positive nodes, or adenocarcinoma subtype. Removal or radiation therapy of the ovaries is indicated in the latter, again after informed consent and full information based on the risk of ovarian recurrence. The same reservations hold in the case of early endometrial cancer (64). Preservation of the ovaries is straightforward when surgery alone is used. When definitive radiation therapy is applied, preservation of the ovary requires high ovarian transposition, which can be performed using laparoscopic techniques (65).

Preservation of the uterus at the time of bilateral oophorectomy is acceptable when the uterus is unaffected at the time of surgery—dilatation and curettage is required to document this—and when later risk of uterine involvement is minimal. Uterine preservation ensures the possibility of pregnancy after in vitro fertilization of donated or cryopreserved oocytes. Preservation of the uterus is always possible in the case of BOT, and is more questionable in the presence of invasive ovarian malignancy, where the limitations to conservative surgery in ovarian cancer apply. Although cryopreservation of ovarian fragments has resulted in pregnancies after pelvic reimplantation of ovarian tissue (66), application of the same technique is a major concern in the case of bilateral ovarian cancer, as ovarian tissue may harbor malignant cells. Future development of techniques allowing successful in vitro follicle and gamete maturation may help overcome the risk of inducing a relapse after reimplantation.

CONCLUSIONS

Preservation or intentional sacrifice of fertility is an essential part of counseling at the time of management of primary gynecologic malignancy in a potentially fertile patient. Upfront radical surgery is not acceptable without informed consent and full exploration of the possibilities of fertility preserving policies is recommended. Gynecologic surgeons and gynecologic oncologists must be aware of all the available techniques. They must also be aware that upfront hysterectomy and/or bilateral salpingo-oophorectomy is faulty in adolescent or young female patients who could be safely managed by using conservative techniques. Careful preoperative workup of any uterine or ovarian mass is the best prevention of unexpected findings and difficult decisions at the time of surgery. In the case of unexpected suspicious ovarian tumors in young patients, comprehensive staging and awaiting the results of definitive pathology, before undertaking the conclusive operation, is standard practice. The limitations of frozen section as a diagnostic test between BOT and invasive ovarian tumors must be known (67).

On the other hand, conservative management seems reasonable only in patients currently or potentially desiring pregnancy. The minimal additional risk of recurrence involved by the conservation of uterus and ovary is not acceptable when pregnancy is not at stake.

Patients managed with fertility preservation deserve active follow-up. Special consideration must be given to the need of annual ultrasound examination of retained ovaries (BOT or ovarian cancer patients), or Pap smears, and MRI in radical trachelectomy patients. Patients with a stable partner should be advised to attempt pregnancy, considering the cumulative risk of recurrence with time. Any infertility factor must be corrected using available techniques including ovarian stimulation, which is not contraindicated even after BOT. Exceptions to the general rule are high-risk conditions, including advanced germ cell tumors that may need additional chemotherapy, knowing that the confounding effect of pregnancy on the levels of markers is a follow-up issue.

It is not clear whether radical surgery is indicated after completion of the desire of pregnancy. It is reasonable to advise total hysterectomy in the case of uterine adenocarcinoma (68) and contralateral oophorectomy in the case of invasive ovarian cancer. In other conditions, such as BOT or conservatively managed cervical cancers, the final decision will be taken with the patient, taking into consideration the risk and curability of recurrence, the accuracy of follow-up in the detection of recurrences, and psychological considerations.

REFERENCES

1. Dargent D, Martin X, Sacchetoni A, et al. Laparoscopic vaginal radical trachelectomy: A treatment to preserve the fertility of cervical carcinoma patients. Cancer 2000; 88:1877–1882.
2. Lanvin D, Elhage A, Henry B, et al. Accuracy and safety of laparoscopic lymphadenectomy. An experimental prospective randomized study. Gynecol Oncol 1997; 67:83–87.
3. Morice P, Sabourin JC, Castaigne D, et al. Frozen section for lymph nodes in uterine cervical carcinoma. Clin Exp Pathol 1999; 47:223–226.
4. Lambaudie E, Collinet P, Narducci F, et al. Laparoscopic identification of sentinel lymph nodes in early stage cervical cancer: Prospective study using a combination of patent blue dye injection and technetium radiocolloid injection. Gynecol Oncol 2003; 89:84–87.
5. Cosson M, Querleu D, Dargent D. Chirurgie Vaginale. Paris: Masson, 2004.
6. Cosson M, Querleu D, Dargent D. Vaginal Surgery. Boca Raton, FL: Taylor and Francis, 2005.
7. Plante M, Renaurd MC, Hoskins IA, et al. Vaginal radical trachelectomy: A valuable fertility-preserving option in the management of early-stage cervical cancer. A series of 50 pregnancies and review of the literature. Gynecol Oncol 2005; 98:3–10.
8. Tanguay C, Plante M, Renaud MC, et al. Vaginal radical trachelectomy in the treatment of cervical cancer: The role of frozen section. Int J Gynecol Pathol 2004; 23:170–175.
9. Allahdin S, Lees DAR, Busby-Earle RMC, et al. Persistent vaginal discharge after radical trachelectomy. J Obstet Gynaecol 2004; 24:941–942.
10. Smith JR, Boyle DC, Corless DJ, et al. Abdominal radical trachelectomy: a new surgical technique for the conservative management of cervical carcinoma. BJOG 1997; 104:1196–1200.
11. Ungar L, Palfalvi L, Hogg R, et al. Abdominal radical trachelectomy: A fertility-preserving option for women with early cervical cancer. BJOG 2005; 112:366–369.
12. Lee CL, Huang KG, Wang CJ, et al. Laparoscopic radical trachelectomy for stage Ib1 cervical cancer. J Am Assoc Gynecol Laparosc 2003; 10:111–115.
13. Cibula D, Ungar L, Palfalvi L, et al. Laparoscopic abdominal radical trachelectomy. Gynecol Oncol 2005; 97:707–709.
14. Rob L, Charvat M, Robova H, et al. Less radical fertility-sparing than radical trachelectomy in early cervical cancer. Int J Gynecol Cancer 2007; 17:304–310.
15. Covens A, Shaw P, Murphy J, et al. Is radical trachelectomy a safe alternative to radical hysterectomy for patients with stage IA-B carcinoma of the cervix. Cancer 1999; 86:2273–2279.
16. Plante M, Renaud MC, François H, et al. Vaginal radical trachelectomy: an oncologically safe fertility-preserving surgery. An updated series of 72 cases and review of the literature. Gynecol Oncol 2004; 94:614–623.
17. Hertel H, Kohler C, Grund D, et al. Radical vaginal trachelectomy (RVT) combined with laparoscopic pelvic lymphadenectomy: Prospective multicenter study of 100 patients with early cervical cancer. Gynecol Oncol 2006: 103:506–511.
18. Piketty M, Barranger E, Najat M, et al. Ovarian recurrence after radical trachelectomy for adenocarcinoma of the cervix. Am J Obstet Gynecol 2005; 193:1382–1383.
19. Chopin N, Covens A, Roy M, et al. Radical vaginal trachelectomy with laparoscopic pelvic lymph node dissection (Dargent's operation): A multicenter collaborative study. Presented at the 11th Biennial Meeting of the International Gynecologic Cancer Society (IGCS), Santa Monica, CA, October 14–18, 2006.
20. Burnett AF. Radical trachelectomy with laparoscopic lymphadenectomy: Review of oncologic and obstetrical outcomes. Curr Opin Obstet Gynecol 2006; 18:8–13.
21. Shepherd JH, Spencer C, Herod J, et al. Radical vaginal trachelectomy as a fertility-sparing procedure in women with early-stage cervical cancer-cumulative pregnancy rate in a series of 123 women. BJOG 2006; 113:719–724.
22. De Hullu JA, Hollema H, Lolkema S, et al. Vulvar carcinoma. The price of less radical surgery. Cancer 2002; 95:2331–2338.
23. Sonoda Y, Abu-Rustum NR, Gemignani ML, et al. A fertility-sparing alternative to radical hysterectomy: How many patients may be eligible? Gynecol Oncol. 2004; 95:534–538.
24. Kobayashi Y, Akiyama F, Hasumi K. A case of successful pregnancy after treatment of invasive cervical cancer with systemic chemotherapy and conization. Gynecol Oncol 2006; 100:213–215.
25. Plante M, Lau S, Brydon L, et al. Neoadjuvant chemotherapy followed by vaginal radical trachelectomy in bulky stage IB1 cervical cancer: Case report. Gynecol Oncol 2006; 101:367–370.

26. Andrade JM, Marana HR, Mangieri LF, et al. Successful preservation of fertility subsequent to a complete pathologic response of a squamous cell carcinoma of the uterine cervix treated with primary systemic chemotherapy. Gynecol Oncol 2000; 71:213–215.
27. Zanetta G, Chiari S, Rota S, et al. Conservative surgery for stage I ovarian carcinoma in women of childbearing age. Br J Obstet Gynaecol 1997; 104:1030–1035.
28. Schilder JM, Thompson AM, DePriest PD, et al. Outcome of reproductive age women with stage IA or IC invasive epithelial ovarian cancer treated with fertility-sparing therapy. Gynecol Oncol 2002; 87:1–7.
29. Morice P, Leblanc E, Rey A, et al. Conservative treatment in epithelial ovarian cancer: Results of a multicenter study of the GLCC and SFOG. Hum Reprod 2005; 20:1379–1385.
30. Querleu D, Leblanc E. Laparoscopic infrarenal lymphadenectomy in the restaging of carcinomas of the ovary and fallopian tube. Cancer 1994; 73:1467–1471.
31. Leblanc E, Querleu D, Narducci F, et al. Laparoscopic restaging of early stage invasive adnexal tumors: A 10 year experience. Gynecol Oncol 2004; 94:624–629.
32. Mantovani G, Gramignano G, Mais V, et al. Use of chemotherapy for ovarian cancer during human pregnancy: Case report and literature review. Eur J Obstet Gynecol Reprod Biol 2007; 131:238–239.
33. Kyser K, Bidus KA, Rodriguez M, et al. Spontaneous pregnancy following cytoreduction with peritonectomy and hyperthermic intraperitoneal chemotherapy. Gynecol Oncol 2006; 100:198–200.
34. Patterson DM, Rustin GJS. Controversies in the management of germ cell tumours of the ovary. Curr Opin Oncol 2006; 18:500–506.
35. Beiner ME, Gotlieb WH, Korach Y. Cystectomy for immature teratoma of the ovary. Gynecol Oncol 2004; 93:381–384.
36. Zanetta G, Bonazzi C, Cantu M, et al. Survival and reproductive function after treatment of malignant germ cell ovarian tumors. J Clin Oncol 2001; 19:1015–1020.
37. Zanetta G, Rota S, Chiari S, et al. Behavior of borderline tumors with particular interest to persistence, recurrence and progression to invasive carcinoma: A prospective study. J Clin Oncol 2001; 19:2658–2664.
38. Cadron I, Amant F, Van Gorp T, et al. The management of borderline tumours of the ovary. Curr Opin Oncol 2006; 18:488–493.
39. Rao GG, Skinner EN, Gehrig PA, et al. Fertility-sparing surgery for ovarian low malignant potential tumors. Gynecol Oncol 2005; 98:263–266.
40. Suh-Burgmann E. Long-term outcomes following conservative surgery for borderline tumor of the ovary: A large population-based study. Gynecol Oncol 2006; 103:841–847.
41. Morice P, Camatte S, Rey A, et al. Prognostic factors for patients with advanced stage serous borderline tumours of the ovary. Ann Oncol 2003; 12:592–598.
42. Querleu D, Papageorgiou T, Lambaudie E, et al. Laparoscopic restaging of borderline ovarian tumours: Results of 30 cases initially presumed as stage IA borderline ovarian tumours. BJOG 2003; 110:201–204.
43. Fortin A, Morice P, Thoury A, et al. Impact of fertility drugs after treatment of borderline ovarian tumors: Results of a retrospective multicenter study. Fertil Steril 2007; 87:591–596.
44. Zhang M, Cheung MK, Shin JY, et al. Prognostic factors responsible for survival in sex cord stromal tumors of the ovary—An analysis of 376 women. Gynecol Oncol 2007; 104:396–400.
45. Abu-Rustum NR, Restivo A, Ivy J, et al. Retroperitoneal nodal metastasis in primary and recurrent granulosa cell tumors of the ovary. Gynecol Oncol 2006; 103:31–34.
46. Ramirez PT, Frumovitz M, Bodurka DC, et al. Hormonal therapy for the management of grade 1 endometrial carcinoma: A literature review. Gynecol Oncol 2004; 95:133–138.
47. Yamazawa K, Hirai M, Fujito A, et al. Fertility-preserving treatment with progestin, and pathological criteria to predict responses, in young women with endometrial cancer. Hum Reprod 2007; 22:1953–1958.
48. Morice P, Fourchotte V, Sideris L, et al. A need for laparoscopic evaluation of patients with endometrial carcinoma selected for conservative treatment. Gynecol Oncol 2005; 96:245–248.
49. Takeshima N, Hirai Y, Tanaka N, et al. Pelvic lymph node metastasis in endometrial cancer with no myometrial invasion. Obstet Gynecol 1996; 88:280–282.
50. Montz FJ, Bristow RE, Bovicelli A, et al. Intrauterine progesterone treatment of early endometrial cancer. Am J Obstet Gynecol 2002; 186:651–657.
51. Lissoni A, Cormio G, Bonazzi C, et al. Fertility-sparing surgery in uterine leiomyosarcoma. Gynecol Oncol 1998; 70:348–350.
52. Martelli M, Oberlin O, Rey A, et al. Conservative treatment for girls with nonmetastatic rhabdomyosarcoma of the genital tract: A report from the Study Committee of the International Society of Pediatric Oncology. J Clin Oncol 1999; 17:2117–2122.
53. Goto S, Iko K, Mitsui T, et al. Survival rates of patients with choriocarcinoma treated with chemotherapy without hysterectomy: Effects of anticancer agents on subsequent births. Gynecol Oncol 2004; 93:529–535.
54. Numnum TM, Kilgore LC, Conner MG, et al. Fertility sparing therapy in a patient with placental site trophoblastic tumor: A case report. Gynecol Oncol 2006; 103:1141–1143.
55. Oehler MK, Wain GV, Brand A. Gynaecological malignancies in pregnancy: A review. Aust N Z J Obstet Gynaecol 2003; 43:414–420.
56. Ghaemmaghami F, Hasanzadeh M. Good fetal outcome of pregnancies with gynaecologic cancer conditions. Int J Gynecol Cancer 2006; 16(S1):225–230.
57. Ungar L, Smith JR, Palfalvi L, et al. Abdominal radical trachelectomy during pregnancy to preserve pregnancy and fertility. Obstet Gynecol 2006; 108:811–814.
58. Caluwaerts S, van Calsteren K, Mertens L, et al. Neoadjuvant chemotherapy followed by radical hysterectomy for invasive cervical cancer diagnosed during pregnancy: Report of a case and review of the literature. Int J Gynecol Cancer 2006; 16:905–908.
59. Tabata T, Nishiura K, Tanida K, et al. Carboplatin chemotherapy in a pregnant patient with undifferentiated ovarian carcinoma: Case report and review of the literature. Int J Gynecol Cancer 2008; 18:181–184.
60. Zhang J, Grifo JA, Del Priore G. Gestational carrier pregnancy with oocytes obtained during surgery for stage IIIc ovarian cancer after controlled ovarian stimulation. Fertil Steril 2005, 83:1547–1549.
61. Azim A, Oktay K. Letrozole for ovulation induction and fertility preservation by embryo cryopreservation in young women with endometrial carcinoma [published online ahead of print Apr 9, 2007]. Fertil Steril.
62. Juretzka MM, O'Hanlan KA, Katz SL, et al. Embryo cryopreservation after diagnosis of stage IIB endometrial cancer and subsequent pregnancy in a gestational carrier. Fertil Steril 2005; 83:1041.
63. Zinger M, Liu JH, Husseinzadeh N, et al. Successful surrogate pregnancy after ovarian transposition, pelvic irradiation and hysterectomy. J Reprod Med 2004; 49:573–574.
64. Lee TS, Jung JY, Kim JW, et al. Feasibility of ovarian preservation in patients with early stage endometrial carcinoma. Gynecol Oncol 2007; 124:52–57.
65. Morice P, Castaigne P, Haie-Meder C, et al. Laparoscopic ovarian transposition for pelvic malignancies: Indications and functional outcomes. Fertil Steril 1998; 70:956–960.
66. Donnez J, Dolmans MM, Demylle D, et al. Livebirth after orthotopic transplantation of cryopreserved ovarian tissue. Lancet 2004; 364:1405–1410.
67. Houck K, Nikrui N, Duska L, et al. Borderline tumors of the ovary: Correlation of frozen and permanent histopathologic diagnosis. Obstet Gynecol 2000; 95:839–843.
68. Ferrandina G, Zannoni GF, Gallotta V, et al. Progression of conservatively treated endometrial carcinoma after full term pregnancy: A case report. Gynecol Oncol 2005; 99:215–217.

26

Ovarian preservation

Jacques Donnez, Marie-Madeleine Dolmans, Anne-Sophie Van Eyck, Anne Van Langendonckt, Pascale Jadoul, and Jean Squifflet

INTRODUCTION

It is now estimated that 1 in every 250 people in the adult population is a childhood cancer survivor. In recent years, around 1,400,000 new cancer cases were expected annually in the United States, approximately half of which were expected to be women. According to previous reports, 8% of these women were predicted to be under 40 years of age.

Advances in the diagnosis and treatment of childhood, adolescent, and adult cancer have greatly increased the life expectancy of premenopausal women with cancer, but have resulted in a growing population of adolescent and adult long-term survivors of childhood malignancies (2), who may experience infertility problems due to induced premature ovarian failure (POF). Aggressive chemotherapy, radiotherapy, and bone marrow transplantation can cure more than 90% of girls and young women affected by such disorders (3,4). However, the ovaries are very sensitive to cytotoxic treatment, especially to alkylating agents (e.g., cyclophosphamide, busulfan, melphalan, chlorambucil, dacarbazine, procarbazine, ifosfamide, thiotepa, and nitrogen mustard), which are classified as high risk for gonadal dysfunction (for review, see Ref. 4).

Cyclophosphamide is the agent most commonly implicated in causing damage to oocytes and granulosa cells in a dose-dependent manner (5). This follicular destruction generally results in the loss of both endocrine and reproductive function, depending on the dose and the age of the patient. Complete amenorrhea was reported after a dose of 5 g of cyclophosphamide in women older than 40 years and after doses of 9 g and 20 g in women of 30 to 40 and 20 to 30 years of age, respectively (6).

Intensive chemotherapy and/or total body irradiation (TBI) required before bone marrow transplantation (BMT) constitute the treatment combination presenting the greatest risk of POF. Indeed, the high doses of chemotherapy (commonly using the highly cytotoxic cyclophosphamide/busulfan regimen) and/or radiotherapy lead to subsequent ovarian failure in almost all cases, children and adults alike (4,7–8).

The different options available for fertility preservation in cancer patients are embryo cryopreservation, oocyte cryopreservation, and ovarian tissue cryopreservation. The choice depends on various parameters: the type and timing of chemotherapy, the type of cancer, the patient's age, and the partner status. Most female cancer patients of reproductive age do not have the option of using established assisted reproductive technologies such as embryo cryopreservation to safeguard their fertility. Indeed, in many cancers, chemotherapy is initiated soon after diagnosis. A promising alternative to prevent fertility loss in these patients is cryopreservation and transplantation of ovarian tissue. Cryopreservation of ovarian tissue is the only option available for prepubertal girls and for women who cannot delay the start of chemotherapy. With the latest advances in cryobiology, ovarian tissue cryopreservation is rapidly becoming a more widely offered technique by many medical centers around the world. The indications for ovarian tissue cryopreservation in case of malignant disease are summarized in Table 1.

Cryopreservation should not be reserved solely for women with malignant disease, however (4). Hematopoietic stem cell transplantation (HSCT) has been increasingly used in recent decades for benign hematological and autoimmune diseases previously unresponsive to immunosuppressive therapy. Other benign diseases, such as recurrent ovarian endometriosis or recurrent ovarian mucinous cysts, are also indications for ovarian cryopreservation. Patients undergoing oophorectomy for prophylaxis may too potentially benefit from ovarian cryopreservation. The indications for cryopreservation of ovarian tissue in case of nonmalignant disease are summarized in Table 2.

In this chapter, we describe the techniques of (*i*) laparoscopic ovarian cortex biopsy with a view to cryopreservation and orthotopic reimplantation, (*ii*) laparoscopic ovariectomy for subsequent whole ovary cryopreservation and transplantation, and (*iii*) ovarian transposition before radiotherapy.

Table 1 Indications for Cryopreservation of Ovarian Tissue in Case of Malignant Disease

Extrapelvic diseases
Bone cancer (osteosarcoma—Ewing's sarcoma)
Thyroid, kidney cancers
Breast cancer
Melanoma
Neuroblastoma
Bowel malignancy
Pelvic diseases
Nongynecological malignancy
Pelvic sarcoma
Sacroblastoma
Rhabdomyosarcoma
Sacral tumors
Rectosigmoid tumors
Gynecological malignancy
Early cervical carcinoma
Early vaginal carcinoma
Early vulvar carcinoma
Selected cases of ovarian carcinoma (stage IA)
Borderline ovarian tumors
Systemic diseases
Hodgkin's disease
Non-Hodgkin's lymphoma
Leukemia
Medulloblastoma

Table 2 Indications for Cryopreservation of Ovarian Tissue in Case of Nonmalignant Disease

Uni-/bilateral oophorectomy
Benign ovarian tumors
Severe and recurrent endometriosis
BRCA-1 or BRCA-2 mutation carriers
Risk of premature menopause
Turner's syndrome
Family history
Benign diseases requiring chemotherapy: autoimmune diseases (systemic lupus erythematosus, rheumatoid arthritis, Behçet's disease, Wegener)
Bone marrow transplantation
Benign hematological diseases: sickle cell anemia, thalassemia major, aplastic anemia
Autoimmune diseases unresponsive to immunosuppressive therapy

CRYOPRESERVATION AND REIMPLANTATION OF OVARIAN CORTEX

Laparoscopic Ovarian Biopsy for Cryopreservation

A laparoscopy is performed under general anesthesia. Three laparoscopic puncture sites, including the umbilicus, are used: 10 mm umbilical, 5 mm right, and 5 mm left lower quadrant, just above the pubic hairline. Ovarian biopsies are taken either with Palmer forceps or laparoscopic scissors, taking care to remove ovarian cortex without provoking extensive bleeding from the medulla.

Biopsy size is determined by the chemotherapeutic or radiotherapeutic regimen to be administered. POF after chemotherapy is dependent on age, drug used, and dose given, and does not occur in all cases. When there is a chance of recovery of ovarian function after treatment, two biopsies—about 12 to 15 mm long and 5 mm wide—are taken from each ovary. When radiotherapy is indicated, the risk of POF is greater and ovariectomy may be proposed. In case of localized radiotherapy, ovarian transposition can be associated.

Ovarian Cortex Cryopreservation

Freezing of ovarian tissue is undertaken according to the protocol described by Gosden and colleagues (9). It was extensively described by our group in the *Lancet* in 2004 (10). We used a slow-freezing protocol with DMSO (dimethyl sulfoxide) as cryoprotectant.

Laparoscopic Frozen-Thawed Ovarian Cortex Reimplantation

In 2004, we reported the first live birth after ovarian cortex cryopreservation and reimplantation. The following technique was used. A first laparoscopy was performed seven days before reimplantation to create a peritoneal window by means of a large incision just beneath the right ovarian hilus, followed by coagulation of the edges of the window (Fig. 1). The goal was to induce angiogenesis and neovascularization in this area. A second laparoscopy was performed seven days after creation of the peritoneal window. A large strip and 35 small cubes of frozen-thawed ovarian tissue were placed into a furrow created by the peritoneal window very close to the ovarian vessels and fimbria on the right side (Fig. 2). No suture was used. An extensive neovascular network was clearly visible in this space (Fig. 3). A third laparoscopy was performed 4 months later to reimplant the remaining ovarian cortical cubes upon the patient's request, as she was now 32 years of age. Indeed, if pregnancy had not ensued from the reimplanted tissue, she would have considered oocyte donation.

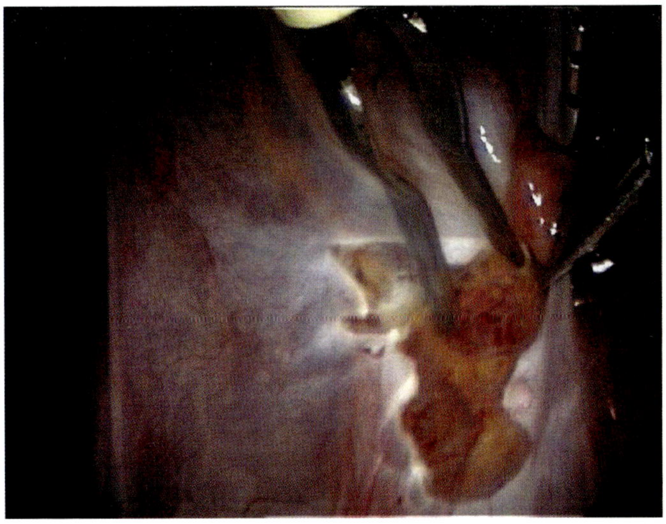

Figure 1 Site of reimplantation. During the first laparoscopy (seven days before transplantation), a peritoneal window was created and the edges of the window were coagulated.

From five to nine months after the first reimplantation, ultrasonography revealed development of a follicle, followed by corpus luteum formation with every menstrual cycle at the site of reimplantation; this corresponded to an estradiol concentration of more than 100 pg/mL and a progesterone level of 12 to 37 ng/mL. Luteinizing hormone (LH) and follicle-stimulating hormone (FSH) levels were lower than those observed before reimplantation. This led to the restoration of consecutive menstrual bleeding every month.

Eleven months after transplantation, the patient was pregnant. Vaginal ultrasonography at eight weeks confirmed a viable intrauterine pregnancy. Triple test evaluation and ultrasonography did not reveal any anomalies. The pregnancy resulted in the live birth of a healthy girl, weighing 3.72 kg, with an Apgar score of 9 at 1 min, 9 at 5 min, and 9 at 10 min.

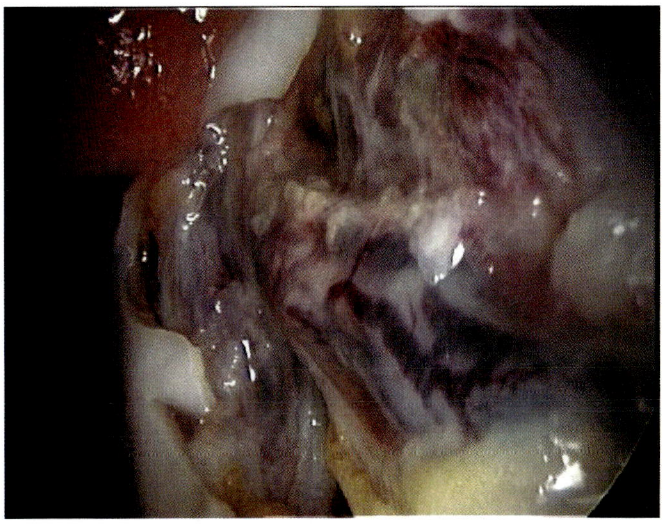

Figure 2 Seven days later (day of reimplantation), an extensive vascular network was clearly visible in this space.

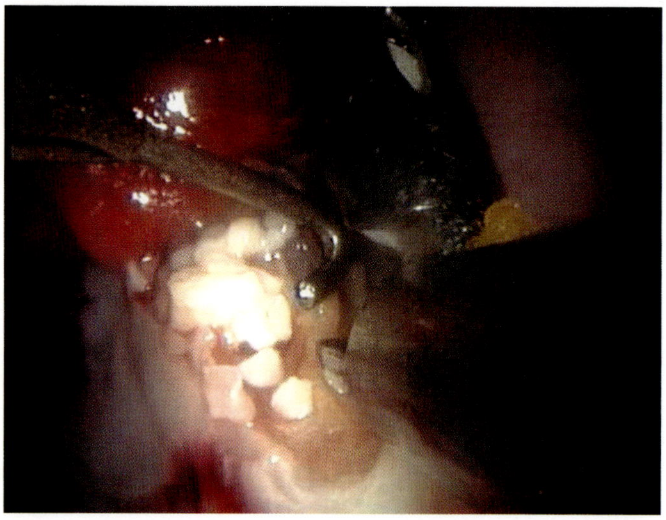

Figure 3 Large strips and small cubes of frozen-thawed ovarian tissue were placed into the furrow created by the peritoneal window very close to the ovarian vessels and fimbria.

Following this first reimplantation of frozen-thawed ovarian cortex, we slightly modified the technique. Since we know from experimental data that the ovary itself, even if atrophic, may be an ideal site for reimplantation, we believe that cortical pieces can be grafted directly onto the ovarian medulla. The remaining ovarian cortex of the atrophic ovary is thus removed and pieces of frozen-thawed ovarian cortex are sutured to the ovarian medulla with nonresorbable stitches (7.0 Prolene) (Fig. 4). This procedure has the advantage of not requiring a first laparoscopy to induce neovascularization. With this technique, the use of small cubes of 2 × 2 mm does not allow easy suturing, so we now prefer to cryopreserve strips of 12 × 5 mm, which are easier to reimplant.

So far, we have performed seven cases of orthotopic ovarian tissue reimplantation.

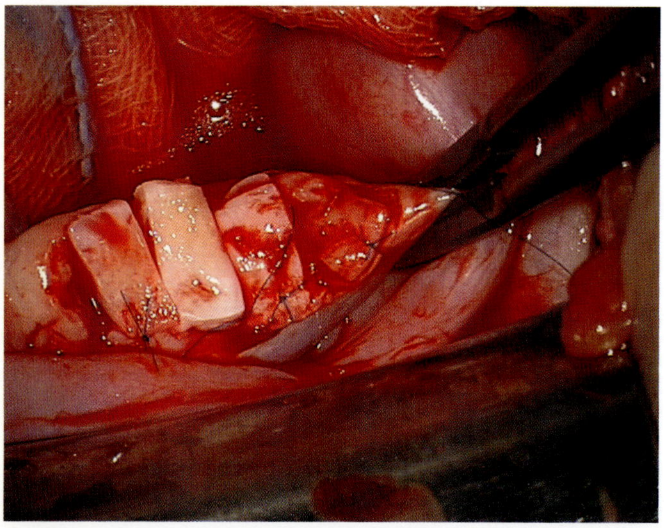

Figure 4 Ovarian cortical pieces were grafted onto the remaining ovary after the cortex of this ovary had been removed and sutured with 7-0 stitches.

Is Ovarian Cortex Transplantation Successful?

To date, ovarian tissue has been successfully cryopreserved and transplanted into rodents, rabbits, sheep, marmoset monkeys, and humans (10–16). Successful fertilization and pregnancy from fresh transplanted ovarian tissue has been described in a primate (17) and humans (18); in both cases, the grafted tissue functioned without any surgical connection to major blood vessels.

Human ovarian tissue can be successfully cryopreserved, showing good survival and function after thawing. Hovatta (19) arrived at this conclusion after reviewing all relevant studies since 1996, when the first case of cryopreservation of human ovarian tissue was reported. The choice of cryoprotectant with maximum permeation capacity but minimum toxicity and ice crystal formation potential is specific to each cell and tissue type (20). In the ovary, it is a compromise between the stroma, follicular cells, and oocytes (19). On the basis of current knowledge, the standard method for human ovarian cryopreservation is slow-programmed freezing, using human serum albumin-containing medium and propanediol, dimethyl sulfoxide, or ethylene glycol as a cryoprotectant, combined or not with sucrose (19).

Reported cases of autotransplantation of cryopreserved ovarian tissue to an orthotopic or heterotopic site (10–13,21–30) were recently reviewed by Donnez *et al.* (4) (Table 3).

In our department, we have performed ovarian cortex reimplantation ($n = 7$ cases) in five women. Of the five women, two underwent unilateral oophorectomy. Removal of the whole ovary is not generally an option because one can never completely exclude recovery of ovarian function after chemotherapy. Indeed, POF after chemotherapy depends on age, drug used, and dose given, and does not happen in all cases (22,31).

Analysis of these seven reimplantation cases raises some important points for discussion. First, in all cases, it took between 4 and 6.5 months after reimplantation before a follicle was seen and a rise in estradiol was detected (Fig. 5). The process of folliculogenesis takes four to six months, during which time the oocyte and surrounding somatic cells undergo a series of changes that eventually result in the development of a large antral follicle, capable of producing a mature oocyte (32). Thus, the appearance of the first follicle originating from the grafted tissue ≥4.5 months after reimplantation is totally consistent with the expected time course. The time interval between implantation of cortical tissue and the first estradiol peak is also consistent with data obtained from sheep (33,34) and human beings (28), although some variations may be observed. Indeed, in the literature, the delay between transplantation and follicular development was found to vary from eight weeks to eight months (2). Such a variation could be partially explained by a difference in follicular reserve at the time of cryopreservation, some women having already received a first regimen of chemotherapy before ovarian biopsy and cryopreservation. In our study, a interval of 5 to 6.5 months was observed in women who had chemotherapy prior to cryopreservation, compared to 4 to 4.5 months in those who underwent tissue cryopreservation before starting chemotherapy.

Another very interesting finding was the persistence of relatively high FSH levels during the follicular phase. FSH levels remained as high as 25 mIU/mL during the follicular phase until ovulation, and then decreased to <15 mIU/mL during the luteal phase if progesterone was more than 5 ng/mL. This may be explained by the relatively low number of surviving primordial follicles in the graft. Such patients should be

Table 3 Autotransplantation of Cryopreserved Human Ovarian Tissue

Reference	Age before freezing	Chemo before freezing	Indication	Graft site	Graft size	Recovery of ovarian function	Outcome
23	29	No	Intractable menometrorrhagia	Orthotopic: pelvic peritoneum	8 pc (5–10 × 2 mm)	16 weeks	↑ E_2, FD after stimulation, ovulation, menses
24	36	Yes	Hodgkin's lymphoma	Orthotopic: ovarian	2 pc (10 × 5 × 1 mm)	8 months	↓ FSH & LH, ↑ E_2, FD, ovulation, menses (1 cycle)
27	47	No	Uterine leiomyoma	Heterotopic: rectus abdominis muscle	40–45 pc (2–3 mm^3)	3–4 months	↑ E_2, FD after stimulation (follicle of 20 mm)
25	37	No	Squamous cell cervical carcinoma (Ib)	Heterotopic: breast (between breast tissue and pectoralis muscle (a)) + abdominal (rectus muscle (b))	40 pc (5 × 5 × 1–2 mm): 20 (a) + 20 (b)	14 weeks	↑ E_2, ↓ FSH, FD (follicle of 11–16 mm) only in (b), ovulation,
29	30	No	Breast cancer	Heterotopic: s. c. abdominal wall	15 pc (from 5 × 5 × 1 to 15 × 5 × 2 mm)	3 months	FD after gonadotropin stimulation, oocyte retrieval, 20 oocytes, 8 IVF-ICSI, 4-cell embryo transfer + 1 aneuploidic embryo
10	25	No	Hodgkin's lymphoma	Orthotopic: ovarian fossa peritoneum	1 pc (12 × 4 × 1 mm) + 67(35 + 32) pc (2 × 2 × 1 mm)	$4^{1/2}$ months	↑ E_2, ↓ FSH & LH, FD (follicle of 22 mm), regular cycles (± 5 weeks), pregnancy, live birth
11	28	Yes	Non-Hodgkin's lymphoma	Orthotopic: ovarian	3 pc (15 × 5 × 1–2 mm) + tiny fragments injected	8 months	↓ FSH, ↑AMH & inhibin B, FD, ovulation, menses, modified natural cycle, oocyte retrieval, 1 metaphase II oocyte IVF-ICSI, 4-cell embryo transfer, pregnancy and live birth
26	28	No	Hodgkin's lymphoma	Orthotopic: ovarian (a) + peritoneum (b) and heterotopic: abdominal wall (c)	12 pc: 4 (a) + 4 (b) + 4 (c)	19/22 weeks	↑ E_2, ↓ FSH, FD (19 weeks), menses (22 weeks), no stimulation, empty follicle (of 20 mm)
	25	No	Hodgkin's lymphoma	Orthotopic: ovarian (a) + peritoneum (b) and heterotopic: abdominal wall (c)	12 pc: 4 (a) + 4 (b) + 4 (c)	18/25 weeks	↑ E_2 ↓ FSH, FD (18 weeks), menses (25 weeks), 2 IVF cycles, 2 metaphase II oocytes, 2-cell embryo
	32	No	Non-Hodgkin's lymphoma	Orthotopic: ovarian	6 pc	8/14 weeks	↑ E_2, ↓ FSH, FD (8 weeks), menses (14 weeks), 1 IVF cycle, 1 metaphase II + 1 GV oocyte, 4-cell embryo
30	30	No	Pure red cell aplasia + BMT	Heterotopic: sc forearm	10 pc (1–2 × 1–2 × 0.5–1 mm)	18 weeks	FD (12.6-mm follicle and 6.7-mm follicle) after local gonadotropin stimulation
4	21	No	Sickle cell anemia + BMT	Orthotopic: ovarian (a) + ovarian fossa peritoneum (b)	69 pc (2×2×1 mm): 45 (a) + 24 (b)	4.5 months	↑ E_2, ↓ FSH and LH, FD (follicle of 20 mm), menses
28	29	Yes	Hodgkin's lymphoma	Heterotopic: subcutaneous abdominal wall	Left ovary in pieces	2 months	↑ E_2, FD, ovulation, 6-week pregnancy and miscarriage, and pregnancy with live birth from native ovary
12	24	Yes	Hodgkin's lymphoma	Orthotopic: ovarian (a) + ovarian fossa peritoneum (b) and heterotopic: sc abdominal wall (c)	18 pc (5 × 5 × 2 mm): 3 (a) + 9 (b) + 6 (c)	4 months	↑inhibin B & E_2 ↓ FSH, FD in all sites: (a): large follicles in ovarian site, (b): only one dominant follicle and (c): follicles <13 mm, 6 ovulations, natural conception, pregnancy, miscarriage at 7 weeks (aneuploidy)
Donnez et al., unpublished data	24	Yes	Non-Hodgkin's lymphoma	Orthotopic: ovarian	5 pc (10 × 4–5 × 1 mm)	5 months	↑ E_2, ↓ FSH, LH, FD (follicle of 21 mm), menses
13	28	No	Hodgkin's lymphoma	Orthotopic: ovarian (a) + peritoneal pocket in right pelvic wall, adjacent to the site of the removed ovary (b) and heterotopic: to a midline subperitoneal pocket on the lower abdominal wall (c)	10 pc (5 × 5 mm): 2 (a) + 4 (b) + 4 (c)	4.5 months	Hormone secretion and FD in all three locations, IVF-ICSI with biochemical pregnancy
77	24	Yes	Hodgkin's lymphoma	Orthotopic: ovarian (a) and heterotopic: sc abdominal wall (b)	8 pc (5 × 5 × 2 mm): 2 (a) + 6 (b)	Second transplantation performed 1 year after the first one	FD (2 follicles of 15 mm in (a)), spontaneous ovulation, ongoing pregnancy
78	-	-	-	Orthotopic: ovarian and heterotopic: abdominal wall	-	20 weeks	↓ FSH, FD, IVF cycles, metaphase II oocytes, embryos, ongoing third trimester pregnancy

FD: follicular development; pc: pieces; E_2: estradiol; sc: subcutaneous.

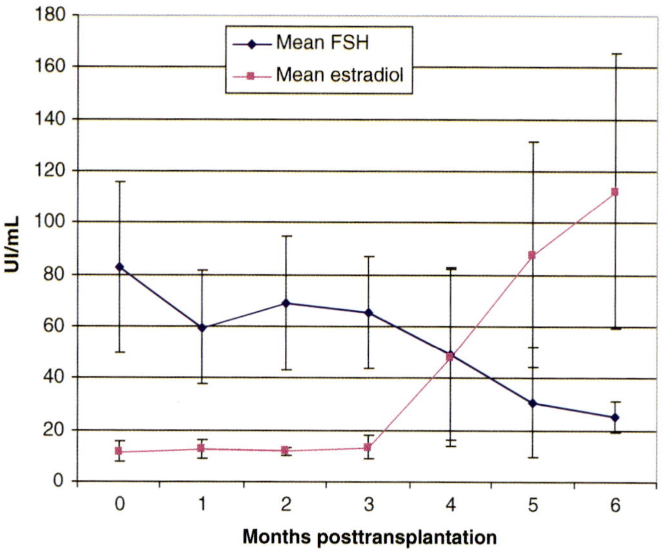

Figure 5 Mean FSH and 17β-estradiol levels (± standard deviation) in the seven cases of frozen-thawed ovarian tissue transplantation. It took between 4 and 6.5 months after transplantation before a rise in estradiol and a drop in FSH were observed. (Note that, in the last four cases, FSH and estradiol values at one month posttransplantation were not taken into account, as the patients were under GnRH agonist downregulation).

considered poor responders, with reduced inhibin B secretion. These results are in line with those obtained in sheep by Campbell *et al.* (35).

A further significant observation was the return to FSH levels of >35 mIU/mL after some menstrual bleeding, which supports the theory suggested by Baird *et al.* (33) that some inhibitory mechanisms, such as inhibin or anti-Müllerian hormones (AMH) normally produced by developing follicles in intact human ovaries, are probably almost nonexistent in transplanted tissue. After transplantation, these patients would have been regarded as poor responders because, out of the 500 to 1000 primordial follicles that would have been transplanted, >50% would have been lost owing to hypoxia (10). Moreover, due to the unequal distribution of primordial follicles in ovarian cortex, as demonstrated by Qu *et al.* (36), Schmidt *et al.* (37), and Gook *et al.* (38), it is quite impossible to clearly evaluate their exact number. The differences in behavior of primordial follicles in grafted tissue could either be due to their unequal distribution or an unequal vascular network resulting in unevenly vascularized areas, alternating with areas of fibrosis, as observed in animal models (34,39,40).

To date, six attempts at oocyte retrieval have been made (three during natural cycles and three during modified natural cycles adding recombinant FSH and GnRH antagonist). In four of them, no eggs were retrieved from aspirated follicles (empty follicle syndrome), while two attempts yielded eggs but they failed to fertilize. Similar data were very recently obtained by Meirow *et al.* (41), who reported recovery of only one egg out of four attempts (25%).

One of our ultrastructural studies (42) of human ovarian follicles after short-term (three weeks) xenografting to nude mice revealed asynchronized development between oocytes and follicular cells during early follicular growth in grafts. Seventy percent of growing human ovarian follicles showed an immature oocyte at the primordial/primary stage, surrounded by granulosa cells normally developing at the secondary stage. However, the presence of well-preserved interdigitations at the oocyte-follicular cell interface suggests maintenance of structural/metabolic cooperation between the different elements of the follicular unit.

This asynchrony identified between the oocyte and follicular cell growth could be due to premature follicular cell activation. An increase in primordial follicular cell growth initiation was indeed observed after xenotransplantation of human ovarian tissue to nude mice. This premature follicular cell activation may result from the stimulation of follicular growth by ischemic and oxidative stress after transplantation via HIF-1 (43) or be due to the removal of some inhibitory mechanisms that normally operate in an intact ovary (34).

Alternatively, primary oocyte development may be delayed because the oocyte is not yet developmentally competent when follicular growth is triggered.

SITE AND SIZE

In the reported series, the peritoneal window created close to the ovarian hilus, as well as the ovarian medulla, were both demonstrated to be equally efficient sites of reimplantation.

Large strips (8–10 mm × 5 mm) or small cubes (2 mm × 2 mm) were reimplanted. Both sizes effectively restored ovarian endocrine function. From a microsurgical point of view, however, it is easier to attach large strips to the medulla than small cubes, which cannot be sutured. Since reimplantation of large strips is easier and just as effective as small cube reimplantation, it is strongly suggested that large strips be taken from the ovarian cortex for cryopreservation purposes.

The maximum follow-up in our series is now four years and the patient is still experiencing follicular development from the grafted tissue.

Safety and Ethics

The transmission of lymphoma via grafts of ovarian tissue from diseased donor mice to healthy recipients was reported by Shaw *et al.* (44). This study highlighted the risks of clinical transplantation of ovarian biopsy samples to women recovering from cancer, especially a blood-borne cancer (44,45). However, there are certain circumstances where the risk of cancerous involvement of the ovary is absent or minimal (31) and where autografting would present little or no danger (46–49). In our series, three women were suffering from malignant disease (Hodgkin's and non-Hodgkin's lymphoma) and two from benign disease (sickle cell anemia and Wegener's disease, both treated by high doses of chemotherapy and ± BMT), but in all cases, the risk of malignant cell transmission was minimal. It is important to stress that no signs of malignant disease recurrence were observed in our study.

In the case of high risk of transmission of malignant cells, future experiments should help us address questions about the relevance of replacing residual malignant cells with grafted tissue. Screening methods must be developed to eliminate the risk of cancer cell transmission with reimplantation. In some diseases, other options must be considered, such as transplantation of isolated follicles (40,50).

Dudzinski (51) conducted a normative analysis of ethical issues in the context of oocyte and ovarian tissue cryopreservation for adolescent cancer survivors and concluded that more research is required before adolescents can ethically be enrolled in clinical trials. We do not fully agree with her conclusions. Indeed, approximately one-third of young women exposed to chemotherapy develop ovarian failure. In 2010, we believe it is our ethical responsibility to propose ovarian tissue cryopreservation, under institutional review board protocols, to all adolescents and young women having to undergo chemotherapy with alkylating agents.

This is why, since 1996, we have systematically proposed cryopreservation to all women under 35 years of age before chemotherapy, when there is a risk of POF. We accept that ovarian tissue cryopreservation is a more innovative and invasive procedure than sperm cryopreservation and that all possible applications in adolescents are ethically complex. However, we firmly believe that ovarian cortex banking should be offered before chemotherapy in all cases where emergency IVF is not possible.

One of the most important ethical issues is ensuring that the intervention does not harm the patient by dangerously delaying cancer treatment and that no remnant cells are reintroduced by subsequent transplantation.

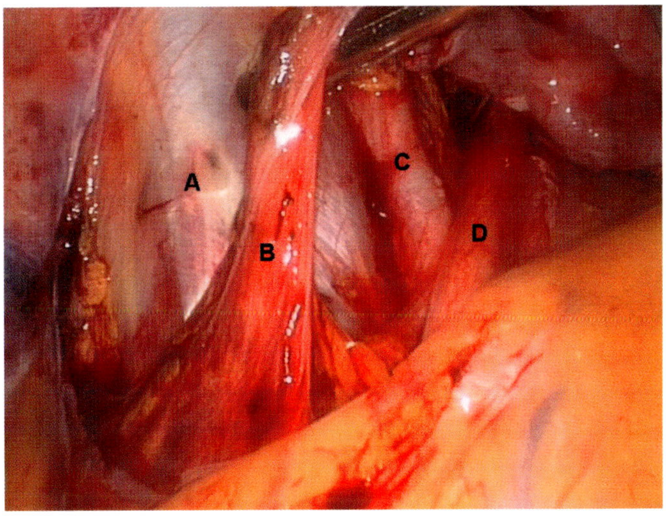

Figure 6 The ovarian pedicle is dissected cranially as high as possible, above the iliac vessels and psoas muscle. **(A)** Psoas muscle. **(B)** Ovarian pedicle. **(C)** Left iliac artery. **(D)** Ureter.

LAPAROSCOPIC OVARIECTOMY FOR WHOLE OVARY CRYOPRESERVATION AND TRANSPLANTATION

Whole ovary cryopreservation has so far been performed in nine patients in our department using the following technique (52,53).

Laparoscopic Ovariectomy

A laparoscopy is performed under general anesthesia. Four laparoscopic puncture sites, including the umbilicus, are used: 10 mm umbilical, 5 mm right, 10 mm medial (allowing the use of 5 mm instruments), and 5 mm left lower quadrant, just above the pubic hairline. Lateral incisions are made next to the deep epigastric vessels. A cannula is placed in the cervix for appropriate uterine mobilization. After inspection of the whole abdominal cavity, biopsies are taken from the right ovary for cryopreservation of ovarian cortex according to a previously described protocol.

The left ovary is then grasped with atraumatic forceps. The ureter and the iliac vessels are identified. If adhesions are found between the sigmoid and the lateral abdominal wall, they are freed. The broad ligament is incised with scissors from the infundibulopelvic ligament to the round ligament, externally to the fallopian tube.

Bipolar coagulation is avoided as far as possible. After dissection of the ureter, the posterior part of the broad ligament is opened with scissors. The ovarian pedicle and the ureter are dissected cranially as high as possible, above the iliac vessels and psoas muscle (Fig. 6). An endobag (Lapsac®, Cook, Limerick, Ireland) is introduced through the inferior medial trocar and opened in the pouch of Douglas.

The proximal isthmic part of the fallopian tube and the utero-ovarian ligament are clamped using two vascular clips (Hem-O-Lok, Weck Closure Systems, Research Triangle Park, North Carolina) and cut. The ovarian pedicle is then clamped using three vascular clips and cut between the two proximal clips (Fig. 7). Care is always taken to place the clips as high as possible on the pedicle leaving, at least 5 to 6 cm of the vascular pedicle attached to the ovary. The freed ovary and fallopian tube are swiftly placed in the endobag and removed from the abdomen through the medial suprapubic incision, which is slightly extended to avoid damage to the ovary. The removed ovary is then immediately handed over to a second team present in the operating room, including a microsurgeon and biologist.

Cryopreservation of the Whole Ovary

The ovary is deposited on a sterile petri dish containing heparinized physiologic solution (100 IU heparin/mL). The petri dish itself is placed on a cooling plate at 4°C. The clip on the ovarian pedicle is removed and the pedicle is dissected with microsurgical instruments under stereomicroscopic visualization. The artery is catheterized with a perfusion catheter, whose size is determined by the size of the main ovarian artery (range 24–18G) (Fig. 8). The catheter is fixed to the artery with nonresorbable 9/0 sutures. The ovarian artery is perfused with heparinized saline solution (52).

A precalibrated pump (Terumo Corporation, Tokyo, Japan) is used to maintain a flow rate of 2.5 mL/min according to the technique described by Martinez et al. This perfusion with heparinized physiologic solution continues until the perfusion liquid draining out of the ovarian veins runs clear and

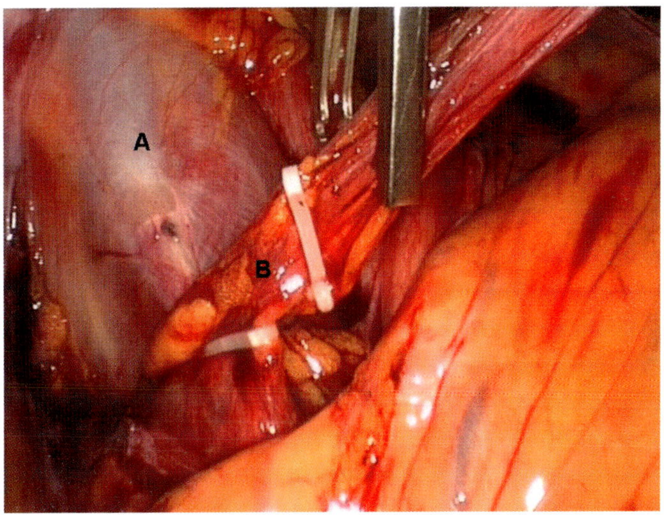

Figure 7 The ovarian pedicle is clamped using three vascular clips. **(A)** Psoas muscle. **(B)** Clipped ovarian pedicle.

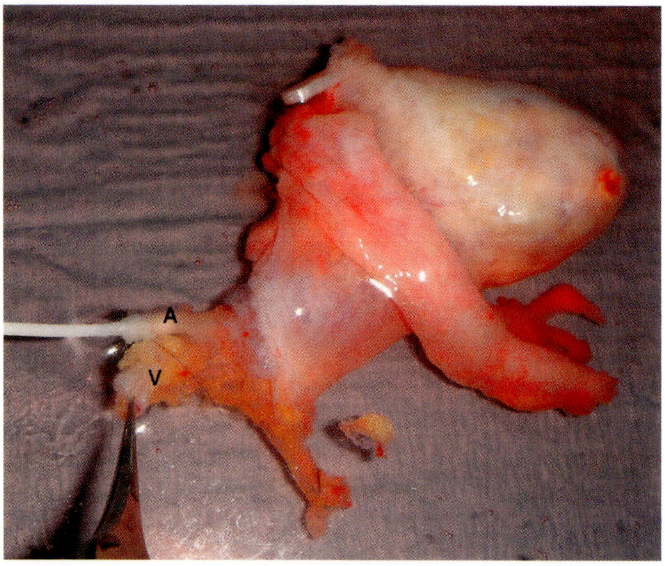

Figure 8 In the operating room, the ovarian artery (A) is catheterized under operative microscopic control and perfused. Liquid outflow allows identification of the ovarian veins (V) and their further microdissection.

all the blood has been evacuated from the ovary, which takes up to 20 minutes.

Thereafter, the ovary is transferred to a second petri dish and perfused and immersed in a cryoprotective solution of HEPES MEM (Gibco, St. Louis, Missouri), supplemented with 10% dimethyl sulfoxide (DMSO; Sigma, St. Louis, Missouri) and 0.4% human serum albumin (Red Cross, Brussels, Belgium) for five minutes at 4°C at a flow rate of 2.5 mL/min, as previously described. The ovary is then placed in a cryovial, where it is pre-equilibrated at 4°C in a bath with the cryoprotectant for 10 minutes, and gently shaken while being transferred to the laboratory. After pre-equilibration, it is placed in a 5100 Cryo 1°C Freezing Container (Nalgene, VWR, Belgium) precooled at 4°C, and deposited in a −80°C freezer. This confers a cooling rate of −1°C/min. After 24 hours in the −80°C freezer, the cryovial containing the ovary is transferred to liquid nitrogen (−196°C).

WHOLE OVARY TRANSPLANTATION: THE CHALLENGE FOR TODAY

In humans, the challenge of whole ovary cryopreservation results from the difficulty of adequate cryoprotective agent diffusion into large tissue masses and the risk of vascular injury caused by intravascular ice formation. Nevertheless, previous studies in our department have demonstrated the feasibility of cryopreservation of intact human ovary with its vascular pedicle using an accessible protocol (52).

We proved high survival rates of follicles, small vessels, and stromal cells, as well as a normal histological structure in all ovarian components after thawing, and observed no signs of apoptosis or ultrastructural alterations in any cell types (53).

In our opinion, when ovariectomy and whole ovary cryopreservation are performed, two technical requirements must be met for subsequent transplantation to be feasible. First, the ovarian pedicle must be long enough to allow the ovarian artery and veins to be individualized and sutured to vessels of similar diameter. Second, the ischemic interval before cryopreservation must be as short as possible to avoid damage to the ovary. We believe laparoscopic removal of the ovary is able to fulfill these two conditions.

Laparoscopic dissection of the ovarian pedicle has been performed for a number of years for the purposes of ovarian transposition and is not a difficult procedure for laparoscopic surgeons. The ovarian pedicle can be easily individualized up to the iliac vessels and above the psoas muscle. The utero-ovarian ligament and the ovarian pedicle may be ligated with sutures. However, as five vascular clips are simpler and faster to place than five sutures, we believe the use of clips reduces the ischemic interval before ovarian artery perfusion with heparinized solution and cryoprotective medium.

Ovarian Transposition Before Radiotherapy

Iatrogenic destruction of the follicular reserve by radiation therapy may be avoided by ovarian transposition to the paracolic gutter. Ovarian transposition by laparotomy was first described by McCall and colleagues in 1958 in patients treated for cervical carcinoma (54). Nowadays, ovarian suspension is generally performed by laparoscopy before irradiation (55–65).

However, it has been demonstrated that ovarian transposition cannot be considered completely infallible because patients receive infradiaphragmatic irradiation (66), often coupled with chemotherapy (66,67). For women who are to receive chemotherapy and/or radiotherapy, ovarian transposition should be associated with proposed cryopreservation of ovarian tissue (68,69), even if *in vitro* maturation of oocytes has not yet proved routinely effective after cryopreservation.

All patients need to be informed of the long-term consequences of cancer and its therapy, even if not all treatments cause infertility.

Surgical Technique

The procedure is performed under general endotracheal anesthesia. After induction of pneumoperitoneum, a 12-mm trocar is inserted subumbilically. The laparoscope is connected to a video camera. Three 5-mm trocars are systematically inserted suprapubically: one in the midline, approximately 3 cm above the symphysis pubis, and the other two a few centimeters on either side, taking care to avoid the epigastric vessels. The surgical procedure of laparoscopic ovarian transposition is identical to that performed by laparotomy. Usually, the right ovary is preferred for transposition because of easier access, as the bowel may be pushed out of the way. But if radiotherapy is localized on the right, the left ovary is transposed. The right adnexa are grasped and mobilized. The isthmic portion of the tube and the utero-ovarian ligament are coagulated using bipolar forceps and cut off at their uterine origin (Fig. 9). The peritoneum is incised along the infundibulopelvic ligament to mobilize the adnexa completely. The course of the ureter is visualized and care is taken to avoid damage to the ureter. Dissection of the infundibulopelvic vessels using bipolar coagulation and scissors is continued until adnexal transposition to the paracolic gutter is achieved, without any traction or torsion to the ovarian vascular pedicle (Fig. 10). Using 1.0 Vicryl, the right ovary is anchored to the peritoneum of the anterior abdominal wall very high in the right paracolic gutter. In order to facilitate fixation of the ovary, a curved needle is inserted into the right lateral flank, in front of the desired anchoring of the ovary.

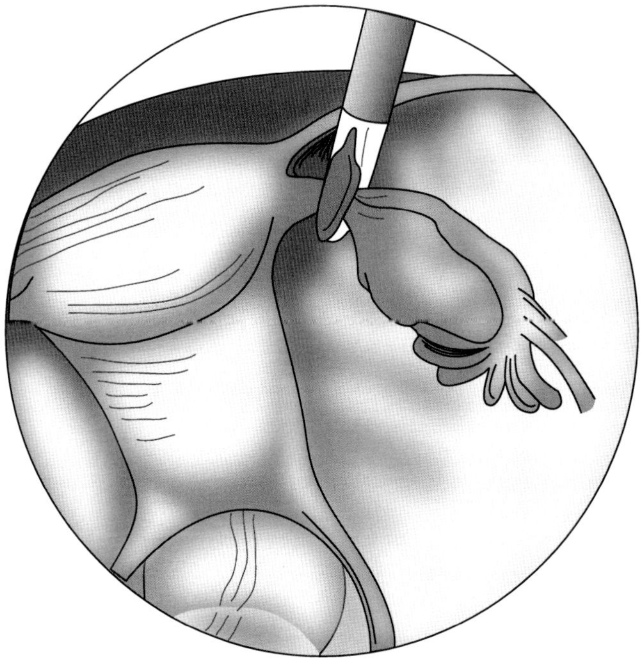

Figure 9 Coagulation of the proximal part of the adnexa.

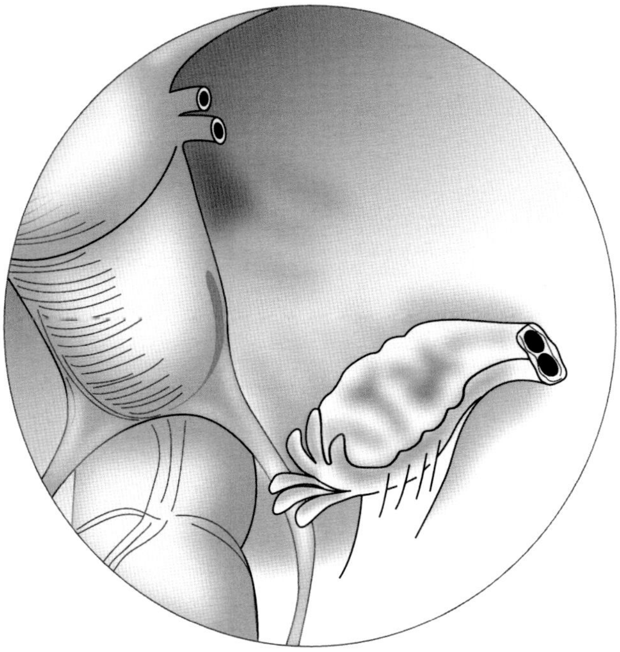

Figure 10 Adnexal transposition avoiding traction to the ovarian vascular pedicle.

Titanium clips are placed on the two opposite borders of the ovary to allow radiological identification prior to radiotherapy (Fig. 11). To avoid bowel incarceration between the transposed ovary and the abdominal wall, the vascular pedicle is attached to the anterolateral abdominal wall with three or four titanium clips.

Indications

The classic indications for ovarian transposition in case of malignant disease are summarized in Table 4. The main indication for ovarian transposition in gynecological malignancy is the detection of early cervical carcinoma. Transposition is usually performed during its surgical treatment.

In case of rectosigmoid tumors in young patients, laparoscopic ovarian transposition is generally performed prior to radiotherapy indicated to decrease tumor size, and before removal of the tumor.

Ovarian Function and Fertility After Ovarian Transposition and Radiotherapy

Haie-Meder and coworkers (70) found that the measured dose of radiotherapy reaching transposed ovaries was 10% of the

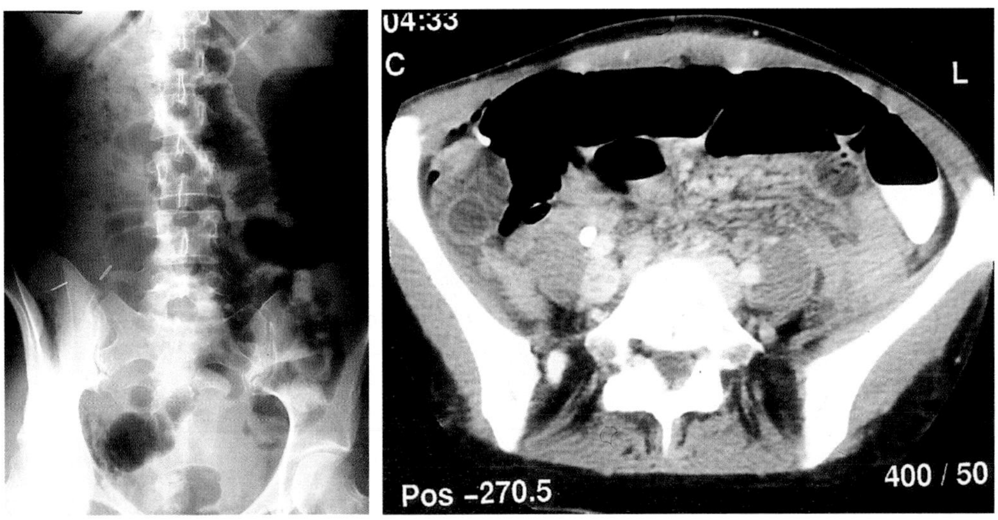

(A) (B)

Figure 11 Postoperative identification of the transposed ovary before radiotherapy using (A) radiography and (B) computerized tomography.

Table 4 Indications for Ovarian Transposition in Case of Malignant Disease

Gynecological malignancy
Early cervical carcinoma
Early vaginal carcinoma
Early vulvar carcinoma
Nongynecological malignancy
Rectosigmoid tumors
Pelvic or extrapelvic sarcoma
Bone cancer (osteosarcoma, Ewing's sarcoma)
Lymphoma
Medulloblastoma

delivered dose when the ovaries were located under shielding blocks, and 4.4% when the ovaries were outside the irradiation field. Nevertheless, results in terms of pregnancy outcome must be evaluated with caution. In their series (70), the pregnancy outcome was just 19%, although ovarian function was apparently preserved. This rate is significantly lower than the rate in the general population. Interpretation is difficult, however, because this low rate could also reflect a patient's personal choice, or an effect of radiotherapy on the uterus itself, which could affect implantation.

A very large prospective series of ovarian transposition in patients with cervical carcinoma treated by a radiosurgical combination was published by Morice (71). Ovarian transposition to the paracolic gutters with radical hysterectomy and lymphadenectomy was performed in 107 patients (bilaterally in 98% of cases). This procedure was recommended for patients under 40 years of age with a small invasive cervical carcinoma ($\leq$3 cm) treated by initial surgery. The rate of ovarian preservation was 90% in patients treated by postoperative vaginal brachytherapy and 60% in patients treated by postoperative external radiation therapy and vaginal brachytherapy.

Abdominal ionizing radiation associated with alkylating agents often induces POF, rendering patients infertile in almost 100% of cases. Indeed, it has been stated that a dose of 5 to 20 Gy administered to the ovary is sufficient to completely impair gonadal function (72), whatever the age of the patient. The dose of radiation required to destroy 50% of the oocyte reserve has been found to be <2 Gy (73). Moreover, uterine irradiation at a young age reduces adult uterine volume (74). Radiation doses between 14 and 30 Gy have been reported to result in uterine dysfunction (32,75,76). The practitioner should be aware of this effect of radiotherapy on the uterus, which could interfere with the implantation capacity of embryos.

In conclusion, there is a place for ovarian transposition in case of radiotherapy exclusively directed at the lowest parts of the pelvis, but there is still a lack of knowledge concerning the effect of radiotherapy on uterine receptivity. All the indications for laparoscopic ovarian transposition should therefore also be indications for ovarian tissue cryopreservation.

CONCLUSIONS

This chapter reviews the indications and surgical procedures for preserving fertility in young patients suffering from cancer or other diseases requiring gonadotoxic therapy. Indeed, advances in the diagnosis and treatment of such diseases have led to increased survival, resulting in a growing population of young women restored to health and wishing to become mothers. The techniques outlined in this chapter give them the opportunity to do so.

REFERENCES

1. Blatt J. Pregnancy outcome in long-term survivors of childhood cancer. Med Pediatr Oncol 1999; 33:29–33.
2. Jemal A, Siegel R, Ward E, et al. Cancer statistics, 2006. CA Cancer J Clin 2006; 56:106–130.
3. Ries LAG, Percy CL, Bunin GR. Introduction. In: Ries LAG, Smith MA, Gurney JG, et al., eds. Cancer Incidence and Survival Among Children and Adolescents: United States SEER Program 1975–1995 [NIH Pub. No. 99–4649]. Bethesda, MD: National Cancer Institute, 1999:1–15.
4. Donnez J, Martinez-Madrid P, Jadoul P, et al. Ovarian tissue cryopreservation and existing alternatives: A review. Hum Reprod Update 2006; 12:519–535.
5. Meirow D, Lewis H, Nugent D, et al. Subclinical depletion of primordial follicular reserve in mice treated with cyclophosphamide: Clinical importance and proposed accurate investigative tool. Hum Reprod 1999; 14:1903–1907.
6. Shalet SM. Effects of cancer chemotherapy on gonadal function of patients. Cancer Treat Rev 1980; 7:141–152.
7. Sanders J, Hawley J, Levy W, et al. Pregnancies following high-dose Cyclophosphamide with or without high-dose Busulfan or total body irradiation and bone marrow transplantation. Blood 1996; 87:3045–3052.
8. Meirow D, Nugent D. The effects of radiotherapy and chemotherapy on female reproduction. Hum Reprod Update 2001; 7:534–543.
9. Gosden RG, Baird DT, Wade JC, et al. Restoration of fertility to oophorectomized sheep by ovarian autografts stored at −196 degrees C. Hum Reprod 1994; 9:597–603.
10. Donnez J, Dolmans MM, Demylle D, et al. Livebirth after orthotopic transplantation of cryopreserved ovarian tissue. Lancet 2004; 364:1405–1410.
11. Meirow D, Levron J, Eldar-Geva T, et al. Pregnancy after transplantation of cryopreserved ovarian tissue in a patient with ovarian failure after chemotherapy. N Engl J Med 2005; 353:318–321.
12. Demeestere I, Simon P, Buxant F, et al. Ovarian function and spontaneous pregnancy after combined hetorotopic and orthotopic cryopreserved ovarian tissue transplantation in a patient previously treated with bone marrow transplantation: case report. Hum Reprod 2006; 21(8):2010–2014.
13. Rosendahl M, Loft A, Byskov AG, et al. Biochemical pregnancy after fertilization of an oocyte aspirated from a heterotopic autotransplant of cryopreserved ovarian tissue: Case report. Hum Reprod 2006; 21(8):2006–2009.
14. Candy CJ, Wood MJ, Whittingham DG. Follicular development in cryopreserved marmoset ovarian tissue after transplantation. Hum Reprod 1995; 10:2334–2338.
15. Candy CJ, Wood MJ, Whittingham DG. Restoration of a normal reproductive lifespan after grafting of cryopreserved mouse ovaries. Hum Reprod 2000; 15:1300–1304.
16. Salle B, Demirci B, Franck M, et al. Normal pregnancies and live births after autograft of frozen-thawed hemi-ovaries into ewes. Fertil Steril 2002; 77:403–408.
17. Lee DM, Yeoman RR, Battaglia DE, et al. Live birth after ovarian tissue transplant. Nature 2004; 428:137–138.
18. Silber SJ, Lenahan KM, Levine DJ, et al. Ovarian transplantation between monozygotic twins discordant for premature ovarian failure. N Engl J Med 2005; 353:58–63.
19. Hovatta O. Methods for cryopreservation of human ovarian tissue. Reprod Biomed Online 2005; 10:729–734.
20. Fuller B, Paynter S. Fundamentals of cryobiology in reproductive medicine. Reprod Biomed Online 2004; 9:680–691.
21. Donnez J, Dolmans MM, Martinez-Madrid B, et al. The role of cryopreservation for women prior to treatment of malignancy. Curr Opin Obstet Gynecol 2005; 17:333–338.
22. Donnez J, Dolmans MM, Demylle D, et al. Restoration of ovarian function after orthotopic (intraovarian and periovarian) transplantation of cryopreserved ovarian tissue in a woman treated by bone marrow transplantation for sickle cell anaemia: Case report. Hum Reprod 2006; 21:183–188.

23. Oktay K, Karlikaya G. Ovarian function after transplantation of frozen, banked autologous ovarian tissue. N Engl J Med 2000; 342:1919.
24. Radford JA, Lieberman BA, Brison D, et al. Orthotopic reimplantation of cryopreserved ovarian cortical strips after high-dose chemotherapy for Hodgkin's lymphoma. Lancet 2001; 357:1172–1175.
25. Kim SS, Hwang IT, Lee HC. Heterotopic autotransplantation of cryobanked human ovarian tissue as a strategy to restore ovarian function. Fertil Stertil 2004; 82:930–932.
26. Schmidt KL, Yding Andersen C, Loft A, et al. Follow-up of ovarian function post-chemotherapy following ovarian cryopreservation and transplantation. Hum Reprod 2005; 20:3539–3546.
27. Callejo J, Salvador C, Miralles A, et al. Long-term ovarian function evaluation after autografting by implantation with fresh and frozen-thawed human ovarian tissue. J Clin Endocrinol Metab 2001; 86:4489–4494.
28. Oktay K. Spontaneous conceptions and live birth after heterotopic ovarian transplantation: Is there a germline stem cell connection? Hum Reprod 2006; 21(6):1345–1348.
29. Oktay K, Buyuk E, Veeck L, et al. Embryo development after heterotopic transplantation of cryopreserved ovarian tissue. Lancet 2004; 363:837–840.
30. Wolner-Hanssen P, Hägglund L, Ploman F, et al. Autotransplantation of cryopreserved ovarian tissue to the right forearm 4½ years after autologous stem cell transplantation. Acta Obstet Gynecol Scand 2005; 84:695–698.
31. Meirow D, Ben Yehuda D, Prus D, et al. Ovarian tissue banking in patients with Hodgkin's disease: Is it safe? Fertil Steril 1998; 69:996–998.
32. Gougeon A. Regulation of ovarian follicular development in primates: Facts and hypotheses. Endocr Rev 1996; 17:121–155.
33. Baird DT, Webb R, Campbell BK, et al. Long-term ovarian function in sheep after ovariectomy and transplantation of autografts stored at −196°C. Endocrinol 1999; 140:462–471.
34. Baird DT, Campbell BK, Souza C, et al. Long-term ovarian function in sheep after ovariectomy and autotransplantation of cryopreserved cortical strips. Eur J Obst Gynecol Reprod Biol 2004; 113:55–59.
35. Campbell BK, Telfer EE, Webb R, et al. Ovarian autografts in sheep as a model for studying folliculogenesis. Mol Cell Endocrinol 2000; 163:131–139.
36. Qu J, Godin PA, Nisolle M, et al. Distribution and epidermal growth factor receptor expression of primordial follicles in human ovarian tissue before and after cryopreservation. Hum Reprod 2000; 15:302–310.
37. Schmidt KL, Byskov AG, Nyboe Andersen A, et al. Density and distribution of primordial follicles in single pieces of cortex from 21 patients and in individual pieces of cortex from three entire human ovaries. Hum Reprod 2003; 18:1158–1164.
38. Gook DA, Edgar DH, Borg J, et al. Diagnostic assessment of the developmental potential of human cryopreserved ovarian tissue from multiple patients using xenografting. Hum Reprod 2005; 20:72–78.
39. Nisolle M, Casanas-Roux F, Qu JP, et al. Histologic and ultrastructural evaluation of fresh and frozen-thawed human ovarian xenografts in nude mice. Fertil Steril 2000; 74:122–129.
40. Dolmans MM, Martinez-Madrid B, Gadisseux E, et al. Short-term transplantation of isolated human ovarian follicles and cortical tissue into nude mice. Reproduction 2007; 134:253–262.
41. Meirow D, Levron J, Eldar-Geva T, et al. Monitoring the ovaries after autotransplantation of cryopreserved ovarian tissue: Endocrine studies, in vitro fertilization cycles and live birth. Fertil Steril 2007; 87(2):418e7–418.e15.
42. Nottola S, Camboni A, Macchiarelli G, et al. Cryopreservation and xenotransplantation of human ovarian tissue: An ultrastructural study. Fertil Steril 2008; 90(1):23–32.
43. Alam H, Maizels ET, Park Y, et al. Follicle stimulating hormone activation of hypoxia-inducible factor-1 by the phosphatidylinositol 3-kinase/AKT/Ras homolog enriched in brain (Rheb)/mammalian target of rapamycin (mTOR) pathway is necessary for induction of select protein markers of follicular differentiation. J Biol Chem 2004; 279:19431–19440.
44. Shaw JM, Bowles S, Koopman P, et al. Fresh and cryopreserved ovarian tissue samples from donors with lymphoma transmit the cancer to graft recipients. Hum Reprod 1996; 11:1668–1673.
45. Shaw JM, Trounson AO. Oncological implications in the replacement of ovarian tissue. Hum Reprod 1997; 12:403–405.
46. Gosden RG, Rutherford AJ, Norfolk D. Ovarian banking for cancer patients: Transmission of malignant cells in ovarian grafts. Hum Reprod 1997; 12:403–405.
47. Moomjy M, Rosenwaks Z. Ovarian tissue cryopreservation: the time is now. Transplantation or in vitro maturation: The time awaits. Fertil Steril 1998; 69:999–1000.
48. Kim SS, Radford J, Harris M, et al. Ovarian tissue harvested from lymphoma patients to preserve fertility may be safe for autotransplantation. Hum Reprod 2001; 16:2056–2060.
49. Seshadri T, Gook D, Lade S, et al. Lack of evidence of disease contamination in ovarian tissue harvested for cryopreservation from patients with Hodgkin lymphoma and analysis of factors predictive of oocyte yield. Br J Cancer 2006; 94(7):1007–1010.
50. Dolmans MM, Michaux N, Camboni A, et al. Evaluation of Liberase, a purified enzyme blend, for the isolation of human primordial and primary ovarian follicles. Hum Reprod 2006; 21(2):413–420.
51. Dudzinski DM. Ethical issues in fertility preservation for adolescent cancer survivors: Oocyte and ovarian tissue cryopreservation. J Pediatr Adolesc Gynecol 2004; 17:97–102.
52. Martinez-Madrid B, Dolmans MM, Van Langendonckt A, et al. Freeze-thawing intact human ovary with its vascular pedicle with a passive cooling device. Fertil Steril 2004; 82:1390–1394.
53. Martinez-Madrid B, Camboni A, Dolmans MM, et al. Apoptosis and ultrastructural assessment after cryopreservation of whole human ovaries with their vascular pedicle. Fertil Steril 2007; 87(5):1153–1165.
54. McCall ML, Keaty EC, Thompson JD. Conservation of ovarian tissue in the treatment of the carcinoma of the cervix with radical surgery. Am J Obstet Gynecol 1958; 75:590–600.
55. Lee C, Lai Y, Soong Y, et al. Laparoscopic ovariopexy before irradiation for medulloblastoma. Hum Reprod 1995; 2:372–374.
56. Covens A, Putten H, Fyles AW, et al. Laparoscopic ovarian transposition. Eur J Gynaecol Oncol 1996; 3:177–182.
57. Clough KB, Goffinet F, Labib A, et al. Laparoscopic unilateral ovarian transposition prior to irradiation: Prospective study of 20 cases. Cancer 1996; 77:2638–2645.
58. Treissman MJ, Miller D, McComb PF. Laparoscopic lateral ovarian transposition. Fertil Steril 1996; 65:1229–1231.
59. Howard FM. Laparoscopic ovarian transposition before radiation: Treatment of Hodgkin's disease. J Am Assoc Gynecol Laparosc 1997; 5:601–604.
60. Tulandi T, Al-Took S. Laparoscopic ovarian suspension before irradiation. Fertil Steril 1998; 70:381–383.
61. Hart R, Sawyer E, Magos A. Case report of ovarian transposition and review of literature. Gynecol Endosc 1999; 8:51–54.
62. Williams RS, Littell RD, Mendenhall NP. Laparoscopic oophoropexy and ovarian function in the treatment of Hodgkin disease. Cancer 1999; 86:2138–2145.
63. Yarali H, Demirol A, Bukulmez O, et al. Laparoscopic high lateral transposition of both ovaries before pelvic irradiation. J Am Assoc Gynecol Laparosc 2000; 7:237–239.
64. Visvanathan DK, Cutner AS, Cassoni AM, et al. A new technique of laparoscopic ovariopexy before irradiation. Fertil Steril 2003; 79:1204–1213.
65. Bisharah M, Tulandi T. Laparoscopic preservation of ovarian function: An underused procedure. Am J Obstet Gynecol 2003; 188:367–370.
66. Baker TG. Radiosensitivity of mammalian oocytes with particular reference to the human female. Am J Obstet Gynecol 1971; 110:746–761.
67. Hodel K, Rich WM, Austin P, et al. The role of ovarian transposition in conservation of ovarian function in radical hysterectomy

followed by pelvic radiation. Gynecol Oncol 1982; 13(2):195–202.

68. Donnez J, Qu J, Nisolle M. Gonadal cryopreservation in the young patient with gynecological malignancy. Curr Opin Obstet Gynecol 2000; 12:1–9.
69. Donnez J, Bassil S. Indications for cryopreservation of ovarian tissue. Hum Reprod Update 1998; 4:248–259.
70. Haie-Meder C, Mlika-Cabanne N, Michel G, et al. Radiotherapy after ovarian transposition: Ovarian function and fertility preservation. Int J Radiat Oncol Biol Phys 1993; 25:419–424.
71. Morice P, Juncker L, Rey A, et al. Ovarian transposition for patients with cervical carcinoma treated by radiosurgical combination. Fertil Steril 2000; 74:743–748.
72. Wallace WH, Thomson AB, Saran F, et al. Predicting age of ovarian failure after radiation to a field that includes the ovaries. Int J Radiat Oncol Biol Phys 2005; 62(3):738–744.
73. Wallace WH, Thomson AB, Kelsey TW. The radiosensitivity of the human oocyte. Hum Reprod 2003; 18(1):117–121.
74. Larsen EC, Schmiegelow K, Rechnitzer C, et al. Radiotherapy at a young age reduces uterine volume of childhood cancer survivors. Acta Obstet Gynecol Scand 2004; 83(1):96–102.
75. Critchley HO. Factors of importance for implantation and problems after treatment for childhood cancer. Med Pediatr Oncol 1999; 33(1):9–14.
76. Critchley HO, Wallace WH. Impact of cancer treatment on uterine function. J Natl Cancer Inst Monogr 2005; (34):64–68.
77. Demeestere I, Simon P, Emiliani S, et al. Ongoing pregnancy after a second cryopreserved ovarian tissue transplantation procedure. Hum Reprod 2007; 22:i43:O109.
78. Andersen C, Loft A, Ernst E, et al. Assisted reproductive techniques after autotransplantation of frozen/thawed ovarian tissue. Hum Reprod 2007; 22:i41:O104.

Index

Note: Page locators in italics indicates figure.